NUTRITION FOR MIDDLE AGED AND ELDERLY

NUTRITION FOR MIDDLE AGED AND ELDERLY

NANCY E. BERNHARDT
AND
ARTUR M. KASKO
EDITORS

Nova Biomedical Books
New York

For permission to use material from this book please contact us:
Telephone 631-231-7269; Fax 631-231-8175
Web Site: http://www.novapublishers.com

NOTICE TO THE READER

The Publisher has taken reasonable care in the preparation of this book, but makes no expressed or implied warranty of any kind and assumes no responsibility for any errors or omissions. No liability is assumed for incidental or consequential damages in connection with or arising out of information contained in this book. The Publisher shall not be liable for any special, consequential, or exemplary damages resulting, in whole or in part, from the readers' use of, or reliance upon, this material.

Independent verification should be sought for any data, advice or recommendations contained in this book. In addition, no responsibility is assumed by the publisher for any injury and/or damage to persons or property arising from any methods, products, instructions, ideas or otherwise contained in this publication.

This publication is designed to provide accurate and authoritative information with regard to the subject matter covered herein. It is sold with the clear understanding that the Publisher is not engaged in rendering legal or any other professional services. If legal or any other expert assistance is required, the services of a competent person should be sought. FROM A DECLARATION OF PARTICIPANTS JOINTLY ADOPTED BY A COMMITTEE OF THE AMERICAN BAR ASSOCIATION AND A COMMITTEE OF PUBLISHERS.

Library of Congress Cataloging-in-Publication Data

Nutrition for the middle aged and elderly / Nancy E. Bernhardt and Artur M. Kasko (editors).
p. ; cm.
ISBN 978-1-60456-146-3 (hardcover)
1. Nutrition disorders in old age. 2. Aged--Nutrition. 3. Middle-aged persons--Nutrition. I. Bernhardt, Nancy E. II. Kasko, Artur M.
[DNLM: 1. Aging. 2. Nutrition Physiology. 3. Aged. 4. Middle Aged. WT 115 N9763 2007]
RC620.6.N877 2007
362.198'9739--dc22 2007048151

Published by Nova Science Publishers, Inc. ✦ New York

Contents

Preface **vii**

Short Communications

Communication A "Coffee or Tea? From the Historically Alleged Curative Properties of Common Beverages to Their Current Evidence-Based Benefits on Human Health" **1**
Andrea A. Conti

Communication B Food Consumption Patterns, Nutrient Intake, and Serum Components among Middle- Aged and Elderly Nepalese **11**
Yoshimi Ohno, Kazuko Hirai, Shiba K. Rai, Jeevan B. Sherchand and Mathura P. Shrestha

Research and Review Articles

Chapter I Relation of Vitamin D, Calcium, and Magnesium to the Risk of Type 2 Diabetes Mellitus **31**
Sara Chacko and Simin Liu

Chapter II A Life-Course Contribution of Nutrition to Future Cognitive Decline **63**
Emanuele Cereda, Alberto Battezzati, Simona Bertoli, Alexis Elias Malavazos and Giulio Testolin

Chapter III The Role of Diet and Nutrition in the Prevention of Cancer **107**
Sa'eed Bawa

Chapter IV The Significance of Diet and Nutrition in the Prevention and Management of Osteoporosis in the Elderly Population **157**
Sa'eed Bawa

Chapter V The Impact of Transtheoretical Model-Based Multiple Behavior Interventions on Nutrition **195**
Sara Johnson, Carol Cummins and Kerry Evers

Chapter VI	The Assessment of Protein-Energy Malnutrition in Elderly People *Roberto Buffa, Giovanni Floris, Paolo Francesco Putzu and Elisabetta Marini*	**213**
Chapter VII	Rationale to Integrate Nutritional Aspect in the Comprehensive Geriatric Assessment *Thierry Pepersack*	**235**
Chapter VIII	I Heard It Through the Grapevine: Beliefs Among College Students and Older Adults Regarding Foods Essential for Building Strength and Muscle *Michael E. Oakes and Heather Leeman*	**253**
Chapter IX	Serum Magnesium and Cancer Mortality *Charles J. Everett, Dana E. King, Brian J. Wells, Ivar L. Frithsen and Arch G. Mainous III*	**271**
Chapter X	Nutrition in Older Adults: An Overview *Rossana Salerno-Kennedy*	**285**
Chapter XI	Fruit and Vegetable Consumption among Mid-Age and Older Women in Australia *Zumin Shi and Julie Byles*	**299**
Chapter XII	Nutrition in the Critically Ill Older Person *Suzie Ferrie*	**319**
Chapter XIII	Magnesium in Aging: Facts or Myths? *Davidovic Mladen, Djurica Snezana, Dragoslav P. Milosevic, Nebojsa Despotovic and Predrag Erceg*	**333**
Chapter XIV	Nutrition for the Middle-Aged and Elderly: Improving Quality of Life over Adulthood *Maria Bernarda Cordeiro and Marly Augusto Cardoso*	**353**
Chapter XV	Bioindicators of Malnutrition and Inflammation in the Elderly *Dana Hrnciarikova, Zdenek Zadak, Bozena Juraskova, Radomir Hyspler and Petr Klemera*	**371**
Chapter XVI	Pulmonary Emphysema: Not Just a Matter of Alveolar Destruction *Simonetta Baldi*	**389**
Chapter XVII	The Role of Dietary Fatty Acids and Acyl-Coa Synthetases in the Development of Colorectal Cancer *Nikolaus Gassler, Andrea Reinartz, Elke Kaemmerer, Dieter Enders and Wolfgang Bettray*	**447**
Index		**459**

Preface

The aging process changes body composition and thus nutritional status changes as one gets older. At the same time the body becomes more susceptible to diseases and diet becomes an even more significant or at least visibly significant than in earlier years.

Moreover, there is frequently socio-economic downward drifting in this age group making nutritious foods more difficult to afford. This new and important book presents the latest research in this vital field.

Short Communication A - Various positive effects on the human body have been attributed through time to diverse beverages commonly consumed in the Western world. The purpose of this paper is to examine the extent to which popular beliefs regarding certain drinks have a scientific basis. A historical description of the putative therapeutic and/or preventive characteristics of four widely consumed beverages will be presented, followed by a discussion of the state-of-the-art biomedical knowledge regarding them. The importance of wine on human health has been affirmed from time immemorial, and today, in an evidence-based nutritional perspective, the beneficial properties on the vascular system of red wine consumed in moderate quantities have been confirmed both on pathophysiological and clinical grounds. The relevance of voices of the past claiming the favourable effects of coffee, tea and chocolate on human health is also examined. Current evidence documents the beneficial effects, not only on the cardiocirculatory system, but also on other human apparati, including the respiratory and the gastrointestinal ones, of the methylxanthines, polyphenols and flavonoids contained in coffee, green tea and chocolate when assumed by healthy subjects in appropriate dosages.

This historical perspective evidences the continuing pertinence of past traditions regarding major beverages, even when compared with up-dated scientific information. The adage that one never learns enough from the past therefore holds true, though the learning may be as easy as drinking a glass of wine, sipping a cup of tea or enjoying a cup of coffee or chocolate.

Chapter I - An increasing body of evidence suggests that low vitamin D status may impair both insulin secretion and action, ultimately increasing the risk of type 2 diabetes mellitus (DM). Experimentally, vitamin D repletion improves insulin sensitivity and insulin secretion in animal studies of rats. Cross-sectional studies in humans suggest an inverse association between circulating vitamin D levels and impaired glucose tolerance, insulin resistance, and risk of type 2 diabetes. Prospective data, albeit limited, also indicate an inverse association between intake of dietary and supplemental vitamin D and type 2 diabetes risk. Calcium and magnesium may exert both independent and interactive effects on the risk of type 2 diabetes through metabolically related pathways. Genetic variants of these pathways, including the vitamin D receptor (VDR) pathway and calcium and magnesium homeostasis related pathways, also appear to play a role in affecting the risk of type 2 diabetes in humans.

Chapter II - Siding the strong association with cardiovascular disease (CVD), growing interest has been recently addressed to other life-course health implications of nutrition, such as that for neuro-degenerative disorders. As the ratio of people aged over 75 years is growing, and since both incidence and prevalence of dementia increase after this age, it has become relevant for health improvement to understand causes and risk factors for dementia. There is growing evidence that both nutritional status and dietary factors significantly contribute to a life-course development of dementia syndromes. With regard to nutritional status, great attention has been paid to obesity and related disorders, such as hypertension, metabolic syndrome and diabetes. Accordingly, also a predominant role of visceral adiposity has been suggested. On the other hand, a great number of studies has investigated the specific role of macronutrients, particularly dietary fats, and some micronutrients (e.g. folic acid, vitamins and various antioxidants) in both positively and negatively affecting the risk of future dementia. Thus, nutritional preventive care is claimed also with regard to diseases other than CV, although an overlapping contribution of vascular factor is recognized in the pathophisiology of cognitive decline. The present review aims to provide a panoramic view on actually existing evidences concerning the interactions between nutritional status, the obesity-related disorders and the dietary factors both in terms of macro and micronutrients. Evidences from clinical trial and prospective cohort studies will be favoured, although animal and in-vitro studies with possible clinical implications will be also considered.

Chapter III - The incidence of cancer in industrialized countries has increased since the early 1970s. It is estimated that more than one-third of cases are associated with factors related to a Western diet. Dietary factors are thought to account for about 30-40% of cancers in industrialized countries and therefore, diet is second only to tobacco as a potentially preventable cause of cancer. The contribution of diet to risk of cancer in developing countries is lower, perhaps around 20% or less. Obesity increases the risk of cancers in the esophagus, colorectum, breast, endometrium, and kidney. Alcohol causes cancers of the oral cavity, pharynx, larynx, esophagus, and liver, and causes a small increase in the risk of breast cancer. The consumption of nutrient sparse foods containing simple sugars brings about the impairment of glucose metabolism consequently leading to insulin resistance. Insulin resistance increases the risk of the development of cancer at many sites. Low intake of fiber, high consumption of red meat, and imbalance of omega-3 and omega-6 fats all increase significantly the risk of cancer. The inclusion to the diet of foods containing phytochemicals, such as flax seed, cruciferous vegetables, particularly broccoli sprouts can significantly decrease cancer risk. Antioxidant vitamins and minerals, such as the carotenoids (α-carotene, β-carotene, lycopene, lutein, and cryptoxanthin), vitamins C and E as well as selenium and zinc have been shown to protect against cancer. Recent scientific trials have shown the importance of pre-, pro- and synbiotics in decreasing the risk of the development of cancer, particularly of the gastrointestinal tract. Milk and dairy products are the good source of calcium and vitamin D. Dairy products are a diverse food group comprising of various factors that could influence risk, e.g., relatively high saturated fat content, growth factors such as IGF-I, and chemical contaminants such as pesticide residues. However, the calcium, vitamin D, and CLA contents of dairy products have been hypothesized to reduce the cancer risk. Adherence to dietary food guidelines can help diminish the incidence of many types of cancers, including breast cancer, colorectal cancer, prostate cancer even by about 50-70%. The relationship between diet, nutrition and the development of cancer are presented in this review. Emphasis will be given to prospective epidemiologic studies because these are less subject to serious problems of confounding that can make cross-cultural comparisons completely misleading, and they avoid the problem of recall bias that can affect typical case-control studies of diet.

Chapter IV - Osteoporosis is defined as a progressive systemic skeletal disease characterized by low bone mass and microarchitectural deterioration of bone tissue, with a consequent increase in bone fragility and susceptibility to fracture. More than one-third of the adult women will suffer one or more osteoporotic fractures in their lifetime. The lifetime risk in men is approximately one-half that in women. The decrease of the bone mineral density is the most important cause of risk fracture. Albeit bone mass and quality is mainly determined genetically, many other factors, including lifestyle (smoking, excess alcohol intake, physical inactivity) and nutrition also have an impact on bone health. Nutrition is the most significant modifiable factor that influences the development and maintenance of bone mass. Adequate intakes of macro- and micronutrients that modulate bone health can help in the prevention and management of osteoporosis. About 80-90% of mineral content in the bone is consisted of calcium and phosphorous. Among other factors, Ca^{2+} and vitamin D deficiencies are important risk factors for a decrease in bone mineral density, consequently inducing osteoporosis. The high prevalence of vitamin D deficiency in healthy elderly people living mainly in southern European countries increase the risk of osteoporotic fractures in these populations above those anticipated for the general elderly population of the European Community. In addition, the ageing of the world population, particularly the European population will double the number of osteoporotic fractures over the next 50 years, unless adequate preventative measures are undertaken. Apart from calcium, phosphorous and vitamin D, other nutrients, such as protein, magnesium, zinc, fluoride, sodium, copper, vitamins B_6, C, K, essential fatty acids from the omega-3 family, and antioxidants are also needed for normal bone turnover. In this paper, each of these nutrients is discussed separately. The efficacy and safety of Ca^{2+} and vitamin D supplements at preventing bone loss and reducing the risk of hip and other fractures are also discussed.

Chapter V - The Transtheoretical Model (TTM), an overview of which will be provided in this chapter, offers a promising intervention framework for nutrition interventions. Several recent applications of the TTM (e.g., Rossi et al., 2005; Prochaska et al., 2005; Prochaska et al., 2004; Campbell et al., 2004; Johnson et al., under review) have included interventions targeting multiple health behaviors such as healthy eating or fruit and vegetable consumption. These interventions will be reviewed, with particular emphasis on how the interventions are effective across the lifespan, including middle-aged and senior populations. Preliminary evidence supporting the notion that co-variation of behavior change can be produced by tailored interventions will be presented. Johnson et al. (under review), for example, reported that a tailored intervention for healthy eating that targeted calorie and fat intake in the context of a weight management intervention had significant effects on an untreated nutrition behavior (i.e., fruit and vegetable intake).

Advantages of multiple behavior approaches will be highlighted and alternative delivery channels for these interventions will be presented. The chapter will conclude with recommendations for maximizing the potential of multiple behavior change interventions that include nutrition targets.

Chapter VI - Protein-energy malnutrition (PEM) refers to an inadequate supply of nutrients and energy with respect to the body's demand. This condition, caused by organic disturbances or by psychological, social and cultural factors, is highly prevalent in the elderly and can lead to a significant increase of morbidity and mortality.

Early detection of individuals at risk for malnutrition is important to prevent a large proportion of chronic diseases.

However, the objective evaluation of malnutrition in the elderly is difficult because of the lack of reference data for comparisons and of the poor standardization of methods and threshold values.

The aim of this chapter is to discuss the different properties of various methods to diagnosis PEM and the concordance among their results.

The techniques differ in portability, expense and invasiveness, and reflect different aspects of PEM. They are: anthropometry (Body Mass Index, BMI); body composition analysis (phase angle and Bioelectrical Impedance Vector Analysis, BIVA); multi-dimensional techniques (Mini Nutritional Assessment, MNA); biochemical markers (albumin).

The authors used literature data and unpublished results for healthy (548 individuals) and pathological (50 individuals with Alzheimer disease) elderly samples from Sardinia (Italy).

The MNA is a valid and suitable method for the global evaluation of the nutritional status, and distinguishes malnourished, at risk of malnutrition, and well nourished individuals.

BMI is an indicator of size, but does not distinguish between changes of body components. Is inexpensive and easy to perform. Clear agreement between MNA and BMI has been shown in many studies and in the healthy and pathological samples from Sardinia. The cut-off of 24 kg/m^2 showed the greater accuracy (73.5%) in the diagnosis of under-nourishment based on the MNA.

Several authors have reported a significant correlation between MNA and albumin; however, this was not found in Alzheimer disease.

The phase angle, a bioelectrical parameter, is considered an applicable indicator of nutritional status. It decreases as the nutritional state worsens. In the Sardinian sample it showed different means between MNA groups, but a weak correlation with MNA.

The application of BIVA demonstrated that the bioelectric characteristics of malnourished individuals or subjects at risk of malnutrition are significantly different from those of people with normal nutrition (MNA$\geq$24). BIVA appears a suitable and promising alternative technique for the nutritional assessment in the elderly.

Chapter VII – The authors first propose a definition of the "geriatric patient" and a holistic management of his multiple dimensions using a "comprehensive geriatric assessment". Then the nutritional status of the geriatric patient was described. The authors review data from the literature which showed that malnutrition represents a cardinal symptom of frailty in older persons. The authors underscored the importance of an early detection of malnutrition and stressed on the fact that geriatricians should increase their vigilance to detect early weight loss and institute-appropriate preventive and health promotion measures. In view of this preoccupant malnutrition, a quality programs are proposed to improve nutritional status of the geriatric patients. A comprehensive screening tool for assessment of nutritional status is needed that is clinically relevant and cost-effective to perform. If malnutrition is suggested by such screening tests, then they should be supplemented by conventional nutritional assessment before treatment is planned.

Chapter VIII - What kinds of messages are the public receiving concerning food intake and potential to build strength/muscle and how have the public assimilated this information? In the present study 132 college students and 109 older respondents were asked to provide information concerning the nutrients that they believe to be important for building strength/muscle as well as the sources for these messages. A second goal involved determining to what degree food names (e.g., an egg) have reputations for building strength/muscle that are congruent with judgements of the nutrient descriptions of those same foods (e.g., the nutrient profile for an egg). Results revealed that both cohorts believed protein to be most important for building strength/muscle and that this information came from the media more than any other source. Interestingly, heightened familiarity with media messages predicted less stereotypical thinking about foods among the older participants. Cohort differences for food names occurred in seven cases but never for descriptions. Wide disparities between a food's name rating for building strength/muscle and ratings of that same food's nutrient description were common. It appears that we have acquired mistaken beliefs about the strength/muscle building potential (and protein content) of foods but the impact of the popular media on these beliefs is not clear.

Chapter IX - The association of serum magnesium with cancer mortality was investigated prospectively using the Atherosclerosis Risk in Communities (ARIC) Study. Black (N=3,898) and nonblack (N=10,534) participants, aged 45-64 at baseline, were analyzed separately. In a Cox's regression adjusted for gender, age, body mass index, exercise, education, number of cigarettes currently smoked, and smoking history, nonblack participants with serum magnesium ≤1.4 meq/l had a hazard ratio of 2.72 (95% CI 1.40-5.29) for all-cancer mortality compared to persons with serum magnesium ≥1.9 meq/l. When nonblack participants were classified as ≤1.6 meq/l versus ≥1.7 meq/l, low serum magnesium had a hazard ratio of 1.53 (95% CI 1.19-1.97) for all-cancer mortality. Significant inverse relationships between nonblack participants' serum magnesium and two types of cancer mortality were found. First, an association with mortality due to malignant neoplasm of respiratory/intrathoracic organs, and second an association with all other types of cancer mortality. For black participants there was no association of serum magnesium and all-cancer mortality. This pattern of a relationship with serum magnesium among nonblack participants, but no association among black participants was similar to previously published research on the development of diabetes and serum magnesium in the ARIC Study.

Chapter X - The aging process alters body composition so that nutritional status changes as one gets older. The nutritional problems of older adults are not only related to physiological decline but also to socio-economic changes and to a multitude of disease processes and the therapeutic regimens prescribed to cure or treat those illnesses. The gap between actual nutrient consumption among older adults and the recommended intakes for diets associated with health promotion and the prevention of chronic disease is large. Undernutrition, which leads to the "anorexia of aging", and obesity are critical factors of disease and death in the middle-aged and elderly.

This article gives a brief overview of the factors which can contribute to malnutrition and suggests strategies for improvement.

Chapter XI - Fruits and vegetables are essential components of a healthy diet. However, only limited information is available about the fruit and vegetable intake of older women. This study describes the socio-demographic and health correlates of intake of fruit and vegetables among two large cohorts of Australian women – one group aged 50-55 years and one aged 79-84 years. Almost all women ate some amount of fruit and vegetables each day. In each cohort, around 8-9% of the women ate five or more serves of vegetables each day, and 30% ate four or more serves each day. In the Mid-age cohort, around 60% of the women ate two or more serves of fruit each day, and the corresponding proportion for the Older cohort was 70%. Around 7-8% of each cohort could be considered to eat the national recommended intake of two serves of fruit and five serves of vegetables. Eating higher levels of fruit and vegetables was associated with country of birth, education, marital status, and with functional abilities and oral health. Longitudinal analyses describe trends in BMI, health-related quality of life and survival according to women's fruit and vegetable intakes.

Chapter XII - Critical illness poses special challenges for the middle-aged or elderly patient. Increasing age correlates with an increased length of stay in intensive care, and older patients are more likely to experience complications that increase morbidity and mortality. There are several key contributing factors. A smaller lean body mass may mean that many older people lack the physical reserve to withstand a prolonged period of critical illness, where more than 1% of body protein may be lost each day even when adequate energy and protein are being provided. Age-related changes in lean body tissue metabolism may mean that the catabolism of critical illness is much greater in older patients, and losses are more difficult to regain, even with optimal nutrition support and intensive rehabilitation. Pre-existing deficiencies, and an increased baseline level of inflammation, may contribute to early depletion of the body's protective antioxidant system and increase demands for particular vitamins, minerals and trace elements. Lastly, changes in absorption and digestion in older people may reduce micronutrient bioavailability, so that deficiencies become more likely, especially with the uniquely altered requirements of critical illness.

In: Nutrition for the Middle Aged and Elderly
Editors: N. E. Bernhardt, A. M. Kasko, pp. 1-10

ISBN: 978-1-60456-146-3

Expert Commentary A

"Coffee or Tea? From the Historically Alleged Curative Properties of Common Beverages to Their Current Evidence-Based Benefits on Human Health"

Andrea A. Conti [*]
Dipartimento di Area Critica Medico Chirurgica,
Università degli Studi di Firenze.
Fondazione Don Carlo Gnocchi, IRCCS Firenze
Centro Italiano per la Medicina Basata sulle Prove,
Firenze, Italy

Abstract

Various positive effects on the human body have been attributed through time to diverse beverages commonly consumed in the Western world. The purpose of this paper is to examine the extent to which popular beliefs regarding certain drinks have a scientific basis. A historical description of the putative therapeutic and/or preventive characteristics of four widely consumed beverages will be presented, followed by a discussion of the state-of-the-art biomedical knowledge regarding them. The importance of wine on human health has been affirmed from time immemorial, and today, in an evidence-based nutritional perspective, the beneficial properties on the vascular system of red wine consumed in moderate quantities have been confirmed both on pathophysiological and clinical grounds. The relevance of voices of the past claiming the favourable effects of coffee, tea and chocolate on human health is also examined. Current evidence documents the beneficial effects, not only on the cardiocirculatory system, but also on other human apparati, including the respiratory and the gastrointestinal ones, of

[*] Author for correspondence: Andrea Alberto Conti, MD, MPH, PhD. Dipartimento di Area Critica Medico Chirurgica, Università degli Studi di Firenze. Viale Morgagni 85, I-50134, Firenze, Italy. Tel.: +39-055-7949357; Fax: +39-055-7947608; E-mail: aa.conti@dac.unifi.it

the methylxanthines, polyphenols and flavonoids contained in coffee, green tea and chocolate when assumed by healthy subjects in appropriate dosages.

This historical perspective evidences the continuing pertinence of past traditions regarding major beverages, even when compared with up-dated scientific information. The adage that one never learns enough from the past therefore holds true, though the learning may be as easy as drinking a glass of wine, sipping a cup of tea or enjoying a cup of coffee or chocolate.

Keywords: *Adults; Cardiovascular System; Chocolate; Coffee; Elderly; Evidence Based Medicine; History of Medicine; Nutrition; Tea; Wine.*

Introduction

Various positive effects on the human body have been attributed through time to diverse beverages commonly consumed in the Western world. The purpose of this paper is to examine the extent to which popular beliefs regarding certain drinks have a scientific basis, and to give a balanced view of the favourable properties of wine, coffee, tea and chocolate. Given that many aliments, if assumed in an excessive way, may be harmful for humans, in this article the positive effects on adult and also elderly healthy subjects of four drinks consumed in moderate quantities will be described. In many cases, these evidence-based beneficial effects interestingly confirm the historically alleged curative properties of the four beverages considered, and, therefore, for each of them, a historical description of the putative therapeutic and/or preventive characteristics is presented, followed by a discussion of the pertinent state-of-the-art biomedical knowledge.

Wine

Wine is an alcoholic beverage derived from the fermentation of the juice of grapes. The importance of wine on human health has been affirmed from time immemorial. The Old Testament documents Noah's knowledge of the fermentation of grapes, while the first miracle of Jesus described in the New Testament is the turning of water into wine. With regard to the Western world, the medical properties of wine were already documented in the Greek epic poems, the *Iliad* and the *Odyssey*. In ancient Egypt, as in many other cultures, the role of wine was central in rites and in religious ceremonies. In the Roman empire wine constituted a fundamental part of the diet, and, given the extent of this empire, the drinking of wine also had enormous impact on the development of viticulture and oenology in Roman-held territories. Furthermore, wine tended to be considered the preferable liquid medium for containing curative substances and, consequently, medicinal wines, meaning wines with different principles added in order to treat different disorders, were already largely in use in Roman times. It may be noted that even today popular medicine continues to make provision for the addition of specific substances to wine for curative purposes (sage for toothache, iron filings for anaemia).

Through time, however, it was essentially the intrinsic positive effects on human health of wine alone that were evidenced. This is confirmed by proverbs, that represent so-called popular wisdom: in Italy, for example, wine is commonly said "to make good blood". In fact, probably because of its appearance as a red fluid, wine was associated to blood in various ways: the common denominator of popular wisdom was that wine assumption, particularly if moderate and during meals, favourably influenced blood composition and circulation [1,2]. It is also important to remember that in Italy as well as in other Mediterranean countries wine has always been considered essential in pharmacopoeia, having been adopted for a wide array of needs, ranging from the cleaning and disinfection of wounds to the procuring of rudimental anaesthesia.

At the present time and in an evidence-based nutritional perspective, granted that an excessive use of wine is dangerous for human health, and that, exactly as for many other substances, wine may become toxic according to its dosage, consistent epidemiological evidence, confirming popular tradition, indicates that regular and moderate red wine intake reduces cardiovascular risk and total mortality in adult and elderly healthy subjects [3,4]. The recommendation of moderation has a clear scientific rationale, since an excess of a level of consumption that has been quantified in one-two glasses of red wine a day for men and one glass of red wine a day for women, has harmful effects on multiple human organs and systems, including the cardiovascular one. Popular recommendations are also correct with regard to the modality of assumption of wine; thus, its parcelled intake with meals has been shown to exert more favourable effects than its autonomous assumption far from meals, and this on account of the tempering effect of food on the rate of its metabolism [5]. With respect to non-drinkers of wine, moderate healthy drinkers usually have higher levels of HDL cholesterol (the so-called "good cholesterol"), lower fibrinogen values and lower PAI-1 (plasminogen activator inhibitor 1) levels [6]. In fact, the pattern of protection of wine on the cardiovascular system is J-shaped, implicating that no and high consumption are less favourable for human health than a moderate intake. The daily regular consumption of 150 ml of wine had been shown to reduce cardiovascular diseases by around 32% [7]. Moreover, today red wine is considered more protective than white wine, as different studies indicate that the positive effects of wine are largely determined by polyphenols, and in particular resveratrol, of which red wine is rich [8]. The neuroprotective, anti-viral and anti-proliferative properties of trans-resveratrol have also been shown [9]. Among other described beneficial effects of resveratrol, mechanisms leading to an increase in nitric oxide, a decrease in the activity of angiotensin II and a decrease in platelet aggregation [6,8] appear interesting. Furthermore, anti-ischemic effects, including the decrease in LDL-oxidation and the enhancement of pro-survival paths, have been documented [10]. Therefore, on evidence-based grounds, it can effectively be said that, for its favourable effects on the cardiovascular and on the coagulation systems, "a little wine makes good blood".

Coffee

Coffee and tea provide further good examples of the relevance of the voices of the past claiming the favourable effects of these beverages on human health. Current evidence well documents the beneficial activity, not only on the cardiocirculatory system but also on other human apparati, including the respiratory and the gastrointestinal ones, of the methylxanthines, polyphenols and flavonoids contained in coffee and green tea assumed by adult and elderly healthy subjects in moderate dosages [11,12].

Coffee originated from Africa, and precisely from Abyssinia, where it was already cultivated in the VII century. By the XI century coffee was widely recognized as a stimulating beverage, sharing with wine the attributed characteristic of producing euphoria. However, since the consumption of wine was forbidden in the Islamic world, coffee there became its substitute and underwent a rapid diffusion. In the XI century the great Persian physician Avicenna described the different positive effects of coffee on the human neurological and cardiovascular systems, and, convinced of its therapeutic value, he prescribed it as a drug. In the XVI century the first coffee shops were opened in Constantinople, from where it was imported to Italy by Venetian merchants. In the first half of the XVII century the first coffee shop was opened in Italy, and, in the course of less than 150 years, more than 200 coffee shops appeared in Venice. At the beginning of the XVIII century the Dutch took coffee to Brazil, and soon after South America became the world's leading area for coffee production.

Although the pharmacological properties of coffee were first described in Europe by the voyager Prospero Alpino at the end of the XVI century (*De plantis Aegypti*, Venice 1592), it was only in the XIX century that the stimulating character of coffee, related to caffeine, was quantitatively defined in Western world. At that time coffee was used both in medical settings and in empirical contexts as an activator drink for the central nervous system, a remedy for headache and a diuretic beverage [2, 13].

Coffee contains caffeine, a methylxanthine, similar to the theofilline characteristic of tea and the theobromine of chocolate. Methylxanthines have various biological effects on different systems and organs, including a positive inotropic and chronotropic influence on the heart. In the cardiovascular system they cause dilation in the coronary, peripheral and renal vessels, and vasoconstriction of the cerebral circulation, a mechanism that partly explains the effective favourable role of caffeine on headaches [11, 12]. Methylxanthines inhibit platelet aggregation, cause bronchodilation, provoke the stimulation of renin release and bring about a general diuretic effect [12]. Coffee therefore not only has activating and stimulating effects on the nervous system, in accordance with popular ideas, but also exerts many other relevant biological actions [14]. It should be stressed that coffee not only contains caffeine, which in effect accounts for merely 2-3% of the total biological activity of this beverage, but also hundreds of different substances with definite effects, including diterpens (fats), magnesium and fenolic acids [11]. Diterpens increase cholesterol, while magnesium increases the sensitivity of human peripheral tissues to insulin. Fenolic acids increase homocysteine, decrease LDL oxidation, platelet aggregation and glucose absorption. The overall importance of coffee in human nutrition is confirmed by the fact that, in many and different populations (Germany, Norway, Spain), coffee is, on a theoretical basis, the single most important dietetic source of precious antioxidants [11, 15].

In synthesis, coffee is a complex aliment, that might be defined as a "variety of beverages", containing numerous and diverse active substances. Their overall action depends on their reciprocal quantitative and qualitative balance, on the method of preparation, on the rhythm and entity of consumption and on the dietetic habits and lifestyle patterns in which the consumption itself is embedded [16]. In past decades coffee has sometimes been accused of being potentially dangerous for the cardiovascular system, and in particular for the heart. A recent comprehensive meta-analysis by our group has on the contrary shown that a moderate daily consumption (1-3 espresso cups a day) in adult and elderly healthy subjects, if included in a correct and balanced diet and within an appropriate lifestyle scheme, does not increase the risk of coronary heart disease [17].

Tea

Camellia sinensis, the technical definition of tea, derives from the Eastern world, as indicated by the adjective "sinensis" (Chinese). Already in the VI century tea was cultivated in China, where it was a very popular beverage, well reputed for its healing and therapeutic qualities. About the middle of the XVI century Giovanbattista Ramusio, the famous Italian humanist, wrote that tea could make fever, headache, stomach ache and joint pain disappear, provided it was assumed as hot as possible. A century later tea was imported into Europe by the Portuguese and Dutch. In Great Britain the consumption of this beverage grew and spread rapidly. Though at first confined to the higher classes, it subsequently gained popularity in every rank of society, becoming the national English drink (as coffee is for Italy). Indeed, it may be said that in England drinking tea became, and still is, almost a ritual. The medical properties of tea had already been observed in the fifteen hundreds, when it was considered a remedy for a wide range of health problems, given that it was retained to accelerate metabolism, to depurate the body, to calm inflammation, to render blood circulation more fluent, and to reduce the sensation of fatigue. In the XIX century its pharmacological effects began to be defined in a precise way, this being particularly true for the diuretic and vasodilatative effects of theophilline, an alkaloid of which tea is rich. If coffee has always been considered a drink useful in activating the human mind, tea has been considered a beverage effective in relaxing the human body. In reality, the alkaloids contained in tea are stimulating substances, and tea contains caffeine as well. It is true, however, as believed in the past, that tea has antioxidant, vasodilatative and diuretic properties, which will now be briefly illustrated [18, 19].

In recent times many biological characteristics of tea, and in particular of green tea, have been documented and their effects with regard to the human organism and human health have been evidenced [20]. The overall positive effects of green tea probably derive from the interaction of polyphenols, and especially of flavonoids and epigallocatechin gallate [21]. Flavonoids have indeed anti-inflammatory, anti-oxidant and anti-thrombogenic properties, which are responsible for their cardioprotective impact [22]. The xanthines and polyphenols contained in tea produce lipolitic and diuretic activity, while catechins have been shown to produce antiatherosclerotic effects. In vitro, in fact, they prevent LDL cholesterol oxidation (the so-called "bad cholesterol") [23].

Evidence is also growing with regard to the fact that tea polyphenols containing a galloyl group may favourably interfere with many different pathways of signal transduction, in particular in cardiovascular system cells. The prompting of pleiotropic effects on the part of green tea may play a key role in the prevention and therapy of cardiovascular diseases, and further extensive research may confirm the impact of tea components on human cells [18]. Green tea catechins also have effects on the molecular mechanisms involved in multi-drug resistance, in the regulation of cellular death and in angiogenesis [24]. Some Japanese researchers have consequently proposed green tea as a preventive beverage for cancer, suggesting the disseminated prophylactic assumption of ten cups per day [25]. However, such a powerful preventive and therapeutic role for tea needs further structured experimentation, as some data need diffuse, in vivo confirmation. Globally, however, up-dated knowledge is extremely promising and confirms many of the alleged properties attributed to tea in the past.

Chocolate

Chocolate is the name given to a drink made by mixing the powder (cocoa) obtained from the crushed seeds of the cacao tree with hot water or milk. It is thought that more than 2,500 years ago Mayans drank chocolate, as suggested by chocolate residues traced in ancient Mayan pots, while the Aztecs linked chocolate with Xochiquetzal, the goddess of fertility. In pre-Columbian America the native populations dried the seeds of the cacao plant, prepared them on the fire, and, after powdering them, mixed this powder with water. They consumed the resulting cocoa as a spicy and bitter drink called xocoatl, seasoned with pepper and vanilla, but not milk. This is interesting, since it has now been established that the maximum positive effects of chocolate on the cardiovascular system are connected to the dark, and not the milk, variety. Spanish conquerors came into contact with the cacao plant in America when the New World was discovered, and the introduction of chocolate into Europe is therefore successive to 1492. In the XVI century in Mexico Fernando Cortez was taken to be the god Quatzcoalt by the natives, and therefore the inhabitants of that region, in his honour, called the cocoa beverage Cacahualt, which later became Chocolatlla, from whence the name.

One of the first documentations in Europe of the use of chocolate as a medical remedy is to be found in the "Ragionamenti del mio viaggio intorno al mondo" ("Reflections on my voyage around the world"), of the Italian voyager Francesco Carletti, who, at the end of the XVI century, wrote that chocolate was then drunk as a real medicine. In a later period, although some exponents of the Catholic Church for some time considered chocolate a voluptuous and transgressive aliment, pope Pius V formally refused to sanction a requested prohibition of chocolate consumption. In effect, it is retained that it was most probably in convents that, at this time, the preparation of chocolate was altered, and its recipe, previously containing hot pepper and spices, was modified in the direction of current taste. Precisely on account of this improvement in flavour, chocolate was also called "theobroma", "the food of the gods". From the word "theobroma" comes the term theobromine, later assigned to the major alkaloid contained in chocolate. The XVII century was the period in which large amounts of chocolate began to be produced in paste form in many European areas, especially in Spain and Flanders, thus testifying to the constantly growing attraction exercised by the substance. In the XIX century, to the generalized recognition of chocolate's pleasing and pleasant qualities, as also of its ability to bring about a good mood and its capacity to cause vasodilation with consequent beneficial effects on the heart and vessels, there was added the scientific confirmation of its diuretic features [2, 26].

As has been said, chocolate derives from the cocoa bean, which is one of the most concentrated sources of flavonoids. The specific antioxidants of chocolate include flavanol molecules, such as catechin and epicatechin, similar to the antioxidants contained in grapes, and consequently in wine, and in tea. Flavonoids reduce platelet activation and aggregation, induce nitric-oxide-dependent vasodilation in healthy humans and prompt the generation of eicosanoids, confirming the historically alleged beneficial effects of chocolate on the vascular apparatus [27]. Flavonoid-rich dark chocolate is a powerful ex vivo and in vivo antioxidant and an anti-atherosclerotic agent in animal models [28]. It may be noted that in the United States chocolate is the third highest individual source of antioxidants, after coffee and tea [29]. Flavonoids also improve the endothelial function by increasing plasma catechins, and decrease vascular cell adhesion molecules in hypercholesterolemic women [30]. These multiple positive effects of chocolate on the cardiovascular system are more specific in dark chocolate and, in general, the darker the chocolate the more likely its favourable effects on the cardiovascular apparatus. In effect, according to the authors of an elegant recent study, the secondary links established between chocolate flavonoids and milk proteins (in milk chocolate) determine a reduced biological availability of flavonoids and an overall reduction of the in vivo antioxidant positive characteristics of chocolate [31]. Recent evidence also indicates that cocoa intake has a favourable effect in reducing arterial pressure [32], thus again confirming popular adages. In elderly individuals with systolic arterial hypertension, 100 mg of dark chocolate a day reduces systolic blood pressure levels by 5.1 mm Hg and diastolic values by 1.8 mm Hg, corresponding to a decrease in cardiovascular events of more than 20% [33]. The mechanisms through which chocolate may decrease blood pressure are likely to be multiple, but, overall, probably linked to its capacity to facilitate the synthesis of nitric oxide. Chocolate has also been proved to lower, at least in animal models, cholesterol and triglycerides. The optimal dosage for the beneficial effects on the cardiovascular system has still to be identified and it currently represents a major area of study for basic and clinical researchers. However, it has already been reported that 50 grams of dark chocolate (1-2 cups a day) may reduce the risk of the insurgence and development of cardiovascular diseases by approximately 10% [34].

Conclusion

This historical perspective evidences the continuing pertinence of past traditions regarding major beverages, even when compared with up-dated scientific information [35]. Although a major challenge for current and future studies consists in identifying the optimal dosage in the assumption of beverages such as tea and chocolate, with regard to wine and coffee dosages, their assumption limits now seem reasonably clear. Best current evidence on wine and coffee indicates that, in adult and elderly healthy people and with specific reference to the cardiovascular system, moderate use is not only better than a higher intake, but also appears more protective than no use at all [36]. The history of medicine thus documents how popular wisdom has proved to be correct and may be summarised by the Latin adage "Est modus in rebus" ("Measure in things") [37].

One therefore never learns enough from the past, though the learning may be as easy as drinking a glass of wine, sipping a cup of tea or enjoying a cup of coffee or chocolate.

Acknowledgements

The Author would like to thank Professor Luisa Camaiora, B.A., M.Phil., for her correction of the English.

References

[1] Foulkes, C. *Larousse Encyclopedia of Wine*. Paris: Larousse; 2001.
[2] Cosmacini, G; Gaudenzi, G; Satolli, R. *Dizionario di storia della salute*. Torino: Einaudi; 1996.
[3] Opie, LH; Lecour, S. The red wine hypothesis: from concepts to protective signalling molecules. *European Heart Journal,* 2007; 28: 1683-93.
[4] Tolstrup, J; Jensen, MK; Tjonneland, A; et al. Prospective study of alcohol drinking patterns and coronary heart disease in women and men. *BMJ*, 2006; 332: 1244-8.
[5] Mukamal, KJ; Jensen, MK; Gronbaek, M; et al. Drinking frequency, mediating biomarkers, and risk of myocardial infarction in women and men. *Circulation*, 2005; 112: 1406-13.
[6] Bradamante, S; Barenghi, L; Piccinini, F; et al. Resveratrol provides late-phase cardioprotection by means of a nitric oxide- and adenosine-mediated mechanism. *Eur. J. Pharmacol.*, 2003; 465: 115-23.
[7] Di Castelnuovo, A; Rotondo, S; Iacoviello, D; Donati, MB; De Gaetano, G. Meta-analysis of wine and beer consumption in relation to vascular risk. *Circulation*, 2002; 105: 2836-44.
[8] Stef, G; Csiszar, A; Lerea, K; et al. Resveratrol inhibits aggregation of platelets from high-risk cardiac patients with aspirin resistance. *J. Cardiovasc. Pharmacol.*, 2006; 48: 1-5.
[9] Palamara, AT; Nencioni, L; Aquilano, K. Inhibition of influenza A virus replication by resveratrol. *J. Infectious. Diseases*, 2005; 191: 1719-29.
[10] Scalbert, A; Manach, C; Morand, C; Remesy, C; Jimenez L. Dietary polyphenols and the prevention of diseases. *Crit. Rev. Food Sci. Nutr.*, 2005; 45: 287-306.
[11] Natella, F; Ghiselli, A; Rossi, L; Sette, S; D'Amicis, A. Caffè e cuore. Roma: INRAN; 2005.
[12] D'Amicis, A; Ghiselli, A; Rossi, L; Sette, S. Caffè e salute. Roma: INRAN; 2005.
[13] Gensini, GF; Conti, AA. Does coffee consumption represent a coronary risk factor? *Recenti Prog. Med.*, 2004; 95: 563-5.
[14] Garattini, S. Caffeine, coffee and health (8th edition). New York: Raven Press; 1993.

[15] Nawrot, P; Jordan, S; Eastwood, J; Rotstein, J; Hugenholtz, A; Feeley, M. Effects of caffeine on human health. *Food Addit. Contam.*, 2003; 20: 1-30.

[16] Tavani, A; Bertuzzi, M; Negri, E; Sorbara, L; La Vecchia, C. Alcohol, smoking, coffee and risk of non-fatal acute myocardial infarction in Italy. *Eur. J. Epidemiol.*, 2001; 17: 1131-7.

[17] Sofi, F; Conti, AA; Gori, AM; Luisi, MLE; Casini, A; Abbate, R; Gensini, GF. Coffee consumption and risk of coronary heart disease: a meta-analysis. *Nutr. Metab. Cardiovasc. Dis.*, 2007; 17: 209-23.

[18] Gensini, GF; Lippi, D; Conti, AA. Past, present and future of green tea: from pleasant beverage to drug in pills? *Recenti Prog. Med.*, 2007; 98: 347-51.

[19] Heiss, ML; Heiss, RJ. *The story of tea: a cultural history and drinking guide*. Ten Speed Press; 2007.

[20] Graham, HN. Green tea composition, consumption, and polyphenol chemistry. *Prev. Med.*, 1992; 21: 334-50.

[21] Cabrera, C; Artacho, R; Gimenez, R. Beneficial effects of green tea. A review. *J. Am. Coll. Nutr.*, 2006; 25: 79-99.

[22] Stangl, V; Dreger, H; Stangl, K; Lorenz, M. Molecular targets of tea polyphenols in the cardiovascular system. *Cardiovasc. Res.*, 2007; 73: 348-58.

[23] Peters, U; Poole, C; Arab, L. Does tea affect cardiovascular disease? A meta-analysis. *Am. J. Epidemiol.*, 2001; 154: 495-503.

[24] Fraser, ML; Mok, GS; Lee, AH. Green tea and stroke prevention: emerging evidence. *Complement. Ther. Med.*, 2007; 15: 46-53.

[25] Fujiki, H; Suganuma, M; Imai, K; Nakachi K. Green tea: cancer preventive beverage and/or drug. *Cancer Letters*, 2002; 188: 9-13.

[26] Coe, SD; Coe, MD. The true history of chocolate. London: Thames and Hudson Ltd.; 1996.

[27] Ding, EL; Hutfless, SM; Ding, X; Girotra S. Chocolate and prevention of cardiovascular disease: a systematic review. *Nutrition and Metabolism*, 2006; 3: 2.

[28] Vinson, JA; Proch, J; Bose, P; et al. Chocolate is a powerful ex vivo and in vivo antioxidant, an anti-atherosclerotic agent in an animal model, and significant contributor to antioxidants in European and American diets. *J. Agric. Food Chem.*, 2006; 54: 8071-6.

[29] Alspach, G. The truth is often bittersweet. Chocolate does a heart good. *Critical Care Nurse*, 2007; 27: 11-5.

[30] Wang-Polagruto, JF; Villablanca, AC; Polagruto, JA; et al. Chronic consumption of flavanol-rich cocoa improves endothelial function and decreases vascular cell adhesion molecules in hypercholesterolemic postmenopausal women. *J. Cardiovasc. Pharmacol.*, 2006; 47 (suppl 2): S177-S186.

[31] Murphy, KJ; Chronopoulos, AK; Singh, I; et al. Dietary flavanols and procyanidin oligomer from cocoa (Theobroma cacao) inhibit platelet function. *Am. J. Clin. Nutr.*, 2003; 77: 1466-73.

[32] Buijsse, B; Feskens, EJM; Kok, FJ; Kromhout D. Cocoa intake, blood pressure and cardiovascular mortality: the Zutphen elderly study. *Arch. Intern. Med.*, 2006; 166: 411-7.

[33] Taubert, D; Berkels, R; Roesen, R; Klaus, W. Chocolate and blood pressure in elderly individuals with isolated systolic hypertension. *JAMA*, 2003; 290: 1029-30.

[34] Franco, OH; Bonneux, L; de Laet, C; Peeters, A; Steyerberg, EW; Mackenbach, JP. The Polymeal: a more natural, safer, and probably tastier (than the Polypill) strategy to reduce cardiovascular disease by more than 75%. *BMJ*, 2004; 329: 1447-50.

[35] Gensini, GF; Conti, AA. From cardiovascular prevention to cardiovascular rehabilitation: statins and Evidence Based Medicine. *Ital. Heart J.*, 2002 Suppl 3: 91-4.

[36] Marcucci, R; Gori, AM; Bertuccioli, M; Gensini, GF; Abbate, R. In vivo effect of Chianti red wine on tissue factor, tissue factor pathway inhibitor and homocysteine levels. *Thromb. Haemost.*, 2005; 94; 689-90.

[37] Conti, AA; Galanti, C; Gensini, GF. Is evidence-based medicine really a craze? Surely it is fashionable to criticize it. A methodologic comment from the Italian Center for Evidence Based Medicine. *Ital. Heart J.*, 2000 Suppl 1(9):1192-5.

In: Nutrition for the Middle Aged and Elderly
Editors: N. E. Bernhardt, A. M. Kasko, pp. 11-29
ISBN: 978-1-60456-146-3

Short Communication B

Food Consumption Patterns, Nutrient Intake, and Serum Components among Middle- Aged and Elderly Nepalese

Yoshimi Ohno[1], Kazuko Hirai[2], Shiba K. Rai[3], Jeevan B. Sherchand[4] and Mathura P. Shrestha[5]
[1]Department of Food Science and Nutrition, School of Human Environmental Sciences, Mukogawa Women's University, Hyogo, Japan
[2]Department of Food and Nutrition, Faculty of Human Life Sciences, Senri Kinran University, Osaka, Japan
[3]Department of Microbiology, Nepal Medical College, Kathmandu, Nepal
[4]Department of Community Medicine and Family Health, Institute of Medicine, Tribhuvan University, Kathmandu, Nepal
[5]Department of Community Health, Institute of Medicine, Tribhuvan University, Kathmandu, Nepal

Introduction

Malnutrition is major public health problem in many developing countries including Nepal [1-5] and is aggravated by a high prevalence of infectious diseases [5, 6]. In view of this situation, we have been evaluating the nutritional status and health of the Nepalese for the past 30 years.

Using the 24-hour recall method, we studied the dietary intake and nutritional serum components of persons aged 10-75 years living in the southern Terai region (an industrial [7-9] and agricultural regions [9-13] at sea level), Bhojpur district (Boya village, a hilly area at an altitude of 1500~2500 m) [14, 15], the Kathmandu valley (an urban area at an altitude of 1330 m) [16], and the northern mountainous area (Jzong village, in a mountainous area at an altitude of 3500 m) [17]. These areas were selected because they were on a geographical belt and included both urban and rural areas.

The Itahari district is an industrial region and the Chitwan district is an agricultural region in the Terai region of southern Nepal. Boya village Development Committee (VDC, area A and B) is a typical remote hilly area and is located in Bhojpur district of eastern Nepal. Dzong village, a small and remote village, is located near Muktinath in the northern mountainous area of the Gandaki region in Nepal.

Fasting venous blood samples were obtained from the subjects, and serum nutritional components were measured using commercial clinical kits [7, 14, 16]. Serum globulin (Glb) levels were obtained by subtracting the albumin (Alb) value from the total protein value, and the Alb/Glb ratio was calculated.

The results described here were obtained from middle-aged and elderly participants (over 30 years of age) of these studies and were compared with each other.

Physical Characteristics of People

The height and body weight were measured for all subjects, and the body mass index (BMI) was calculated as weight/height^2 (kg/m^2). The systolic (SBP) and the diastolic blood pressure (DBP) were measured. The physical characteristics of the subjects are shown in Table 1. The mean values of the height and body weight for males were higher than those for females. Among males, the mean values of height for the subjects in the Itahari tended to be high, and those for the people in Boya village tended to be low. The mean heights of females in area B, Boya village, were lower compared with those of the others. The mean level of BMI varied from 16.7$\pm$0.9 (30-39-year-old females in the Chitwan) to 24.8$\pm$3.7 (40-49-year-old males in the Itahari); however, the BMI values mostly averaged from 18 to 20. These BMI values were lower than 22, the value considered to indicate the lowest morbidity due to diseases in Japanese people between 30 and 59 years of age [18]; however, rural 19-year-old Bangladeshi women had the lowest mortality rate with a BMI of 16.37-20.71 [19]. Therefore, the mean BMI value of the subjects seemed to be adequate although the most of them were rather lean, and not overweight. The mean values of SBP were between 147$\pm$15 mmHg (50-72-year-old males in the Itahari) and 107$\pm$8 mmHg (30-39-year-old group in the Itahari), and five age groups showed SBP of over 130 mmHg, which indicated borderline high blood pressure [20]. Concerning DBP, five age groups showed DBP of over 85 mmHg. People living in the Terai region tended to have higher blood pressure than those in the other areas.

Table 1. Physical characteristics of the middled-aged and elderly Nepalese

Area	Sex	Age group	Subjects	Height	Weight	Body mass index	Blood pressure (mmHg)	
			(n)	(cm)	(kg)	(kg/m^2)	SBP	DBP
Itahari	Male	30-39	7	169±6	58.9±7.9	20.6±2.2	117±11	81±8
		40-49	3	166±4	69.0±12.5	24.8±3.7	120±0	88±3
		50-72	5	164±4	66.0±13.5	24.5±5.4	147±15	95±5
	Female	30-39	11	151±4	52.0±9.5	22.8±3.7	107±8	77±5
		40-49	5	152±6	50.2±7.6	21.7±2.8	140±36	93±12
Chitwan	Male	30-39	12	165±6	50.7±5.9	18.6±1.2	130±13	86±7
		40-49	5	163±8	49.2±1.7	18.5±1.5	113±8	77±6
		50-68	6	162±3	53.2±5.1	20.3±2.6	132±3.2	81±8
	Female	30-39	9	151±5	38.2±3.7	16.7±0.9	120±10	79±8
		40-49	8	147±5	39.8±2.6	18.3±1.2	127±12	80±8
		50-59	4	152±7	42.0±43.0	18.3±1.4	130±0	84±4
Area A	Male	30-39	8	156±7	48.8±4.1	20.2±2.0	114±16	81±11
		40-49	6	159±6	50.0±6.2	20.0±2.6	120±21	80±6
		50-73	14	160±10	45.5±4.9	18.1±2.6	113±16	79±10
	Female	30-39	15	150±5	46.4±3.6	20.8±2.1	110±10	74±7
		40-49	13	151±8	40.8±7.6	18.0±3.7	106±11	70±14
		50-72	17	149±7	42.8±4.2	19.3±1.9	123±18	85±14

Table 1. (Continued)

Area	Sex	Age group	Subjects (n)	Height (cm)	Weight (kg)	Body mass index (kg/m^2)	Blood pressure (mmHg)	
							SBP	DBP
Area B	Male	30-39	12	152±9	52.8±6.0	22.9±3.4	118±12	76±10
		40-49	7	161±9	49.6±10.1	19.0±2.3	112±8	79±5
		50-73	14	155±8	47.8±6.5	20.0±2.3	113±16	78±10
	Female	30-39	10	147±5	44.1±5.0	20.3±2.3	109±13	71±11
		40-49	17	148±7	45.8±7.1	20.9±2.8	111±10	71±11
		50-72	14	145±6	44.9±4.6	21.3±1.5	119±15	79±13
Dzong	Male	30-39	9	165±4	53.9±4.0	19.8±1.4	125±20	80±6
		40-49	3	162±2	54.1±2.5	20.6±1.2	115±6	72±9
		50-76	17	160±7	53.0±9.0	20.7±2.4	130±26	77±13
	Female	30-39	17	151±6	48.0±5.4	20.9±1.8	121±10	77±9
		40-49	4	154±5	49.7±2.5	20.9±0.3	128±24	82±11
		50-75	16	151±5	44.7±4.5	19.7±1.2	129±25	82±22
Kathmandu	Male	30-39	25	164±5	56.6±7.2	20.9±2.5	132±16	83±13
		40-49	6	157±8	51.0±4.0	20.8±1.1	125±13	79±11
		50-84	21	160±7	53.5±8.4	20.8±2.5	129±27	78±15
	Female	30-39	23	152±6	48.9±7.5	21.2±3.1	121±13	77±9
		40-49	6	154±5	53.0±7.9	22.3±3.7	127±17	82±8
		50-75	18	150±7	44.1±4.7	19.7±1.7	125±25	79±22

Values are mean±SD. Abbreviations: SBP, systolic blood pressure; DBP, diastolic blood pressure.

Table 2.1. Mean daily food consumption of the middled-aged and elderly Nepalese in the Terai region and the Kathmandu valley

Food group (g/day)	Itahari			Chitwan			Kathmandu valley		
	30-39	40-49	50≦	30-39	40-49	50≦	30-39	40-49	50≦
Male: number	7	3	5	12	5	6	25	6	21
Total cereals	328±185	401±105	494±122	450±83	460±121	423±106	406±96	310±155	368±105
Rice	300±191	360±133	363±150	430±61	460±121	410±113	318±134	196±199	166±77
Wheat	28±64	41±37	115±258	11±26	0±0	0±0	28±66	72±85	143±86
Potatoes	133±34	149±85	78±64	64±84	92±174	64±88	139±102	110±153	153±107
Sugar and sweetening	25±22	12±12	24±14	6±7	11±11	6±4	6±4	5±3	7±7
Fats and oils	25±15	29±12	31±30	8±6	7±2	6±4	11±5	13±5	15±8
Pulses	31±18	46±13	44±43	10±18	0±0	6±6	34±31	60±41	29±18
Vegetables: Colored	83±172	52±20	23±51	216±101	144±163	139±92	34±31	52±37	49±28
Others	68±56	79±65	153±37	40±75	52±69	80±75	72±54	64±33	67±33
Fruits	10±19	69±117	0±0	13±35	0±0	0±0	5±8	47±100	19±42
Meats	10±26	12±20	7±16	19±65	0±0	0±0	78±68	64±29	34±27
Eggs	0±0	0±0	10±22	0±0	0±0	20±40	4±20	17±26	5±15
Fishes	12±32	0±0	17±38	26±49	20±45	0±0	0±0	0±0	3±13
Milk and dairy products	262±239	313±133	330±228	149±266	106±164	202±186	45±71	23±52	24±55
Alcoholic beverages	86±227	0±0	100±224	157±247	20±45	229±185	63±156	407±440	213±249

Table 2.1. (Continued)

Food group (g/day)	Itahari			Chitwan			Kathmandu valley		
	30-39	40-49	50≦	30-39	40-49	50≦	30-39	40-49	50≦
Females: number	11	5	0	9	8	4	23	6	18
Total cereals	500±142	455±163	*	355±154	424±86	328±58	384±114	368±127	333±98
Rice	406±200	377±186	*	326±147	424±86	322±66	212±132	145±95	165±64
Wheat	94±165	58±104	*	18±36	0±0	0±0	92±79	87±88	119±76
Potatoes	93±70	165±122	*	13±20	111±86	145±172	146±93	145±129	150±112
Sugar and sweetening	29±24	31±16	*	5±8	2±3	3±3	11±6	12±13	11±12
Fats and oils	20±13	21±13	*	9±5	13±13	11±5	16±7	11±7	15±10
Pulses	50±31	64±84	*	8±12	3±9	13±10	46±29	33±20	39±22
Vegetables: Colored	57±75	36±59	*	283±112	96±84	152±176	78±39	59±8	48±25
Others	102±92	96±59	*	70±156	100±128	51±50	57±41	51±39	71±26
Fruits	8±11	9±18	*	0±0	0±0	0±0	10±9	14±15	19±25
Meats	0±0	0±0	*	17±35	0±0	13±25	38±32	21±19	32±29
Eggs	0±0	0±0	*	0±0	8±21	0±0	0±0	0±0	0±0
Fishes	0±0	17±38	*	18±53	13±35	0±0	4±21	0±0	0±0
Milk and dairy products	293±439	262±74	*	212±287	156±204	204±281	19±38	15±30	7±28
Alcoholic beverages	6±21	48±107	*	29±47	28±78	0±0	41±63	50±63	86±84

Values are mean±SD.

Table 2.2. Mean daily food consumption of the middled-aged and elderly Nepalese in the hilly and mountainous areas

Food group (g/day)	Boya village (A)			Boya village (B)			Dzong village		
	30-39	40-49	50≦	30-39	40-49	50≦	30-39	40-49	50≦
Male: number	11	6	15	11	7	19	9	3	17
Total cereals	435±197	451±161	340±70	436±135	414±64	328±93	423±81	301±102	373±109
Rice	314±153	357±146	252±64	282±109	256±106	226±95	232±153	72±63	143±46
Maize*	121±121	55±79	82±91	149±101	151±48	89±68	96±93	144±52	177±55
Potatoes	73±58	100±152	77±70	86±80	177±101	144±103	242±63	203±177	185±91
Sugar and sweetening	*	*	*	*	*	*	8±3	6±3	7±7
Fats and oils	3±2	4±2	4±2	2±1	3±1	3±2	12±6	17±5	16±7
Pulses	44±22	22±30	24±30	9±15	31±25	18±18	50±31	72±58	35±14
Vegetables: Colored	36±35	40±62	26±39	40±28	40±30	53±39	55±26	74±34	52±29
Others	25±30	9±14	45±44	36±29	62±33	47±23	87±20	77±37	79±24
Fruits	*	*	*	*	*	*	19±11	9±0	23±46
Meats	33±55	18±29	20±33	29±49	35±58	40±69	35±22	54±41	34±24
Eggs	0±0	0±0	0±0	0±0	0±0	100[a)]	0±0	0±0	0±0
Fishes	11±26	18±29	0±0	0±0	0±0	3±14	0±0	0±0	0±0
Milk and dairy products	213±212	80±196	119±180	76±123	19±49	211±245	3±10	0±0	2±7
Alcoholic beverages	351±378	338±301	570±336	461±399	455±253	401±343	207±231	647±510	264±252

Table 2.2. (Continued)

Food group	Boya village (A)			Boya village (B)			Dzong village		
(g/day)	30-39	40-49	50≦	30-39	40-49	50≦	30-39	40-49	50≦
Females: number	10	9	9	9	13	10	17	4	16
Total cereals	448±105	407±71	408±110	404±93	363±111	337±73	407±101	369±170	304±76
Rice	315±112	280±110	257±90	220±117	229±82	235±59	177±70	140±49	146±54
Maize*	126±116	126±99	138±113	150±79	112±103	97±81	139±74	138±71	125±72
Potatoes	107±67	72±94	107±81	167±112	125±102	135±72	191±71	181±73	141±106
Sugar and sweetening	*	*	*	*	*	*	15±6	11±5	7±6
Fats and oils	3±2	3±2	5±3	4±3	3±1	3±3	19±7	17±8	13±8
Pulses	23±22	27±33	33±38	25±21	31±26	17±13	51±18	39±11	31±17
Vegetables: Colored	28±32	46±26	43±41	37±38	49±60	28±27	67±29	61±8	46±20
Others	49±37	82±78	78±63	44±34	47±32	61±65	81±22	76±16	67±28
Fruits	*	*	*	*	*	*	21±19	16±9	10±10
Meats	16±30	0±0	26±59	28±35	38±79	11±23	45±23	38±20	30±25
Eggs	0±0	0±0	0±0	0±0	0±0	20[b)]	0±0	0±0	0±0
Fishes	0±0	7±14	0±0	0±0	0±0	0±0	0±0	0±0	0±0
Milk and dairy products	101±169	209±285	57±91	144±189	229±267	65±140	21±40	11±23	3±8
Alcoholic beverages	248±296	312±250	369±305	111±116	327±319	283±295	52±62	50±41	115±77

Values are mean±SD. Buckwheat instead of maize in mountains area. a),b): n=1.

Table 3.1. Mean daily nutrient intake of the middled-aged and elderly Nepalese in the Terai region and the Kathmandu valley

Nutrient	Itahari			Chitwan			Kathmandu valley		
(per day)	30-39	40-49	50≦	30-39	40-49	50≦	30-39	40-49	50≦
Male: number	7	3	5	12	5	6	25	6	21
Energy (kcal)	2010±585	2391±467	2700±296	2282±458	2045±566	2070±457	2021±454	1916±781	1968±540
Protein (g)	50.3±10.8	61.6±14.1	72.5±16.4	54.5±15.8	45.3±15.2	45.9±11.0	54.0±16.2	50.0±15.5	50.4±14.2
Animal protein (g)	12.1±7.6	11.5±0.2	15.2±7.2	11.2±14.8	7.1±7.3	7.3±4.4	15.9±4.8	14.3±4.4	8.4±2.4
Fat (g)	43.7±18.2	54.5±1.4	50.8±9.5	25.5±13.1	21.2±6.0	22.3±8.5	30.5±12.2	32.4±8.0	29.9±9.6
Carbohydrate (g)	336.0±123.1	398.3±99.1	474.3±59.2	427.5±69.0	399.5±111.7	391.8±93.3	355.1±79.6	288.2±143	322.9±87.1
Dietary fiber (g)	6.0±3.0	7.2±2.7	8.5±4.3	4.8±1.1	4.4±0.8	4.7±1.3	12.0±6.0	13.4±7.8	16.8±6.5
Ca (mg)	557±269	649±316	726±305	499±329	404±174	452±162	174±80	209±111	195±63
P (mg)	1258±381	1458±417	1927±572	1222±320	1112±310	1195±244	998±255	1037±402	1211±329
Fe (mg)	10.5±3.8	13.3±2.2	15.3±6.2	8.6±3.2	6.0±1.8	7.0±1.8	8.8±2.3	9.4±2.9	10.2±3.0
Vitamin A (μgRe)	439±603	400±169	351±167	548±281	407±349	443±267	255±199	366±293	349±200
Vitamin B_1 (mg)	1.62±0.62	1.99±0.59	2.49±0.79	1.88±0.29	1.78±0.58	1.65±0.40	1.28±0.3	1.20±0.5	1.46±0.4
Vitamin B_2 (mg)	0.97±0.40	1.09±0.35	1.25±0.33	0.84±0.37	0.66±0.17	0.79±0.21	0.61±0.2	0.70±0.2	0.69±0.2
Niacin (mg)	14.4±4.2	16.0±4.9	20.3±7.2	16.1±5.1	13.4±3.9	13.8±2.8	14.4±4.5	14.9±6.8	15.8±6.2
Vitamin C (mg)	103±98	167±166	63±44	143±47	100±64	105±33	88±44	86±56	96±44
Female: number	11	5	0	9	8	4	23	6	18
Energy (kcal)	2545±593	2564±887	*	1695±597	1966±313	1566±243	1921±498	1767±545	1746±531
Protein (g)	63.2±14.6	66.3±27.7	*	44.0±15.0	43.3±10.1	38.3±7.4	50.7±14.3	44.1±18.2	45.6±16.3

Table 3.1. (Continued)

Nutrient	Itahari			Chitwan			Kathmandu valley		
(per day)	30-39	40-49	50≦	30-39	40-49	50≦	30-39	40-49	50≦
Animal protein (g)	5.4±6.3	9.0±8.0	*	11.5±8.9	7.1±8.3	8.3±8.6	8.1±2.4	4.3±1.8	5.9±2.1
Fat (g)	42.2±16.2	41.3±19.1	*	26.4±14.5	27.6±17.3	21.3±8.8	30.6±10.5	23.3±9.8	27.1±15.0
Carbohydrate (g)	466.4±113.2	455.4±163.7	*	303.7±44.3	367.5±44.3	93.2±41.3	341.8±95.3	328.0±95.7	305.2±87.4
Dietary fiber (g)	8.5±3.5	9.5±5.0	*	5.0±1.6	4.2±1.0	4.4±1.4	17.6±6.8	15.3±7.4	16.4±5.9
Ca (mg)	500±266	614±370	*	544±347	361±239	384±168	228±77	184±49	173±76
P (mg)	1633±458	1703±664	*	1019±438	1075±319	935±185	920±337	750±312	814±219
Fe (mg)	13.5±5.0	13.9±5.4	*	6.5±1.3	5.7±1.3	6.0±2.2	2.8±9.8	8.1±4.0	9.3±3.2
Vitamin A (μgRe)	321±290	365±260	*	741±300	312±241	402±386	507±265	463±261	419±223
Vitamin B_1 (mg)	2.40±0.59	2.26±1.03	*	1.66±0.28	1.47±0.22	1.94±0.41	1.34±0.40	1.22±0.52	1.30±0.39
Vitamin B_2 (mg)	0.85±0.29	0.95±0.35	*	0.80±0.38	0.64±0.40	0.73±0.45	0.66±0.24	0.62±0.24	0.67±0.23
Niacin (mg)	19.7±6.3	19.5±6.5	*	12.6±3.1	12.9±2.0	12.3±2.2	14.2±5.2	13.4±6.2	14.9±4.8
Vitamin C (mg)	74±60	90±50	*	156±57	96±53	116±76	102±42	98±47	95±43

Values are mean±SD.

Table 3.2. Mean daily nutrient intake of the middled-aged and elderly Nepalese in the hilly and mountainous areas

Nutrient	Boya village (A)			Boya village (B)			Dzong village		
(per day)	30-39	40-49	50≦	30-39	40-49	50≦	30-39	40-49	50≦
Male: number	11	6	15	11	7	19	9	3	17
Energy (kcal)	2185±629	2044±458	1682±327	1974±447	2046±331	1771±362	2232±402	2088±902	2061±525
Protein (g)	61.8±21.7	50.3±8.5	41.2±16.4	46.4±14.2	53.1±17.0	49.1±14.9	54.2±10.1	53.9±19.5	52.1±14.3
Animal protein (g)	14.6±5.1	9.0±1.5	7.4±2.9	7.6±2.3	6.9±4.6	14.5±4.6	6.4±1.2	9.7±3.5	6.2±1.7
Fat (g)	24.7±6.0	19.8±5.0	17.4±9.7	18.9±5.3	23.2±6.3	20.5±16.1	26.9±9.8	33.2±12.5	30.2±10.2
Carbohydrate (g)	397.7±143	382.6±103.2	294.7±47.8	363.9±98.6	370.1±53.4	307.5±69.5	89.0±54.4	93.2±112.5	34.7±84.2
Dietary fiber (g)	22.8±12.6	15.6±9.7	15.2±9.3	20.3±9.5	27.1±6.4	17.6±7.4	19.3±4.3	19.2±5.6	19.2±4.3
Ca (mg)	353±222	195±224	227±223	197±124	170±83	358±250	289±53	254±121	183±52
P (mg)	1426±549	1236±268	1018±316	1263±384	1281±244	1131±326	1191±255	1194±385	1302±289
Fe (mg)	11.0±4.2	9.1±2.3	7.5±3.2	8.6±2.4	10.5±2.6	7.9±2.0	10.8±1.9	10.5±3.0	11.0±2.5
Vitamin A (μgRe)	218±188	144±123	114±100	187±100	188±128	235±93	398±254	527±359	363±216
Vitamin B_1 (mg)	1.68±0.63	1.50±0.23	1.19±0.33	1.39±0.37	1.50±0.20	1.26±0.30	1.54±0.21	1.36±0.39	1.56±0.34
Vitamin B_2 (mg)	0.89±0.38	0.57±0.34	0.61±0.37	0.63±0.29	0.63±0.21	0.84±0.39	0.66±0.18	0.78±0.23	0.70±0.19
Niacin (mg)	15.3±3.8	14.4±3.9	13.5±3.7	15.1±5.4	16.7±5.1	14.3±4.7	16.6±4.4	19.3±7.1	17.4±5.6
Vitamin C (mg)	46±37	48±33	42±26	51±27	83±25	80±42	131±25	130±43	110±34
Female: number	10	9	9	9	13	10	17	4	16
Energy (kcal)	2006±336	1990±349	2070±273	1946±370	1898±448	1654±378	2123±462	1899±527	1603±415
Protein (g)	47.5±12.0	54.1±15.8	51.3±14.4	50.4±10.8	54.1±15.5	36.5±10.6	57.7±12.7	52.9±10.6	42.3±12.7

Table 3.2. (Continued)

Nutrient	Boya village (A)			Boya village (B)			Dzong village		
(per day)	30-39	40-49	50≦	30-39	40-49	50≦	30-39	40-49	50≦
Animal protein (g)	6.1±1.5	7.9±2.3	6.5±1.8	9.6±2.1	14.1±4.0	4.1±1.2	8.8±1.9	7.2±1.4	5.5±1.7
Fat (g)	21.5±10.6	23.9±10.8	29.2±22.2	30.9±16.2	26.5±19.1	17.4±8.7	35.2±10.4	32.4±6.3	24.9±12.6
Carbohydrate (g)	391.2±63.9	364.5±55.6	363.8±66.5	354.5±66.2	331.5±89.8	303.7±66.6	72.9±75.9	35.2±117.4	73.7±62.9
Dietary fiber (g)	21.0±11.1	24.6±12.1	24.5±12.0	24.4±7.3	21.4±12.4	17.2±8.3	20.9±5.0	18.9±3.4	14.8±4.4
Ca (mg)	203±163	376±333	262±221	280±185	389±302	165±150	231±66	204±17	158±53
P (mg)	1212±338	1349±278	1259±379	1212±238	1245±372	952±295	1293±319	1199±296	1040±308
Fe (mg)	9.2±2.6	10.5±4.1	10.0±3.4	9.7±2.3	9.5±3.0	7.3±1.9	11.3±2.7	10.3±2.2	9.0±2.6
Vitamin A (μgRe)	140±112	240±184	183±157	163±114	219±160	184±139	606±245	562±244	348±163
Vitamin B_1 (mg)	1.47±0.37	1.59±0.37	1.45±0.39	1.51±0.25	1.46±0.43	1.18±0.30	1.56±0.36	1.40±0.37	1.25±0.35
Vitamin B_2 (mg)	0.60±0.26	0.81±0.41	0.71±0.35	0.69±0.23	0.87±0.41	0.50±0.23	0.81±0.16	0.78±0.03	0.62±0.18
Niacin (mg)	13.0±3.4	12.5±2.5	13.6±2.9	12.4±2.0	14.0±4.4	11.1±3.2	17.7±3.8	16.8±2.4	14.3±4.2
Vitamin C (mg)	54±27	46±28	63±36	80±47	70±45	64±29	117±31	106±30	88±39

Values are mean±SD.

Food Consumption and Nutrient Intake

Table 2 shows the mean food consumption of the subjects (Table 2-1 for subjects in the Terai region and the Kathmandu valley; Table 2-2 for those in Boya and Dzong villages). The main food items consumed were rice, potatoes and vegetables for all subjects. The mean daily consumption of total amounts of cereals was lower than that of Japanese people over 30 years of age [21], and higher than that of nomads in Inner Mongolia, China [22].

Some of the consumed food items varied from area to area, although the dietary patterns were found to be very simple and similar. People living in the Terai region and the Kathmandu valley consumed wheat, while those in Boya and Dzong villages consumed maize and buckwheat, respectively. People in the Terai region and Boya village consumed more milk and dairy products than the others. The consumption of meat, fish, and egg was low, but it varied from area to area. Egg and fish consumption was not generally frequent, even in the urban areas in the Kathmandu valley. Alcoholic beverages were consumed by most subjects regardless of sex, especially in Boya village.

Food consumption seemed to be greatly influenced by food habits, food availability, and socioeconomic conditions.

Table 3 shows the mean nutrient composition of diets (Table 3-1 for subjects in the Terai region and the Kathmandu valley, Table 3-2 for those in Boya and Dzong villages). The mean energy intakes ranged from 1566±243 kcal for females over 50 years of age in the Chitwan to 2700±296 kcal for males over 50 years of age in the Itahari. Very elderly subjects had lower energy intakes, with a few exceptions. The estimated energy intake requirement for the Nepalese is 2250 kcal/person/ day [23]. Most subjects, except for the people in the Itahari, had lower intakes than the recommended value. As explained earlier, the proportion of animal proteins were very low. In general, of all nutrients, the mean carbohydrate intake was high and was the main contributors to the total energy intake. The calcium (Ca) intake was related to the consumption of milk and dairy products; a higher consumption of milk and dairy products resulted in a higher intake of Ca (Table 2 and 3). The subjects' iron intake was close to that of the Japanese (7.7-9.5 mg/person/day in individuals over 30 years of age) [21] and lower than that of nomads [22] with a few exceptions. The vitamin A intake of subjects living in Boya village was lower than that of the others. The mean intakes of vitamin B_1 were 1.18±0.30-2.49±0.79 mg/person/day, which was sufficient for the subjects due to the consumption of under-milled rice. The mean vitamin C intake depended on the amounts of potatoes, vegetables, and fruits consumed.

Table 4 shows the contribution of nutrients to the total energy intake. The energy contribution of carbohydrate to the total energy intake was very high, about 70 % or more for both sexes, and higher than that for subjects in the Chitwan and Boya villages. There was a report that the contribution to protein, fat and carbohydrate to the total energy intake for the Tibetan immigrants living in the suburban district of Kathmandu was 12, 20-23 and 65-68 %, respectively [24]. The energy contribution of fat to the total energy intake was related with the consumption of food of animal origin, such as meat and milk and dairy products.

Table 4. Contribution of nutrients to the total energy intake

Subjects	n	Source of energy (%)		
		Protein	Fat	Carbohydrate
Itahari				
Male	15	10.6±0.3	19.5±2.0	69.9±1.7
Female	16	10.3±0.6	15.2±0.1	74.5±0.4
Chitwan				
Male	23	9.7±0.5	10.3±0.5	80.0±0.9
female	21	10.1±0.8	13.6±1.0	76.3±1.4
Area A				
Male	32	11.3±0.8	10.3±0.8	78.4±1.5
Female	28	10.6±0.9	11.6±1.9	77.8±2.3
Area B				
Male	37	11.4±1.0	10.8±1.1	77.9±2.0
Female	32	10.9±1.3	12.8±2.3	76.3±3.2
Dzong				
Male	29	11.4±1.0	14.3±2.9	74.3±3.9
Female	37	11.4±0.1	15.4±0.4	73.3±0.5
Kathmandu				
Male	52	11.4±0.6	15.1±1.7	73.4±2.2
Female	47	11.0±0.6	14.5±1.5	74.5±1.8

Values are mean±SD, and are caluculated using the amounts of protein, fat and carbohydrate in Table 2.

3. Serum Nutritional Components

Recently, blood profiles are used as one of the methods for the evaluation of nutrient status of people. As shown in Table 5, the mean values of serum components were approximately within the normal ranges for the Japanese (total protein, 6.5-7.9 g/dl; albumin, 4.0-5.0 g/dl; total cholesterol, TC, 150-230 mg/dl for both sexes; triacylglycerol, TG, 80-150 mg/dl for males, 70-130 mg/dl for females) [25]. However, the mean TC level was in the low-normal range, whereas the mean TG level was in the high-normal range with a few exceptions. The relatively large proportion of carbohydrate-laden cereals relative to all food consumed may have contributed to the higher serum TG level because excess carbohydrates are converted to fat in the human body. Other reports also support the view that high-carbohydrate diets increase serum TG [26, 27].

Table 5. Serum protein, albumin/globulin ratio and lipids of the middled-aged and elderly Nepalese

Area	Sex	Age group	Subjects (n)	Total protein (g/dl)	Albumin g/dl)	Alb/Glb ratio (kg/m^2)	Total cholesterol (mg/dl)	Triacylglycerol (mg/dl)
Itahari	Male	30-39	10	8.2±0.4	4.6±0.2	1.3±0.2	155±32	175±78
		40-49	3	7.8±0.5	4.6±0.3	1.4±0.3	193±11	228±110
		50-72	5	7.8±0.4	4.3±0.2	1.2±0.2	147±35	112±67
	Female	30-39	12	7.8±0.4	4.5±0.3	1.4±0.1	118±25	99±46
		40-49	5	8.4±0.8	4.5±0.6	1.2±0.1	147±49	156±69
Chitwan	Male	30-39	12	8.7±0.4	4.8±0.3	1.2±0.1	167±31	134±65
		40-49	9	8.6±0.7	4.6±0.2	1.2±0.2	131±23	106±64
		50-68	10	8.3±0.5	4.4±0.4	1.1±0.2	146±31	95±47
	Female	30-39	12	8.6±0.6	4.6±0.3	1.2±0.1	149±36	79±26
		40-49	6	8.7±0.4	4.5±0.3	1.1±0.1	151±34	94±27
		50-59	10	8.7±0.5	4.5±0.2	1.1±0.1	152±35	136±63
Area A	Male	30-39	8	7.6±0.5	4.3±0.5	1.3±0.3	136±32	165±75
		40-49	6	7.0±0.7	3.9±0.2	1.3±0.3	126±29	151±66
		50-73	14	7.3±0.5	4.1±0.4	1.3±0.3	129±28	121±70
	Female	30-39	15	7.3±0.5	4.1±0.4	1.4±0.3	139±28	132±52
		40-49	12	7.3±0.5	4.1±0.3	1.3±0.2	137±25	113±35
		50-72	16	7.5±0.5	4.3±0.3	1.3±0.2	159±26	158±84

Table 5. (Continued)

Area	Sex	Age group	Subjects	Total protein	Albumin	Alb/Glb ratio	Total cholesterol	Triacylglycerol
			(n)	(g/dl)	g/dl)	(kg/m^2)	(mg/dl)	(mg/dl)
Area B	Male	30-39	12	7.3±0.4	4.4±0.4	1.5±0.5	152±33	117±54
		40-49	7	7.3±0.3	4.0±0.5	1.3±0.3	138±20	137±64
		50-73	14	7.5±0.4	4.4±0.4	1.4±0.2	153±25	117±56
	Female	30-39	10	7.3±0.4	4.4±0.3	1.5±0.1	129±22	121±94
		40-49	17	7.4±0.3	4.2±0.3	1.4±0.2	141±30	122±56
		50-72	12	7.6±0.3	4.4±0.3	1.4±0.2	156±24	140±55
Dzong	Male	30-39	9	8.5±0.7	5.1±0.5	1.5±0.3	168±40	156±83
		40-49	3	8.0±0.6	4.9±0.2	1.6±0.2	145±10	77±47
		50-76	17	8.3±0.6	4.5±0.7	1.2±0.3	175±59	144±95
	Female	30-39	17	7.5±0.5	4.5±0.5	1.5±0.3	140±28	89±50
		40-49	4	7.9±0.4	4.6±0.1	1.4±0.1	147±36	77±41
		50-75	16	8.3±0.4	4.5±0.4	1.2±0.2	165±45	131±52
Kathmandu	Male	30-39	25	8.2±0.6	5.1±0.3	1.7±0.2	168±29	128±67
		40-49	6	7.8±1.2	4.8±0.5	1.6±0.3	170±35	80±30
		50-84	21	8.2±0.7	4.5±0.6	1.3±0.3	172±54	151±115
	Female	30-39	23	7.7±0.5	4.6±0.4	1.5±0.2	136±28	83±40
		40-49	6	8.1±0.4	4.6±0.2	1.3±0.1	134±21	87±49
		50-75	18	8.1±0.5	4.5±0.4	1.3±0.3	157±47	123±56

Values are mean±SD. Abbreviations: Alb/Glb ratio, albumin/globulin ratio.

Another reason for the higher TG level in the Nepalese may be the lower intake of lipids, especially polyunsaturated fatty acids (PUFA). Replacing fats with carbohydrates increases the fasting TG serum level, whereas n-3 PUFA from fish oils decreases them [28, 29]. As the subjects in the present study did not consume fish frequently, the amounts of n-3 PUFA intake seemed not to be sufficient for those people. The subjects' high-carbohydrate, low-fat, and low-protein diets, in addition to their poor eating habits, may have caused their rather high serum TG. Subjects of both sexes in Boya village consumed a significant amount of alcoholic beverages and showed higher TG levels than all other subjects of both sexes in other areas. It is also well known that alcohol consumption causes higher TG level.

Conclusion

All of these findings suggest the important role of eating patterns, such as excessive or deficient or appropriate food intake. In general, the subjects' nutritional status was acceptable despite a possible latent deficiency of some nutrients in some areas due to a lack of animal origin food groups or vegetables, as reported by Brown et al. [30]. Although it is generally difficult to modify people's eating habits, the subjects in this study should be encouraged to consume a sufficient amount of food from animal origin as well as nutritional supplements (which could be added to foods). It is necessary to encourage the Nepalese to consume higher-quality food and to provide educational programs to raise their awareness about proper food intake and nutrition.

References

[1] Chen LC, Chowdhury AKMA, and Huffman SA: Anthropometric assessment of energy-protein malnutrition and subsequent risk of mortality among preschool-aged children. *Am. J. Clin. Nutr.,* 33, 1836-1845, 1980.

[2] Ramalingaswami V: New global perspectives on overcoming malnutrition. *Am. J. Clin. Nutr.*, 61, 259-263, 1995.

[3] Forman MR, Hundt GL, Berendes HW, Abu-Saad K, Zangwill L, Chang D, Bellmaker I, Abu-Saad I, and Graubard B: Undernutrition among Bedouin Arab children: A follow-up of the Bedouin infant feeding study. *Am. J. Clin. Nutr.*, 61, 495-500, 1995.

[4] Underwood BA, and Arthur P: The contribution of vitamin A to public health. *Fed. Am. Societ Exper. Biol. J.*, 10, 1040-1048, 1996.

[5] Rai KS, Rai G, Hirai K, Abe A, and Ohno Y: The health system in Nepal-An introduction. *Environ. Health Preventive Med.*, 6, 1-8, 2001.

[6] Rai SK, Hirai K, Abe A, and Ohno Y: Infectious diseases and malnutrition status in Nepal: an overview. *Mal. J. Nutr.*, 8, 191-200, 2002.

[7] Hirai K, Okuno Y, Nagata K, Tamura T, Ohno Y, Nakayama J, Rai SK, Sakya HN, and Shrestha MP: Nutritional survey on the serum status of lipids, protein, and calcium levels in Nepalese. *J. Clin. Biochem. Nutr.*, 9, 205-213, 1990.

[8] Hirai K, Nakayama J, Sonoda M, Ohno Y, Okuno Y, Nagata K, Tamura T, Sakya HN, and Shrestha MP: Food consumption and nutrient intake and their relationship among Nepalese. *Nutr. Res.,* 13, 987-994, 1993.

[9] Ohno Y, Hirai K, Nagata K, Tamura T, Rai SK, Onta S, Devkota M, and Shreestha MP: Evaluation of the iron status in Nepalese living in southern Nepal. *Nutr. Res.*, 18, 1847-1855, 1998.

[10] Ohno Y, Hirai K, Sato N, Ito M, Yamamoto T, Tamura T, and Shrestha MP: Food consumption pattern and nutrient intake among Nepalese living in the southern rural Terai region. *Asia Pacific J. Clin. Nutr*., 6, 251-255, 1997.

[11] Ohno Y, Hirai K, Nagata K, Tamura T, and Shrestha MP: Serum mineral levels among Nepalese living in the southern agricultural Terai region. *Envirn. Health Preventive* Med, 5, 1-5, 2000.

[12] Ohno Y, Shibata H, Hirai K, Nakanishi M, Nagata K, Tamura T, Rai SK, and Shrestha MP: Study on physical and some serum parameters of inhabitants living in agricultural Terai region, Nepal. *Nepal Med. College J*., 5, 105, 2003.

[13] Hirai K, Ohno Y, Jindai M, Aoki Y, Hayashi E, Higuchi H, Mizuno S, Nagata K, Tamura T, Rai SK, and Shrestha MP: Serum nutritional status of tocopherol and retinol normalized to lipids of persons living in the southern rural Terai region in Nepal. *EnvirOn. Health Prev. Med*., 9, 13-21, 2004.

[14] Rai SK, Hirai K, Ohno Y, and Matsumura T: Village health and sanitary profile from eastern hilly region, Nepal. Kobe *J. Med. Sci*., 43, 121-133, 1997.

[15] Ohno Y, Hirai K, Higuchi H, Sakai K, Nagata K, Tamura T, Rai CK, and Rai SK: Serum nutritional components and dietary food intake of people living in a remote hilly village in eastern Nepal. *J. Clin. Biochem. Nutr*., 35, 71-80, 2004.

[16] Ohno Y, Hirai K, Sakata S, Shimizu S, Akai Y, Ogoshi K, Sherchand S, Gurung R, Sherchand JB, and Shrestha MP: Food consumption and serum nutritional status of people living in the Kathmandu valley in Nepal. *Envirn. Health Preventive Med*., 10, 78-85, 2005.

[17] Ohno Y, Hirai K, Sakata S, Shimizu S, Akai Y, Ogoshi K, Sherchand S, Gurung R, Sherchand JB, and Shrestha MP: Nutritional status of people living in Dzong village, in the northern mountainous area of Nepal. *Asia Pacific J. Public Health*, 18, 20-29, 2006.

[18] Tokunaga K, Matsuzawa Y, Kotani K, Keno Y, Kobatake T, Fujioka S, and Tarui S: Ideal body weight estimated from the body mass index with the lowest morbidity. *Int. J. Obesity,* 15, 1-5, 1991.

[19] Hosegood V, and Cambell OMR: Body mass index, height, weight arm circumference, and mortality in rural Bangladeshi women: A 19-y longitudinal study. *Am. J. Clin. Nutr.*, 77, 341-347, 2003.

[20] Bujo H: Metabolic syndrome-Pathogenesis and treatment from the view of obesity and adipocyte. *Jpn. J. Nutr. Diet*, 64, 299-307, 2006.

[21] National Nutrition Survey: 2003, Section of Nutrition, Bureau of Public Health, Ministry of Health and Welfare. *Jpn. J. Nutr. Diet,* 63, 157-167, 2005.

[22] Ohno Y, Hirai K, Sowa S, Oka S, and Murai Y: Food and nutrient intakes among nomads living in three different areas of Inner Mongolia, China. *Asia Pacific J. Clin. Nutr*., 14, 7-18, 2005.

[23] Ali A: Status of Health in Nepal. *Resource Center for Primary Health Care*, Nepal and South-South Solidarity, India, pp. 39-40, 1991.

[24] Itoh K, Kawasaki T, Ogaki T, Yoshimizu Y, Funatsu S, Khakya NS, Ghimire PK, and Acharya GP: Nutritional investigation in the Tibetan immigrants living in suburban district of Nepal. *J. Health Sci.*, 15, 21-27, 1993.

[25] Shiina S, Hosoya K, and Kamei S: The serum parameters and their pathology for patient care and dietary guidelines. In: Shiina S, Ishiyaku Publishing Co, Tokyo, Jpn, pp47-49 (TP and Alb), p23 (TC), p26 (TG), 1996 (in Japanese).

[26] Parks EJ: Dietary carbohydrate's effects on lipogenesis and the relationship of lipogenesis to blood insulin and glucose concentration. *Bri. J. Nutr.,* 87 (suppl 2), S247-S253, 2002.

[27] Treuth MS, Sunehag AL, Trautwein LM, Bier DM, Haymond MW, and Butte N: Metabolic adaptation to high-fat and high-carbohydrate diets in children and adolescents. *Am. J. Clin. Nutr.*, 479-489, 2003.

[28] Harris WS: n-3 Fatty acids and serum lipoproteins: Human studies. *Am. J. Clin. Nutr.*, 65 (suppl), 1645S-1654S, 1997.

[29] Mensink RP, Zock PL, Kester ADM, and Katan MB: Effects of dietary fatty acids and carbohydrates on the ratio of serum total to HDL cholesterol and on serum lipids and apolipoproteins: A meta-analysis of 60 controlled trials. *Am. J. Clin. Nutr.*, 65 (suppl), 1628S-1644S, 1997.

[30] Brown ML, Worth RM, and Shah NK: Food habits and food intake in Nepal. *Trop. Geogr. Med.*, 20, 217-224, 1967.

In: Nutrition for the Middle Aged and Elderly
Editors: N. E. Bernhardt, A. M. Kasko, pp. 31-61
ISBN: 978-1-60456-146-3

Chapter I

Relation of Vitamin D, Calcium, and Magnesium to the Risk of Type 2 Diabetes Mellitus

Sara Chacko[1] and Simin Liu[2]
[1]Department of Epidemiology, University of California, Los Angeles
[2]Departments of Epidemiology and Medicine, University of California, Los Angeles

Abstract

An increasing body of evidence suggests that low vitamin D status may impair both insulin secretion and action, ultimately increasing the risk of type 2 diabetes mellitus (DM). Experimentally, vitamin D repletion improves insulin sensitivity and insulin secretion in animal studies of rats. Cross-sectional studies in humans suggest an inverse association between circulating vitamin D levels and impaired glucose tolerance, insulin resistance, and risk of type 2 diabetes. Prospective data, albeit limited, also indicate an inverse association between intake of dietary and supplemental vitamin D and type 2 diabetes risk. Calcium and magnesium may exert both independent and interactive effects on the risk of type 2 diabetes through metabolically related pathways. Genetic variants of these pathways, including the vitamin D receptor (VDR) pathway and calcium and magnesium homeostasis related pathways, also appear to play a role in affecting the risk of type 2 diabetes in humans.

I. Introduction

Several lines of evidence support the hypothesis that low vitamin D status is associated with impaired β-cell function, insulin resistance, impaired glucose tolerance, and type 2 diabetes. Experimental studies have identified vitamin D receptors (VDR) on the pancreatic β-cells that may promote transcription of genes (human insulin gene) necessary for insulin secretion[1]. Low bioavailability of vitamin D can therefore negatively impact insulin production and potentially lead to impaired glucose tolerance and type 2 diabetes, although the exact mechanism of this action and the extent of influence on β-cell function and insulin resistance are not fully understood.

The vitamin D endocrine system is complex, involving multiple pathways and interactions, and it is possible that the effects of vitamin D on insulin and glucose metabolism are mediated by metabolically related minerals. Vitamin D is principally responsible for calcium and phosphorus homeostasis and may play a role in magnesium absorption. Accumulating evidence suggests that calcium and magnesium may exert independent and interactive effects on insulin secretion, insulin resistance, and type 2 diabetes, although the extent of influence and interaction with vitamin D is uncertain.

This chapter will review and summarize the physiology and metabolism of vitamin D in the body and consider potential interactions with calcium, magnesium, and other minerals. Animal and epidemiologic evidence linking low vitamin D status to insulin secretion, insulin resistance, and type 2 diabetes will also be assessed. We will also explore potential biological mechanisms and future research directions with a special emphasis on genetic polymorphisms of the vitamin D receptors (VDR) and magnesium and calcium homeostasis related pathways.

II. A Brief Overview of the Vitamin D Endocrine System

A. Overview

Vitamin D consists of a group of fat-soluble steroid prohormones that are essential for healthy body functioning. There are two main forms of vitamin D, cholecalciferol (vitamin D_3), and ergocalciferol (vitamin D_2). Vitamin D_3 can be obtained in small amounts from fatty fish such as salmon, mackerel, tuna, and cod. In addition, some dairy and cereal products are fortified with vitamin D_3 in the U.S. Yet, the major source of vitamin D in the body is still synthesized in the skin after direct exposure to sunlight or ultraviolet light whereby 7-dehydrocholestrol in the plasma membrane of the epidermal cells is converted to cholecalciferol. The amount of cholecalciferol the skin produces depends on the duration of exposure, time of day, season, latitude of the location, sunscreen use and skin pigmentation [2]. Vitamin D_2 is produced by ultraviolet irradiation of plant sterols and is added to some foods. After consumption of vitamin D containing food or endogenous production in the body, vitamin D is further metabolized by the liver and the kidney into the hormonally active form of the vitamin, 1,25-dihydroxyvitamin D ($25(OH)_2D$). (Hereinafter, vitamin D refers to both cholecalciferol [vitamin D_3] and ergocalciferol [vitamin D_2] unless otherwise specified). The first step in vitamin D metabolism is transport to the liver where it is hydroxylated into 25-hydroxyvitamin D (25(OH)D) and released into the blood stream. If there are adequate stores of 25(OH)D circulating in the bloodstream, it is then converted into the vitamin D hormone 1,25-dihydroxyvitamin D (1,25 $(OH)_2D$), or calcitriol, in the kidney. The production of 1,25 $(OH)_2D$ in the kidney is homeostatically regulated through a negative feedback loop controlled by parathyroid hormone (PTH). When serum calcium (Ca^{2+}) levels drop, PTH is secreted from the parathyroid gland and directly stimulates 1,25 $(OH)_2D$ production in the kidney to increase Ca^{2+} absorption and ensure the maintenance of calcium homeostasis. Conversely, 1,25 $(OH)_2D$ synthesis is suppressed in states of hypercalcemia due to low secretion of PTH (Figure 1)[3].

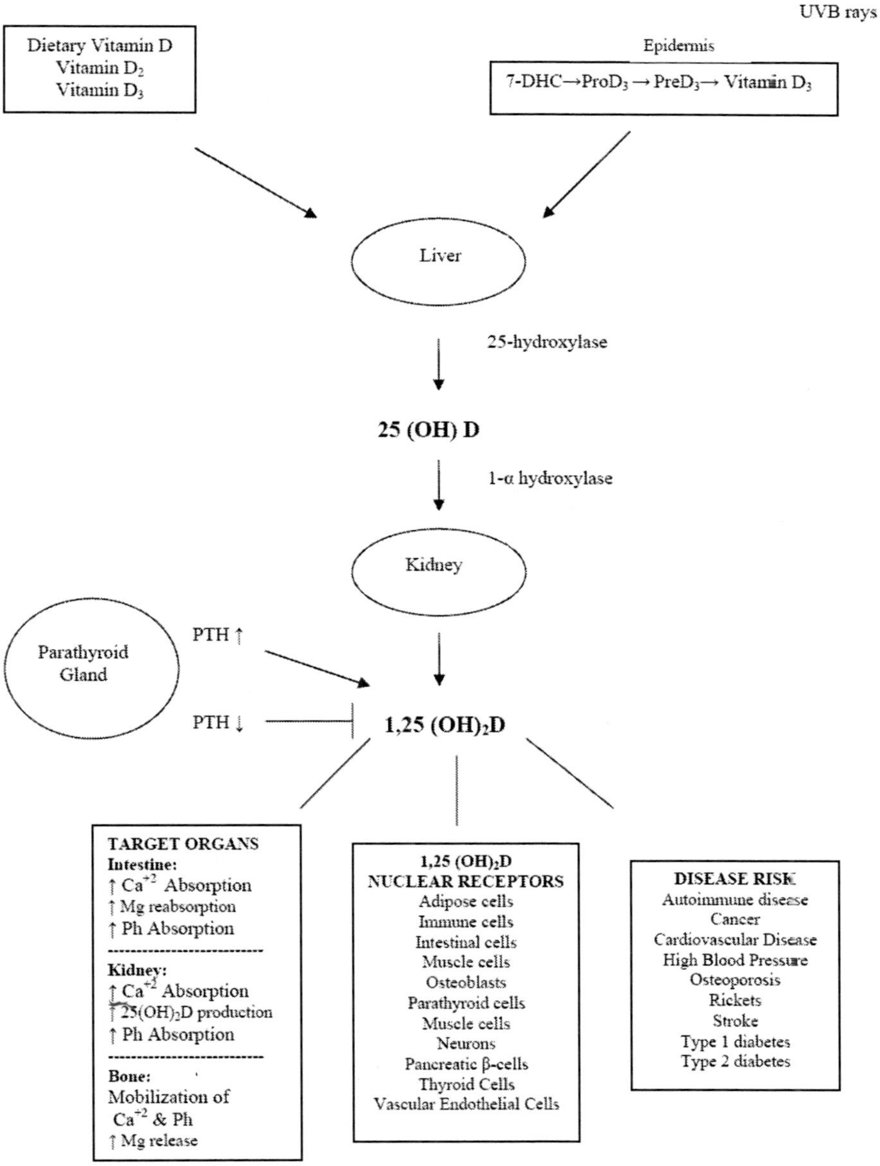

Figure 1. Vitamin D Endocrine System.

1,25 $(OH)_2D$ is a potent steroid hormone with strong regulatory effects on calcium homeostasis, and it is considered the active metabolite of vitamin D in the body. 1,25 $(OH)_2D$ binds to vitamin D receptors (VDR) which can be found in more than thirty cell types throughout the body, including intestinal cells, muscle cells, osteoblasts, parathyroid cells, epidermal cells, vascular endothelial cells, neurons, immune cells, and pancreatic β-cells [4]. VDR acts as a transcription factor to regulate the rate of gene transcription in many cell types throughout the body, exerting effects on calcium homeostasis, cell proliferation and differentiation, immune function, and various endocrine functions including insulin resistance [5].

B. Interaction with Calcium and Phosphorous

The major physiologic functions of vitamin D in the body include the regulation of calcium and phosphorous homeostasis in the blood and the promotion of bone mineralization and growth. Target organs of the system include the intestine, bone, and kidney[6]. Homeostatic control of extracellular calcium (Ca^{2+}) is essential for numerous cellular and tissue functions, and a feedback system involving vitamin D controls the balance of intra- and extracellular calcium[7]. Levels of extracellular Ca^{2+} must be maintained within the range of 7 mgCa/100 ml to 12 mg/100 ml for optimal physiological functioning[8]. When Ca^{2+} concentrations fall below the optimal level, 1,25 $(OH)_2D$ acts to increase Ca^{2+} through increasing the absorption of calcium from the gastrointestinal tract and reabsorption of calcium into the kidney. 1,25 $(OH)_2D$ binds to nuclear receptors in the intestinal cells which stimulate the synthesis of messenger RNA molecules that code for calcium binding protein (CaBP), a protein responsible for transporting calcium into the bloodstream. Synthesis of CaBP is dependent on the presence of 1,25 $(OH)_2D$ in the blood. Therefore, if circulating serum vitamin D falls below the optimal level (80 nmol/L; 32 ng/dL)[9-12], dietary calcium absorption is impaired and stores of calcium from the bones must be mobilized to maintain normal functioning of the neuromuscular system.

Phosphorous is an essential mineral required by the body for bone and teeth mineralization, ATP production, utilization of macronutrients for growth, and cell and tissue repair[13]. Excessive serum phosphate can inhibit the production of 1,25 $(OH)_2D$ in the kidneys, reduce extracellular Ca^{2+} concentrations, and increase the production of parathyroid hormone (PTH)[14], which may lead to secondary hyperparathyroidism, a condition associated with osteoporosis and bone degradation. 1,25 $(OH)_2D$ acts to maintains normal phosphorous levels in the blood through a mechanism similar to the control of extracellular Ca^{2+}. 1,25 $(OH)_2D$ increases absorption of dietary phosphorus in the gut, reabsorption in the kidney, and mobilization of phosphate from the bone through stimulation of osteoclastic activity[5].

C. Interaction with Calciotropic Hormones

Calcium homeostasis is principally mediated by the actions of the calciotropic hormones including 1,25 $(OH)_2D$, PTH, and calcitonin. 1,25 $(OH)_2D$ interacts with PTH and calcitonin to exert direct and indirect effects on hundreds of physiological processes. PTH, released in response to low extracellular levels of calcium (Ca^{2+}), is an important endocrine regulator of calcium homeostasis and stimulates the production of 1,25 $(OH)_2D$ in the kidney. A negative feedback loop exists between calcium, PTH, and 1,25 $(OH)_2D$ that ensures that extracellular calcium levels (Ca^{2+}) are maintained within the narrow limits required for cellular function. PTH works to maintain Ca^{2+} levels through several mechanisms including the stimulation of the production of 1,25 $(OH)_2D$ in the kidney and subsequent absorption of calcium in the small intestine, the mobilization of calcium from the bone, and suppression of calcium loss in urine [15]. Calcitonin, a calciotropic hormone produced primarily in the C cells of the thyroid gland, is also involved in the endocrine control of calcium. Calcitonin exerts effects on the bone and kidney to decrease elevated extracellular Ca^{2+} levels in the blood and maintain calcium balance in the body [16].

Calcium homeostasis is essential for numerous physiological functions including proper functioning of the neuromuscular system, secretion of hormones and enzymes, blood clotting, and the mineralization of bone and teeth. Given the close metabolic interconnections of the hormones involved in the homeostatic control of calcium, it is imperative to consider the joint and interactive effects when discussing the physiological effects of vitamin D.

D. Interaction with Magnesium

Vitamin D may also play an important role in magnesium absorption[17], although the extent of influence is not completely understood. Magnesium, an essential intracellular cation that acts as a co-factor in hundreds of enzymatic reactions in the body, has been shown to interact with calciotropic hormones and is highly involved in calcium homeostasis [18]. Just as PTH is secreted in response to low extracellular concentrations of Ca^{2+}, PTH is released in response to low extracellular concentrations of Mg [19]. PTH stimulates Mg reabsorption in the Loop of Henle and the distal tubule [20, 21], releases Mg from the bone [18], and increases intestinal absorption[22, 23]. In addition, PTH leads to increased production of 1,25 $(OH)_2D$ in the kidney which may mediate this process further enhancing Mg absorption in the intestine (Figure 2) [24, 25].

III. Vitamin D Status

Serum levels of 25(OH)D are currently the best marker of vitamin D bioavailability in humans and are used to measure vitamin D status [26]. There is currently no clear consensus among researchers as to what constitutes a deficiency in vitamin D. One proposed categorization includes deficiency (0-25 nmol/l; 0-10ng/ml), insufficiency (<25-50.0 nmol/l; <10-20ng/ml), hypovitaminosis D (<50-100 nmol/l; <20-40 ng/ml), adequacy (70-100 to 250 nmol/l; 28-40 to 100 ng/ml), and toxicity (>250 nmol/l; >100 ng/ml) [27]. Recent work in the field suggests that higher levels of vitamin D may have beneficial effects on a number of adverse health outcomes. It has been suggested that the optimal physiologic level of serum vitamin D for calcium absorption, PTH concentration, and a number of other health outcomes including bone health, lower-extremity function, dental health, and colorectal cancer prevention falls between 75 nmol/L (30 ng/mL) to 100 nmol/L (40 ng/dL)[9-12, 28, 29].

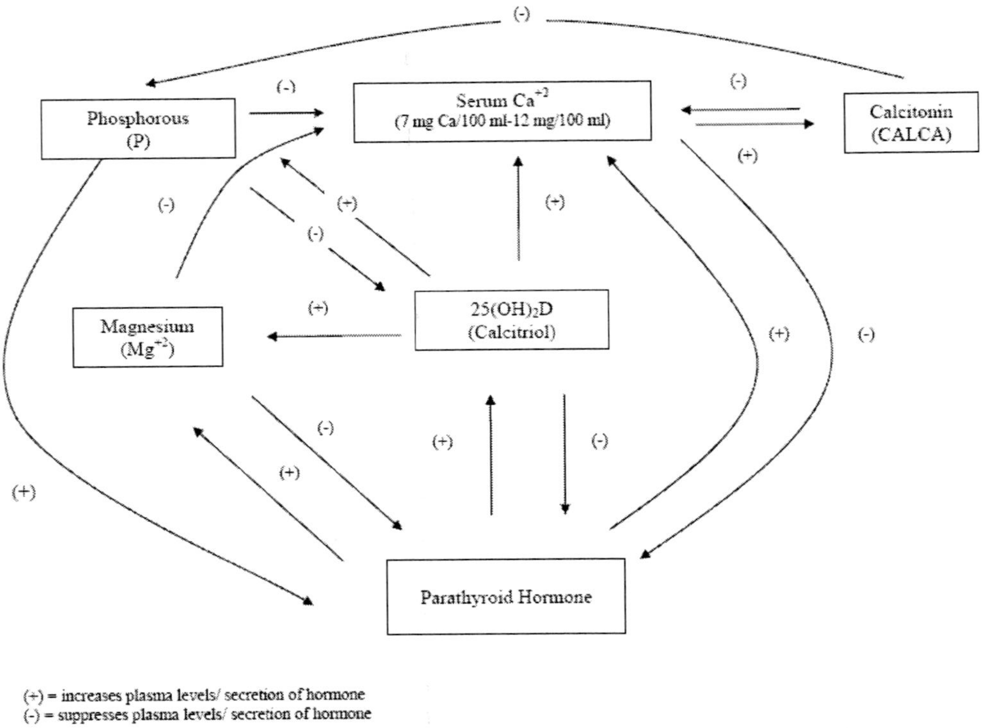

Figure 2. The Interaction between Vitamin D, Calcium, Phosporous, Magnesium and Capciotropic Hormones.

Low vitamin D status is an increasingly recognized problem worldwide, and recently it has been identified as an "epidemic" in the United States. [11]. A number of factors, including limited sun exposure, dark skin pigmentation, lack of dietary vitamin D, and obesity have been identified as risk factors for low vitamin D status. High risk groups for low vitamin D status include the elderly, especially those living in nursing homes [30]; the obese [31, 32]; and dark skinned individuals who do not produce adequate amounts of cholecalciferol from sunlight exposure due to high skin pigmentation [2, 33, 34]. However, increasing evidence suggests low vitamin D status is also common among apparently healthy populations, especially in the winter time. One cross-sectional study assessing serum vitamin D levels in Boston found a 36% prevalence of vitamin D insufficiency among healthy young adults aged 18-29 (n=69) at the end of winter [35].

A. Vitamin D Status and the Elderly

Low vitamin D status among the elderly is a well-documented problem and may lead to decreased bone and muscle strength and the increased incidence of bone fractures due to impaired calcium absorption [30]. Several serological studies have found a high prevalence of vitamin D deficiency among older populations [36, 37]. This may be partially explained by a decrease in the concentration of important vitamin D precursors, including 7-dehydrocholesterol and previtamin D_3, in the skin of older individuals. A reduction in these vitamin D precursors can potentially result in the decreased production of vitamin D_3. McLaughlin et al.[38] found a strong negative association (r = -0.89) between age and levels of 7-dehydrocholesterol in the skin independent of the total mass of the epidermis. Furthermore, the production of previtamin D_3 in the epidermis and dermis was more than two times greater among 8-year-olds (442 ng/cm^2 preD-3) than among 82-year-olds (183 ng/cm^2 preD-3) after exposure to ultraviolet radiation. These findings suggest that aging affects the ability of skin to produce the necessary precursors for vitamin D synthesis, making elderly individuals more susceptible to low vitamin D status. The elderly may also increase their risk of vitamin D deficiency by staying indoors longer or consuming a diet poor in vitamin D[2].

B. Vitamin D Status and Obesity

Overweight and obese individuals are also at high-risk for low vitamin D status. Although this association is not completely understood, one possible explanation is that overweight individuals have inadequate exposure to UV radiation in sunlight due to clothing choices or limited mobility[39]. Alternatively, it is possible that increased production of 1,25 $(OH)_2D$ in obese individuals exerts negative feedback on hepatic synthesis of 25(OH)D[40].

It has also been suggested that vitamin D may accumulate in excess adipose tissue in obese individuals resulting in reduced bioavailability of the vitamin in the bloodstream, and several recent reports indicate that total adiposity may be an important predictor of low vitamin D status. In a study of the cutaneous synthesis of vitamin D_3 in response to UV-B irradiation (n=13 controls, BMI: 22.2±0.04; n=13 obese participants, BMI: 38 ± 1.7), basal concentrations of 7-dehydrocholesterol and vitamin D_3 were not significantly different between obese and control participants. However, 24 hours after exposure to whole body irradiation (wavelength 260-330 nm), the increase in circulating vitamin D_3 concentrations was significantly less in obese participants than in controls (Difference between basal and post-irradiation vitamin D_3 concentrations: Controls: 38.3 ± 5.5 nmol/L vs obese participants: 17.4 ± 3.6 nmol/L; p=0.0029)[41]. These findings support the hypothesis that vitamin D synthesized by the skin is not readily available in the bloodstream in obese individuals, perhaps due to excessive storage in body fat. In addition, total body fat percentage measured with dual-energy x-ray absorptiometry (DXA) was negatively associated with circulating levels of 25(OH)D (r= -0.13, p=.013) in a cross-sectional study of healthy women (n=410, aged 20-80 years old, BMI ranging from 17-30 kg/m^2) after controlling for race, age, season, and dietary vitamin D intake [42]. More recently, DXA total body fat percentage was negatively associated with 25(OH)D levels in a sample of men and women (n=453) aged 65 years and older (r= -0.261, p< 0.001). The association was attenuated with the use of anthropometric measures (i.e BMI, waist circumference, waist-to-hip ratio) indicating that fat mass, not total body weight, is the most important factor driving the inverse relation between obesity and circulating 25(OH)D concentrations [43].

However, it is also possible that obesity is the consequence of low vitamin D status. Excess parathyroid hormone (PTH), released in response to low circulating 25(OH)D concentrations, stimulates the production of 1,25 $(OH)_2D$ in the kidney to increase extracellular calcium (Ca^{2+}) concentrations and maintain calcium homeostasis. However, excess 1,25 $(OH)_2D$ also stimulates the influx of extracellular Ca^{2+} into the adipocytes, and thus may enhance lipogenesis and weight gain [44, 45]. Several studies have reported an inverse relation between calcium levels and obesity [46-49].

Irrespective of the underlying biological mechanism, cross-sectional studies of obese individuals consistently show decreased serum vitamin D levels in overweight and obese individuals [31, 32, 39, 43, 50-53]. A small cross-sectional study (n=13 obese white participants; n=13 nonobese white participants) showed that serum 25(OH)D levels were significantly lower in obese white subjects than non obese subjects (Mean 25(OH)D levels in obese 11 ± 1 ng/ml vs. Nonobese: 16 ± 2 ng/ml; $p< 0.05$) [32]. Among morbidly obese females (n=60) tested for vitamin D deficiency, 62% were found to be below the "normal" range (defined as 16-74 ng/ml). In addition, serum vitamin D levels were negatively correlated to BMI ($r=-0.49$; $p<0.001$) [31]. Among middle-aged Caucasian subjects from the 1958 British birth cohort (n=1,798), serum 25(OH)D levels decreased with increasing BMI (25(OH)D <75 nmol/l among 80% of obese participants vs 68% of nonobese subjects; p for trend < 0.001)[54]. Results from the Third National Health and Nutrition Examination Survey (NHANES III, 1988-1994) were consistent with these findings. After controlling for multiple risk factors, the odds of abdominal obesity increased linearly across decreasing quintiles of serum concentrations of 25(OH)D [25(OH)D ≥96.4 nmol/l: OR= 0.30 (0.21,0.42); 78.2-96.3 nmol/l: OR=0.55 (0.41, 0.72); 63.5-78.1 nmol/L: OR=0.65 (0.52,0.81); 48.5-63.4 nmol/l: OR=0.78 (0.61,0.98); p for trend < .0001) [53]. Furthermore, among 10,066 women aged ≥45 years in the Women's Health Study, means of waist circumference and BMI increased significantly across decreasing quintiles of total vitamin D intake [Waist circumference: Highest quintile of vitamin D intake (511-2369 IU/day): 39.7 inches; Lowest quintile (6.0-159 IU/day): 43.5 inches, p for trend = 0.0004; BMI: Highest quintile: 14.4 kg/m^2; Lowest quintile: 20.2 kg/m^2, p for trend < 0.0001][55].

C. Vitamin D Status and Ethnicity

Ethnic, cultural, and geographic factors such as skin color, dress, diet, and latitude influence vitamin D status, and substantial variation in vitamin D status is observed across ethnic groups and countries. Ethnic groups with dark skin pigmentation, especially African Americans, are at increased risk for low vitamin D status due to high levels of melanin in the skin. Research suggests that melanin in the skin competes with 7-dehydrocholesterol (7-DHC) for UVB rays, thereby limiting the synthesis of vitamin D-3 in individuals with dark skin [56]. Observational studies assessing vitamin D status in humans show that African-Americans have lower circulating levels of 25(OH)D and are more likely to be vitamin D deficient that other ethnic groups [33, 50, 56-58]. Mean levels of 25(OH)D were found to be lower in African Americans than in Caucasians in a clinical intervention study (n=26) assessing the vitamin D endocrine system [6±1 vs 20±2 ng/ml, $p<0.001$][57]. Likewise, in a cross-sectional study of 379 obese African American and Caucasian adults, 43% of African Americans had 25(OH)D levels ≤ 37.5 nmol/L as compared with 11.7% of the Caucasians. [50]. Furthermore, results from NHANES III (1988-1994) suggest that almost 50% of African

American women of reproductive age in the United States have 25(OH)D levels ≤ 37.5 nmol/L, indicating high levels of vitamin D deficiency [33].

Low vitamin D status is also common in many Asian countries and the Middle East [59]. In a cross-sectional survey of adolescent girls in Beijing (n=1,277),[60] more than 40% of girls had 25(OH)D concentrations of <12.5 nmol/L. The latitude of Beijing and the lack of sunlight in the winter may partially explain this high prevalence of low vitamin D status. Similarly, low serum concentrations of vitamin D were reported in a young adult population of Japanese women[61], with 42.1% of the population having serum 25(OH)D concentrations < 30 nmol/L. Low vitamin D status is prevalent among Indian populations as well. In a study of postmenopausal women living in south India (n=164) [62], varying degrees of low vitamin D status were reported in approximately 82% of the women. Likewise, in a population of pregnant women in northern India (n=207) [63], 43% of the population had serum 25(OH)D concentrations <10 ng/ml, and 67% had concentrations <15 ng/ml. Middle Eastern populations such as the Lebanese[64], Turkish[65, 66], Jordanians[67], Iranians[68], and Saudi Arabians[69] also exhibit low vitamin D status. Prevailing patterns of dress among Muslims may explain the high prevalence of low vitamin D status in India and the Middle East where many women wear the traditional veil covering most of the body. Cross-sectional studies [64, 65, 67] suggest a higher prevalence of low vitamin D status among veiled females when compared with non-veiled females and males, indicating that culture and dress may be an important predictor of vitamin D status.

D. Health Effects of Low Vitamin D Status

Severe vitamin D deficiency was first defined as a serious health problem in Europe and North America during the late 19th and early 20th century when infants began developing rickets, a disease characterized by weakening of the bones and muscles, due to lack of sunlight exposure[3]. This disorder is now rare in the United States, although it can be found in developing countries and among some high-risk groups. Milder forms of low vitamin D status, however, are now endemic across all areas of the world and are related to an increasing number of illnesses and disorders, including cardiovascular disease, hypertension, inflammatory and autoimmune diseases, and type 2 diabetes [4].

Vitamin D is essential for the absorption of calcium and phosphorous in the body, and inadequate levels of vitamin D can result in impaired intestinal absorption of calcium and phosphorous leading to decreased bone mineral density, bone fragility, and bone loss [70]. This increases the risk of bone fractures and falls, especially in the elderly [30]. In addition, low levels of calcium in the blood can lead to secondary hyperparathyroidism, the overproduction of parathyroid hormone in the body, further worsening deleterious effects on the bone.

Given that vitamin D may play a role in the intestinal absorption of magnesium, it is possible that low vitamin D status may also lead to number of health effects mediated by the effects of low intracellular Mg concentrations [$(Mg^{2+})_i$]. Previous reports indicate that $(Mg^{2+})_i$ levels are frequently low in diabetic and hypertensive patients[71-74], and it is possible that $(Mg^{2+})_i$ plays an important role in insulin-mediated glucose uptake and vascular tone. In addition, dietary magnesium intake is associated with a number of health conditions including cardiovascular disease[75], stroke[76], hypertension[77], and type 2 diabetes[74, 78], suggesting that magnesium exerts a range of health effects that could potentially be associated with low vitamin D status and impaired Mg absorption.

In recent years, research attention has shifted toward the investigation of the role of vitamin D in the pathogenesis of chronic diseases, including type 2 diabetes. An accumulating body of research suggests that the role of vitamin D in the human body extends far beyond calcium absorption and bone mineralization, although the interactions with calcium, magnesium, and other minerals remain an essential part of inquiry in this area. The identification of VDR in numerous tissues throughout the body has generated much research interest in a wide range of potential health effects of vitamin D. Increasing evidence indicates that vitamin D influences the immune system and response to infections, the development of inflammatory and autoimmune diseases, and chronic diseases such as cancer, cardiovascular disease, and diabetes mellitus. It has even been suggested that fluctuating vitamin D levels are responsible for the seasonality of epidemic flu [79]. The evidence for these relationships has been reviewed extensively elsewhere [4, 11, 70]. Hereinafter, we will focus our discussion on the role of vitamin D in the development of type 2 diabetes, the animal and epidemiologic evidence examining this association, and potential biological mechanisms including possible interactions with calcium, magnesium, and other minerals.

IV. Vitamin D and Type 2 Diabetes

A. Animal Evidence

The discovery of VDR in the pancreatic β-cells in chicks over 25 years ago provided evidence that vitamin D may affect insulin secretion [80, 81]. This finding, combined with the identification of vitamin D-dependent calcium-binding protein (CaBP) in the pancreas of several other animals [82-84] prompted a host of depletion and repletion studies of vitamin D in animals that consistently demonstrate the importance of vitamin D in the pancreatic secretion of insulin.

Vitamin D repletion significantly improved insulin secretion in an *in vitro* study of isolated perfused pancreases from vitamin D-deficient rats [85]. Over a 30 minute period of glucose and arginine perfusion, insulin secretion was reduced by 48% in those pancreases not replenished with vitamin D. Kadowaki and Norman [86] reported similar effects in a series of *in vitro* experiments in isolated perfused rat pancreases controlling for the effects of caloric intake and serum calcium levels. In the first experiment, vitamin D deficient (-D) and vitamin D sufficient (+D) rats were pair-fed, receiving identical quantities of food, to assure equal caloric intake. After treatment with arginine-glucose, the +D rats exhibited significantly higher insulin secretion than the –D rats, suggesting that vitamin D status, not caloric intake, was responsible for the insulin response. The second experiment investigated the effects of varying calcium levels on the insulin response. Results indicated that serum calcium levels did not influence arginine-glucose-induced insulin secretion in rats [86].

In vivo studies have reported comparable findings regarding the effects of vitamin D on insulin secretion. Vitamin D deficient rats injected with 1,25 $(OH)_2D$ exhibited over an 100% increase in peripheral blood levels of insulin (17 microunits/ml increase) as compared with the control group[87]. Similarly, among live +D rats and -D rats, glucose-mediated insulin secretion and glucose tolerance declined significantly in the -D rats as compared with the +D rats after a glucose load. Additionally, repletion with vitamin D recovered insulin function and improved glucose tolerance in the –D rats [88]. Findings from an intervention study of the effects of vitamin D-deficiency on insulin secretion and glucose tolerance in rabbits were consistent. Rabbits on a vitamin D-deficient diet exhibited a significant reduction in insulin secretion and glucose tolerance after only 2 months on the diet. Furthermore, repletion with an injection of vitamin D restored normal insulin function [89].

It has been suggested that reductions in insulin secretion observed in –D rats can be explained, at least partially, by the difference in caloric intake between the –D and +D rats. In a study assessing the effects of decreased food intake and vitamin D-deficiency on impaired glucose secretion in rats, Chertow et al. [90] observed an association between vitamin D-deficiency and inhibition of insulin release, but only in the rats were not pair-fed. When +D and –D rats were pair fed, there was no significant difference in insulin secretion. This study suggests that total caloric intake, not vitamin D deficiency, is responsible for impaired insulin secretion. However, subsequent studies explored this possibility with similar methods and concluded that the effect of caloric intake on insulin secretion was secondary to the effect of vitamin D status [86]. Overall, the totality of the evidence supports the role of vitamin D in pancreatic insulin secretion.

Little is known about the direct effects of vitamin D on insulin resistance in animals, and scant animal research has investigated this topic. In several *in vitro* studies of rat adipocytes, pre-treatment with 100 nM 1,25 $(OH)_2D$ suppressed insulin-induced glucose uptake via activation of the PKCβ pathway[91, 92]. These findings suggest that excess calcitriol in insulin-responsive cells can lead to hyperglycemia and insulin resistance. Elevated levels of 1,25 $(OH)_2D$ are generally the result of low circulating 25(OH)D levels and impaired calcium absorption, and excess 1,25 $(OH)_2D$ has been shown to stimulate the influx of intracellular free calcium $[Ca^{2+}]$ into adipocytes, leading to weight gain, insulin resistance, and the development of type 2 diabetes in humans[44].

B. Evidence from Studies in Humans

In addition to animal studies, numerous clinical and epidemiologic studies have investigated the association of serum and dietary vitamin D with insulin secretion, impaired glucose tolerance, insulin resistance and type 2 diabetes in humans.

Cross-Sectional Evidence

A number of cross-sectional studies have reported inverse associations between vitamin D and risk factors for type 2 diabetes, including decreased insulin secretion, glucose intolerance, insulin resistance, as well as established type 2 diabetes (Table 1).

Table 1. Cross-sectional studies of Vitamin D and Type 2 Diabetes

Reference	Study Population	Outcome	Outcome Measurement	Results
Scragg et al. 1995	5,677 men and women aged 40-64 yrs: New Zealand	IGT Type 2 Diabetes	Fasting & 2-hr plasma glucose/ Serum insulin level T2D	Inverse association btw 25(OH)D and T2D/IGT [Mean (SD) of cases vs controls: 69(31) vs 76(34) nmol/l; p=.001]
Baynes et al. 1997	142 elderly Dutchmen aged 70-88: Seven Countries Study	IGT Type 2 Diabetes	Fasting and 2-hr plasma glucose	Inverse association btw 25(OH)D and insulin secretion & glucose [Insulin concentration AUC: r= -0.23, p<0.05; Glucose AUC: r=-0.23, p<0.01]
Isaia et al. 2001	799 postmenopausal white women: Italy	Type 2 Diabetes	Self-report of T2D	Inverse association btw 25(OH)D and T2D (Mean (SD) of cases vs controls (11(9.8) vs 9(11.3) ng/ml, p<0.01)
Chiu et al. 2004	126 healthy glucose-tolerant subjects (Mean age 26): California	IGT β-cell function Insulin Sensitivity	Fasting & 2-hr plasma glucose / 1st and 2nd phase insulin response (Hyperglycemic clamp)	Inverse association btw 25(OH)D and fasting glucose [OGTT: β_{120min}= -0.52]; Positive association btw 25(OH)D and insulin sensitivity (r=0.46, p<.0001)
Scragg et al. 2004	6,228 adults aged ≥20yrs: NHANES III	IGT Type 2 Diabetes	T2D: Fasting and 2 hr plasma glucose	Inverse association btw 25(OH)D & IR: Whites [$\beta_{LOG\ HOMA\ IR}$ (SE) = -0.009 (0.004); p=0.058]; Mex Amer [$\beta_{LOG\ HOMA\ IR}$ (SE) = -0.016 (0.005); =.0024]
Ford et al. 2005	8,421 adults aged ≥20yrs: NHANES III	Metabolic Syndrome	NCEP criteria	Inverse association btw 25(OH)D and hyperglycemia [Highest quartile of 25(OH)D: OR=.44 (0.29, 0.68)]
Need et al. 2005	753 postmenopausal white women	IGT	Fasting plasma glucose	Inverse association btw 25(OH)D and fasting glucose (r=-0.15, p<0.01)
Hyponnen and Power 2006	7,189 Caucasians aged 45 years: British birth Cohort	IGT	HbA1C (%)	Inverse association btw 25(OH)D and A1C [25(OH)D ≥75 nmol/l: HbA1C = 5.12%; 25(OH)D <25 nmol/l: HbA1C = 5.37%; p for trend <0.0001)
Hahn et al. 2006	120 female patients with polycystic ovarian syndrome (Mean age: 28): Germany	IGT Insulin Sensitivity	Fasting & 2-hr plasma glucose and insulin	Inverse association btw 25(OH)D and insulin resistance (r=-0.19, p=0.03) and hyperinsulinemia (r=-0.19, p=0.04)

IGT= Impaired glucose tolerance; OGTT= Oral glucose tolerance test; IR= Insulin resistance.

Table 2. Prospective cohort studies of Vitamin D and Type 2 Diabetes

Reference	Study Population	Outcome	Outcome Measurement	Results
Liu et al. 2005	10,066 female health professionals ≥45 years: Women's Health Study	Type 2 Diabetes	Self-report	Inverse association btw total and dietary vitamin D and metabolic syndrome [Highest total quartile: OR=0.89 (0.72-1.09); Highest dietary quartile: OR=0.85 (0.70-1.02)] ; No association after controlling for dietary Ca
Pittas et al. 2006	83,779 female nurses aged 30-55 years: Nurses Health Study	Type 2 Diabetes	Self-report	Inverse association btw total vitamin D and risk of T2DM [Highest total quartile: OR=0.77 (0.63-0.94); Highest dietary quartile: OR=0.81 (0.64-1.01)]; No association after controlling for Mg and Ca

Table 3. Clinical Intervention studies of Vitamin D and Type 2 Diabetes

Reference	Study Population	Treatment	Follow-up	Outcome	Results
Gedik et al. 1986	4 severe vitamin D-deficient females 10 healthy controls	2,000 IU vitamin D3/d	6 months	Insulin Secretion	Improved insulin secretion after treatment [Insulin AUC (mu/min) Pre-treat: 9.09 ± .07 Post-treat:13.6 ±0.5; P<0.05]
Orwoll et al. 1994	35 established type 2 diabetics	1 ug/d calcitriol for 4 days	1 month	IGT Insulin Secretion	No improvement in insulin secretion or glucose among established diabetics; Improvement in diabetics [Change in insulin AUC: <3 yrs: 337 ±301 pmol/L vs. >6yrs: 0.7±93 pmol/L]
Boucher et al. 1995	44 "at risk" (IGT) cases and 15 "low" controls	Single bolus injection of 100,000 IU vitamin D3	12 weeks	IGT Type 2 Diabetes	Improved insulin secretion in IGT group [Specific insulin (mIU/l): Pre-treat: 36.8±24.4; Post-treat: 96.2±82.4; p<0.01] Abnormal glucose tolerance unchanged
Fliser et al. 1997	18 healthy males (mean age 26±3yrs)	1.5 ug/d calcitriol	7 days	Fasting plasma glucose	No significant change in mean glucose or insulin
Borissova et al. 2003	10 postmenopausal females with T2DM 17 matched controls	1332 IU vitamin D	1 month	Insulin Secretion IGT	Baseline FPIS: 34.7±12.9 mU/l vs. Post-treat FPIS: 46.6±16.1 mU/l; p<0.05
Pittas 2007	314 adults aged 65 years and over	Combined vitamin D and Ca (700IU vitamin D3 & 500mg Ca)	3 years	IGT Insulin resistance	Increases in FPG & IR smaller in treated than placebo group [Increases: Treatment FPG: 0.02 ± 0.09 nmol/L vs. Placebo FPG: 0.34 ± 0.11 nmol/L; Treatment IR: 0.05± 0.19; Placebo: 0.91 ± 0.31, p=0.031).

IGT= Impaired glucose tolerance; IR= Insulin resistance; Insulin AUC= Insulin area under the curve; FPG= Fasting plasma glucose.

With regard to insulin secretion and glucose metabolism, 25(OH)D concentrations were inversely associated with insulin secretion and OGTT glucose concentrations (Insulin concentration AUC: r= -0.23, $p<0.05$; Glucose AUC: r=-0.23, $p<0.01$) among elderly Dutchmen (n=142) aged 70-88 years[93]. Similarly, Need et al[94] reported an inverse association between serum 25(OH)D levels and fasting glucose (r=-0.150, $p<0.001$) among postmenopausal white women (n=753; aged 34-94 years). Among 8,421 men and nonpregnant women ≥20 years who had fasted ≥8 hours (NHANES III, 1988-1994), a test for a linear trend indicated increasing risk for hyperglycemia across decreasing quintiles of vitamin D intake [25(OH)D ≥ 96.4 nmol/l: OR of hyperglycemia = 0.44 (0.29,0.68); 25(OH)D: 48.5-63.4 nmol/l: OR of hyperglycemia = 0.92 (0.69, 1.23) p<.001][53]. In this same population, Vitamin D status was inversely associated with fasting and 2-hr glucose in non-Hispanic whites [25(OH)D: ≥ 80.0 nmol/l: Fasting glucose OR= 0.25 (0.11,0.60); 2-hr glucose OR=0.25 (0.11, 0.60)] and Mexican Americans [25(OH)D: ≥ 80.0 nmol/l: Fasting glucose OR= 0.17 (0.08, 0.37); 2-hr glucose OR= 0.45(0.15, 1.38)], but not in non-Hispanic blacks[58]. The lack of inverse association among non-Hispanic blacks may possibly be explained by the small numbers of African Americans within the highest quartile of serum vitamin D, although it has been suggested that African Americans metabolize vitamin D and other related hormones differently that other ethnic groups[57].

Long term measures of glucose metabolism (i.e. HbA1C) were also associated with vitamin D status. In the 1958 British birth cohort (n=7,189), as 25(OH)D levels decreased, HbA1C levels increased [25(OH)D ≥75 nmol/l: HbA1C = 5.12%; 25(OH)D <25 nmol/l: HbA1C = 5.37%; p for trend <0.0001)[54]. The effect was strongest for 25(OH)D concentrations ≤65 nmol/L, suggesting an interaction between 25(OH)D and glucose levels. In addition, adjustment for BMI and waist circumference weakened the negative association between 25(OH)D and HbA1C [Unadjusted percentage change in A1C per 10-unit increase in 25(OH)D: -0.49 (-0.58, -0.40); vs Adjusted for BMI and A1C: -0.16 (-0.22, -0.10), indicating that BMI may mediate the relation between 25(OH)D concentration and glucose metabolism.

Inverse associations between 25(OH)D concentrations and insulin resistance have also been reported. Among healthy, glucose-tolerant subjects living in California (n=126), 25(OH)D concentrations were positively associated with insulin sensitivity (r=0.4600, p<.0001), first-phase insulin response (r=-0.2513, p=.0045), and second-phase insulin response (r=-0.3487, p=0.0001) measured with the hyperglycemic clamp. No association was reported between 25(OH)D concentration and β-cell function. However, the significant inverse association between 25(OH)D levels and fasting glucose concentrations [Regression coefficients: $\beta_{fasting}$= -0.114; β_{30min}= -0.092; β_{60min}= -0.698; β_{90min}= -0.605; β_{120min}= -0.52] indicates that low 25(OH)D levels do exert effects on β-cell function. If β-cell function was optimal, then glucose concentrations would be expected to remain normal even with low circulating 25(OH)D. Among the NHANES III population[58], insulin resistance was inversely associated with vitamin D levels among non-Hispanic whites [$\beta_{LOG\ HOMA\ IR}$ (SE) = -0.009 (0.004); p=0.058] and Mexican Americans [$\beta_{LOG\ HOMA\ IR}$ (SE) = -0.016 (0.005); p=0.0024]. Consistent with these findings, 25(OH)D was inversely associated with insulin resistance among German women with polycystic ovarian syndrome (PCOS)[52].

In addition to risk factors for type 2 diabetes, cross-sectional studies suggest an association between low 25(OH)D concentrations and prevalent type 2 diabetes. Scragg et al[95] assessed serum 25(OH)D levels among workforce members aged 40-64 years in New Zealand (n=5,677). After adjustment for potential confounders, serum 25(OH)D levels were significantly lower in both newly diagnosed diabetics and impaired glucose tolerant cases when compared with controls matched on sex, age, ethnicity, and date of interview [Mean (SD): 69 (31) vs 76 (34) nmol/l; p=0.0016). Adjusted odds ratios associated with serum 25(OH)D levels showed a decreased risk of type 2 diabetes among the middle [OR=.57 (0.32, 1.02), p=0.059] and highest [OR=.36, (0.19,0.71), p=0.003) tertiles of 25(OH)D concentrations when compared with the lowest. Similarly, among 799 postmenopausal Italian women (n=66 diabetics)[96], mean levels of serum 25(OH)D were significantly lower in diabetic patients than in controls (Means of 25(OH)D ± SD: 11 ± 9.8 vs. 9 ± 11.3 ng/ml, $p<0.008$) and the prevalence of vitamin D-deficiency was higher among this group (Diabetics: 39% vs. Controls: 25%).

Prospective Cohort Evidence

Several prospective cohort studies have investigated the long-term effects of vitamin D on insulin secretion, glucose metabolism, insulin resistance, and incident type 2 diabetes (Table 2). Liu et al[55] reported an inverse association between total and dietary vitamin D and the metabolic syndrome over an average of 8.8 years of follow-up in the Women's Health Study (n=10,066) [Highest total vitamin D quartile: OR=0.89 (0.72,1.09); Highest dietary vitamin D quartile: OR=0.85 (0.70,1.02)]. After controlling for calcium however, the association between total and dietary vitamin D and metabolic syndrome disappeared, suggesting calcium as a potential mediator of this relation. Similarly, total and dietary vitamin D intake were inversely associated with risk of type 2 diabetes over a 20-year follow up period in the Nurses Health Study[97] (n=83,779) [Highest total quartile: OR=0.77 (0.63, 0.94); Highest dietary quartile: OR=0.81 (0.64, 1.01)], but the linear trend was not significant after controlling for both dietary calcium and magnesium intake, indicating that the effects of vitamin D may be mediated by these metabolically related micronutrients.

Clinical Intervention Trials

Although the majority of research exploring the role of vitamin D in the pathophysiology of diabetes thus far has been cross-sectional in nature, several clinical trials have explored the effects of vitamin D supplementation on type 2 diabetes with varied results (Table 3).

Insulin secretion, but not glucose levels, improved significantly after vitamin D treatment in several small clinical trials[98-100]. After 6 months of treatment with 2,000 IU vitamin D3 daily (n=4 female patients with severe vitamin D deficiency; n=10 healthy volunteers), insulin secretion in the vitamin D-deficient group improved significantly [Insulin AUC (mu/min) Pre-treat: 9.09 ± .07 vs. Post-treat:13.6 ±0.5; $P<0.05$], surpassing baseline levels in the healthy group. Insulinogenic indices followed a similar pattern and rose significantly after treatment in the vitamin D-deficient group [Pre-treatment: 1.71±0.4 vs. Post-treatment: 2.48±0.3]. Plasma glucose levels remained unchanged after treatment[98]. Consistent findings were reported in a trial of East London Asians [n=44 subjects "at risk" for diabetes (spot blood glucose level > 6.0 mmol/l < 2 hr post cibum, or > 4.6 mmol/l > 2 hr post cibum on two separate occasions), n=15 age and sex-matched "low risk" controls]. Eight to twelve weeks after a single bolus injection of 100,000 IU of vitamin D, insulin secretion, but not glucose levels improved significantly [Specific insulin (mIU/l): Pre-treatment: 36.8±24.4; Post-treatment: 96.2±82.4; p<0.01][99]. Similarly, first phase insulin secretion (FPIS) improved significantly in diabetics (n=10 postmenopausal females with type 2 diabetes, n=17 age- and BMI-matched controls) after treatment with 1332 IU vitamin D daily for 1 month [Baseline FPIS: 34.7±12.9 mU/l vs. Post-treatment FPIS: 46.6±16.1 mU/l; p<0.05]. In addition, there was a strong correlation between the change in FPIS and the change in 25(OH)D levels (r=0.7234, p=0.018), indicating a role of vitamin D in insulin secretion[100].

With regard to insulin resistance, two trials[100, 101] have reported positive effects of vitamin D supplementation. In the largest double-blinded, randomized controlled trial to date (n=314 Caucasian adults aged 65 years and over)[101], participants were randomly assigned to a combined calcium-vitamin D supplement (700 IU vitamin D3, 500 mg CA) or placebo for 3 years. Among impaired glucose tolerant participants, increases in fasting plasma glucose and insulin resistance (measured by HOMA-IR) over the study period were significantly smaller than those increases in the placebo group [Increases: Treatment Fasting Plasma Glucose (FPG): 0.02 ± 0.09 nmol/L vs. Placebo FPG: 0.34 ± 0.11 nmol/L; Treatment IR: 0.05± 0.19; Placebo: 0.91 ± 0.31, p=0.031). In a smaller trial of type 2 diabetics[100], HOMA-IR decreased after one month of treatment with vitamin D [Post-treatment: 7.82±2.31 mU/l.mmol/l vs. Pretreatment: 6.15 mU/l.mmol/l; p>0.8], although the change was not significant.

However, several clinical trials have observed no effect on insulin secretion, glucose homeostasis, and insulin resistance[102, 103]. In a randomized, placebo-controlled, crossover trial of 1,25 dihydroxyvitamin D3 treatment (1 μg/day for 4 days) in established diabetics (n=35, aged 40-70 years)[102], no effect on fasting insulin or glucose concentrations was reported. However, those subjects with a shorter duration of diabetes showed greater improvements in insulin secretion after administration of vitamin D [Change in insulin area under the curve for diabetics <3 yrs duration: 337 ±301 pmol/L vs. 3-6 yrs: 3.6± 122 pmol/l vs. >6 yrs: 0.7±93 pmol/l], suggesting that vitamin D does not influence insulin secretion in established diabetics, but may exert effects earlier in the development of the disease. Similarly, in a randomized, placebo-controlled study of 1,25 $(OH)_2D_3$ treatment (1.5 *u*g/ day for seven days) in healthy white males (n=18)[103], there were no significant changes in mean glucose, insulin, or insulin sensitivity after treatment [Pre-treatment mean glucose disposal rate: 7.0±1.4 $mgkg^{-1}min^{-1}$; Post-treatment: 7.2±1.4 $mgkg^{-1}min^{-1}$). However, mean PTH levels decreased [Pre-treatment: 2.6± 0.9 $pmol/l^{-1}$ vs. Post-treatment: 1.7±0.9] and urinary excretion increased [Pre-treatment: 4.3±1.5 vs. Post-treatment: 6.0±2.2 pmol/l] after treatment, indicating biological actions of 1,25 $(OH)_2D_3$.

Taken together, these studies suggest that vitamin D supplementation may have beneficial effects on type 2 diabetes. Diverse study populations, vitamin D supplements, doses, and follow-up periods make comparisons difficult; however, the majority of the evidence seems to support the advantageous role of vitamin D supplementation in improving markers of type 2 diabetes, especially when given in larger doses for longer durations of time.

V. Potential Biological Mechanisms

A. Insulin Secretion

Independent Effects of Vitamin D

Vitamin D is necessary for normal pancreatic secretion of insulin, and animal models consistently show an improved insulin response to glucose stimulation after treatment with vitamin D_3[85-87]. Reports from studies in humans described earlier in this review support this model[54, 58, 95, 98-100, 102, 104]. The presence of specific vitamin D receptors on the pancreatic β-cells and evidence of involvement in gene transcription provides a plausible biological explanation for this association.

Joint Effects of Vitamin D and Calcium

Several lines of evidence suggest that calcium may be a potential mediator of the relation between vitamin D and insulin secretion. In an *in vitro* study of rat pancreatic islets, Kikuchi et al examined the role of intracellular calcium ($[Ca^{2+}]_i$)stores on insulin release. Control islets were those with normal $[Ca^{2+}]_i$ levels, and a second set of islets was loaded with $[Ca^{2+}]_i$. Glucose-stimulated first-phase insulin release was 3.5 times greater in the islets loaded with $[Ca^{2+}]_i$. These findings suggest that calcium may play a role in first phase insulin release in rats [105]. Similarly, in a study assessing the respective role of vitamin D and calcium on insulin response, calcium repletion alone normalized glucose tolerance and insulin secretion in vitamin D-depleted rats [106].

Insulin secretion is dependent on the balance between extracellular and intracellular calcium levels[107], and evidence that intracellular Ca^{2+} ($[Ca^{2+}]_i$) levels in various cell types rise with the administration of vitamin D provides additional support for the mediating role of calcium in insulin secretion[108-110]. It is possible that vitamin D stimulates the entry of extracellular (Ca^{2+}) into the β-cells through voltage dependent Ca^{2+} channels and leads to the activation of second messenger systems involving protein kinase A and cAMP [111]. A vitamin D induced influx of $[Ca^{2+}]_i$ into the β-cells may potentially affect the balance between intra- and extracellular calcium levels and affect insulin secretion through a nongenomic pathway. However, the role of vitamin D and calcium in insulin secretion is still disputed due to animal models demonstrating the independent role of vitamin D[86, 88, 89] combined with evidence from clinical intervention studies in humans demonstrating improved insulin secretion after treatment with vitamin D[98-100]. Based on the totality of the evidence, it is likely that vitamin D and calcium exert both independent and interactive effects on insulin secretion. However, further research assessing the independent effects of each on insulin secretion is essential to further our understanding of the role of vitamin D in the development of type 2 diabetes.

Joint Effects of Vitamin D and Magnesium

Vitamin D plays a role in the absorption of magnesium, and it is well-established that magnesium is a key regulator of insulin and glucose metabolism[71, 78]. Clinical and prospective studies in humans[112, 113] suggest that dietary magnesium may improve insulin secretion and glucose response. However, the direct effects of magnesium on insulin secretion are not completely understood. Magnesium is required for insulin secretion from the pancreatic β-cells, and a deficiency in magnesium has been shown to lead to impaired insulin secretion and disturbances in glucose homeostasis in animal models[114, 115]. *In vitro* studies[116, 117] suggest that the balance of extra- and intracellular Mg^{2+} in the pancreatic β-cells may regulate the secretion of insulin. Given that intracellular Mg^{2+} is dependent upon the influx of extracellular Mg^{2+} through the voltage dependent Ca^{2+} channels, it is possible that extracellular Mg^{2+} competitively inhibits this pathway and in turn, inhibits the secretion of insulin which is dependent on this pathway[117]. Another possible mechanism through which the balance of intra- and extracellular Mg^{2+} may affect insulin secretion is the hypothesis that extracellular Mg^{2+} plays a role in ATP-sensitive potassium channels involved in insulin secretion[116]. However, the role of magnesium in the pancreatic secretion of insulin is still unclear, and it is possible that the effects of magnesium on glucose metabolism are mediated via effects on insulin sensitivity[71, 78, 118, 119].

B. Insulin Resistance

Independent Effects of Vitamin D

Vitamin D receptors (VDR) identified on numerous cell types throughout the body, including insulin responsive tissues such as muscle cells[120], suggest that vitamin D may affect insulin responsiveness and glucose uptake. Vitamin D may regulate insulin receptor gene expression at the genomic level by increasing the total insulin receptor number through an increase in the levels of mRNA of the insulin receptor gene. An increase in insulin receptors may potentially increase the binding of insulin, stimulating the cascade of intracellular events leading to the translocation of GLUT-4 transporter to the plasma membrane and greater influx of glucose into cell[121, 122]. This effect has been demonstrated in human promonocytic cells, generally considered to be a good *in vitro* model to study insulin receptors, and it is possible that this same biological process occurs in other insulin responsive cells, such as muscle and adipose tissue.

Joint Effects of Vitamin D and Calcium

Vitamin D may also indirectly affect insulin resistance by influencing intracellular free calcium ($[Ca^{2+}]_i$) levels in insulin responsive target tissues. 1,25 $(OH)_2D$ stimulates the influx of calcium into insulin responsive cells such as adipocytes[46] and can lead to elevated $[Ca^{2+}]_i$ levels. An optimal range of $[Ca^{2+}]_i$ is required for insulin-stimulated glucose transport in skeletal muscle and adipose tissue[123, 124], and high levels of $[Ca^{2+}]_i$ in adipocytes can contribute to insulin resistance [125, 126]. It is possible that elevated levels of $[Ca^{2+}]_i$ inhibit the dephosphorylation of the glucose transporter, Glut4, and decrease insulin-stimulated glucose tranport[127]. Increased $[Ca^{2+}]_i$ may also affect insulin sensitivity via protein kinase C activation and inactivation of the insulin receptor[128]. Inverse associations between vitamin D status and insulin resistance observed in several cross-sectional studies[52, 53, 58, 104] support the role of vitamin D in insulin resistance. However, the inverse association was not independent of calcium intake in the Women's Health Study[55], suggesting a possible mediating role of calcium. Results from intervention trials are limited and report inconsistent findings[100, 103]. Based on this evidence, it seems reasonable to conclude that vitamin D and insulin resistance are inversely associated, although the exact causal mechanism, and whether the association is driven by low vitamin D status or a related mineral such as calcium, remains to be determined.

Joint Effects of Vitamin D and Magnesium

Intracellular Mg^{2+} concentrations are known to be an important mediator of insulin action and glucose homeostasis, and depletion of intracellular Mg^{2+} is a well-recognized characteristic of type 2 diabetes [73, 118, 119]. Insulin has been shown to regulate influx of Mg^{2+} into the intracellular space [129], and Mg^{2+} also influences the action of insulin. Decreased intracellular Mg^{2+} concentrations are associated with an impairment in insulin action and glucose uptake in insulin sensitive tissues such as skeletal muscle tissue[130], heart muscles[131], and adipocytes[132]. Animal models[133] suggest that a defect in the tyrosine kinase activity of insulin receptors may be responsible for the decrease in insulin sensitivity associated with decreased intracellular Mg^{2+} concentrations, a plausible explanation given the critical role of intracellular Mg^{2+} in the Mg-ATP complex and phosphorylation reactions, including phosphorylation of the insulin receptor [134]. Although the connection between vitamin D and magnesium is not fully characterized, vitamin D may possibly influence the balance of intra- and extra-cellular Mg^{2+} in insulin-responsive tissues through its effects on the absorption of Mg in the small intestine, thereby exerting effects on insulin resistance via alterations in Mg^{2+} concentrations.

VI. Genetic Variants

A. Vitamin D Receptor (VDR) Polymorphisms

Biological actions of vitamin D are mediated by the vitamin D receptor (VDR), a ligand-activated member of the steroid/thyroid hormone-receptor superfamily[3]. Vitamin D influences gene transcription through a series of steps involving high affinity and highly selective bonds to the VDR. 1,25 $(OH)_2$ D binds to retinoid X receptor (RXR), forming a heterodimer which binds to specific DNA sequence elements in the promoter regions of hormone responsive genes called Vitamin D Response Elements (VDRE)[6]. The VDR gene is located on chromosome 12cen-q12 and contains 14 exons[135]. Genetic variations in the VDR may potentially lead to deleterious effects on gene expression, including the dysregulation of insulin and glucose levels in the body and the development of type 2 diabetes.

Genetic polymorphisms, or common genetic variants that appear in more than 1% of the population, have been identified on the VDR gene in humans[3]. Examples of polymorphisms identified in the VDR gene include *Tru*9I, *Fok*I, *Taq*I, *Bsm*I, *Eco*RV, and *Apa*I[136]. The effects of VDR polymorphisms on type 1 diabetes have been studied extensively in varied populations, and published findings have been conflicting[137-141]. The b allele of the *Bsm*I polymorphism was associated with susceptibility to Type 1 diabetes in a population of South Indians (53/84; p=0.016) [139]. *Bsm*I and *Apa*I were linked to Type

1 diabetes in a Taiwanese population [*BsmI*: BB OR=6.74 (4.54, 8.94); *Apa*I: AA OR=2.46 (1.68,3.24)][141]. No such associations were found in Finnish[138] and Chilean[140] populations. In a recent meta-analysis of the studies in this area, little evidence was found to suggest an association between VDR polymorphisms, including *Apa*I, *Bsm*I, *Fok*I, and *Taq*, and type 1 diabetes[142]. However, it is plausible that there are alternative VDR polymorphisms other than those well-studied that may play a role in type 1 diabetes.

The role of VDR polymorphisms in insulin secretion, glucose homeostasis, insulin resistance, and risk of type 2 diabetes has been explored in several studies, and findings have been inconsistent. In a study of healthy Bangladeshi Asians (n=171)[143], the *Apa*I, *Bsm*I, and *Taq*I polymorphisms were positively associated with insulin secretion but not insulin resistance [Insulin secretion Index (ISI): *Apa*I: AA genotype = 146.8 (112.8, 191.0); aa = 68.5 (48.9-95.8); *Bsm*I: BB = 120.5(89.0, 163.1); bb = 80.7 (64.6, 100.7); *Taq*I: TT = 87.5 (72.2, 106.0); tt = 173.3 (102.0, 294.4)]. In the Rancho Bernardo Study[144], a community-based study of nondiabetic Caucasians (n=1,545), the *Apa*I polymorphism was associated with the prevalence of glucose intolerance [AA genotype: 30.9%; aa: 39.9%, p for trend <0.05], and fasting plasma glucose was significantly higher in individuals with the aa genotype compared to those with the AA genotype (5.43 ± 0.56 mmol/L vs. 5.35 ± 0.57 mmol/L, p<0.05]. The *Bsm*I polymorphism was associated with insulin resistance, with higher insulin resistance reported among individuals with the bb genotype [HOMA IR: BB genotype: 2.8 ± 1.5 vs bb: 3.2 ± 2.2, p<0.05].

With regard to prevalent type 2 diabetes, several studies reported no association with VDR polymorphisms[144-146]. Specifically, *Bsm*I, *Tru9*I, and *Apa*I were not associated with prevalent type 2 diabetes in a population of French Caucasians (n=309 diabetic patients; 143 healthy controls)[145], and the *Fok*I, *Apa*I, *Bsm*I, and *Taq*I were not associated with type 2 diabetes in a homogenous Polish population (n=308 diabetic patients, 240 healthy controls)[146]. However, the B allele of the *Bsm*I polymorphism was associated with increased odds of having prevalent type 2 diabetes [BB genotype: OR=3.64 (1.53, 8.55), p=0.002] in a population of German patients at high risk for coronary artery disease (n=293)[147].

Further research is required to unravel the role of VDR polymorphisms in the development of type 2 diabetes. It is likely that conflicting findings in this area stem from inadequate power to detect associations, a common problem among genetic association studies, combined with tight linkage disequilibrium between several of the selected polymorphisms (i.e. ApaI, BsmI, TaqI, EcoRV). In addition, most of the VDR polymorphisms studied thus far are located in nonfunctional introns of the VDR gene.

Observed associations may reflect linkage disequilibrium with a functional variant elsewhere in the VDR gene that has not been considered[135]. Further exploration of these selected polymorphisms and other potential candidate genes in larger studies is essential to deepen our understanding of the molecular impact of genetic variants of the VDR in the development of Type 2 diabetes.

B. Magnesium and Calcium Homeostasis-Related Genetic Variants

Magnesium and calcium homeostasis in the body is tightly regulated, and imbalances in intra- and extracellular levels of these ions can disrupt a number of cellular and systemic processes that may play a role in the pathogenesis of disease, including type 2 diabetes. Recently, several genes encoding proteins responsible for Mg^{2+} cellular influx have been identified, including members of the transient receptor potential (TRP) family of cation channels[148-150]. TRPM6, an Mg^{2+} and Ca^{2+} channel permeable channel localized in the kidney tubules and intestinal epithelia, has been shown to play a critical role in intestinal and renal Mg^{2+} absorption[151]. Mutations in TRPM6 lead to hypomagnesemia with secondary hypocalcemia, an autosomal recessive disorder characterized by impaired intestinal Mg^{2+} absorption, decreased PTH, and decreased serum Ca^{2+} levels[148, 149]. TRPM7, a closely related intracellular ligand-gated ion channel, may interact with TRPM6 to form channel complexes regulating the influx of Mg^{2+} into the cell[150, 152]. These findings suggest that TRPM6 and TRPM7 play a crucial role in intracellular Mg levels, a key factor in insulin and glucose metabolism[71, 78]. Similarly, TRP channels play an important role in Ca^{2-} signaling and may exert effects on a range of Ca^{2+} dependent functions including the balance of intra- and extracellular calcium, known to affect insulin secretion[107] and insulin resistance[124, 125]. Given the close interconnection between TRP channels and mineral absorption and homeostasis, defects in these ion channels are critically important to examine in future research into the pathogenesis of type 2 diabetes. It is possible that genetic variation in these channels may help to explain variations in risk of type 2 diabetes in the general population.

Conclusion

The link between low vitamin D status and type 2 diabetes is of critical public health importance due to the severity of the diabetes epidemic and the urgent need for prevention efforts. An extensive body of literature suggests the potential important role of low vitamin D status in the development of type 2 diabetes. However, the vitamin D endocrine system is an elaborate system, involving a complex interplay of interactions between calcium, phosphorus, magnesium, and other minerals and hormones. Disentangling the independent and interactive effects of these factors is of critical importance, and further research is essential in this area. To date, the majority of the human research in this area has been cross-sectional in design, hindering the ability to make causal inferences. Future research should therefore focus on assessing the effects of vitamin D supplementation in prospective studies of large and diverse populations with careful assessment of vitamin D status as well as in randomized controlled settings in diverse populations. In addition, mechanistic and interaction studies assessing the role of metabolically related minerals are needed to understand the interrelations among vitamin D and insulin secretion, insulin resistance, and type 2 diabetes. Consideration of gene-environment interactions, including genetic variants of the vitamin D receptor and other pathways involved in mineral homeostasis should also be investigated further. Research of this nature is essential to further our understanding of the pathophysiology of type 2 diabetes and the potential use of vitamin D and other minerals in primary prevention and treatment.

References

[1] Boucher, B.J., Inadequate vitamin D status: does it contribute to the disorders comprising syndrome 'X'? *Br. J. Nutr.*, 1998. 79(4): p. 315-27.

[2] Holick, M.F., McCollum Award Lecture, 1994: vitamin D--new horizons for the 21st century. *Am. J. Clin. Nutr.*, 1994. 60(4): p. 619-30.

[3] Feldman, D., F.H. Glorieux, and J.W. Pike, eds. *Vitamin D*. 1997, Academic Press: San Diego.

[4] Zittermann, A., Vitamin D in preventive medicine: are we ignoring the evidence? *Br. J. Nutr.*, 2003. 89(5): p. 552-72.

[5] Dusso, A.S., A.J. Brown, and E. Slatopolsky, Vitamin D. *Am. J. Physiol. Renal. Physiol.*, 2005. 289(1): p. F8-28.

[6] Holick, M.F., Vitamin D: *Physiology, Molecular Biology, and Clinical Applications*. 1999, Totowa: Humana Press Inc. 458.

[7] Hurwitz, S., Homeostatic control of plasma calcium concentration. *Crit. Rev. Biochem. Mol. Biol.*, 1996. 31(1): p. 41-100.

[8] Norman, A.W., The vitamin D endocrine system. *Physiologist*, 1985. 28(4): p. 219-32.

[9] Vieth, R., Why the optimal requirement for Vitamin D3 is probably much higher than what is officially recommended for adults. *J. Steroid. Biochem. Mol. Biol.*, 2004. 89-90(1-5): p. 575-9.

[10] Vieth, R., et al., The urgent need to recommend an intake of vitamin D that is effective. *Am. J. Clin. Nutr.*, 2007. 85(3): p. 649-50.

[11] Holick, M.F., The vitamin D epidemic and its health consequences. *J. Nutr.*, 2005. 135(11): p. 2739S-48S.

[12] Hollis, B.W., Circulating 25-hydroxyvitamin D levels indicative of vitamin D sufficiency: implications for establishing a new effective dietary intake recommendation for vitamin D. *J. Nutr.*, 2005. 135(2): p. 317-22.

[13] Takeda, E., et al., Inorganic phosphate homeostasis and the role of dietary phosphorus. *J. Cell Mol. Med.*, 2004. 8(2): p. 191-200.

[14] Amato, D., et al., Acute effects of soft drink intake on calcium and phosphate metabolism in immature and adult rats. *Rev. Invest Clin.*, 1998. 50(3): p. 185-9.

[15] Poole, K.E. and J. Reeve, Parathyroid hormone - a bone anabolic and catabolic agent. *Curr. Opin. Pharmacol.*, 2005. 5(6): p. 612-7.

[16] Huang, C.L., et al., Molecular physiology and pharmacology of calcitonin. *Cell Mol. Biol.* (Noisy-le-grand), 2006. 52(3): p. 33-43.

[17] Moon, J., The role of vitamin D in toxic metal absorption: a review. *J. Am. Coll Nutr.*, 1994. 13(6): p. 559-64.

[18] Zofkova, I. and R.L. Kancheva, The relationship between magnesium and calciotropic hormones. *Magnes Res.*, 1995. 8(1): p. 77-84.

[19] Loughead, J.L., et al., A role for magnesium in neonatal parathyroid gland function? *J. Am. Coll Nutr.*, 1991. 10(2): p. 123-6.

[20] Bailly, C., N. Roinel, and C. Amiel, Stimulation by glucagon and PTH of Ca and Mg reabsorption in the superficial distal tubule of the rat kidney. *Pflugers Arch.*, 1985. 403(1): p. 28-34.

[21] Morel, F., Sites of hormone action in the mammalian nephron. *Am. J. Physiol.*, 1981. 240(3): p. F159-64.
[22] Hulter, H.N. and J.C. Peterson, Renal and systemic magnesium metabolism during chronic continuous PTH infusion in normal subjects. *Metabolism*, 1984. 33(7): p. 662-6.
[23] Rude, R.K., Magnesium metabolism and deficiency. *Endocrinol. Metab. Clin. North Am.*, 1993. 22(2): p. 377-95.
[24] Miller, E.R., et al., Mineral Balance Studies with the Baby Pig: Effects of Dietary Vitamin D2 Level Upon Calcium, Phosphorus and Magnesium Balance. *J. Nutr.*, 1965. 85: p. 255-9.
[25] Karbach, U. and K. Ewe, Calcium and magnesium transport and influence of 1,25-dihydroxyvitamin D3. In vivo perfusion study at the colon of the rat. *Digestion*, 1987. 37(1): p. 35-42.
[26] Hollis, B.W., Assessment of vitamin D nutritional and hormonal status: what to measure and how to do it. *Calcif Tissue Int.*, 1996. 58(1): p. 4-5.
[27] Zittermann, A., Vitamin D and disease prevention with special reference to cardiovascular disease. *Prog. Biophys. Mol. Biol.*, 2006. 92(1): p. 39-48.
[28] Bischoff-Ferrari, H.A., et al., Estimation of optimal serum concentrations of 25-hydroxyvitamin D for multiple health outcomes. *Am. J. Clin. Nutr.*, 2006. 84(1): p. 18-28.
[29] Heaney, R.P., The Vitamin D requirement in health and disease. *J. Steroid Biochem. Mol. Biol.,* 2005. 97(1-2): p. 13-9.
[30] Lips, P., Vitamin D deficiency and secondary hyperparathyroidism in the elderly: consequences for bone loss and fractures and therapeutic implications. *Endocr. Rev.*, 2001. 22(4): p. 477-501.
[31] Buffington, C., et al., Vitamin D Deficiency in the Morbidly Obese. *Obes. Surg.*, 1993. 3(4): p. 421-424.
[32] Liel, Y., et al., Low circulating vitamin D in obesity. *Calcif Tissue Int.*, 1988. 43(4): p. 199-201.
[33] Nesby-O'Dell, S., et al., Hypovitaminosis D prevalence and determinants among African American and white women of reproductive age: third National Health and Nutrition Examination Survey, 1988-1994. *Am. J. Clin. Nutr.*, 2002. 76(1): p. 187-92.
[34] Willis, C.M., et al., A prospective analysis of plasma 25-hydroxyvitamin D concentrations in white and black prepubertal females in the southeastern United States. *Am. J. Clin. Nutr.,* 2007. 85(1): p. 124-30.
[35] Tangpricha, V., et al., Vitamin D insufficiency among free-living healthy young adults. *Am. J. Med.,* 2002. 112(8): p. 659-62.
[36] Gloth, F.M., 3rd, et al., Vitamin D deficiency in homebound elderly persons. *Jama*, 1995. 274(21): p. 1683-6.
[37] LeBoff, M.S., et al., Occult vitamin D deficiency in postmenopausal US women with acute hip fracture. *Jama*, 1999. 281(16): p. 1505-11.
[38] MacLaughlin, J. and M.F. Holick, Aging decreases the capacity of human skin to produce vitamin D3. *J. Clin. Invest*, 1985. 76(4): p. 1536-8.

[39] Compston, J.E., et al., Vitamin D status and bone histomorphometry in gross obesity. *Am. J. Clin. Nutr.*, 1981. 34(11): p. 2359-63.

[40] Bell, N.H., S. Shaw, and R.T. Turner, Evidence that 1,25-dihydroxyvitamin D3 inhibits the hepatic production of 25-hydroxyvitamin D in man. *J. Clin. Invest.*, 1984. 74(4): p. 1540-4.

[41] Wortsman, J., et al., Decreased bioavailability of vitamin D in obesity. *Am. J. Clin. Nutr.*, 2000. 72(3): p. 690-3.

[42] Arunabh, S., et al., Body fat content and 25-hydroxyvitamin D levels in healthy women. *J. Clin. Endocrinol. Metab.*, 2003. 88(1): p. 157-61.

[43] Snijder, M.B., et al., Adiposity in relation to vitamin D status and parathyroid hormone levels: a population-based study in older men and women. *J. Clin. Endocrinol. Metab.*, 2005. 90(7): p. 4119-23.

[44] Zemel, M.B., Regulation of adiposity and obesity risk by dietary calcium: mechanisms and implications. *J. Am. Coll. Nutr.*, 2002. 21(2): p. 146S-151S.

[45] McCarty, M.F. and C.A. Thomas, PTH excess may promote weight gain by impeding catecholamine-induced lipolysis-implications for the impact of calcium, vitamin D, and alcohol on body weight. *Med. Hypotheses.*, 2003. 61(5-6): p. 535-42.

[46] Zemel, M.B., et al., Regulation of adiposity by dietary calcium. *Faseb J.*, 2000. 14(9): p. 1132-8.

[47] Heaney, R.P., Normalizing calcium intake: projected population effects for body weight. *J. Nutr.*, 2003. 133(1): p. 268S-270S.

[48] Davies, K.M., et al., Calcium intake and body weight. *J. Clin. Endocrinol. Metab.*, 2000. 85(12): p. 4635-8.

[49] Drapeau, V., et al., Modifications in food-group consumption are related to long-term body-weight changes. *Am. J. Clin. Nutr.*, 2004. 80(1): p. 29-37.

[50] Yanoff, L.B., et al., The prevalence of hypovitaminosis D and secondary hyperparathyroidism in obese Black Americans. *Clin. Endocrinol.* (Oxf), 2006. 64(5): p. 523-9.

[51] Parikh, S.J., et al., The relationship between obesity and serum 1,25-dihydroxy vitamin D concentrations in healthy adults. *J. Clin. Endocrinol. Metab.*, 2004. 89(3): p. 1196-9.

[52] Hahn, S., et al., Low Serum 25-Hydroxyvitamin D Concentrations are Associated with Insulin Resistance and Obesity in Women with Polycystic Ovary Syndrome. *Exp. Clin. Endocrinol. Diabetes,* 2006. 114(10): p. 577-83.

[53] Ford, E.S., et al., Concentrations of serum vitamin D and the metabolic syndrome among U.S. adults. *Diabetes Care*, 2005. 28(5): p. 1228-30.

[54] Hypponen, E. and C. Power, Vitamin D status and glucose homeostasis in the 1958 British birth cohort: the role of obesity. *Diabetes Care*, 2006. 29(10): p. 2244-6.

[55] Liu, S., et al., Dietary calcium, vitamin D, and the prevalence of metabolic syndrome in middle-aged and older U.S. women. *Diabetes Care*, 2005. 28(12): p. 2926-32.

[56] Clemens, T.L., et al., Increased skin pigment reduces the capacity of skin to synthesise vitamin D3. *Lancet*, 1982. 1(8263): p. 74-6.

[57] Bell, N.H., et al., Evidence for alteration of the vitamin D-endocrine system in blacks. *J. Clin. Invest.*, 1985. 76(2): p. 470-3.

[58] Scragg, R., M. Sowers, and C. Bell, Serum 25-hydroxyvitamin D, diabetes, and ethnicity in the Third National Health and Nutrition Examination Survey. *Diabetes Care*, 2004. 27(12): p. 2813-8.
[59] Lips, P., Vitamin D status and nutrition in Europe and Asia. *J. Steroid. Biochem. Mol. Biol.,* 2007. 103(3-5): p. 620-5.
[60] Fraser, D.R., Vitamin D-deficiency in Asia. *J. Steroid. Biochem. Mol. Biol*., 2004. 89-90(1-5): p. 491-5.
[61] Nakamura, K., et al., Low serum concentrations of 25-hydroxyvitamin D in young adult Japanese women: a cross sectional study. *Nutrition,* 2001. 17(11-12): p. 921-5.
[62] Harinarayan, C.V., Prevalence of vitamin D insufficiency in postmenopausal south Indian women. *Osteoporos Int*., 2005. 16(4): p. 397-402.
[63] Sachan, A., et al., High prevalence of vitamin D deficiency among pregnant women and their newborns in northern India. *Am. J. Clin. Nutr.,* 2005. 81(5): p. 1060-4.
[64] Gannage-Yared, M.H., et al., Hypovitaminosis D in a sunny country: relation to lifestyle and bone markers. *J. Bone Miner Res*., 2000. 15(9): p. 1856-62.
[65] Alagol, F., et al., Sunlight exposure and vitamin D deficiency in Turkish women. *J. Endocrinol. Invest*, 2000. 23(3): p. 173-7.
[66] Atli, T., et al., The prevalence of Vitamin D deficiency and effects of ultraviolet light on Vitamin D levels in elderly Turkish population. *Arch. Gerontol. Geriatr*., 2005. 40(1): p. 53-60.
[67] Mishal, A.A., Effects of different dress styles on vitamin D levels in healthy young Jordanian women. *Osteoporos Int.,* 2001. 12(11): p. 931-5.
[68] Hashemipour, S., et al., *Vitamin D deficiency and causative factors in the population of Tehran.* BMC Public Health, 2004. 4: p. 38.
[69] Sedrani, S.H., A.W. Elidrissy, and K.M. El Arabi, Sunlight and vitamin D status in normal Saudi subjects. *Am. J. Clin. Nutr.,* 1983. 38(1): p. 129-32.
[70] Lips, P., Vitamin D physiology. *Prog. Biophys. Mol. Biol*., 2006. 92(1): p. 4-8.
[71] Paolisso, G. and M. Barbagallo, Hypertension, diabetes mellitus, and insulin resistance: the role of intracellular magnesium. *Am. J. Hypertens.,* 1997. 10(3): p. 346-55.
[72] Resnick, L.M., Cellular ions in hypertension, insulin resistance, obesity, and diabetes: a unifying theme. *J. Am. Soc. Nephrol.,* 1992. 3(4 Suppl): p. S78-85.
[73] Resnick, L.M., et al., Intracellular and extracellular magnesium depletion in type 2 (non-insulin-dependent) diabetes mellitus. *Diabetologia,* 1993. 36(8): p. 767-70.
[74] Ma, J., et al., Associations of serum and dietary magnesium with cardiovascular disease, hypertension, diabetes, insulin, and carotid arterial wall thickness: the ARIC study. Atherosclerosis Risk in Communities Study. *J. Clin. Epidemiol.,* 1995. 48(7): p. 927-40.
[75] Arsenian, M.A., Magnesium and cardiovascular disease. *Prog. Cardiovasc. Dis.,* 1993. 35(4): p. 271-310.
[76] Ascherio, A., et al., Intake of potassium, magnesium, calcium, and fiber and risk of stroke among US men. *Circulation,* 1998. 98(12): p. 1198-204.
[77] Mizushima, S., et al., Dietary magnesium intake and blood pressure: a qualitative overview of the observational studies. *J. Hum. Hypertens.,* 1998. 12(7): p. 447-53.

[78] Barbagallo, M. and L.J. Dominguez, Magnesium metabolism in type 2 diabetes mellitus, metabolic syndrome and insulin resistance. *Arch. Biochem. Biophys.,* 2007. 458(1): p. 40-7.

[79] Cannell, J.J., et al., Epidemic influenza and vitamin D. *Epidemiol. Infect.*, 2006. 134(6): p. 1129-40.

[80] Pike, J.W., L.L. Gooze, and M.R. Haussler, Biochemical evidence for 1,25-dihydroxyvitamin D receptor macromolecules in parathyroid, pancreatic, pituitary, and placental tissues. *Life Sci.,* 1980. 26(5): p. 407-14.

[81] Christakos, S. and A.W. Norman, Studies on the mode of action of calciferol. XXIX. Biochemical characterization of 1,25-dihydroxyvitamin D3 receptors in chick pancreas and kidney cytosol. *Endocrinology,* 1981. 108(1): p. 140-9.

[82] Arnold, B.M., et al., Radioimmunoassay studies of intestinal calcium-binding protein in the pig. II. The distribution of intestinal CaBP in pig tissues. *Can. J. Physiol. Pharmacol.,* 1975. 53(6): p. 1135-40.

[83] Christakos, S., et al., Studies on the mode of action of calciferol. XIII. Development of a radioimmunoassay for vitamin D-dependent chick intestinal calcium-binding protein and tissue distribution. *Endocrinology*, 1979. 104(5): p. 1495-503.

[84] Morrissey, R.L., et al., Calcium-binding protein: its cellular localization in jejunum, kidney and pancreas. *Proc. Soc. Exp. Biol. Med.,* 1975. 149(1): p. 56-60.

[85] Norman, A.W., et al., Vitamin D deficiency inhibits pancreatic secretion of insulin. *Science*, 1980. 209(4458): p. 823-5.

[86] Kadowaki, S. and A.W. Norman, Dietary vitamin D is essential for normal insulin secretion from the perfused rat pancreas. *J. Clin. Invest.*, 1984. 73(3): p. 759-66.

[87] Clark, S.A., W.E. Stumpf, and M. Sar, Effect of 1,25 dihydroxyvitamin D3 on insulin secretion. *Diabetes,* 1981. 30(5): p. 382-6.

[88] Cade, C. and A.W. Norman, Vitamin D3 improves impaired glucose tolerance and insulin secretion in the vitamin D-deficient rat in vivo. *Endocrinology*, 1986. 119(1): p. 84-90.

[89] Nyomba, B.L., R. Bouillon, and P. De Moor, Influence of vitamin D status on insulin secretion and glucose tolerance in the rabbit. *Endocrinology*, 1984. 115(1): p. 191-7.

[90] Chertow, B.S., et al., Cellular mechanisms of insulin release: the effects of vitamin D deficiency and repletion on rat insulin secretion. *Endocrinology*, 1983. 113(4): p. 1511-8.

[91] Huang, Y., et al., Effect of 1 alpha,25-dihydroxy vitamin D3 and vitamin E on insulin-induced glucose uptake in rat adipocytes Dominant negative protein kinase Cbeta improves 1alpha, 25-dihydroxy vitamin D3-induced insulin resistance. *Diabetes Res. Clin. Pract.*, 2002. 55(3): p. 175-83.

[92] Natsume, Y., et al., Dominant negative protein kinase Cbeta improves 1alpha, 25-dihydroxy vitamin D3-induced insulin resistance. *Endocr. Res.*, 2003. 29(4): p. 457-64.

[93] Baynes, K.C., et al., Vitamin D, glucose tolerance and insulinaemia in elderly men. *Diabetologia,* 1997. 40(3): p. 344-7.

[94] Need, A.G., et al., Relationship between fasting serum glucose, age, body mass index and serum 25 hydroxyvitamin D in postmenopausal women. *Clin. Endocrinol.* (Oxf), 2005. 62(6): p. 738-41.

[95] Scragg, R., et al., Serum 25-hydroxyvitamin D3 levels decreased in impaired glucose tolerance and diabetes mellitus. *Diabetes Res. Clin. Pract.*, 1995. 27(3): p. 181-8.

[96] Isaia, G., R. Giorgino, and S. Adami, High prevalence of hypovitaminosis D in female type 2 diabetic population. *Diabetes Care,* 2001. 24(8): p. 1496.

[97] Pittas, A.G., et al., Vitamin D and calcium intake in relation to type 2 diabetes in women. *Diabetes Care*, 2006. 29(3): p. 650-6.

[98] Gedik, O. and S. Akalin, Effects of vitamin D deficiency and repletion on insulin and glucagon secretion in man. *Diabetologia,* 1986. 29(3): p. 142-5.

[99] Boucher, B.J., et al., Glucose intolerance and impairment of insulin secretion in relation to vitamin D deficiency in east London Asians. *Diabetologia*, 1995. 38(10): p. 1239-45.

[100] Borissova, A.M., et al., The effect of vitamin D3 on insulin secretion and peripheral insulin sensitivity in type 2 diabetic patients. *Int. J. Clin. Pract.*, 2003. 57(4): p. 258-61.

[101] Pittas, A.G., et al., The Effects of Calcium and Vitamin D Supplementation on Blood Glucose and Markers of Inflammation in Non-diabetic Adults. *Diabetes Care*, 2007.

[102] Orwoll, E., M. Riddle, and M. Prince, Effects of vitamin D on insulin and glucagon secretion in non-insulin-dependent diabetes mellitus. *Am. J. Clin. N*utr., 1994. 59(5): p. 1083-7.

[103] Fliser, D., et al., No effect of calcitriol on insulin-mediated glucose uptake in healthy subjects. *Eur. J. Clin. Invest.,* 1997. 27(7): p. 629-33.

[104] Chiu, K.C., et al., Hypovitaminosis D is associated with insulin resistance and beta cell dysfunction. *Am. J. Clin. Nutr.,* 2004. 79(5): p. 820-5.

[105] Kikuchi, M., et al., Biphasic insulin release in rat islets of Langerhans and the role of Intracellular Ca++ stores. *Endocrinology*, 1979. 105(4): p. 1013-9.

[106] Beaulieu, C., et al., Calcium is essential in normalizing intolerance to glucose that accompanies vitamin D depletion in vivo. *Diabetes,* 1993. 42(1): p. 35-43.

[107] Milner, R.D. and C.N. Hales, The role of calcium and magnesium in insulin secretion from rabbit pancreas studied in vitro. *Diabetologia,* 1967. 3(1): p. 47-9.

[108] Farach-Carson, M.C., I. Sergeev, and A.W. Norman, Nongenomic actions of 1,25-dihydroxyvitamin D3 in rat osteosarcoma cells: structure-function studies using ligand analogs. *Endocrinology*, 1991. 129(4): p. 1876-84.

[109] Tornquist, K. and A.H. Tashjian, Jr., Dual actions of 1,25-dihydroxycholecalciferol on intracellular Ca2+ in GH4C1 cells: evidence for effects on voltage-operated Ca2+ channels and Na+/Ca2+ exchange. *Endocrinology*, 1989. 124(6): p. 2765-76.

[110] Civitelli, R., et al., Nongenomic activation of the calcium message system by vitamin D metabolites in osteoblast-like cells. *Endocrinology*, 1990. 127(5): p. 2253-62.

[111] de Boland, A.R. and A.W. Norman, Influx of extracellular calcium mediates 1,25-dihydroxyvitamin D3-dependent transcaltachia (the rapid stimulation of duodenal Ca2+ transport). *Endocrinology,* 1990. 127(5): p. 2475-80.

[112] Paolisso, G., et al., Dietary magnesium supplements improve B-cell response to glucose and arginine in elderly non-insulin dependent diabetic subjects Impaired insulin-induced erythrocyte magnesium accumulation is correlated to impaired insulin-mediated glucose disposal in type 2 (non-insulin-dependent) diabetic patients. *Acta Endocrinol.* (Copenh), 1989. 121(1): p. 16-20.

[113] Song, Y., et al., Dietary magnesium intake in relation to plasma insulin levels and risk of type 2 diabetes in women. *Diabetes Care*, 2004. 27(1): p. 59-65.

[114] Gueux, E. and Y. Rayssiguier, The effect of magnesium deficiency on glucose stimulated insulin secretion in rats. *Horm. Metab. Res.*, 1983. 15(12): p. 594-7.

[115] Matsunobu, S., et al., Insulin secretion and glucose uptake in hypomagnesemic sheep fed a low magnesium, high potassium diet. *J. Nutr. Biochem.*, 1990. 1(3): p. 167-71.

[116] Ishizuka, J., et al., In vitro relationship between magnesium and insulin secretion. *Magnes. Res.,* 1994. 7(1): p. 17-22.

[117] Murakami, M., et al., Role of extracellular magnesium in insulin secretion from rat insulinoma cells. *Proc. Soc. Exp. Biol. Med.,* 1992. 200(4): p. 490-4.

[118] Yajnik, C.S., et al., Fasting plasma magnesium concentrations and glucose disposal in diabetes. *Br. Med.* J. (Clin Res Ed), 1984. 288(6423): p. 1032-4.

[119] Takaya, J., H. Higashino, and Y. Kobayashi, Intracellular magnesium and insulin resistance. *Magnes. Res.*, 2004. 17(2): p. 126-36.

[120] Simpson, R.U., G.A. Thomas, and A.J. Arnold, Identification of 1,25-dihydroxyvitamin D3 receptors and activities in muscle. *J. Biol. Chem.*, 1985. 260(15): p. 8882-91.

[121] Leal, M.A., et al., The effect of 1,25-dihydroxyvitamin D3 on insulin binding, insulin receptor mRNA levels, and isotype RNA pattern in U-937 human promonocytic cells. *Exp. Cell Res.*, 1995. 217(2): p. 189-94.

[122] Maestro, B., et al., Stimulation by 1,25-dihydroxyvitamin D3 of insulin receptor expression and insulin responsiveness for glucose transport in U-937 human promonocytic cells. *Endocr. J.,* 2000. 47(4): p. 383-91.

[123] Zemel, M.B., Insulin resistance vs. hyperinsulinemia in hypertension: insulin regulation of Ca2+ transport and Ca(2+)-regulation of insulin sensitivity. *J. Nutr.*, 1995. 125(6 Suppl): p. 1738S-1743S.

[124] Draznin, B., et al., The existence of an optimal range of cytosolic free calcium for insulin-stimulated glucose transport in rat adipocytes. *J. Biol. Chem.,* 1987. 262(30): p. 14385-8.

[125] Draznin, B., et al., Possible role of cytosolic free calcium concentrations in mediating insulin resistance of obesity and hyperinsulinemia. *J. Clin. Invest.*, 1988. 82(6): p. 1848-52.

[126] Segal, S., et al., Postprandial changes in cytosolic free calcium and glucose uptake in adipocytes in obesity and non-insulin-dependent diabetes mellitus. *Horm. Res.,* 1990. 34(1): p. 39-44.

[127] Begum, N., et al., GLUT-4 phosphorylation and its intrinsic activity. Mechanism of Ca(2+)-induced inhibition of insulin-stimulated glucose transport. *J. Biol. Chem.,* 1993. 268(5): p. 3352-6.

[128] Zemel, M.B., Nutritional and endocrine modulation of intracellular calcium: implications in obesity, insulin resistance and hypertension. *Mol. Cell Biochem.,* 1998. 188(1-2): p. 129-36.

[129] Hwang, D.L., C.F. Yen, and J.L. Nadler, Insulin increases intracellular magnesium transport in human platelets. *J. Clin. Endocrinol. Metab.*, 1993. 76(3): p. 549-53.

[130] Naitoh, T., et al., Intracellular Ca2+ and Mg2+ regulation for insulin-stimulated glucose uptake into mouse diaphragm muscles. *Jpn. J. Pharmacol.,* 1991. 56(2): p. 241-4.

[131] Paxton, R. and L. Ye, Regulation of heart insulin receptor tyrosine kinase activity by magnesium and spermine. *Mol. Cell Biochem*., 2005. 277(1-2): p. 7-17.

[132] Nadler, J. and S. Scott, Evidence that pioglitazone increases intracellular free magnesium concentration in freshly isolated rat adipocytes. *Biochem. Biophys. Res. Commun.*, 1994. 202(1): p. 416-21.

[133] Suarez, A., et al., Impaired tyrosine-kinase activity of muscle insulin receptors from hypomagnesaemic rats. *Diabetologia*, 1995. 38(11): p. 1262-70.

[134] Barbagallo, M., et al., Altered ionic effects of insulin in hypertension: role of basal ion levels in determining cellular responsiveness. *J. Clin. Endocrinol. Me*tab., 1997. 82(6): p. 1761-5.

[135] Zmuda, J.M., J.A. Cauley, and R.E. Ferrell, Molecular epidemiology of vitamin D receptor gene variants. *Epidemiol. Rev*., 2000. 22(2): p. 203-17.

[136] Reis, A.F., O.M. Hauache, and G. Velho, Vitamin D endocrine system and the genetic susceptibility to diabetes, obesity and vascular disease. *A review of evidence. Diabetes Metab*., 2005. 31(4 Pt 1): p. 318-25.

[137] Skrabic, V., et al., Vitamin D receptor polymorphism and susceptibility to type 1 diabetes in the Dalmatian population. *Diabetes Res. Clin. Pract*., 2003. 59(1): p. 31-5.

[138] Turpeinen, H., et al., Vitamin D receptor polymorphisms: no association with type 1 diabetes in the Finnish population. *Eur. J. Endocrinol*., 2003. 149(6): p. 591-6.

[139] McDermott, M.F., et al., Allelic variation in the vitamin D receptor influences susceptibility to IDDM in Indian Asians. *Diabetologia,* 1997. 40(8): p. 971-5.

[140] Angel, B., et al., Vitamin D receptor polymorphism and susceptibility to type 1 diabetes in Chilean subjects: a case-parent study. *Eur. J. Epidemiol.,* 2004. 19(12): p. 1085-7.

[141] Chang, T.J., et al., Vitamin D receptor gene polymorphisms influence susceptibility to type 1 diabetes mellitus in the Taiwanese population. *Clin. Endocrinol.* (Oxf), 2000. 52(5): p. 575-80.

[142] Guo, S.W., et al., Meta-analysis of vitamin D receptor polymorphisms and type 1 diabetes: a HuGE review of genetic association studies. *Am. J. Epidemiol.,* 2006. 164(8): p. 711-24.

[143] Hitman, G.A., et al., Vitamin D receptor gene polymorphisms influence insulin secretion in Bangladeshi Asians. *Diabetes,* 1998. 47(4): p. 688-90.

[144] Oh, J.Y. and E. Barrett-Connor, Association between vitamin D receptor polymorphism and type 2 diabetes or metabolic syndrome in community-dwelling older adults: the Rancho Bernardo Study. *Metabolism,* 2002. 51(3): p. 356-9.

[145] Ye, W.Z., et al., Vitamin D receptor gene polymorphisms are associated with obesity in type 2 diabetic subjects with early age of onset. *Eur. J. Endocrinol.,* 2001. 145(2): p. 181-6.

[146] Malecki, M.T., et al., Vitamin D receptor gene polymorphisms and association with type 2 diabetes mellitus in a Polish population. *Exp. Clin. Endocrinol. Diabetes*, 2003. 111(8): p. 505-9.

[147] Ortlepp, J.R., et al., The vitamin D receptor gene variant is associated with the prevalence of type 2 diabetes mellitus and coronary artery disease. *Diabet. Med.,* 2001. 18(10): p. 842-5.
[148] Schlingmann, K.P., et al., Hypomagnesemia with secondary hypocalcemia is caused by mutations in TRPM6, a new member of the TRPM gene family. *Nat. Genet.,* 2002. 31(2): p. 166-70.
[149] Walder, R.Y., et al., Mutation of TRPM6 causes familial hypomagnesemia with secondary hypocalcemia. *Nat. Genet.,* 2002. 31(2): p. 171-4.
[150] Nadler, M.J., et al., LTRPC7 is a Mg.ATP-regulated divalent cation channel required for cell viability. From worm to man: three subfamilies of TRP channels. *Nature,* 2001. 411(6837): p. 590-5.
[151] Voets, T., et al., TRPM6 forms the Mg2+ influx channel involved in intestinal and renal Mg2+ absorption. TRP channels in disease TRPM7: channeling the future of cellular magnesium homeostasis? *J. Biol. Chem.,* 2004. 279(1): p. 19-25.
[152] Chubanov, V., et al., Disruption of TRPM6/TRPM7 complex formation by a mutation in the TRPM6 gene causes hypomagnesemia with secondary hypocalcemia. *Proc. Natl. Acad. Sci. USA,* 2004. 101(9): p. 2894-9.

In: Nutrition for the Middle Aged and Elderly
Editors: N. E. Bernhardt, A. M. Kasko, pp. 63-106
ISBN: 978-1-60456-146-3

Chapter II

A Life-Course Contribution of Nutrition to Future Cognitive Decline

Emanuele Cereda*[*1], *Alberto Battezzati*[1], *Simona Bertoli*[1], *Alexis Elias Malavazos*[1] and *Giulio Testolin*[2]
[1]International Center for the Assessment of Nutritional Status (ICANS), University of Milan, Italy
[2]Endocrinology Unit, Department of Medical and Surgical Sciences, University of Milan, IRCCS Policlinico San Donato, Milan, Italy

Abstract

Siding the strong association with cardiovascular disease (CVD), growing interest has been recently addressed to other life-course health implications of nutrition, such as that for neuro-degenerative disorders. As the ratio of people aged over 75 years is growing, and since both incidence and prevalence of dementia increase after this age, it has become relevant for health improvement to understand causes and risk factors for dementia. There is growing evidence that both nutritional status and dietary factors significantly contribute to a life-course development of dementia syndromes. With regard to nutritional status, great attention has been paid to obesity and related disorders, such as hypertension, metabolic syndrome and diabetes. Accordingly, also a predominant role of visceral adiposity has been suggested. On the other hand, a great number of studies has investigated the specific role of macronutrients, particularly dietary fats, and some micronutrients (e.g. folic acid, vitamins and various antioxidants) in both positively and negatively affecting the risk of future dementia. Thus, nutritional preventive care is claimed also with regard to diseases other than CV, although an overlapping contribution of vascular factor is recognized in the pathophisiology of cognitive decline. The present review aims to provide a panoramic view on actually existing evidences concerning the interactions between nutritional status, the obesity-related disorders and the dietary

* Corresponding author: Dr. Emanuele Cereda, International Center for the Assessment of Nutritional Status (ICANS), University of Milan, via Botticelli 21, 20133 Milan, Italy. phone: +39 02 503.16079 - Fax: +39 02 503.16077, e-mail: emanuele.cereda@virgilio.it

factors both in terms of macro and micronutrients. Evidences from clinical trial and prospective cohort studies will be favoured, although animal and in-vitro studies with possible clinical implications will be also considered.

Introduction

The term "age-related cognitive decline" was recently proposed to indicate a deterioration of cognitive functioning due to normal physiological aging processes or to pre-dementia stage, but within normal limits given the person's age [1,2]. Accordingly, it is still difficult to establish whether dementia represents a distinct clinical entity or it is the expression of normal ageing [3]. Recent longitudinal studies, using more sophisticated and detailed diagnostic instruments for the assessment of cognitive functions, suggested that it is possible to distinguish different degrees of functioning impairment [4,5]. Thus, understanding the timing and how risk and protective factors act throughout life is relevant. In fact, animal studies have shown that atherosclerotic degeneration can appear early in youth and are associated with fat intake, as well as Alzheimer's disease (AD) lesions can develop as early as during the third decade but before the development of pre-clinical and clinical dementia symptoms [6]. Along with this, the classification of clinical dementia subtypes is still debated in terms of the underlying pathologies [Table 1] and no precise boundaries can be defined to distinguish AD from the other forms of dementias. A definitive diagnosis of AD can be made only post mortem, when demonstration of pathological signs (deposits of extracellular amyloid-beta peptide in diffuse plaques and in plaques containing elements of degenerating neurons, known as neuritic plaques; intracellular deposits of abnormally hyperphosphorylated tau protein, a microtubule assembly protein, in the form of neurofibrillary tangles) is provided [7], while a diagnosis of probable or possible AD by clinical criteria is made only in absence or in presence of other contributing disorders respectively [8]. It is in this scenario that potential interactions between AD and different disorders as well as the existence of overlapping syndromes have also considered [9].

Thus, it seems more appropriate to define dementia as a clinical state of severe cognitive impairment that likely reflects the summed effects of multiple pathological processes associated with advanced aging.

With the growth in the elderly population, it is expected that the incidence of dementia will increase 400% in the next 20 years and that prevalence will reach epidemic-like diffusion [10-12].

Unfortunately, treatment options are still limited. Therefore, the prevention of dementia syndromes through identification and management of modifiable risk factors is of public health importance [Figure 1].

A progressively larger number of prospective evaluations is becoming available and different insights on a life-course approach to the aetiology of late-onset dementias have been provided. Though, a widely acceptable causal model is difficult to design. Moreover, existing literature is far from being free of controversial results and conflicting reports. Genetic and environmental factors strongly interact with ageing and variously contribute to dementia syndromes. Thus, associations between cognitive development, education, socio-economic status, occupation, lifetime nutrition (nutritional status and diet) and other lifestyles (e.g. physical activity) and adult disease (e.g. diabetes, insulin resistance, hypertension) cannot be considered independently [13-26].

Table 1. Etiologic classification of dementia syndromes

Primary

- Alzheimer's disease
- Pick's disease

Secondary

- Vascular dementia (diffuse small-vessel disease, multi infarct dementia)
- Degenerative (Parkinson's disease, Huntington's disease, Wilson's disease, cortico-basal degeneration, progressive myoclonic epilepsy)
- Endocrine and metabolic
- Nutritional (alcoholic, Wernicke-Korsakoff's syndrome, vitamin deficiency – B12, folate, thiamine, niacin)
- Toxic (anoxia, carbon monoxide or heavy metal poisoning)
- Neoplastic (primary cerebral tumours)
- 'Normal Pressure' hydrocephalus
- Traumatic (chronic subdural haematoma, post-head injury, hypoxia, punch-drunk syndrome)
- Infective (HIV, Syphilis, prion diseases, chronic meningitis, post-encephalitic, multiple sclerosis)
- Others (minor and overlapping syndromes)

Among this plethora of protective/risk factors, diet, in terms of the adequacy of both energy and specific nutrients, together with nutritional status, above all in term of weight accumulation (body mass index), are possibly the best studied environmental influences on brain development and ageing [19,27-29]. For decades, the role of these factors has engaged scientific and lay interest. The hope is that by identifying healthy lifestyles and consuming set of nutrients, we can promote longevity and prevent diseases. Both positive and negative longitudinal links have been described and different plausible biological mechanisms have been proposed. Some may actually be antagonistic and the real effects are difficult to detect, particularly because too many years are required to evaluate a nutrition model. In addition, the existing studies have more frequently investigated the role of single nutrients rather than of a dietary pattern. Thus, much more needs to be done to generalise the present findings, according to the etherogeneity of population studied, duration of observational period and inclusion of covariates. The aim of this review is to summarise present knowledge concerning the effects of nutritional status, obesity-related disorders and dietary factors on the aging and maintenance of the brain, as well as their implication in pathophysiologic pathways of cognitive decline.

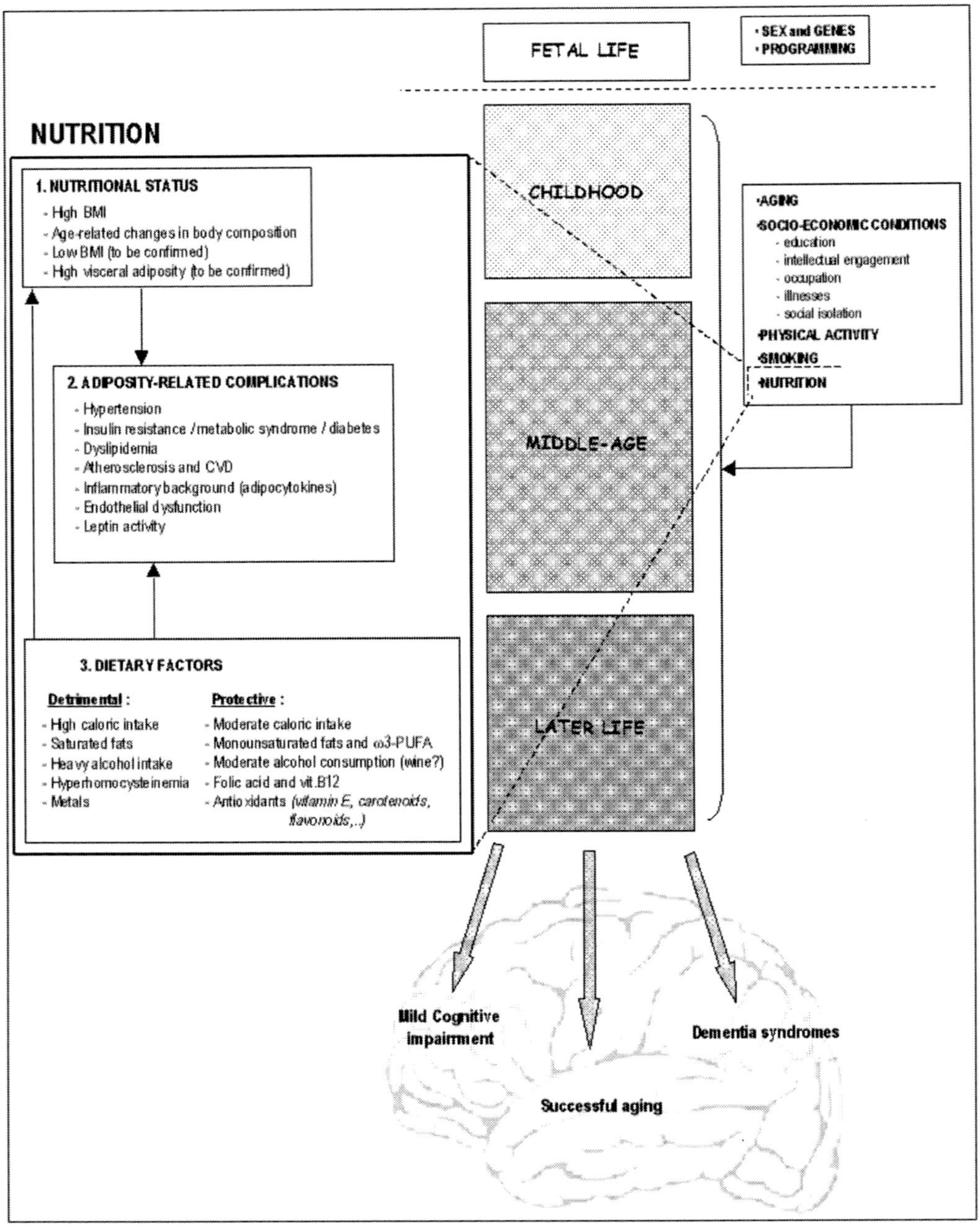

Figure 1. Life-course model of cognitive development and decline with aging.

Nutritional Status and Cognitive Decline

Estimating mortality, morbidity attributable to nutritional status in the population raises complex methodological issues. On the other hand, as the prevalence of malnutrition and obesity continues to increase among older adults, the search of a causal link and the debate about the potential hazards have received growing attention [30, 31].

Malnutrition is a widespread problem in elderly persons and poor nutrition is associated with more doctors' visits, more hospitalizations, more health costs and reduced survival rates [32, 33]. However, the impact of poor nutritional status on functional and cognitive declines is not well known in elderly people, but suggestion for risk increasing have been presented [34, 35].

Alarmingly, obesity affects about 30% of adults in industrialised countries and among those aged over 65 years, the number of overweight and obese adults has been increasing from 39 and 16.6%, respectively, in 1998, to 40.3 and 22%, respectively, in 2006 [36]. Siding this, the risk of death from all and individual (cardiovascular disease, cancer, or other diseases) causes increases throughout the range of moderate and severe overweight for both sexes and in all age groups [30,31] and there is a prevailing assumption that obesity is an independent risk factor for age-related cognitive decline [37].

Body Mass Index (BMI)

The most common and simple measure of nutritional status used in population-based and clinical studies is BMI, which is calculated as weight (kg)/height (m^2). The BMI has been found by the National Research Council's Committee on Diet and Health and the NSI as a useful descriptor of body weight accumulation (over- and underweight) [38] and is considered to be interpretable in terms of body composition according its capacity to predict total adipose tissue with an error of 10% or less when compared with imaging techniques [39].

In the last decades, particular attention has been focused on the existence of a longitudinal link between middle-age adiposity and the decline of cognitive function [29,34,35,37,40-43]. However, the relationship between dementia and later-life obesity is less clear, as in some cases an association with normal-/under-weight has been reported [35,44]. With this regard, we remind that BMI is not a perfect measure of adiposity and is affected by factors such as ethnicity and age. Particularly, among older individuals, BMI may underestimate adiposity because lean body mass is replaced by fat on aging [45]. The aging process also causes a pseudo-increase in BMI due to a shortened stature secondary to compression of the intravertebral disks, osteoporosis, and other pathologies. Moreover, among some individuals, weight loss may be a potential pre-clinical marker for dementia, above for AD and particularly when measured 6–10 years before a clinical diagnosis [35,46,47]. In fact, the neurodegeneration of hypothalamus accompanying AD may be responsible of disruptions in energy metabolism homoeostasis which is regulated through the control of hunger and satiety, the regulation of energy expenditure, and the release of hormones that increase use of energy stores [48].

According to this background of considerations, it reasonable to argue that the association of BMI to dementia may be more accurately assessed at midlife than in the older years. Although there is considerable evidence that middle-age weight excess should be considered an independent risk factor for late-onset cognitive decline [29,34,35,37,40-43,49], recent analyses suggest that the relationship is not a simple one and most likely a J-shaped curve where also a low BMI may represent a risk factor [34,35,49]. As suggested above, this association may be sometimes the result of weight loss [35, 46, 47] and, although no certain cause has been already demonstrated, weight loss preceding hyperinsulinemia has been singled out as a possible contributor [50,51].

In fact, increased insulin, along with insulin resistance, has been included among those modifiable factors through which overall adiposity may directly affect cognitive functions [52-55]. Moreover, a link with the pathogenesis of neurodegenerative disorders such as AD and Parkinson's disease has been demonstrated [56, 57]. This implies that excess insulin could be directly toxic to the brain, rather than just increasing cardiovascular risk. Along with this, a very recent study has demonstrated that reduced insulin signaling in aging brains of overweight and insulin resistant mices is able to promote healthy metabolism and to extend life span [58].

Obesity is nowadays stigmatised as a disease whose adverse effects lie in its enlarged fat cells and their secreted products, including neurochemical mediators (e.g. leptin), procoaugulant proteins, inflammatory peptides, and cytokines [59-61].

Nowadays, it is well accepted that the fundamental cause of progressive overweight is a chronic imbalance between energy intake and energy expenditure in whose regulation leptin, an adipocyte-produced hormone directly related to body fat, represents the coupling factor [62]. Accordingly, obesity has been also proposed as a "chronic, relapsing neurochemical disease", with adipose tissue talking to the brain [63]. With this regard, it has been demonstrated that this peptide is involved not only in hypothalamic integration of energy homeostasis, but also in the modulation of memory performance and neuron's activity in the hippocampus [64-67]. Thus, the disruption of the meurochemical pathways occurring along with weight excess could probably lead also to functional modifications of cognitive processes.

Similarly to cardiovascular disease, also an inflammatory atherosclerotic model has been proposed to explain the higher cognitive impairment of those elders with higher serum levels of inflammatory markers, such as C-reactive protein (CRP), interleukin-6 (IL-6), and tumor necrosis factor-alpha (TNF-α) [68-71], and pro-thrombotic proteins affecting platelet aggregation and endothelial function, such as fibrinogen and intercellular adhesion molecule 1 [72,73]. In fact, adipose tissue is properly considered a dynamic endocrine organ that secretes in the blood stream a number of factors that are increasingly recognized to contribute to vascular systemic inflammation as well as to chronic degenerative diseases [59, 74-78].

Cardiovascular Disease (CVD) and Obesity-Related Disorders

Hippocrates wrote "Corpulence is not only a disease itself, but the harbinger of others", recognising that obesity is a medical disorder that also leads to many comorbidities.

According to the inflammatory atherosclerotic model, longitudinal analyses have demonstrated that vascular disease may significantly contribute to accelerated cognitive decline. Probably, this may pass through multiple asymptomatic brain injuries related to peripheral vascular disease [79-82].

Coronary heart disease, stroke as well as peripheral vascular disease are different expressions of the same pathology [83, 84], whose link with obesity has been timely underscored [85]. In fact, according to adipose tissue-related metabolic dysregulations, obese patients frequently presents a cohort of vascular risk factors: dyslipidemia, insulin resistance (from normal blood glucose to diabetes) and hypertension [85,86].

With regard to the role of blood lipids, we report that studies have supported the hypothesis that apolipoprotein E (APOE), upon the APOE genotype (subtype epsilon-4), imparts risk for both an atherogenic lipid profile and dementia syndromes [87-90]. Furthermore, longitudinal studies have suggested that high serum total and LDL cholesterol at midlife could be considered independent risk factors too [42,90-95].

On the contrary, no meaningful association has been found for HDL [88,95], with the exception of when inserted in the context of a favourable lipid profile secondary to a longevity genotype of cholesterol ester transfer protein (lower levels of CETP, higher HDL levels, and larger lipoprotein particles) [96].

Along with this, treatment by lipid lowering drugs seem to positively affect both risk and progression [93-95].

Dyslipidemia is frequently secondary to concomitant insulin resistance and diabetes [85,86,97,98], conditions that have been included among the cohort of pathophysiologic contributors [71,99-101] due to direct insulin action on brain, detrimental effects of protracted impaired glucose, accelerated atherosclerosis and associated cerebral infarctions [52-54,102-104]. Thus, considering that poor metabolic control is a deranging factor for tissue/organ damage in diabetics, a tighter glycemic control and careful follow-up of treatment would profit to both vascular disease progression and cognitive decline prevention [105-107].

Another factor that should be cited in discussion is blood pressure. Hypertension (systolic blood pressure ≥140 mmHg, diastolic blood pressure of 90 mm Hg or more at rest) is a risk factor for stroke, ischemic white-matter lesions, cardiovascular disorders, and vascular dementia because also of its frequent clustering with other vascular risk factors Hypertension may also lead to vessel wall changes in the brain, leading to hypoperfusion, ischemia and hypoxia which may initiate the pathological process of AD. Up today, the association between blood pressure and dementia is still debated [108,109]. Findings from longitudinal studies suggest an association between high blood pressure and dementia [42,110,111], probably due to artery stiffness and severe atherosclerosis. In turn the use of antihypertensives (particularly ACE inhibitors with or without diuretics) from double-blind placebo-controlled trials has suggested to reduce incidence of dementia, but mainly that stroke-related [109,112,113].

However, other studies have described an inverse association [114,115], perhaps related to poor cerebral perfusion. Accordingly, higher blood pressure levels are probably required to maintain an adequate cerebral perfusion and treatment of hypertension contraindicated.

Suggested Role of Visceral Adiposity

According to different theories and hypothesis that have been put forward to explain the association between obesity, CVD and dementia syndromes, a central pathophysiologic role has been addressed to adipose tissue nature [29,43]. In fact, it is now well accepted that adipose tissue act as an endocrine organ rather than only as a fat-storage depot [116,117]. However, the metabolic and inflammatory dysregulatory proprieties depend on body-fat compartment localization and, with this regard, the detrimental profile of visceral fat has been emphasized [59,97,117,118]. Along with this, recent reports progressively support that visceral adipose tissue (VAT) is more likely implicated in cognitive decline than overall weight excess, as depicted by BMI [35,44,70,71,100,111,119-122]. Accordingly, pathophysiologic theories (atherosclerotic, inflammatory and neurochemical) and related determinants (insulin resistance, dyslipidemia, hypertension, leptin, homocysteine, cytokines) have shown stronger association with trunkal obesity [59, 78, 87, 116, 117, 123-127].

We have previously described the involvement of leptin on cognition [64-67]. Free leptin increases with BMI, but for individuals with the same BMI, the leptin circulating levels can vary by 1 order of magnitude, suggesting that leptin is regulated by factors other than the size of the adipose tissue depot, such as nutritional and hormonal factors related also to visceral adiposity [117]. Leptin mRNA expression is greater in subcutaneous than in omental adipocytes and increases with the dimension of adipocytes [128]. On the other hand, aging is accompanied by a change in both body composition and fat distribution [129,130], thus explaining a progressive reduction of leptin activity.

Raised triglycerides concentration, low HDL cholesterol, high levels of small dense LDL particles, raised blood pressure, insulin resistance (with or without impaired/elevated fasting glucose), pro-thrombotic state are key elements of the metabolic syndrome, whose anatomic precondition is intra-abdominal fat deposition [97,117,118,123,131]. VAT has been singled out as the most important predictor of arterial hypertension, independently from age, gender and race [132-134] and a synergistic influence cognitive function has been nighlighted [135]. Moreover, adding information about abdominal disposal of adipose tissue gives stronger prediction also of glucose control impairment [136,137]. With this regard, there is also some support for increased inflammation [138-140], which in turn have shown to be independently associated with both visceral adiposity and systemic complications [75,77,78,97,116,118,128,141,142].

Another possible factor recently invoked is homocysteine (Hcy). With interest in VAT implications, we report significant associations between Hcy and both waist-hip ratio [143] and quantitative measurements of this compartment (by computed tomography), but not with subcutaneous adipose tissue, thus suggesting the latter as an important determinant of Hcy circulating levels [144].

Finally, we remind that all the above indicated factors significantly contribute to the development of a vascular burden whose role in cognitive decline has been considered and linking to visceral adiposity supported [123-127].

Thus, there is convincing evidence for VAT's contribution but recent results need to be replicated and supported further [35, 44, 119, 121, 122]. Unfortunately, imaging techniques are unlikely to be applicable on a routine basis, but anthropometric surrogates would be helpful in spite of their incapacity in discriminating VAT from subcutaneous fat [118]. Moreover, BMI has been widely used as nutritional status indicator for many decades. It will take a long time before appropriate data will be available.

Diet and Cognitive Decline

In the 1950s and 60s Ancel Keys for the first time indicated that people living in the Greek island of Crete was very healthy. Particularly, the finding that coronary heart disease mortality is lower in the countries bordering the Mediterranean Sea than in Northern Europe appeared to be largely due to a safe and protective dietary profile which is mainly based on cereals, legumes, vegetables, fresh and dried fruit, fish and more rarely meat, olive oil, and wine consumed only with meals [146]. Since then, this pattern has come to be termed 'Mediterranean diet'. However, at the beginning, attention has more frequently been focused on single food category or nutrient just to find the strongest associations with survival and diseases and to define links of causality. Unfortunately, to define causality, replication of findings, specificity of the association, temporal and dose-response relations, and biological plausibility are required [147]. Thus, despite the still important role in nutritional epidemiology for the study of individual nutrients and foods, and the extensive observational evidence that individual nutrients might be associated with disease risk, large randomised controlled trials have not been very successful in showing the hypothesized effects of single nutrients [148,149]. Then, interest has concentrated on dietary patterns, because they can accommodate the complex interplay of nutrients within a diet [150]. Moreover, an approach based on cluster analysis allow to place individuals from different countries into similar pattern risk groups, finally providing higher substantiality to evidences provided [150-152]. If this progress has been successfully obtained in epidemiological investigation addressing CV disease and related mortality, the role of dietary habits in cognitive decline, however, has not been extensively investigated. Up today, most of prospective studies have been conducted with interest on individual dietary components nutrients or at least food categories (e.g. fruit, vegetables, fish) [153-155]. In addition, other caveats of the evidence relating diet to cognitive decline have been pointed out: 1) error in estimation due to error in the measurement of nutrient; 2) reduced length of latency period of dementia when recruiting people age over 65 years; 3) possibility that dietary pattern reported may reflect the consequence of a pre-clinical cognitive decline; 4) the fact that the participants, not the investigators, choose their exposures which can results in uncontrolled confounding [21,156,157].

It is only recent the attempt of research into diet and dementia to deal with whole foods and dietary pattern [158,159]. Preliminary investigations appear promising in opening new insights. Once again Mediterranean diet has captured the attention and studies conclude that higher adherence is associated with risk reduction [158,159]. Probably, this is the result of favorable effects on lipoprotein levels, endothelium dysfunction, insulin resistance, metabolic syndrome, antioxidant capacity, inflammatory molecules and widely cardiovascular disease [160-163]. However, further experimental research is needed to evaluate the underlying mechanisms.

Caloric Intake and Nutritional Status

Caloric intake is an important confounder usually considered in nutritional epidemiology [164]. Alternatively, it has been also studied as independent factor [165-167]. One of the possible mechanism through which Mediterranean diet positively acts in risk reduction is probably due to its association with caloric intake [159,160]. Prospective studies have raised the possibility that higher consumption of calories in middle age may accelerate the decline in cognitive function seen with aging, as apparently occurs in some animals [160,165-167]. Alternatively, there is evidence supporting a potential neuroprotective role of caloric restriction in the brain [168], probably mediated by a lower oxidative damage of reactive oxygen species produced during respiration [168-171]. Moreover, reduced caloric intake is associated with decreased neuronal death, increased expression of neurotrophic factors in the brain and higher capacity for plasticity and repair in neurodegenerative disorders [171,172]. Along with these molecular considerations, we also remind the importance of feeding in negatively affecting overall adiposity. Although physical activity and both environmental and genetic factors undoubtedly all contribute to the development of obesity, there is in fact evidence that quality of diet, in both terms of calorie intake (over-nutrition) and dietary factors (e.g. sweets, snacks, condiments, entrées, and carbohydrates coupled with a low variety of vegetable, promote long-term increases in body fatness [173-175]. Particularly, recent reports have suggested that a low glycemic index (how much a food raises blood glucose levels when compared to a solution of glucose or to white bread) diet may have a role in the management of obesity through its ability to increase the satiety value of food and modulate appetite, thus reducing caloric intake and achieving long-term weight control [176,177]. In addition, also body fat distribution (gynoid vs abdominal), a better predictor of obesity-related metabolic and CV complications, has been demonstrated to mirror time trends in reported food consumption [174].

However, preliminary reports do not support an association between glycemic load and AD's risk and the popular practice of low carbohydrate diets for the prevention of AD in the elderly [179].

Specific Implications of Macronutrients (Dietary Fats)

Although the implication total calorie intake in affecting oxidative stress has been reported [168-170], there is also evidence that the balance of nutrients, particularly high intake of fats, may also play an independent role [180]. The relationship between macronutrient intake and cognitive decline is not well understood. Very few data are available and, when looking to those existing, we must also consider the possibility of unmeasured confounders.

According to the consistent association with risk of CVD, including stroke and coronary heart disease [181-184], only the effect of dietary fats has drawn significant interest. It is in this sense believed that low intake of hydrogenated and saturated fats, low intake of cholesterol, intake of non-hydrogenated unsaturated fats (monounsaturated fatty acids – MUFA), and high intake of n-3 polyunsaturated fatty acids (PUFA), such as eicosapentaenoic and docosahexaenoic acids (EPA and DHA) and α-linolenic acid (α-LA), can positively affect the risk through vascular mechanisms.

Recent reports from prospective analyses have shown that the risk of global cognitive decline is increased by greater energy intakes from both saturated and trans-hydrogenated fats [185-187], while MUFA (the principal source of fat in Mediterranean diet) are significantly associated with a better cognitive performance [188]. In addition, also PUFA may exert a protective role, particularly those belonging to n-3 family (EPA, DHA, α-LA) which are mainly related to fish consumption [183,186,189-191]. However, studies addressing dietary intakes and plasma levels (good reflection of long-term dietary intakes) of n-6 PUFA have shown discordant associations, with studies describing a protective role of moderate-to-high intake or concentrations and other finding an inverse association [185,186,191,192]. This was probably related to the fact among the n-6 PUFA family we can find components, the arachidonic and the linoleic acid, with opposite properties and health implications (eicosanoid biosynthesis). Thus, as shown by data analyses from the cohort of EVA and ARIC studies, arachidonic acid and LA should be probably considered separately [191,192]. Therefore, as suggested in the prevention of CVD (optimal value <5:1) [193,194], also the ratio of dietary n-3/n-6 PUFA intake may influence the potential role of PUFA [191,192].

Along with the contribution of fats to overall oxidative stress [180], other mechanisms have been also proposed. We have previously underscored that hypercholesterolemia (total cholesterol and LDL) in middle age appears associated with cognitive decline [42,90-95]. Moreover, in animal model a high intake of cholesterol brings to enhanced neuronal damage [195]. Along with these, a genetic predisposition (APOE genotype) to an unfavourable response to intakes of fats [196] represents an independent risk factor [87-90].

In man, dietary pattern analyses have shown that a Western diet (characterized by high intakes of processed meats, eggs, red meats, and high-fat dairy products) is more likely to be associated with CV risk factors (total, HDL and LDL cholesterol) and both markers of inflammation and endothelial dysfunction [197,198]. Consumption of dietary hydrogenated and saturated fatty acids is associated with an increase in small, dense LDL, and an adverse lipoprotein profile [199-201], but also with insulin resistance [202] which in turn may be related to dementia [52-57].

On the contrary, dietary n-3 PUFA are linked with a lower inflammatory background, greater insulin sensitivity, hypocoagulability , and with a better lipid profile [202-204], even in presence of an adverse genetic predisposition (APOE) [205]. Similarly to n-3 PUFA, also intake of MUFA is associated with favourable alterations of insulin sensitivity, coagulation and lipoproteins, particularly of LDL particles size [206,207]. In addition, both MUFA and PUFA could be related to the integrity and the fluidity of neuronal membranes, thus affecting cell longevity and neuronal transmission [208,209].

Finally, we remind that the percentage of energy from dietary fat has received particular attention also for its possible consequences on overweight and obesity [202,210,211]. However, an expert panel recently concluded that dietary fat may not be the sole dietary determinant of body fatness it has widely been assumed to be [212].

Alcohol Consumption

Apart from the existence of a true alcoholic dementia, several prospective studies have explored the relation between alcoholic drinks and cognitive decline and, although different methodological approaches have been used, there is general agreement in addressing a risk lowering effect to moderate consumption [213-219].

Alcohol may have paradoxical and competing effects in the brain. On the one hand it acts as a neurotoxin, mainly through an oxidative mechanism, but the type of damage induced (e.g. neuronal mitochondrial dysfunction end degeneration) will depend on the amount and developmental timing of exposure, along with other genetic factors [220,221].

On the other hand, siding the inverse association with risk of coronary heart disease [222], it seems able to lower the risk of cerebrovascular disease. In fact, imaging studies in human have shown that, in spite of being related to greater brain atrophy, moderate alcohol consumption (1 to 5 drinks/day or 7 to 15 drinks/week) is also associated with fewer silent brain infarcts, less white-matter disease, and a lower risk of clinical stroke. However, heavy drinkers (>5 drinks/day or >15 drinks/week) present both higher brain damage and stroke risk [223-226].

Although the mechanisms relating alcohol and cognitive decline still remain unknown, some hypotheses have suggested potential benefit deriving from lower vascular damage (atherosclerotic model) and the non-alcohol effects of wine [227-229].

Alcohol intake is strongly positively associated with large and medium-sized HDL particles, which have been included among cardioprotective factors. In addition, U-shaped associations with both dimension and number of LDL particles have been observed, with light consumers (<7 drinks/week) having the highest number of large particles and moderate consumers (7-13 drinks/week) showing the lowest number of small LDL. Furthermore, a favourable influence on endothelial function, platelet adhesiveness, and haemostatic/fibrinolytic cascade have been considered [227-230].

Some investigators have also claimed the additional benefits of wine [213-216], the significant factor explaining the French paradox (low incidence of ischemic heart disease in France despite the traditionally high intake of saturated fat) [228]. Wine may contain considerable amounts of antioxidants (polyphenols) not present in beer and spirits, which may have a protective effect on the progression of dementia [228,230].

Accordingly, while some prospective studies have shown that moderate consumers (1 to 3 servings/day or ethanol: 15-30 g/day), irrespective of type of alcoholic beverage, present a lower risk [217-219], others, in which type of alcohol source was investigated, have underscored the additional potentialities of wine consumption [213-216]. Most of these studies produced data suggesting that heavy alcohol intake (≥4 servings/day or ethanol >35 g/day) was related to a high risk of dementia, but frequently the results were not statistically significant given the small number of elderly people who reported heavy intakes.

In addition, the coexistence of an APOE genotype seems to modify the relationship by progressively increasing risk along with midlife alcohol consumption. Finally, also in abstainers (up to 1 serving/day or ethanol <12 g/day) the risk appears to be slightly increased, thus suggesting that limited intake might benefit, but not indicating that people should start drinking or increase wine consumption to avoid dementia. In fact, there are no available randomised trials of the effects of alcoholic drinks on these outcomes and no recommendations can be made. Nowadays, only moderation is suggested (less than three servings of wine a day).

The epidemiological studies of vascular disease consistently reveal associations with alcohol consumption, sometimes positive and sometimes negative, but the assessment of quantity, frequency, and duration of alcohol intake is commonly limited. Future studies would benefit from more thorough assessment of alcohol use, including a lifetime consumption history.

Specific Implications of Micronutrients

The metabolic effects of micronutrients have been widely investigated in the last century. Particularly, deficiency states, such that of iodine for goitre and cretinism, have clearly underscored their essentiality for growth and function. In this context, some minerals and vitamins were found to affect brain function and there is general believe and somewhat evidence that appropriate intakes of certain micronutrients may be beneficial in reducing the risk of cognitive decline. In addition, studies have in some cases suggested (epidemiology) and in other demonstrated (basic science) a pathogenic involvement. Though, several mechanisms seem to interact. Moreover, micronutrients should be considered in the wider context of a balanced diet, situation that makes even more difficult the evaluation of a life long-lasting exposition. Several steps must be done towards explanation, but there is a strong suggestion that preventive effects against pathogenesis of CVD are likely to be effective also against neuro-degenerative diseases [231,232].

Vitamins B6, B9 (folic acid), B12 and homocysteine - Homocysteine (Hcy) is a risk factor for a variety of conditions that afflict the elderly, both in the cardiovascular and nervous systems and the skill of Hcy to induce cell death in its own right is well established [233]. Hcy is a non-essential sulfur-containing amino acid that is derived from methionine metabolism and its catabolism is related to folate, vitamin B12, and vitamin B6. The intracellular levels of Hcy are highly regulated and any increased production is met by export from cells. Consequently, plasma concentrations of Hcy reflect intracellular concentrations of Hcy and homeostasis of the enzymes involved in methionine metabolism to ensure a supply of methyl groups for essential reactions in all cells. Hcy transport in the brain has not been wholly investigated and various recent findings suggests that its can be shifted from the plasma into the brain and vice versa probably via specific, bi-directional cellular transporters in addition to simple diffusion mechanism [234]. Morever, human neuronal cells are able to produce Hcy under normal conditions [235]. In the brain, Hcy is remethylated to form methionine accepting a methyl group from methyl-tetrahydrofolate, with vitamin B12 involved as a cofactor, whereas vitamin B6 is necessary for the conversion of Hcy to cysteine [236]. Particularly, the latter reaction is fundamental because numerous methylation reactions take place in the brain including synthesis and degradation of neurotransmitters, membrane phospholipids and controlled DNA-methylation [237]. Moreover, the Hcy trans-sulfuration pathway is the major source of glutathione, an important cytosolic antioxidant agent [235,236].

The neurotoxic actions of homocysteine has been considered in several in vivo and in vitro models of neuronal loss which have evidenced that animals exposed to Hcy suffer from restricted growth, neural or cognitive dysfunction [235,238,239] and impaired brain energy metabolism [240]. The available data suggest numerous possible mechanisms whereby Hcy damages and kills neurons. In particular, Hcy induces DNA breakage by a mechanism that may involve impaired transmethylation of DNA and increased oxidative stress [235,241,242] Moreover, Hcy may affect oxidative stress by other mechanisms including the modulation of the activity of endothelial nitric oxide synthase and cytoplasmic calcium influx [242], which in turn can cause metabolic aberrations and modulate gene transcription with subsequent cell death [243].

Hcy plasma concentration increases with age and numerous studies in recent years have investigated its role in aging brain damage not only as neurotoxin but also as a risk factor for vascular disease [79-82]. Particularly, high serum Hcy levels and low intake of folate are related to an increased risk of stroke [244-247], and prospective studies suggest that a 25% reduction of Hcy achieved with folate supplementation is associated with about a 20% lower risk of stroke [247]. Along with this, hyperHcy has shown a significant association with volumetric changes in white matter of patients with small vessels disease as well as with brain atrophy on MRI of non-demented elderly [248,249].

Epidemiological and longitudinal studies have suggested a causal link between high plasma Hcy and both the incidence of dementia and the worsening in some measures of cognitive function [250-256]. However, when addressing to Hcy metabolism and the implication of B vitamins and folate status, there are conflicting data on the association with dementia and cognition [252-260], although some studies have shown that folate, vitamin B12, and/or B6 deficiencies are frequent in demented elderly persons [261].

Other studies have also considered a different approach to the relationship between B vitamins and future cognitive decline by investigating eventual associations with oral intake of these compounds. Unfortunately, data are still inconsistent and preliminary reports suggest a protective action only for high folate intake [262-264]. On the other hand, we might presume that the positive association between Mediterranean dietary pattern and successful brain aging is partly related to the increased intake of B vitamins by fruits and vegetables consumption [153,155,158-160].

Although, in vitro and in vivo studies strongly suggested a causal role for Hcy and B vitamins status in the neurological diseases, clinical studies are not convincing. All these findings take together suggest that the relation between Hcy and aging brain damage is a promising field of research for the prevention of the age-related neurodegenerative diseases, but the causal role of Hcy would be probably cleared only by vitamin supplementation studies.

Vitamins/antioxidants and oxidative stress - Oxidative stress may be related in several ways to dementia. Firstly, it increases with ageing, which is itself a risk factor for dementia. Secondly, it is related to vascular disease leading to stroke, another important risk factor for dementia. Even more interestingly, the pathogenic lesions of AD, i.e. the amyloid beta peptide deposition in neuritic plaques, is associated to oxidative stress [265,266].

Oxidative stress and inflammation are secondary events to amyloid deposition causing the reduction in iron and copper concentrations in brain tissue, leading to the formation of hydrogen peroxide [267]. That, conversely, inflammation and oxidative stress can initiate the neuronal damage leading to amyloid deposition is theoretically possible but currently not demonstrated. In any case, the modulation of oxidative stress by local antioxidant systems in the brain should affect the development of the AD lesions.

Therefore, the dietary intakes of vitamin C, carotenes, vitamin E and non vitamin dietary antioxidants (flavonoids) have been studied for their ability to prevent or slow down the progression of AD, or for their ability to affect cognition [21].

Several [268,269] but not all studies [270] found that peripheral concentrations of antioxidants are reduced in people with mild cognitive impairment or AD. Specifically, elderly who ingest vitamin C seem to be more protected by cognitive impairment [271,272], but an effect of circulating vitamin C on intelligence quotient has already been found in adolescents [273].

Vitamin E shows an antioxidant and antiinflammatory effect in vitro by reducing lipid peroxidation promoted by amyloid deposition [274]. Furthermore, in transgenic animal models of AD, vitamin E supplementation reduces the rate of amyloid deposition [275].

The risk of dementia is higher in the subjects with the lowest vitamin E concentrations [276] and vitamin E is among the vitamin supplements whose use is claimed to reduce the risk of Alzheimer disease [277], although several studies suggested that dietary vitamin E and not vitamin E supplements can reduce the risk of AD [278,279]. This discrepancy raises the problem of the heterogeneity of vitamin E, that is found in 4 different tocopherol forms (alpha, beta, gamma and delta) and corresponding tocotrienols in the diet, whereas supplements contain alpha-tocopherol only. Corn and soybean oil are major dietary sources of gamma-tocopherol, that shows greater anti-inflammatory [280-282] and antioxidant [281] power than the alpha form. When vitamin E dietary intakes were broken down in the various tocopherol forms, a slower rate of cognitive decline was associated with intakes of alpha-tocopherol equivalents, and alpha- and gamma-tocopherols [283].

It is worth appreciating how these observations underscore major problems inherent to the evaluation of single micronutrient intakes in observational studies.

Beyond the protective effects of vitamin C and tocopherols intakes, evidence that an high intake of carotene or flavonoids, is associated to a lower than expected risk of AD among smokers has been provided by the Rotterdam study [279]. One prospective study found a reduced risk of dementia associated to an higher intake of flavonoids [284], possibly contributing to the protective effect of wine consumption discussed above [285].

Suggested role of metals - The hypothetical involvement of some heavy metals, both physiological (Iron, Copper, Zinc), and toxic (Aluminium, Manganese), in the etio-pathogenesis of cognitive decline, particularly AD, has been suggested decades ago and interest has grown stronger in recent years with the advent of modern cellular and molecular techniques and their expanding use in neuroscience. Although neuronal function can be assessed experimentally, in-use experimental procedures (chemical, cellular, physiological, hystochemical and epidemiological) clearly present advantages and disadvantages [286]. In addition, it should be underscored that by now different dementia syndromes have been identified. However, only AD, the major cause of cognitive decline, has been widely investigated.

The possible involvement of aluminium (Al) in AD was first suggested in experimental animal studies of neurofibrillary degeneration [287,288]. Though, animal species (e.g. transgenic mice versus rabbit) present different degree of sensitivity to Al neurotoxicity, thus yielding to contradictory results [287]. On the other hand, its role has been further accredited by studies showing the accumulation of aluminium in neurofibrillary tanglebearing neurons from AD brains [289]. Along with this, dietary Al has been well demonstrated to modulate *in-vivo* neuronal degeneration by oxidative and inflammatory pathways, while treatment with Al chelating agents abrogates the intraneuronal protein accumulations following the administration of Al [287,290,291].

So far, the most of human epidemiological studies on Al intake have focused on exposure through drinking water, as it is present naturally and is widely used in water treatment to reduce the number of small particles and improve the colour, and only a few have investigated intake through foods. Though, results are still inconsistent. Moreover, studies are more or less open to critique, but the positive relationship cannot be totally dismissed [292].

Other metals have been also linked to brain functioning and AD. Of particular interest is the role of Iron (Fe), Copper (Cu) and Zinc (Zn). Similarly to Al, there is evidence indicating that Zn, Cu and Fe are significantly elevated in the AD brain [293], and drugs with metal chelating properties could produce a protective action against neuronal degeneration [288, 294].

Although in-vitro studies have suggested dual effects of Zn on toxicity, this metal is more likely to be protective against cognitive decline. In fact, Zn is necessary to maintain the integrity of all biological membranes and DNA-handling system. Moreover, it seems to inhibit neurotoxicity by displacing Cu and Fe-mediated cell-free peroxide production. On the other hand, zinc is fairly redox inert and should be considered as indirect antioxidant [295]. With regard to diet study, sub-optimal zinc nutriture may lead to increase transfer of aluminium and other toxins to the brain [296]. Finally, it has been recently suggested that a n-3 PUFA enriched diet may improve brain Zn metabolism by increasing a specific transporter expression in neurons [297].

As Al, Cu enhances neurofibrillary degeneration (by metal-protein associations leading to pathogenetic protein aggregation and by metal-catalysed protein oxidation resulting in protein damage), thus supporting a role for copper homeostasis [288,293]. In addition, Cu has been shown to interact adversely through an oxidative mechanism by the production of hydrogen peroxide [295]. In patients affected by Wilson's disease (genetic disorder characterized by Cu accumulation due to incapacity in eliminating excess of intake), neurologic disorders are very common [297]. Several case-control studies have reported that patients with AD present high serum Cu levels when compared with patients with vascular dementia or mild cognitive impairment or normal cognitive function [298,299]. In addition, a very recent prospective study have shown a marginally statistically significant association between Cu intake and cognitive change only in subjects whose diet was rich in saturated fats [187].

Like Cu, also Fe has been implicated in the pathogenesis of dementia via the similar mechanisms [288-290,292,293,296]. In addition, Fe deficiency due to altered homeostasis have been associated with changes in the synthesis of heme, thus affecting brain cells functioning and damage through mitochondrial dysfunction, reduced nitric oxide synthase activity, modifications in zinc homeostasis [300, 301].

Finally, although selenium (Se) is an important key trace element for antioxidant enzymes, there is little information addressing its protective role [187,302]. Of more interest is probably the interaction between Se and mercury (Hg), as they share the same cellular transport mechanisms [187]. Thus, low dietary Se levels may expose to higher Hg loads, but epidemiologic studies fails to confirm an association with cognitive functions [303].

In conclusion, basic-science studies have shown that metal ions such as Al, Zn, Cu and Fe play a role in neurons degeneration. Moreover, a possible application for drugs with metal chelating properties is consistent with its beneficial effects in modulating neurodegeneration [304]. However, with regard to Zn, it remains debatable whether its supplementation is beneficial.

All these considerations support a possible implication for low-dose chronic exposure. Though, different epidemiological studies fail in confirming this, while others suggest that metals are more likely to act as cofactors rather than independent factors [187,231,297]. In fact, when addressing to possible oxidative action of metals it should be considered that many free radical scavengers are present in food, particularly in fresh fruit and vegetable (eg, as carotenoids and flavonoids). Vegetables also contain variable amounts of chelating molecules (e.g. phytic acid), which can inhibit trace elements and mineral absorption and bio-availability, particularly of Fe, Zn, calcium and manganese but not Cu [305]. In addition, metals and micronutrients frequently shares common mechanisms of transport and absorption, thus resulting in absorption and availability modulation.

Supplements and Cognitive Decline

Giving a close look at the existing cross-sectional and longitudinal studies, we can find several suggestions that diet or nutrient supplements could delay or reduce cognitive decline in later life. Though, the evidence [306-337] is still inconsistent and large randomised-controlled trial are required to have the hypothesized effects of single nutrients confirmed. By contrast, most of preliminary intervention studies (randomised-controlled trial) with supplements provide no evidence for a beneficial effect, while only a few found a significant benefit [306,312,318-321].

Different trials have investigated the benefit of folic acid supplementation, alone [306-313] or in combination with other nutrients [314-317], but only two found an improvement on cognitive functions, respectively in a selected adult population with raised homocysteine levels (>13 μmol/L) [306] and in a group of community dwelling elderly with a high prevalence of hyperhomocysteinemia [312].

However, little attention has been paid to the possible protective role of n-3 long-chain PUFA. Up today only four trials have been performed, two addressing the progression of disease in patients with mild to moderate AD undergoing EPA and DHA supplementation [318,322], and three investigating the efficacy of ethyl-EPA in Huntington's disease (HD) [319-321]. Positive outcome on both motor and neuropsychological functions in HD and AD progression have been univocally reported but further studies are clearly warranted. With this regard, a large population study (Older People And n-3 Long-chain polyunsaturated fatty acids - OPAL - study) on cognitively-normal elderly has been recently designed [322] and results will be available in the next years.

A possible role of vitamin E has been also pointed out [323-328]. Unfortunately, among the completed trials only one showed that high dose vitamin E in mild to moderate AD patients is associated with a slower progression of disease, while others, including one on similar series [324], did not provide any overall benefit [323,325-328]. With interest in the physiopatholgic oxidative pathway, others antioxidants, such as those derived from *Ginkgo biloba* and *Theobroma cacao*, have been considered [329-334] but results with potential clinical significance and of sufficient magnitude to be recognized by the caregivers were reported only in few cases [330,331]. Also short-term supplementation by soy-derived antioxidant fractions (isoflavones) provided similar results, with some trials describing potential gains [335,336] and not supporting the hypothesized effect [337,338].

Only three studies have considered the possible role of a multivitamin and multimineral fortification of diet but the reported results do not provide enthusiasm [314-317]. However, greater attention and expectations should be addressed to the results from Project FACT, in which the efficacy of supplements treatment will be tested when coupled to the effect of a walking program. In fact, this is the first study that more likely aims to reproduce a suggested life-course approach to cognitive functions and to investigate the role of lifestyles on the rate of cognitive decline [315].

Finally, in some cases the effect on cognitive functioning of a whole diet formula has been also tested, but the absence of improvements could be generally explained by the short intervention time and by the severe baseline mental impairment of the patients recruited [339-341].

Although we did not perform an extensive and systematic literature review, a critical evaluation of the above indicated trials offers the possibility to focus on several discrepancies in study designs that could be taken into account when planning future interventions.

Most of the trials reviewed clearly address an important limitation in the populations recruited, ranging from patient with normal cognitive function to those with severe disease. Moreover, those reporting positive effects have generally included subjects at risk of nutritional deficiencies, or with nutritional risk (e.g. hyperhocysteinemia) or with overt dementia (e.g. mild to severe AD). Age was frequently over 65 years, fact that obviously puts in doubt the preventive role of supplements against a life-course deterioration of cognitive functions. With this regard, also the extremely variable duration of trials, varying from few months to 3-years, must be considered when critically evaluating the overall benefits of treatments.

Another weakness of these experimental studies addresses the cognitive function tests used. In most of cases only some cognitive domains have been investigated (e.g. attention, concentration, memory, executive function) by targeted battery of neuropsychological testes and only in a few the variation associated with the individual tests was decreased by clustering raw test scores for several tests in compound performance measures.

Finally, the trials here analysed have dealt with the effects of variable dosages of a specific nutrient, which is very far from the possibility to identify a protective dietary pattern. Only recent studies have considered the potentialities of a multiple supplementation and an integrated approach with a physical activity or a nutritional education program [315,342], but restricted data are available. However, results of the Mediterranean diet in cardiovascular disease secondary prevention, in spite of disclosing the underlying mechanisms, emphasize the need to undertake additional research also in the areas of primary prevention of both cardiovascular disease and cognitive impairment [343]. Unfortunately, changing a group of persons to a particular dietary profile or lifestyle is hard to achieve and particularly difficult to maintain for a long time. In addition, there is also some support for the effectiveness and durability of a concomitant cognitive training intervention in improving targeted cognitive abilities [344,345].

In conclusion, current results provide no evidence for a beneficial effect of daily supplements, which are likely to act as cofactors. Moreover, systematic use with preventive meaning seems highly unlikely to be considered cost effective [346]. However, the possibility of beneficial effects in already cognitively-compromised older people and those at greater risk of nutritional deficiency deserves further attention, at least in slowing the rate of decline.

Conclusion

Substantial progress has been made in the understanding of the neurobiology of cognitive decline, but comprehensive causal models are not available. On the basis of reviewed findings, reasons exist to believe that both nutritional status and diet significantly contribute to its occurrence and prevention. However, it is unlikely to consider a single nutrient, or a food group or dietary pattern is the only responsible. Nutrition should be included in a multi-factorial physiopathologic model and its individual role is still difficult to quantify. Only a lifetime pattern of risk factors acting together with a genetic vulnerability might help to explain cognitive decline.

Recommendation on caloric moderation, adherence to a healthy eating behaviour and weight loss should be made in case of comorbidities (e.g. hypertension, diabetes, CVD) but randomised trials are needed to obtain specific suggestion to change macronutrients and micronutrients intakes [21].

In addition, aggressive pharmacological treatment of vascular risk factors such as diabetes, hypercholestrolemia, hypertension could also convey to a better health in later life [9]. A potential therapeutic role on systemic complications might be also addressed to inflammatory background unlocking [347,348]. Finally, a possible reversibility of cognitive deterioration cannot be excluded at all but further data are needed before substantial evolution of knowledge will be provided.

References

[1] American Psychiatric Association, Committee on Nomenclature and Statistics. *Diagnostic and Statistical Manual of Mental Disorders, Fourth Edition, Text Revision (DSM-IV-TR)*. Washington, DC: American Psychiatric Association, 2000.

[2] Levy R. Aging-associated cognitive decline. Working Party of the International Psychogeriatric Association in collaboration with the World Health Organization. *International Psychogeriatrics* 1994;6:63–68.

[3] Brayne, C; Calloway, P. Normal ageing, impaired cognitive function and senile dementia of Alzheimer type: a continuum? *Lancet* 1988;1:1265–1267.

[4] O'Connor, DW; Pollitt, PA; Hyde, JB; Fellows, JL; Miller, ND; Brook, CP; Reiss, BB; Roth, M. The prevalence of dementia as measured by the Cambridge Mental Disorders of the Elderly Examination. *Acta Psychiatrica Scandinavica* 1989;79:190-198.

[5] Hendrie, HC; Hall, KS; Brittain, HM; Austrom, MG; Farlow, M; Parker, J; Kane, M. The CAMDEX: a standardized instrument for the diagnosis of mental disorder in the elderly: a replication with a US sample. *Journal of the American Geriatrics Society* 1988;36:402-408.

[6] Finch CE. Developmental origins of aging in brain and blood vessels: an overview. *Neurobiology of Aging* 2005;26:281–291.

[7] Dickson, TC; Vickers, JC. The morphological phenotype of beta-amyloid plaques and associated neuritic changes in Alzheimer's disease. *Neuroscience* 2001;105: 99–107.

[8] McKhann, G; Drachman, D; Folstein, M; Katzman, R; Price, D; Stadlan, EM. Clinical diagnosis of Alzheimer's disease: report of the NINCDS-ADRDA Work Group under the auspices of Department of Health and Human Services Task Force on Alzheimer's Disease. *Neurology* 1984;34: 939–44.

[9] Decarli, C. Vascular factors in dementia: an overview. *Journal of the Neurological Sciences* 2004;226:19-23.

[10] Borjesson-Hanson, A; Edin, E; Gislason, T; Skoog, I. The prevalence of dementia in 95 year olds. *Neurology* 2004;63:2436–2438.

[11] Ravaglia, G; Forti, P; Maioli, F; Martelli, M; Servadei, L; Brunetti, N; Dal monte, E; Bianchin, M; Mariani, E. Incidence and etiology of dementia in a large elderly Italian population. *Neurology* 2005;64:1525-1530.

[12] Brookmeyer, R, Gray, S. Methods for projecting the incidence and prevalence of chronic diseases in aging populations: application to Alzheimer's disease. *Statistics in Medicine* 2000;19:1481-1493.

[13] Whalley, LJ; Dick, FD; McNeill, G. A life-course approach to the aetiology of late-onset dementias. *Lancet Neurology* 2006;5:87–96.

[14] Lynch, JW; Kaplan, GA; Shema, SJ. Cumulative impact of sustained economic hardship on physical, cognitive, psychological, and social functioning. *New England Journal of Medicine* 1997;337:1889-1895.

[15] Turrell, G; Lynch, JW; Kaplan, GA, Everson SA, Helkala EL, Kauhanen J, Salonen JT. Socioeconomic position across the lifecourse and cognitive function in late middle age. *The Journal of Gerontology Series B: Psychological Sciences and Social Sciences* 2002;57:S43-51.

[16] Bennett, DA; Wilson, RS; Schneider, JA; Evans, DA; Mendes de Leon, CF; Arnold, SE; Barnes, LL; Bienias, JL. Education modifies the relation of AD pathology to level of cognitive function in older persons. *Neurology* 2003;60:1909–1915.

[17] Staff, RT; Murray, AD; Deary, IJ; Whalley, LJ. What provides cerebral reserve? *Brain* 2004;127:1191–1199.

[18] Neuropathology Group. Medical Research Council Cognitive Function and Aging Study. Pathological correlates of late-onset dementia in a multicentre, community-based population in England and Wales. Neuropathology Group of the Medical Research Council Cognitive Function and Ageing Study (MRC CFAS). *Lancet* 2001; 357:169–75.

[19] Marmot, MG; Shipley, MJ. Do socioeconomic differences in mortality persist after retirement? 25 year follow up of civil servants from the first Whitehall study. *British Medical Journal* 1996;313:1177–1180.

[20] Sturman, MT; Morris, MC; Mendes de Leon, CF; Bienias, JL; Wilson, RS; Evans, DA. Physical activity, cognitive activity, and cognitive decline in a biracial community population. *Archives of Neurology* 2005;62:1750-1754.

[21] Luchsinger, JA; Mayeux, R. Dietary factors and Alzheimer's disease. *Lancet Neurology* 2004;3:579-587.

[22] Qiu, C; Winblad, B; Fratiglioni, L. The age-dependent relation of blood pressure to cognitive function and dementia. *Lancet Neurology* 2005;4:487-499.

[23] Arvanitakis, Z; Wilson, RS; Bennett, DA. Diabetes mellitus, dementia, and cognitive function in older persons. *Journal of Nutrition, Health and Aging* 2006;10:287-291.

[24] Messier, C. Impact of impaired glucose tolerance and type 2 diabetes on cognitive aging. *Neurobiology of Aging* 2005;26 Suppl 1:26-30.

[25] Hofman, A; Ott, A; Breteler, MM; Bots, ML; Slooter, AJ; van Harskamp, F; van Duijn, CN; Van Broeckhoven, C; Grobbee, DE. Atherosclerosis, apolipoprotein E, and prevalence of dementia and Alzheimer's disease in the Rotterdam Study. *Lancet* 1997;349:151-154.

[26] Kivipelto, M; Helkala, EL; Hanninen, T; Laakso, MP; Hallikainen, M; Alhainen, K; Soininen, H; Tuomilehto, J; Nissinen, A. Midlife vascular risk factors and late-life mild cognitive impairment: A population-based study. *Neurology* 2001;56:1683–1689.

[27] Bourre, JM. Effects of nutrients (in food) on the structure and function of the nervous system: update on dietary requirements for brain. Part 1: micronutrients. *Journal of Nutrition, Health and Aging* 2006;10:377-385.

[28] Bourre, JM. Effects of nutrients (in food) on the structure and function of the nervous system: update on dietary requirements for brain. Part 2 : macronutrients. *Journal of Nutrition, Health and Aging* 2006;10:386-399.

[29] Gustafson, D. Adiposity indices and dementia. *Lancet Neurology* 2006;5:713-720.

[30] Calle, EE; Thun, MJ; Petrelli, JM; Rodriguez, C; Heath, CW Jr. Body-mass index and mortality in a prospective cohort of U.S. adults. *New England Journal of Medicine* 1999;341:1097-1105.

[31] Flegal, KM; Graubard, BI; Williamson, DF; Gail, MH. Excess deaths associated with underweight, overweight, and obesity. *Journal of the American Medical Association* 2005;293:1861-1867.

[32] Volkert, D; Berner, YN; Berry, E; Cederholm, T; Coti Bertrand, P; Milne, A; Palmblad, J; Schneider, S; Sobotka, L; Stanga, Z; DGEM (German Society for Nutritional Medicine); Lenzen-Grossimlinghaus R, Krys U, Pirlich M, Herbst B, Schutz T, Schroer W, Weinrebe W, Ockenga J, Lochs H; ESPEN (European Society for Parenteral and

Enteral Nutrition). ESPEN Guidelines on Enteral Nutrition: Geriatrics. *Clinical Nutrition* 2006;25:330-360.

[33] Elia, M; Zellipour, L; Stratton, RJ. To screen or not to screen for adult malnutrition? *Clinical Nutrition* 2005;24:867-884.

[34] Whitmer, RA; Gunderson, EP; Barrett-Connor, E; Quesenberry, CP Jr; Yaffe, K. Obesity in middle age and future risk of dementia: a 27 year longitudinal population based study. *British Medical Journal* 2005;330:1360.

[35] Luchsinger, JA; Patel, B; Tang, MX; Schupf, N; Mayeux, R. Measures of adiposity and dementia risk in elderly persons. *Archives of Neurology* 2007;64:392-398.

[36] Centers for Disease Control CDC's Behavioral Risk Factor Surveillance System (BRFSS).; Accessed May 12, 2007 from *http://apps.nccd.cdc.gov/**

[37] Gorospe, EC; Dave, JK. The risk of dementia with increased body mass index: a systematic review. *Age Ageing* 2007;36:23-29.

[38] Committee on Diet and Health, Food and Nutrition Board, Commission on Life Sciences, National Research Council Diet and Health. *Implications for reducing chronic disease risk.* Washington DC: National Academy Press, 1989.

[39] Sjostrom, L. A CT-based multi-compartment body composition technique and anthropometric predictions of lean body mass, total and subcutaneous adipose tissue. *International Journal of Obesity* 1991;15:19.

[40] Gustafson, D; Rothenberg, E; Blennow, K; Steen, B; Skoog I. An 18-year follow-up of overweight and risk of Alzheimer disease. *Archives of Internal Medicine* 2003;163:1524–1528.

[41] Gustafson, D; Lissner, L; Bengtsson, C; Bjorkelund, C; Skoog, I. A 24-year follow-up of body mass index and cerebral atrophy. *Neurology* 2004;63:1876–1881.

[42] Kivipelto, M; Ngandu, T; Fratiglioni, L; Viitanen, M; Kareholt, I; Winblad, B; Helkala, EL; Tuomilehto, J; Soininen, H; Nissinen, A. Obesity and vascular risk factors at midlife and the risk of dementia and Alzheimer disease. *Archives of Neurology* 2005;62:1556-1560.

[43] Cournot, M; Marquie, JC; Ansiau, D; Martinaud, C; Fonds, H; Ferrieres, J; Ruidavets, JB. Relation between body mass index and cognitive function in healthy middle-aged men and women. *Neurology* 2006;67:1208-1214.

[44] Razay, G; Vreugdenhil, A; Wilcock, G. Obesity, abdominal obesity and Alzheimer disease. *Dementia and Geriatric Cognitive Disorders* 2006;22:173-176.

[45] Baumgartner, RN; Heymsfield, SB; Roche, AF. Human body composition and the epidemiology of chronic disease. *Obesity Research* 1995;3:73–95.

[46] Barrett-Connor, E ; Edelstein, SL ; Corey-Bloom, J ; Wiederholt, WC. Weight loss precedes dementia in community-dwelling older adults. *Journal of the American Geriatrics Society* 1996;44:1147–1152.

[47] Stewart, R; Masaki, K; Xue, QL; Peila, R; Petrovitch, H; White, LR; Launer, LJ. A 32-year prospective study of change in body weight and incident dementia: the Honolulu-Asia Aging Study. *Archives of Neurology* 2005;62:55–60.

[48] Schwartz, MW; Woods, SC; Porte, D; Seeley, RJ; Baskin, DG. Central nervous system control of food intake. *Nature* 2000; 404:661–671.

[49] Rosengren, A; Skoog, I; Gustafson, D; Wilhelmsen, L. Body mass index, other cardiovascular risk factors, and hospitalization for dementia. *Archives of Internal Medicine* 2005;165:321-326.

[50] Wedick, NM; Mayer-Davis, EJ; Wingard, DL; Addy, CL; Barrett-Connor, E. Insulin resistance precedes weight loss in adults without diabetes: the Rancho Bernardo Study. *American Journal of Epidemiology* 2001;153:1199-1205.

[51] Young, SE; Mainous, AG 3rd; Carnemolla, M. Hyperinsulinemia and cognitive decline in a middle-aged cohort. *Diabetes Care* 2006;29:2688-2693.

[52] Gerozissis, K. Brain insulin: regulation, mechanisms of action and functions. *Cellular and Molecular Neurobiology* 2003;23:1–25.

[53] Freychet, P. Insulin receptors and insulin actions in the nervous system. *Diabetes/Metabolism Research and Reviews* 2000;16:390–392.

[54] Kern, W; Born, J; Schreiber, H; Fehm, HL. Central nervous system effects of intranasally administered insulin during euglycemia in men. *Diabetes* 1999;48:557-563.

[55] Stolk, RP; Breteler, MM; Ott, A; Pols, HA; Lamberts, SW; Grobbee, DE; Hofman, A. Insulin and cognitive function in an elderly population. The Rotterdam Study. *Diabetes Care* 1997;20:792-795.

[56] Frolich, L; Blum-Degen, D; Bernstein, HG; Engelsberger, S; Humrich, J; Laufer, S; Muschner, D; Thalheimer, A; Turk, A; Hoyer, S; Zochling, R; Boissl. KW; Jellinger, K; Riederer, P. Brain insulin and insulin receptors in aging and sporadic Alzheimer's disease. *Journal of Neural Transmisson* 1998;105:423-438.

[57] Takahashi, M; Yamada, T; Tooyama, I; Moroo, I; Kimura, H; Yamamoto, T; Okada, H. Insulin receptor mRNA in the substantia nigra in Parkinson's disease. *Neuroscience Letters* 1996;204:201-204.

[58] Taguchi, A; Wartschow, LM; White, MF. Brain IRS2 signaling coordinates life span and nutrient homeostasis. *Science* 2007; 317:369-372.

[59] Tilg, H; Moschen, AR. Adipocytokines: mediators linking adipose tissue, inflammation and immunity. *Nature Reviews Immunology* 2006;6:772-783.

[60] Hauner, H. Secretory factors from human adipose tissue and their functional role. *Proceedings of Nutrition Society* 2005;64:163-169.

[61] Trayhurn, P; Beattie, JH. Physiological role of adipose tissue: white adipose tissue as an endocrine and secretory organ. *Proceedings of Nutrition Society* 2001;60:329-339.

[62] Zhang, Y; Proenca, R; Maffei, M; Barone, M; Leopold, L; Friedman, JM. Positional cloning of the mouse obese gene and its human homologue. *Nature* 1994;372:425-432.

[63] Bray, GA. Obesity is a chronic, relapsing neurochemical disease. *International Journal of Obesity* 2004;28:34-38.

[64] Ueno, N; Dube, MG; Inui, A; Kalra, PS; Kalra, SP. Leptin modulates orexigenic effects of ghrelin and attenuates adiponectin and insulin levels and selectively the dark-phase feeding as revealed by central leptin gene therapy. *Endocrinology* 2004;145:4176-4184.

[65] Funahashi, H; Yada, T; Suzuki, R; Shioda S. Distribution, function, and properties of leptin receptors in the brain. *International Review of Cytology* 2003;224:1-27.

[66] Harvey, J. Novel actions of leptin in the hippocampus. *Annals of Medicine* 2003;35:197-206.

[67] Boghossian, S; Ueno, N; Dube, MG; Kalra, P; Kalra, S. Leptin gene transfer in the hypothalamus enhances longevity in adult monogenic mutant mice in the absence of circulating leptin. *Neurobiology of Aging* 2007; doi:10.1016/j.neurobiolaging.2006.08.010 – In Press.

[68] Engelhart, MJ; Geerlings, MI; Meijer, J; Kiliaan, A; Ruitenberg, A; van Swieten, JC; Stijnen, T; Hofman, A; Witteman, JC; Breteler, MM. Inflammatory proteins in plasma and the risk of dementia: the Rotterdam study. *Archives of Neurology* 2004;61:668-672.

[69] van Dijk, EJ; Prins, ND; Vermeer, SE; Vrooman, HA; Hofman, A; Koudstaal, PJ; Breteler, MM. C-reactive protein and cerebral small-vessel disease: the Rotterdam Scan Study. *Circulation* 2005;112:900-905.

[70] Yaffe, K; Lindquist, K; Penninx, BW; Simonsick, EM; Pahor, M; Kritchevsky, S; Launer, L; Kuller, L; Rubin, S; Harris, T. Inflammatory markers and cognition in well-functioning African-American and white elders. *Neurology* 2003;61:76-80.

[71] Yaffe, K; Kanaya, A; Lindquist, K; Simonsick, EM; Harris, T; Shorr, RI; Tylavsky, FA; Newman, AB. The metabolic syndrome, inflammation, and risk of cognitive decline. *Journal of the American Medical Association* 2004;292:2237-2242.

[72] Rafnsson, SB; Deary, IJ; Smith, FB; Whiteman, MC; Rumley, A; Lowe, GD; Fowkes, FG. Cognitive decline and markers of inflammation and hemostasis: the Edinburgh artery study. *Journal of the American Geriatrics Society* 2007;55:700-707.

[73] van Oijen, M; Witteman, JC; Hofman, A; Koudstaal, PJ; Breteler, MM. Fibrinogen is associated with an increased risk of Alzheimer disease and vascular dementia. *Stroke* 2005;36:2637-2641.

[74] Hotamisligil, GS. Inflammation and metabolic disorders. *Nature* 2006;444:860-867.

[75] Malavazos, AE; Corsi, MM; Ermetici, F; Coman, C; Sardanelli, F; Rossi, A; Morricone, L; Ambrosi, B. Proinflammatory cytokines and cardiac abnormalities in uncomplicated obesity: relationship with abdominal fat deposition. *Nutrition Metabolism and Cardiovascular Diseases* 2007;17:294-302.

[76] Cereda, E; Malavazos, AE. A possible role of visceral fat-related inflammation in linking obstructive sleep apnea to left ventricular hypertrophy. *Hypertension* 2007;49:e23.

[77] Malavazos, AE; Cereda, E; Morricone, L; Coman, C; Corsi, MM; Ambrosi, B. Monocyte chemoattractant protein 1: a possible link between visceral adipose tissue-associated inflammation and subclinical echocardiographic abnormalities in uncomplicated obesity. *European Journal of Endocrinology* 2005;153:871-877.

[78] Malavazos, AE; Cereda, E; Morricone, L; Corsi, MM; Ambrosi, B. Monocyte chemoattractant protein-1 in adipose tissue. *Journal of Clinical Endocrinology and Metabolism* 2005;90:3128.

[79] Vermeer, SE; Prins, ND; den Heijer, T; Hofman, A; Koudstaal, PJ; Breteler, MM. Silent brain infarcts and the risk of dementia and cognitive decline. *New England Journal of Medicine* 2003;348:1215-1222.

[80] Prins, ND; van Dijk, EJ; den Heijer, T; Vermeer, SE; Koudstaal, PJ; Oudkerk, M; Hofman, A; Breteler, MM. Cerebral white matter lesions and the risk of dementia. *Archives of Neurology* 2004;61:1531-1534.

[81] Kovari, E; Gold, G; Herrmann, FR; Canuto, A; Hof, PR; Bouras, C; Giannakopoulos, P. Cortical microinfarcts and demyelination affect cognition in cases at high risk for dementia. *Neurology* 2007;68:927-931.

[82] Liem, MK; van der Grond, J; Haan, J; van den Boom, R; Ferrari, MD; Knaap, YM; Breuning, MH; van Buchem, MA; Middelkoop, HA; Lesnik Oberstein, SA. Lacunar infarcts are the main correlate with cognitive dysfunction in CADASIL. *Stroke* 2007;38:923-928.

[83] Atherosclerotic disease of the aortic arch as a risk factor for recurrent ischemic stroke. The French Study of Aortic Plaques in Stroke Group. *New England Journal of Medicine* 1996;334:1216-1221.

[84] Iribarren, C; Sidney, S; Sternfeld, B; Browner, WS. Calcification of the aortic arch: risk factors and association with coronary heart disease, stroke, and peripheral vascular disease. *Journal of the American Medical Association* 2000;283:2810-2815.

[85] Musaad, S; Haynes, EN. Biomarkers of Obesity and Subsequent Cardiovascular Events. *Epidemiologic Reviews* 2007; doi:10.1093/epirev/mxm005 - In Press.

[86] Schneider, HJ; Glaesmer, H; Klotsche, J; Bohler, S; Lehnert, H; Zeiher, AM; Marz, W; Pittrow, D; Stalla, GK; Wittchen, HU; DETECT Study Group. Accuracy of anthropometric indicators of obesity to predict cardiovascular risk. *Journal of Clinical Endocrinology and Metabolism* 2007;92:589-594.

[87] Davidson, Y; Gibbons, L; Purandare, N; Byrne, J; Hardicre, J; Wren, J; Payton, A; Pendleton, N; Horan, M; Burns, A; Mann, DM. Apolipoprotein E epsilon4 allele frequency in vascular dementia. *Dementia and Geriatric Cognitive Disorders* 2006;22:15-19.

[88] Li, G; Shofer, JB; Kukull, WA; Peskind, ER; Tsuang, DW; Breitner, JC; McCormick, W; Bowen, JD; Teri, L; Schellenberg, GD; Larson, EB. Serum cholesterol and risk of Alzheimer disease: a community-based cohort study. *Neurology* 2005;65 1045-1050.

[89] Kukull, WA; Higdon, R; Bowen, JD; McCormick, WC; Teri, L; Schellenberg, GD; van Belle, G; Jolley, L; Larson, EB. Dementia and Alzheimer disease incidence: a prospective cohort study. *Archives of Neurology* 2002;59:1737-1746.

[90] Hall, K; Murrell, J; Ogunniyi, A; Deeg, M; Baiyewu, O; Gao, S; Gureje, O; Dickens, J; Evans, R; Smith-Gamble, V; Unverzagt, FW; Shen, J; Hendrie, H. Cholesterol, APOE genotype, and Alzheimer disease: an epidemiologic study of Nigerian Yoruba. *Neurology* 2006;66:223-227.

[91] Kivipelto, M; Helkala, EL; Laakso, MP; Hanninen, T; Hallikainen, M; Alhainen, K; Soininen, H; Tuomilehto, J; Nissinen, A. Midlife vascular risk factors and Alzheimer's disease in later life: longitudinal, population based study. *British Medical Journal* 2001;322:1447-1451.

[92] Moroney, JT; Tang, MX; Berglund, L; Small, S; Merchant, C; Bell, K; Stern, Y; Mayeux, R. Low-density lipoprotein cholesterol and the risk of dementia with stroke. *Journal of the American Medical Association* 1999;282:254-260.

[93] Bernick, C; Katz, R; Smith, NL; Rapp, S; Bhadelia, R; Carlson, M; Kuller, L; Cardiovascular Health Study Collaborative Research Group. Statins and cognitive function in the elderly: the Cardiovascular Health Study. *Neurology* 2005;65:1388-1394.

[94] Sparks, DL; Sabbagh, MN; Connor, DJ; Lopez, J; Launer, LJ; Browne, P; Wasser, D; Johnson-Traver, S; Lochhead, J; Ziolwolski, C. Atorvastatin for the treatment of mild to moderate Alzheimer disease: preliminary results. *Archives of Neurology* 2005;62:753-757.

[95] Miida, T; Takahashi, A; Ikeuchi, T. Prevention of stroke and dementia by statin therapy: experimental and clinical evidence of their pleiotropic effects. *Pharmacology and Therapeutics* 2007;113:378-393.

[96] Barzilai, N; Atzmon, G; Derby, CA; Bauman, JM; Lipton, RB. A genotype of exceptional longevity is associated with preservation of cognitive function. *Neurology* 2006;67:2170-2175.

[97] Despres, JP; Lemieux, I. Abdominal obesity and metabolic syndrome. *Nature* 2006;444:881-887.

[98] Chahil, TJ; Ginsberg, HN. Diabetic dyslipidemia. *Endocrinology and Metabolism Clinics of North America* 2006;35:491-510, VII-VIII.

[99] Young, SE; Mainous, AG 3rd; Carnemolla M. Hyperinsulinemia and cognitive decline in a middle-aged cohort. *Diabetes Care* 2006;29:2688-2693.

[100] Elias, MF; Elias, PK; Sullivan, LM; Wolf, PA; D'Agostino, RB. Obesity, diabetes and cognitive deficit: the Framingham Heart Study. *Neurobiology of Aging* 2005;26 (Suppl 1):11-16.

[101] Xiong, GL; Plassman, BL; Helms, MJ; Steffens, DC. Vascular risk factors and cognitive decline among elderly male twins. *Neurology* 2006;67:1586-1591.

[102] 102 Messier, C; Awad, N; Gagnon, M. The relationships between atherosclerosis, heart disease, type 2 diabetes and dementia. *Neurological Research* 2004;26:567-572.

[103] Knopman, DS; Mosley, TH; Catellier, DJ; Sharrett, AR; Atherosclerosis Risk in Communities (ARIC) Study. Cardiovascular risk factors and cerebral atrophy in a middle-aged cohort. *Neurology* 2005;65:876-881.

[104] Mosley, TH Jr; Knopman, DS; Catellier, DJ; Bryan, N; Hutchinson, RG; Grothues, CA; Folsom, AR; Cooper, LS; Burke, GL, Liao, D; Szklo, M. Cerebral MRI findings and cognitive functioning: the Atherosclerosis Risk in Communities study. *Neurology* 2005;64:2056-2062.

[105] Epidemiology of Diabetes Interventions and Complications (EDIC). Design, implementation, and preliminary results of a long-term follow-up of the Diabetes Control and Complications Trial cohort. *Diabetes Care* 1999;22:99-111.

[106] Abbatecola, AM; Rizzo, MR; Barbieri, M; Grella, R; Arciello, A; Laieta, MT; Acampora, R; Passariello, N; Cacciapuoti, F; Paolisso, G. Postprandial plasma glucose excursions and cognitive functioning in aged type 2 diabetics. *Neurology* 2006;67:235-240.

[107] Diabetes Control and Complications Trial/Epidemiology of Diabetes Interventions and Complications Study Research Group; Jacobso,n AM; Musen, G; Ryan, CM; Silvers, N; Cleary, P; Waberski, B; Burwood, A; Weinger, K; Bayless, M; Dahms, W; Harth, J.

Long-term effect of diabetes and its treatment on cognitive function. *New England Journal of Medicine* 2007;356:1842-1852.

[108] Skoog, I; Gustafson, D. Update on hypertension and Alzheimer's disease. *Neurological Research* 2006;28:605-611.

[109] Kehoe, PG; Wilcock, GK. Is inhibition of the renin-angiotensin system a new treatment option for Alzheimer's disease? *Lancet Neurology* 2007;6:373-378.

[110] Qiu, C; von Strauss, E; Fastbom, J; Winblad, B; Fratiglioni, L. Low blood pressure and risk of dementia in the Kungsholmen project: a 6-year follow-up study. *Archives of Neurology* 2003;60:223-228.

[111] Elias, MF; Elias, PK; Sullivan, LM; Wolf, PA; D'Agostino, RB. Lower cognitive function in the presence of obesity and hypertension: the Framingham heart study. *International Journal of Obesity* 2003;27:260–268.

[112] Forette, F; Seux, ML; Staessen, JA; Thijs, L; Babarskiene, MR; Babeanu, S; Bossini, A; Fagard, R; Gil-Extremera, B; Laks, T; Kobalava, Z; Sarti, C; Tuomilehto, J; Vanhanen, H; Webster, J; Yodfat, Y; Birkenhager, WH; Systolic Hypertension in Europe Investigators. The prevention of dementia with antihypertensive treatment: new evidence from the Systolic Hypertension in Europe (Syst-Eur) study. *Archives of Internal Medicine* 2002;162:2046-2052.

[113] Fransen, M; Anderson, C; Chalmers, J; Chapman, N; Davis, S; MacMahon, S; Neal, B; Sega, R; Terent, A; Tzourio, C, Woodward, M; PROGRESS. Effects of a perindopril-based blood pressure-lowering regimen on disability and dependency in 6105 patients with cerebrovascular disease: a randomised controlled trial. *Stroke* 2003;34:2333-2338.

[114] Ruitenberg, A; Skoog, I; Ott, A; Aevarsson, O; Witteman, JC; Lernfelt, B; van Harskamp, F; Hofman, A; Breteler, MM. Blood pressure and risk of dementia: results from the Rotterdam study and the Gothenburg H-70 Study. *Dementia and Geriatric Cognitive Disorders* 2001;12:33-39.

[115] Morris, MC; Scherr, PA; Hebert, LE; Glynn, RJ; Bennett, DA; Evans, DA. Association of incident Alzheimer disease and blood pressure measured from 13 years before to 2 years after diagnosis in a large community study. *Archives of Neurology* 2001;58:1640-1646.

[116] You, T; Yang, R; Lyles, MF; Gong, D; Nicklas, BJ. Abdominal adipose tissue cytokine gene expression: relationship to obesity and metabolic risk factors. *American Journal of Physiology Endocrinology and Metabolism* 2005;288:E741-747.

[117] Wajchenberg, BL. Subcutaneous and visceral adipose tissue: their relation to the metabolic syndrome. *Endocrine Reviews* 2000; 21:697-738.

[118] Klein, S; Allison, DB; Heymsfield, SB; Kelley, DE; Leibel, RL; Nonas, C; Kahn, R. Waist Circumference and Cardiometabolic Risk: A Consensus Statement from Shaping America's Health: Association for Weight Management and Obesity Prevention; NAASO, The Obesity Society; the American Society for Nutrition; and the American Diabetes Association. *Obesity* 2007;15:1061-1067.

[119] Jagust, W; Harvey, D; Mungas, D; Haan, M. Central obesity and the aging brain. *Archives of Neurology* 2005;62:1545-1548.

[120] Kuo, HK; Jones, RN; Milberg, WP; Tennstedt, S; Talbot, L; Morris, JN; Lipsitz, LA. Effect of blood pressure and diabetes mellitus on cognitive and physical functions in

older adults: a longitudinal analysis of the advanced cognitive training for independent and vital elderly cohort. *Journal of the American Geriatrics Society* 2005;53:1154–1161.

[121] Wolf, PA; Beiser, A; Elias, MF; Au, R; Vasan, RS; Seshadri, S. Relation of obesity to cognitive function: importance of central obesity and synergistic influence of concomitant hypertension. The Framingham Heart Study. *Current Alzheimer Research* 2007;4:111-116.

[122] Cereda, E; Sansone, V; Meola, G; Malavazos, AE. Increased visceral adipose tissue rather than BMI as a risk factor for dementia. *Age and Aging* 2007, - In Press.

[123] Montague, CT; O'Rahilly, S. The perils of portliness: causes and consequences of visceral adiposity. *Diabetes* 2000;49:883-888.

[124] Seidell, JC; Perusse, L; Despres, J-P; Bouchard, C. Waist and hip circumferences have independent and opposite effects on cardiovascular disease risk factors: The Quebec Family Study. *American Journal of Clinical Nutrition* 2001;74:315–321.

[125] Rexrode, KM; Carey, VJ; Hennekens, CH; Walters, EE; Colditz, GA; Stampfer, MJ; Willett, WC; Manson, JE. Abdominal adiposity and coronary heart disease in women. *Journal of the American Medical Association* 1998;280:1843-1848.

[126] Rexrode, KM; Buring, JE; Manson, JE. Abdominal and total adiposity and risk of coronary heart disease in men. *International Journal of Obesity* 2001;25:1047-1056.

[127] Onat, A; Avci, GS; Barlan, MM; Uyarel, H; Uzunlar, B; Sansoy, V. Measures of abdominal obesity assessed for visceral adiposity and relation to coronary risk. *International Journal of Obesity* 2004;28:1018-1025.

[128] Hamilton, BS; Paglia, D; Kwan, AYM; Deitel, M. Increased obese mRNA expression in omental fat cells from massively obese humans. *Nature Medicine* 1995;1:953–956.

[129] St-Onge, MP. Relationship between body composition changes and changes in physical function and metabolic risk factors in aging. *Current Opinion in Clinical Nutrition and Metabolic Care* 2005;8:523-528.

[130] Elia, M. Obesity in the elderly. *Obesity Research* 2001;9 Suppl 4:S244-248.

[131] Carr, DB; Utzschneider, KM; Hull, RL; Kodama, K; Retzlaff, BM; Brunzell, JD; Shofer, JB; Fish, BE; Knopp, RH; Kahn, SE. Intra-abdominal fat is a major determinant of the National Cholesterol Education Program Adult Treatment Panel III criteria for the metabolic syndrome. *Diabetes* 2004;53:2087-2094.

[132] Ding J, Visser M, Kritchevsky SB, Nevitt M, Newman A, Sutton-Tyrrell K, Harris TB. The association of regional fat depots with hypertension in older persons of white and African American ethnicity. *American Journal of Hypertension* 2004;17:971-976.

[133] Feldstein, CA; Akopian, M; Olivieri, AO; Kramer, AP; Nasi, M; Garrido, D. A comparison of body mass index and waist-to-hip ratio as indicators of hypertension risk in an urban Argentine population: a hospital-based study. *Nutrition Metabolism and Cardiovascular Diseases* 2005;15:310-315.

[134] Rahmouni, K; Correia, ML; Haynes, WG; Mark, AL. Obesity-associated hypertension: new insights into mechanisms. *Hypertension* 2005;45:9-14.

[135] Wolf, PA; Beiser, A; Elias, MF; Au, R; Vasan, RS; Seshadri, S. Relation of obesity to cognitive function: importance of central obesity and synergistic influence of

concomitant hypertension. The Framingham Heart Study. *Current Alzheimer Research* 2007;4:111-116.

[136] Goodpaster, BH; Krishnaswami, S; Harris, TB; Katsiaras, A; Kritchevsky, SB; Simonsick, EM; Nevitt, M; Holvoet, P; Newman, AB. Obesity, regional body fat distribution, and the metabolic syndrome in older men and women. *Archives of Internal Medicine* 2005;165:777-783.

[137] Wang, Y; Rimm, EB; Stampfer, MJ; Willett, WC; Hu, FB. Comparison of abdominal adiposity and overall obesity in predicting risk of type 2 diabetes among men. *American Journal of Clinical Nutrition* 2005;81:555-563.

[138] Sartipy, P; Loskutoff, DJ. Monocyte chemoattractant protein 1 in obesity and insulin resistance. *Proceedings of the National Academy of Sciences U.S.A.* 2003; 100:7265–7270.

[139] Weisberg, SP; McCann, D; Desai, M; Rosenbaum, M; Leibel, RL; Ferrante, AW. Obesity is associated with macrophage accumulation in adipose tissue. *Journal of Clinical Investigation* 2003; 112:1796–1808.

[140] Xu, H; Barnes, GT; Yang, Q; Tan, G; Yang, D; Chou, CJ; Sole, J; Nichols, A; Ross, JS; Tartaglia LA; Chen H. Chronic inflammation in fat plays a crucial role in the development of obesity-related insulin resistance. *Journal of Clinical Investigation* 2003;112:1821-1830.

[141] Curat, CA; Wegner, V; Sengenes, C; Miranville, A; Tonus, C; Busse, R; Bouloumie, A. Macrophages in human visceral adipose tissue: increased accumulation in obesity and a source of resistin and visfatin. *Diabetologia* 2006;49:744-747.

[142] Bruun, JM; Lihn, AS; Pedersen, SB; Richelsen, B. MCP-1 release is higher in visceral than subcutaneous human adipose tissue. Implication of macrophages resident in the adipose tissue. *Journal of Clinical Endocrinology and Metabolism* 2005.4:2282–2289.

[143] Uysal, O; Arikan, E; Cakir, B. Plasma total homocysteine level and its association with carotid intima-media thickness in obesity. *Journal of Endocrinological Investigation* 2005;28:928-934.

[144] Malavazos, AE; Ermetici, F; Corsi, MM; Tufano, A; Morricone, L; Ambrosi, B. Relation of visceral adiposity, homocysteine levels and left ventricular morphology. *Journal of Endocrinological Investigation* 2006;29:573-4.

[145] Liu KH, Chan YL, Chan WB, Chan JC, Chu CW. Mesenteric fat thickness is an independent determinant of metabolic syndrome and identifies subjects with increased carotid intima-media thickness. *Diabetes Care* 2006;29:379-384.

[146] Keys A et al. Coronary heart disease in seven countries. *Circulation* 1970;41 – 4th Supplement.

[147] Gordis, L. *Epidemiology. 2nd ediition.* Philadelphia: WB Saunders Company, 2000.

[148] Hennekens, CH; Buring, JE; Manson, JE; Stampfer, M; Rosner, B; Cook, NR; Belanger, C; LaMotte, F; Gaziano, JM; Ridker, PM; Willett, W; Peto, R. Lack of effect of long-term supplementation with beta carotene on the incidence of malignant neoplasms and cardiovascular disease. *New England Journal of Medicine* 1996;334:1145-149.

[149] Schatzkin, A; Lanza, E; Corle, D; Lance, P; Iber, F; Caan, B; Shike, M; Weissfeld, J; Burt, R; Cooper, MR; Kikendall, JW; Cahill, J. Lack of effect of a low-fat, high-fiber

diet on the recurrence of colorectal adenomas. Polyp Prevention Trial Study Group. *New England Journal of Medicine* 2000;342:1149-1155.

[150] Jacques, PF; Tucker, KL. Are dietary patterns useful for understanding the role of diet in chronic disease? *American Journal of Clinical Nutrition* 2001;73:1-2.

[151] Trichopoulou, A; Orfanos, P; Norat, T; Bueno-de-Mesquita, B; Ocke, MC; Peeters, PH; van der Schouw, YT; Boeing, H; Hoffmann, K; Boffetta, P; Nagel, G; Masala, G; Krogh, V; Panico, S; Tumino, R; Vineis, P; Bamia, C; Naska, A; Benetou, V; Ferrari, P; Slimani, N; Pera, G; Martinez-Garcia, C; Navarro, C; Rodriguez-Barranco, M; Dorronsoro, M; Spencer, EA; Key, TJ; Bingham, S; Khaw, KT; Kesse, E; Clavel-Chapelon, F; Boutron-Ruault, MC; Berglund, G; Wirfalt, E; Hallmans, G; Johansson, I; Tjonneland, A; Olsen, A; Overvad, K; Hundborg, HH; Riboli, E; Trichopoulos, D. Modified Mediterranean diet and survival: EPIC-elderly prospective cohort study. *British Medical Journal* 2005;330:991.

[152] Cereda, E; Malavazos, AE; Favaro, C; Pagani, AM. Modified Mediterranean diet and survival: evidence for diet linked longevity is substantial. *British Medical Journal* 2005;330:1329.

[153] Morris, MC; Evans, DA; Tangney, CC; Bienias, JL;Wilson, RS. Associations of vegetable and fruit consumption with age-related cognitive change. *Neurology* 2006;67:1370-1376.

[154] van Gelder, BM; Tijhuis, M; Kalmijn, S; Kromhout, D. Fish consumption, n-3 fatty acids, and subsequent 5-y cognitive decline in elderly men: the Zutphen Elderly Study. *American Journal of Clinical Nutrition* 2007;85:1142-1147.

[155] Borek, C. Garlic reduces dementia and heart-disease risk. *Journal of Nutrition* 2006;136(3 Suppl):S810-812.

[156] Grimes, DA; Schulz, KF. Cohort studies: marching towards outcomes. *Lancet* 2002;359:341-345.

[157] Grimes, DA; Schulz, KF. Bias and causal associations in observational research. *Lancet* 2002;359:248-252.

[158] Scarmeas, N; Stern, Y; Mayeux, R; Luchsinger, JA. Mediterranean diet, Alzheimer disease, and vascular mediation. *Archives of Neurology* 2006;63:1709-1717.

[159] Scarmeas, N; Stern, Y; Tang, MX; Mayeux, R; Luchsinger, JA. Mediterranean diet and risk for Alzheimer's disease. *Annals of Neurology* 2006;59:912-921.

[160] Serra-Majem, L; Roman, B; Estruch, R. Scientific evidence of interventions using the Mediterranean diet: a systematic review. *Nutrition Reviews* 2006;64(2 Pt 2):S27-47.

[161] Fung, TT; Rimm, EB; Spiegelman, D; Rifai, N; Tofler, GH; Willett, WC; Hu, FB. Association between dietary patterns and plasma biomarkers of obesity and cardiovascular disease risk. *American Journal of Clinical Nutrition* 2001;73:61-67.

[162] Kerver, JM; Yang, EJ; Bianchi, L; Song, WO. Dietary patterns associated with risk factors for cardiovascular disease in healthy US adults. *American Journal of Clinical Nutrition* 2003;78:1103-1110.

[163] Lopez-Garcia, E; Schulze, MB; Fung, TT; Meigs, JB; Rifai, N; Manson, JE; Hu, FB. Major dietary patterns are related to plasma concentrations of markers of inflammation and endothelial dysfunction. *American Journal of Clinical Nutrition* 2004;80:1029-1035.

[164] Willett, W; Stampfer, MJ. Total energy intake: implications for epidemiologic analyses. *American Journal of Epidemiology* 1986;124:17–27.

[165] Fraser, GE; Singh, PN; Bennett, H. Variables associated with cognitive function in elderly California Seventh-day Adventists. *American Journal of Epidemiology* 1996;143:1181-1190.

[166] Huijbregts, PP; Feskens, EJ; Rasanen, L; Fidanza, F; Alberti-Fidanza, A; Nissinen, A; Giampaoli, S; Kromhout, D. Dietary patterns and cognitive function in elderly men in Finland, Italy and The Netherlands. *European Journal of Clinical Nutrition* 1998;52:826-831.

[167] Luchsinger, JA; Tang, MX; Shea, S; Mayeux, R. Caloric intake and the risk of Alzheimer disease. *Archives of Neurology* 2002;59:1258-1263.

[168] Wang, J; Ho, L; Qin, W; Rocher, AB; Seror, I; Humala, N; Maniar, K; Dolios, G; Wang, R; Hof, PR; Pasinetti, GM. Caloric restriction attenuates beta-amyloid neuropathology in a mouse model of Alzheimer's disease. *The FASEB Journal* 2005;19:659-661.

[169] Sohal, RS; Weindruch, R. Oxidative stress, caloric restriction, and aging. *Science* 1996;273:59-63.

[170] Wolf, G. Calorie restriction increases life span: a molecular mechanism. *Nutrition Reviews* 2006;64(2 Pt 1):89-92.

[171] Lee, J; Duan, W; Long, JM; Ingram, DK; Mattson, MP. Dietary restriction increases the number of newly generated neural cells, and induces BDNF expression, in the dentate gyrus of rats. *Journal of Molecular Neuroscience* 2000;15:99-108.

[172] Mattson, MP. Neuroprotective signaling and the aging brain: take away my food and let me run. *Brain Research* 2000;886:47-53.

[173] McCrory, MA; Fuss, PJ; McCallum, JE ; Yao, M ; Vinken, AG; Hays, NP; Roberts, SB. Dietary variety within food groups: association with energy intake and body fatness in men and women. *American Journal of Clinical Nutrition* 1999;69:440-447.

[174] Paul, DR; Novotny, JA; Rumpler, WV. Effects of the interaction of sex and food intake on the relation between energy expenditure and body composition. *American Journal of Clinical Nutrition* 2004;79:385-389.

[175] Raynor, HA; Jeffery, RW; Tate, DF; Wing, RR. Relationship between changes in food group variety, dietary intake, and weight during obesity treatment. *International Journal of Obesity* 2004;28:813-820.

[176] Warren, JM; Henry, CJ; Simonite, V. Low glycemic index breakfasts and reduced food intake in preadolescent children. *Pediatrics* 2003;112:e414.

[177] Ball, SD; Keller, KR; Moyer-Mileur, LJ; Ding, YW; Donaldson, D; Jackson, WD. Prolongation of satiety after low versus moderately high glycemic index meals in obese adolescents. *Pediatrics* 2003;111:488-494.

[178] Krachler, B; Eliasson, M; Stenlund, H; Johansson, I; Hallmans, G; Lindahl, B. Reported food intake and distribution of body fat: a repeated cross-sectional study. *Nutrition Journal* 2006;5:34.

[179] Luchsinger, JA; Tang, MX; Mayeux, R. Glycemic load and risk of Alzheimer's disease. *Journal of Nutrition, Health and Aging* 2007;11:238-241.

[180] Jacob, RA. Evidence that diet modification reduces in vivo oxidant damage. *Nutrition Reviews* 1999;57:255-258.

[181] He, K; Song, Y; Daviglus, ML; Liu, K; Van Horn, L; Dyer, AR; Greenland, P. Accumulated evidence on fish consumption and coronary heart disease mortality: a meta-analysis of cohort studies. *Circulation* 2004;109:2705-2011.

[182] He, K; Song, Y; Daviglus, ML; Liu, K; Van Horn, L; Dyer, AR; Goldbourt, U; Greenland, P. Fish consumption and incidence of stroke: a meta-analysis of cohort studies. *Stroke* 2004;35:1538-1542.

[183] Whelton, SP; He, J; Whelton, PK; Muntner, P. Meta-analysis of observational studies on fish intake and coronary heart disease. *American Journal of Cardiology* 2004;93:1119 –1123.

[184] Hu, FB; Stampfer, MJ; Manson, JE; Rimm, E; Colditz, GA; Rosner, BA; Hennekens, CH; Willett, WC. Dietary fat intake and the risk of coronary heart disease in women. *New England Journal of Medicine* 1997;337:1491-1499.

[185] Laitinen, MH; Ngandu, T; Rovio, S; Helkala, EL; Uusitalo, U; Viitanen, M; Nissinen, A; Tuomilehto, J; Soininen, H; Kivipelto, M. Fat intake at midlife and risk of dementia and Alzheimer's disease: a population-based study. *Dementia and Geriatric Cognitive Disorders* 2006;22:99-107.

[186] Morris, MC; Evans, DA; Bienias, JL; Tangney, CC; Wilson, RS. Dietary fat intake and 6-year cognitive change in an older biracial community population. *Neurology* 2004;62:1573-9157.

[187] Morris, MC; Evans, DA; Tangney, CC; Bienias, JL; Schneider, JA; Wilson, RS; Scherr, PA. Dietary copper and high saturated and trans fat intakes associated with cognitive decline. *Archives of Neurology* 2006;63:1085-1088.

[188] Solfrizzi, V; Colacicco, AM; D'Introno, A; Capurso, C; Torres, F; Rizzo, C; Capurso, A; Panza, F. Dietary intake of unsaturated fatty acids and age-related cognitive decline: a 8.5-year follow-up of the Italian Longitudinal Study on Aging. *Neurobiology of Aging* 2006;27:1694-1704.

[189] Morris, MC; Evans, DA; Bienias, JL; Tangney, CC; Bennett, DA; Wilson, RS; Aggarwal, N; Schneider, J. Consumption of fish and n-3 fatty acids and risk of incident Alzheimer disease. *Archives of Neurology* 2003;60:940-946.

[190] van Gelder, BM; Tijhuis, M; Kalmijn, S; Kromhout, D. Fish consumption, n-3 fatty acids, and subsequent 5-y cognitive decline in elderly men: the Zutphen Elderly Study. *American Journal of Clinical Nutrition* 2007;85:1142-7114.

[191] Heude, B; Ducimetiere, P; Berr, C. Cognitive decline and fatty acid composition of erythrocyte membranes—the EVA Study. *American Journal of Clinical Nutrition* 2003;77:803– 8.

[192] Beydoun, MA; Kaufman, JS; Satia, JA; Rosamond, W; Folsom, AR. Plasma n-3 fatty acids and the risk of cognitive decline in older adults: the Atherosclerosis Risk in Communities Study. *American Journal of Clinical Nutrition* 2007;85:1103-1111.

[193] Wijendran, V; Hayes, KC. Dietary n-6 and n-3 fatty acid balance and cardiovascular health. *Annual Review of Nutrition* 2004;24:597-615.

[194] Hibbeln, JR; Nieminen, LR; Blasbalg, TL; Riggs, JA; Lands, WE. Healthy intakes of n-3 and n-6 fatty acids: estimations considering worldwide diversity. *American Journal of Clinical Nutrition* 2006;83(6 Suppl):S1483-1493.

[195] Hardy, JA; Higgins, GA. Alzheimer's disease: the amyloid cascade hypothesis. *Science* 1992;256:184-185.

[196] Berglund, L. The APOE gene and diets--food (and drink) for thought. *American Journal of Clinical Nutrition* 2001;73:669-670.

[197] Lopez-Garcia, E; Schulze, MB; Fung, TT; Meigs, JB; Rifai, N; Manson, JE; Hu, FB. Major dietary patterns are related to plasma concentrations of markers of inflammation and endothelial dysfunction. *American Journal of Clinical Nutrition* 2004;80:1029-1035.

[198] Kerver, JM; Yang, EJ; Bianchi, L; Song, WO. Dietary patterns associated with risk factors for cardiovascular disease in healthy US adults. *American Journal of Clinical Nutrition* 2003;78:1103-1110.

[199] Mauger, JF; Lichtenstein, AH; Ausman, LM; Jalbert, SM; Jauhiainen, M; Ehnholm, C; Lamarche, B. Effect of different forms of dietary hydrogenated fats on LDL particle size. *American Journal of Clinical Nutrition* 2003;78:370-375.

[200] Lichtenstein, AH; Ausman, LM; Jalbert, SM; Schaefer, EJ. Effects of different forms of dietary hydrogenated fats on serum lipoprotein cholesterol levels. *New England Journal of Medicine* 1999;340:1933-1940.

[201] Matthan, NR; Welty, FK; Barrett, PH; Harausz, C; Dolnikowski, GG; Parks, JS; Eckel, RH; Schaefer, EJ; Lichtenstein, AH. Dietary hydrogenated fat increases high-density lipoprotein apoA-I catabolism and decreases low-density lipoprotein apoB-100 catabolism in hypercholesterolemic women. *Arteriosclerosis, Thrombosis, and Vascular Biology* 2004;24:1092-1097.

[202] Bray, GA; Lovejoy, JC; Smith, SR; DeLany, JP; Lefevre, M; Hwang, D; Ryan, DH; York, DA. The influence of different fats and fatty acids on obesity, insulin resistance and inflammation. *Journal of Nutrition* 2002;132:2488-2491.

[203] Carpentier, YA; Portois, L; Malaisse, WJ. n-3 fatty acids and the metabolic syndrome. *American Journal of Clinical Nutrition* 2006 Jun;83(6 Suppl):S1499-1504.

[204] Shahar, E; Folsom, AR; Wu, KK; Dennis, BH; Shimakawa, T; Conlan, MG; Davis, CE; Williams, OD. Associations of fish intake and dietary n-3 polyunsaturated fatty acids with a hypocoagulable profile. The Atherosclerosis Risk in Communities (ARIC) Study. *Arteriosclerosis and Thrombosis* 1993;13:1205-1212.

[205] Anil, E. The impact of EPA and DHA on blood lipids and lipoprotein metabolism: influence of apoE genotype. *Proceedings of Nutrition Society* 2007;66:60-68.

[206] Vessby, B; Unsitupa, M; Hermansen, K; Riccardi, G; Rivellese, AA; Tapsell, LC; Nalsen, C; Berglund, L; Louheranta, A; Rasmussen, BM; Calvert, GD; Maffetone, A; Pedersen, E; Gustafsson, IB; Storlien, LH; KANWU Study. Substituting dietary saturated for monounsaturated fat impairs insulin sensitivity in healthy men and women: The KANWU Study. *Diabetologia* 2001;44:312-319.

[207] Allman-Farinelli, MA; Gomes, K; Favaloro, EJ; Petocz, P. A diet rich in high-oleic-acid sunflower oil favorably alters low-density lipoprotein cholesterol, triglycerides,

and factor VII coagulant activity. *Journal of the American Dietetic Association* 2005;105:1071-1079.

[208] Uauy, R; Dangour, AD. Nutrition in brain development and aging: role of essential fatty acids. *Nutrition Reviews* 2006;64(5 Pt 2):S24-33.

[209] Jones, CR ; Arai, T ; Rapoport, SI. Evidence for the involvement of docosahexaenoic acid in cholinergic stimulated signal transduction at the synapse. *Neurochemical Research* 1997;22:663-670.

[210] Willett, WC. Is dietary fat a major determinant of body fat? *American Journal of Clinical Nutrition* 1998;67(Suppl):S556–562.

[211] Lissner, L; Heitmann, BL. Dietary fat and obesity: evidence from epidemiology. *European Journal of Clinical Nutrition* 1995;49:79–80.

[212] Roberts, SB; Pi-Sunyer, FX; Dreher, M; Hahn, R; Hill, JO; Kleinman, RE; Peters, JC; Ravussin, E; Rolls, BJ; Yetley, E; Booth, SL. Physiology of fat replacement and fat reduction: effects of dietary fat and fat substitutes on energy regulation. *Nutrition Reviews* 1998;56(Part 2):S29-41.

[213] Lindsay, J; Laurin, D; Verreault, R. Risk Factors for Alzheimer's disease: a prospective analysis from the Canadian Study of Health and Aging. *American Journal of Epidemiology* 2002;156:445–53.

[214] Luchsinger, JA; Tang, MX; Siddiqui, M; Shea, S; Mayeux R. Alcohol intake and risk of dementia. *Journal of the American Geriatrics Society* 2004;52:540-546.

[215] Solfrizzi, V; D'Introno, A; Colacicco, AM; Capurso, C; Del Parigi, A; Baldassarre, G; Scapicchio, P; Scafato, E; Amodio, M; Capurso, A; Panza, F; Italian Longitudinal Study on Aging Working Group. Alcohol consumption, mild cognitive impairment, and progression to dementia. *Neurology* 2007;68:1790-1799.

[216] Truelsen, T; Thudium, D; Gronbaek, M; Copenhagen City Heart Study. Amount and type of alcohol and risk of dementia: the Copenhagen City Heart Study. *Neurology* 2002;59:1313-1319.

[217] Ruitenberg, A; van Swieten, JC; Witteman, JC; Mehta, KM; van Duijn, CM; Hofman, A, Breteler MM. Alcohol consumption and risk of dementia: the Rotterdam Study. *Lancet* 2002;359:281-286.

[218] Stampfer, MJ; Kang, JH; Chen, J; Cherry, R; Grodstein, F. Effects of moderate alcohol consumption on cognitive function in women. *New England Journal of Medicine* 2005;352:245-253.

[219] Anttila, T; Helkala, EL; Viitanen, M; Kareholt, I; Fratiglioni, L; Winblad, B; Soininen, H; Tuomilehto, J; Nissinen, A; Kivipelto, M. Alcohol drinking in middle age and subsequent risk of mild cognitive impairment and dementia in old age: a prospective population based study. *British Medical Journal* 2004;329:539.

[220] Harper, C; Matsumoto, I. Ethanol and brain damage. *Current Opinion in Pharmacology* 2005;5:73-78.

[221] Pascual, M; Blanco, AM; Cauli, O; Minarro, J; Guerri, C. Intermittent ethanol exposure induces inflammatory brain damage and causes long-term behavioural alterations in adolescent rats. *European Journal of Neuroscience* 2007;25:541-550.

[222] Rimm, EB; Williams, P; Fosher, K; Criqui, M; Stampfer, MJ Moderate alcohol intake and lower risk of coronary heart disease: meta-analysis of effects on lipids and haemostatic factors. *British Medical Journal* 1999;319:1523-8.

[223] den Heijer, T; Vermeer, SE; van Dijk, EJ; Prins, ND; Koudstaal, PJ; van Duijn, CM; Hofman, A; Breteler, MM. Alcohol intake in relation to brain magnetic resonance imaging findings in older persons without dementia. *American Journal of Clinical Nutrition* 2004;80:992-997.

[224] Mukamal, KJ; Longstreth, WT Jr; Mittleman, MA; Crum, RM; Siscovick, DS. Alcohol consumption and subclinical findings on magnetic resonance imaging of the brain in older adults: the cardiovascular health study. *Stroke* 2001;32:1939-1946.

[225] Pfefferbaum, A. Alcoholism damages the brain, but does moderate alcohol use? Lancet Neurology 2004;3:143-144.

[226] Sacco, RL; Elkind, M; Boden-Albala, B; Lin, IF; Kargman, DE; Hauser, WA; Shea, S; Paik, MC. The protective effect of moderate alcohol consumption on ischemic stroke. *Journal of the American Medical Association* 1999;281:53-60.

[227] Mukamal, KJ; Mackey, RH; Kuller, LH; Tracy, RP; Kronmal, RA; Mittleman, MA; Siscovick, DS. Alcohol Consumption and Lipoprotein Subclasses in Older Adults. *Journal of Clinical Endocrinology and Metabolism* 2007; doi: 10.1210/jc.2006-2422 – In Press.

[228] Belleville, J. The French paradox: possible involvement of ethanol in the protective effect against cardiovascular diseases. *Nutrition* 2002;18:173–77.

[229] Vasdev, S; Gill, V; Singal, PK. Beneficial effect of low ethanol intake on the cardiovascular syst6em: possible biochemical mechanisms. *Vascular Health and Risk Management* 2006;2:263-276.

[230] Zern, TL; Fernandez, ML. Cardioprotective effects of dietary polyphenols. *Journal of Nutrition* 2005;135:2291-2294.

[231] Staehelin, HB. Micronutrients and Alzheimer's disease. *Proceedings of Nutrition Society* 2005;64:565-570.

[232] Bates, CJ; Benton, D; Biesalski, HK; Staehelin, HB; van Staveren, W; Stehle, P; Suter, PM; Wolfram, G. Nutrition and aging: a consensus statement. *Journal of Nutrition, Health and Aging* 2002;6:103-116.

[233] Clarke, R; Lewington, S; Sherliker, P; Armitage, J. Effects of B-vitamins on plasma homocysteine concentrations and on risk of cardiovascular disease and dementia. *Current Opinion in Clinical Nutrition and Metabolic Care* 2007;10:32-39.

[234] Griffiths, R; Grieve, A; Allen, S; Olverman, HJ. Neuronal and glial plasma membrane carrier-mediated uptake of L-homocysteate is not selectively blocked by beta-p-chlorophenylglutamate. *Neuroscience Letters* 1992;147:175-178.

[235] Ho, PI; Ashline, D; Dhitavat, S; Ortiz, D; Collins, SC; Shea, TB; Rogers, E. Folate deprivation induces neurodegeneration: roles of oxidative stress and increased homocysteine. *Neurobiology of Disease* 2003;14:32-42.

[236] Leboeuf, R. Homocysteine and Alzheimer's disease. *Journal of the American Dietetic Association* 2003;103:304-307.

[237] Scott, JM; Molloy, AM; Kennedy, DG; Kennedy, S; Weir, DG. Effects of the disruption of transmethylation in the central nervous system: an animal model. *Acta Neurologica Scandinavica -Supplementum* 1994;154:27-31.

[238] Streck, EL; Bavaresco, CS; Netto, CA; Wyse, AT. Chronic hyperhomocysteinemia provokes a memory deficit in rats in the Morris water maze task. *Behavioural Brain Research* 2004;153:377-381.

[239] Algaidi, SA; Christie, LA; Jenkinson, AM; Whalley, L; Riedel, G; Platt, B. Long-term homocysteine exposure induces alterations in spatial learning, hippocampal signalling and synaptic plasticity. *Experimental Neurology* 2006;197:8-21.

[240] Streck, EL; Delwing, D; Tagliari, B; Matte, C; Wannmacher, CM; Wajner, M; Wyse, AT. Brain energy metabolism is compromised by the metabolites accumulating in homocystinuria. *Neurochemistry International* 2003;43:597-602.

[241] Kruman, II; Culmsee, C; Chan, SL; Kruman, Y; Guo, Z; Penix, L; Mattson, MP. Homocysteine elicits a DNA damage response in neurons that promotes apoptosis and hypersensitivity to excitotoxicity. *The Journal of Neuroscience* 2000;20:6920-6926.

[242] Ho, PI; Ortiz, D; Rogers, E; Shea, TB. Multiple aspects of homocysteine neurotoxicity: glutamate excitotoxicity, kinase hyperactivation and DNA damage. *Journal of Neuroscience Research* 2002;70:694-702.

[243] Ermak, G; Davies, KJ. Calcium and oxidative stress: from cell signaling to cell death. *Molecular Immunology* 2002;38:713-721.

[244] Clarke, R; Daly, L; Robinson, K, Naughten, E; Cahalane, S; Fowler, B; Graham, I. Hyperhomocysteinemia: an independent risk factor for vascular disease. *New England Journal of Medicine* 1991;324:1149-1155.

[245] Boushey, CJ; Beresford, SA; Omenn, GS; Motulsky, AG. A quantitative assessment of plasma homocysteine as a risk factor for vascular disease. Probable benefits of increasing folic acid intakes. *Journal of the American Medical Association* 1995;274:1049-1057.

[246] Homocysteine Studies Collaboration. Homocysteine and risk of ischemic heart disease and stroke: a meta-analysis. *Journal of the American Medical Association* 2002;288:2015-2022.

[247] Wang, X; Qin, X; Demirtas, H; Li, J; Mao, G; Huo, Y; Sun, N; Liu, L; Xu, X. Efficacy of folic acid supplementation in stroke prevention: a meta-analysis. *Lancet* 2007;369:1876-1882.

[248] den Heijer, T; Vermeer, SE; Clarke, R; Oudkerk, M; Koudstaal, PJ; Hofman, A; Breteler, MM. Homocysteine and brain atrophy on MRI of non-demented elderly. *Brain* 2003;126(Pt 1):170-175.

[249] Wong, A; Mok, V; Fan, YH; Lam, WW; Liang, KS; Wong, KS. Hyperhomocysteinemia is associated with volumetric white matter change in patients with small vessel disease. *Journal of Neurology* 2006;253:441-447.

[250] Seshadri, S; Beiser, A; Selhub, J; Jacques, PF; Rosenberg, IH; D'Agostino, RB; Wilson, PW; Wolf, PA. Plasma homocysteine as a risk factor for dementia and Alzheimer's disease. *New England Journal of Medicine* 2002;346:476-483.

[251] Quadri, P; Fragiacomo, C; Pezzati, R; Zanda, E; Forloni, G; Tettamanti, M; Lucca, U. Homocysteine, folate, and vitamin B-12 in mild cognitive impairment, Alzheimer

disease, and vascular dementia. *American Journal of Clinical Nutrition* 2004;80:114-122.

[252] Nurk, E; Refsum, H; Tell, GS; Engedal, K; Vollset, SE; Ueland, PM; Nygaard, HA; Smith, AD. Plasma total homocysteine and memory in the elderly: the Hordaland Homocysteine Study. *Annals of Neurology* 2005;58:847-857.

[253] Ravaglia, G; Forti, P; Maioli, F; Martelli, M; Servadei, L; Brunetti, N; Porcellini, E; Licastro, F. Homocysteine and folate as risk factors for dementia and Alzheimer disease. *American Journal of Clinical Nutrition* 2005;82:636-643.

[254] Tucker, KL; Qiao, N; Scott, T; Rosenberg, I; Spiro, A 3rd. High homocysteine and low B vitamins predict cognitive decline in aging men: the Veterans Affairs Normative Aging Study. *American Journal of Clinical Nutrition* 2005;82:627-635.

[255] Kado, DM; Karlamangla, AS; Huang, MH; Troen, A; Rowe, JW; Selhub, J; Seeman, TE. Homocysteine versus the vitamins folate, B6, and B12 as predictors of cognitive function and decline in older high-functioning adults: MacArthur Studies of Successful Aging. *American Journal of Medicine* 2005;118:161-167.

[256] Haan, MN; Miller, JW; Aiello, AE; Whitmer, RA; Jagust, WJ; Mungas, DM; Allen, LH; Green, R. Homocysteine, B vitamins, and the incidence of dementia and cognitive impairment: results from the Sacramento Area Latino Study on Aging. *American Journal of Clinical Nutrition* 2007;85:511-517.

[257] Tettamanti, M; Garri, MT; Nobili, A; Riva, E; Lucca, U. Low folate and the risk of cognitive and functional deficits in the very old: the Monzino 80-plus study. *Journal of the American College of Nutrition* 2006;25:502-508.

[258] Crystal, HA; Ortof, E; Frishman, WH; Gruber, A; Hershman, D; Aronson, M. Serum vitamin B12 levels and incidence of dementia in a healthy elderly population: a report from the Bronx Longitudinal Aging Study. *Journal of the American Geriatrics Society* 1994;42:933-936.

[259] Wang, HX; Wahlin, A; Basun, H; Fastbom, J; Winblad, B; Fratiglioni, L. Vitamin B(12) and folate in relation to the development of Alzheimer's disease. *Neurology* 2001;56:1188-1194.

[260] Kang, JH; Irizarry, MC; Grodstein, F. Prospective study of plasma folate, vitamin B12, and cognitive function and decline. *Epidemiology* 2006;17:650-657.

[261] Selhub, J; Bagley, LC; Miller, J; Rosenberg, IH. B vitamins, homocysteine, and neurocognitive function in the elderly. *American Journal of Clinical Nutrition* 2000;71:614S-620S.

[262] Morris, MC; Evans, DA; Bienias, JL; Tangney, CC; Hebert, LE; Scherr, PA; Schneider, JA. Dietary folate and vitamin B12 intake and cognitive decline among community-dwelling older persons. *Archives of Neurology* 2005;62:641-645.

[263] Morris, MC; Evans, DA; Schneider, JA; Tangney, CC; Bienias, JL; Aggarwal, NT. Dietary folate and vitamins B-12 and B-6 not associated with incident Alzheimer's disease. *Journal of Alzheimer's Disease* 2006;9:435-443.

[264] Luchsinger, JA; Tang, MX; Miller, J; Green, R; Mayeux, R. Relation of higher folate intake to lower risk of Alzheimer disease in the elderly. *Archives of Neurology* 2007;64:86-92.

[265] Markesbery, WR. Oxidative stress hypothesis in Alzheimer's disease. *Free Radical Biology and Medicine* 1997; 23:134–47.

[266] Christen, Y. Oxidative stress and Alzheimer disease. *American Journal of Clinical Nutrition* 2000; 71 (Suppl):S621–29.

[267] Nagano, S; Huang, X; Moir, RD; Payton, SM; Tanzi, RE; Bush, AI. Peroxidase activity of cyclooxygenase-2 (COX-2) cross-links {beta}-amyloid (A{beta}) and Generates A{beta}-COX-2 hetero-oligomers that are increased in Alzheimer's disease. *Journal of Biological Chemistry* 2004;279:14673–78.

[268] Berr, C; Richard, MJ; Roussel, AM; Bonithon-Kopp, C. Systemic oxidative stress and cognitive performance in the population-based EVA study. Free Radic Biol Med 1998;24:1202–08.

[269] Rinaldi, P; Polidori, MC; Metastasio, A; Mariani, E; Mattioli, P; Cherubini, A; Catani, M; Cecchetti, R; Senin, UM; Mecocci, P. Plasma antioxidants are similarly depleted in mild cognitive impairment and in Alzheimer's disease. *Neurobiology of Aging* 2003;24:915–19.

[270] Launer, LJ. Is there epidemiologic evidence that antioxidants protect against disorders in cognitive function? *Journal of Nutrition, Health and Aging* 2000;4:197–201.

[271] Paleologos, M; Cumming, R; Lazarus, R. Cohort study of vitamin C intake and cognitive impairment. *American Journal of Epidemiology* 1998;148:45-50.

[272] Wengreen, HJ; Munger, RG; Corcoran, CD; Zandi, P; Hayden, KM; Fotuhi, M; Skoog, I; Norton, MC; Tschanz, J; Breitner, JC; Welsh-Bohmer, KA. Antioxidant intake and cognitive function of elderly men and women: the Cache County Study. *Journal of Nutrition, Health and Aging* 2007;11:230-7.

[273] Southon, S; Wright, A; Finglas, P; Bailey, A; Loughridge, J; Walker, A. Dietary intake and micronutrient status in adolescents: effect of vitamin and trace element supplementation on indices of status and performance tests of verbal an non-verbal intelligence. *British Journal of Nutrition* 1994;71:897-918.

[274] Butterfield, DA; Castegna, A; Drake, J; Scapagnini, G; Calabrese, V. Vitamin E and neurodegenerative disorders associated with oxidative stress. *Nutritional Neuroscience* 2002;5:229–39.

[275] Sung, S; Yao, Y; Uryu, K; Yang, H; Lee, VM; Trojanowski, JQ. and Pratico D. Early vitamin E supplementation in young but not aged mice reduces Abeta levels and amyloid deposition in a transgenic model of Alzheimer's disease. *FASEB Journal* 2004; 18: 323-325.

[276] Larrieu S., Letenneur L., Helmer C., Dartigues J.F. and Barberger-Gateau P. Nutritional factors and risk of incident dementia in the PAQUID longitudinal cohort. *Journal of Nutrition, Health and Aging* 2004; 8 : 150-154.

[277] Zandi, PP; Anthony, JC; Khachaturian, AS; Stone, SV; Gustafson, D; Tschanz, JT., Norton M.C., Welsh-Bohmer K.A. and Breitner J.C. Reduced risk of Alzheimer disease in users of antioxidant vitamin supplements: the Cache County Study. *Archives of Neurology* 2004;61:82-88.

[278] Morris, MC; Evans, DA; Bienias, JL; Tangney, CC; Bennett, DA; Aggarwal, N; Wilson, RS; Scherr, PA. Dietary intake of antioxidant nutrients and the risk of incident

Alzheimer's disease in a biracial community study. *Journal of the American Medical Association* 2002;287:3230 –7.

[279] Engelhart, MJ; Geerlings, MI; Ruitenberg, A; van Swieten, JC; Hofman, A; Witteman, JC; Breteler, MM. Dietary intake of antioxidants and risk of Alzheimer disease. *Journal of the American Medical Association* 2002;287:3223–9.

[280] Jiang, Q; Ames, BN. Gamma-tocopherol, but not alphatocopherol, decreases proinflammatory eicosanoids and inflammation damage in rats. *FASEB Journal* 2003;17:816 –22.

[281] Williamson, KS; Gabbita, SP; Mou, S; West, M; Pye, QN; Markesbery, WR; Cooney, RV; Grammas, P; Reimann-Philipp, U; Floyd, RA; Hensley, K. The nitration product 5- nitrogamma- tocopherol is increased in the Alzheimer brain. *Nitric Oxide* 2002;6:221–7.

[282] Morton, LW; Ward, NC; Croft, KD; Puddey, IB. Evidence for the nitration of gamma-tocopherol in vivo: 5-nitro-gamma-tocopherol is elevated in the plasma of subjects with coronary heart disease. *Biochemical Journal* 2002;364:3–8.

[283] Morris, MC; Evans, DA; Tangney, CC; Bienias, JL; Wilson, RS. Aggarwal, NT; Scherr, PA Relation of the tocopherol forms to incident Alzheimer disease and to cognitive change. *American Journal of Clinical Nutrition* 2005;81:508–14.

[284] Commenges, D; Scotet, V; Renaud, S; Jacqmin-Gadda, H; Barberger-Gateau, P; Dartigues, JF. Intake of flavonoids and risk of dementia. *European Journal of Epidemiology* 2000;16:357-363.

[285] Heinonen, IM; Lehtonen, PJ; Hopia, AI. Antioxidant activity of berry and fruit wines and liquors. *Journal of Agricultural and Food Chemistry* 1998; 46: 25–31.

[286] Platt, B. Experimental approaches to assess metallotoxicity and ageing in models of Alzheimer's disease. *Journal of Alzheimer's Disease* 2006;10:203-213.

[287] Savory, J; Herman, MM; Ghribi, O. Mechanisms of aluminum-induced neurodegeneration in animals: Implications for Alzheimer's disease. *Journal of Alzheimer's Disease* 2006;10:135-144.

[288] House, E; Collingwood, J; Khan, A; Korchazkina, O; Berthon, G; Exley, C. Aluminium, iron, zinc and copper influence the in vitro formation of amyloid fibrils of Abeta42 in a manner which may have consequences for metal chelation therapy in Alzheimer's disease. *Journal of Alzheimer's Disease* 2004;6:291-301.

[289] Good, PF; Perl, DP; Bierer, LM; Schmeidler, J. Selective accumulation of aluminum and iron in the neurofibrillary tangles of Alzheimer's disease: a laser microprobe (LAMMA) study. *Annals of Neurology* 1992;31:286-292.

[290] Domingo, JL. Aluminum and other metals in Alzheimer's disease: a review of potential therapy with chelating agents. *Journal of Alzheimer's Disease* 2006;10:331-341.

[291] Campbell, A. The role of aluminum and copper on neuroinflammation and Alzheimer's disease. *Journal of Alzheimer's Disease* 2006;10:165-172.

[292] Solfrizzi, V; Colacicco, AM; D'Introno, A; Capurso, C; Parigi, AD; Capurso, SA; Torres, F; Capurso, A; Panza, F. Macronutrients, aluminium from drinking water and foods, and other metals in cognitive decline and dementia. *Journal of Alzheimer's Disease* 2006;10:303-330.

[293] Lovell, MA; Robertson, JD; Teesdale, WJ; Campbell, JL; Markesbery, WR. Copper, iron and zinc in Alzheimer's disease senile plaques. *Journal of the Neurological Sciences* 1998;158:47-52.

[294] Cherny, RA; Atwood, CS; Xilinas, ME; Gray, DN; Jones, WD; McLean, CA; Barnham, KJ; Volitakis, I; Fraser, FW; Kim, Y; Huang, X; Goldstein, LE; Moir, RD; Lim, JT; Beyreuther, K; Zheng, H; Tanzi, RE; Masters, CL; Bush, AI. Treatment with a copper-zinc chelator markedly and rapidly inhibits beta-amyloid accumulation in Alzheimer's disease transgenic mice. *Neuron* 2001;30:665-676.

[295] Huang, X; Cuajungco, MP; Atwood, CS; Hartshorn, MA; Tyndall, JD; Hanson, GR; Stokes, KC; Leopold, M; Multhaup, G; Goldstein, LE; Scarpa, RC; Saunders, AJ; Lim, J; Moir, RD; Glabe, C; Bowden, EF; Masters, CL; Fairlie, DP; Tanzi, RE; Bush, AI. Cu(II) potentiation of alzheimer abeta neurotoxicity. Correlation with cell-free hydrogen peroxide production and metal reduction. *Journal of Biological Chemistry* 1999;274:37111-37116.

[296] Yokel, RA. Blood-brain barrier flux of aluminum, manganese, iron and other metals suspected to contribute to metal-induced neurodegeneration. *Journal of Alzheimer's Disease* 2006;10:223-253.

[297] Jayasooriya, AP; Ackland, ML; Mathai, ML; Sinclair, AJ; Weisinger, HS; Weisinger, RS; Halver, JE; Kitajka, K; Puskas, LG. Perinatal omega-3 polyunsaturated fatty acid supply modifies brain zinc homeostasis during adulthood. *Proceedings of the National Academy of Sciences U.S.A.* 2005;102:7133-7138.

[298] Squitti, R; Pasqualetti, P; Cassetta, E; Dal Forno, G; Cesaretti, S; Pedace, F; Finazzi-Agro, A; Rossigni, PM. Elevation of serum copper levels discriminates Alzheimer's disease from vascular dementia. *Neurology* 2003;60:2013-2014.

[299] Squitti, R; Lupoi, D; Pasqualetti, P; Dal Forno, G; Verzieri, F; Chiovenda, P; Rossi, L; Cortesi, M; Cassetta, E; Rossigni, PM. Elevation of serum copper levels in Alzheimer's disease. *Neurology* 2002;59:1153-1161.

[300] Atamna, H; Frey, WH 2nd. A role for heme in Alzheimer's disease: heme binds amyloid beta and has altered metabolism. *Proceedings of the National Academy of Sciences U.S.A.* 2004;101:11153-11158.

[301] Atamna, H; Liu, J; Ames, BN. Heme deficiency selectively interrupts assembly of mitochondrial complex IV in human fibroblasts: revelance to aging. *Journal of Biological Chemistry* 2001;276:48410-48416.

[302] Akbaraly, NT; Hininger-Favier, I; Carriere, I; Arnaud, J; Gourlet, V; Roussel, AM; Berr, C. Plasma selenium over time and cognitive decline in the elderly. *Epidemiology* 2007;18:52-58.

[303] Weil, M; Bressler, J; Parsons, P; Bolla, K; Glass, T; Schwartz, B. Blood mercury levels and neurobehavioral function. *Journal of the American Medical Association* 2005;293:1875-1882.

[304] Fisher, AE; Naughton, DP. Why nutraceuticals do not prevent or treat Alzheimer's disease. *Nutrition Journal* 2005;4:14.

[305] Hurrell, RF. Influence of vegetable protein sources on trace element and mineral bioavailability. *Journal of Nutrition* 2003;133:S2973-2977.

[306] Durga, J; van Boxtel, MP; Schouten, EG; Kok, FJ; Jolles, J; Katan, MB; Verhoef, P. Effect of 3-year folic acid supplementation on cognitive function in older adults in the FACIT trial: a randomised, double blind, controlled trial. *Lancet* 2007;369:208-216.

[307] McMahon, JA; Green, TJ; Skeaff, CM; Knight, RG; Mann, JI; Williams, SM. A controlled trial of homocysteine lowering and cognitive performance. *New England Journal of Medicine* 2006;354:2764-2772.

[308] Eussen, SJ; de Groot, LC; Joosten, LW; Bloo, RJ; Clarke, R; Ueland, PM; Schneede, J; Blom, HJ; Hoefnagels, WH; van Staveren, WA. Effect of oral vitamin B-12 with or without folic acid on cognitive function in older people with mild vitamin B-12 deficiency: a randomized, placebo-controlled trial. *American Journal of Clinical Nutrition* 2006;84:361-370.

[309] Stott, DJ; MacIntosh, G; Lowe, GD; Rumley, A; McMahon, AD; Langhorne, P; Tait, RC; O'Reilly, DS; Spilg, EG; MacDonald, JB; MacFarlane, PW; Westendorp, RG. Randomized controlled trial of homocysteine-lowering vitamin treatment in elderly patients with vascular disease. *American Journal of Clinical Nutrition* 2005;82:1320-1326.

[310] Toole, JF; Malinow, MR; Chambless, LE; Spence, JD; Pettigrew, LC; Howard, VJ; Sides, EG; Wang, CH; Stampfer, M. Lowering homocysteine in patients with ischemic stroke to prevent recurrent stroke, myocardial infarction, and death: the Vitamin Intervention for Stroke Prevention (VISP) randomized controlled trial. *Journal of the American Medical Association* 2004;291:565-575.

[311] Clarke, R; Harrison, G; Richards, S; Vital Trial Collaborative Group. Effect of vitamins and aspirin on markers of platelet activation, oxidative stress and homocysteine in people at high risk of dementia. *Journal of Internal Medicine* 2003;254:67-75.

[312] Lewerin, C; Matousek, M; Steen, G; Johansson, B; Steen, B; Nilsson-Ehle, H. Significant correlations of plasma homocysteine and serum methylmalonic acid with movement and cognitive performance in elderly subjects but no improvement from short-term vitamin therapy: a placebo-controlled randomized study. *American Journal of Clinical Nutrition* 2005;81:1155-1162.

[313] Bryan, J; Calvaresi, E; Hughes, D. Short-term folate, vitamin B-12 or vitamin B-6 supplementation slightly affects memory performance but not mood in women of various ages. *Journal of Nutrition* 2002;132:1345-1356.

[314] Wolters, M; Hickstein, M; Flintermann, A; Tewes, U; Hahn, A. Cognitive performance in relation to vitamin status in healthy elderly German women-the effect of 6-month multivitamin supplementation. *Preventive Medicine* 2005;41:253-259.

[315] van Uffelen, JG; Hopman-Rock, M; Chin, A; Paw, MJ; van Mechelen, W. Protocol for Project FACT: a randomised controlled trial on the effect of a walking program and vitamin B supplementation on the rate of cognitive decline and psychosocial well-being in older adults with mild cognitive impairment [ISRCTN19227688]. *BMC Geriatrics* 2005;5:18.

[316] Planas, M; Conde, M; Audivert, S; Perez-Portabella, C; Burgos, R; Chacon, P; Rossello, J; Boada, M; Tarraga, LL. Micronutrient supplementation in mild Alzheimer disease patients. *Clinical Nutrition* 2004;23:265-272.

[317] McNeill, G ; Avenell, A ; Campbell, MK ; Cook, JA ; Hannaford, PC ; Kilonzo, MM ; Milne, AC ; Ramsay, CR ; Seymour, DG ; Stephen, AI ; Vale, LD. Effect of multivitamin and multimineral supplementation on cognitive function in men and women aged 65 years and over: a randomised controlled trial. *Nutrition Journal* 2007;6:10.

[318] Freund-Levi, Y; Eriksdotter-Jonhagen, M; Cederholm, T; Basun, H; Faxen-Irving, G; Garlind, A; Vedin, I; Vessby, B; Wahlund, LO; Palmblad, J. Omega-3 fatty acid treatment in 174 patients with mild to moderate Alzheimer disease: OmegAD study: a randomized double-blind trial. *Archives of Neurology* 2006;63:1402-1408.

[319] Puri, BK; Bydder, GM; Counsell, SJ; Corridan, BJ; Richardson, AJ; Hajnal, JV; Appel, C; Mckee, HM; Vaddadi, KS; Horrobin, DF. MRI and neuropsychological improvement in Huntington disease following ethyl-EPA treatment. *Neuroreport* 2002;13:123-126.

[320] Puri, BK; Leavitt, BR; Hayden, MR; Ross, CA; Rosenblatt, A; Greenamyre, JT; Hersch, S; Vaddadi, KS; Sword, A; Horrobin, DF; Manku, M; Murck, H. Ethyl-EPA in Huntington disease: a double-blind, randomized, placebo-controlled trial. *Neurology* 2005;65:286-292.

[321] Vaddadi, KS; Soosai, E; Chiu, E, Dingjan, P. A randomised, placebo-controlled, double blind study of treatment of Huntington's disease with unsaturated fatty acids. *Neuroreport* 2002;13:29-33.

[322] Alan, DD; Clemens, F; Elbourne, D; Fasey, N; Fletcher, AE; Hardy, P; Holder, GE; Huppert, FA; Knight, R; Letley, L; Richards, M; Truesdale, A; Vickers, M, Uauy, R. A randomised controlled trial investigating the effect of n-3 long-chain polyunsaturated fatty acid supplementation on cognitive and retinal function in cognitively healthy older people: the Older People And n-3 Long-chain polyunsaturated fatty acids (OPAL) study protocol [ISRCTN72331636]. *Nutrition Journal* 2006;5:20.

[323] Petersen, RC; Thomas, RG; Grundman, M; Bennett, D; Doody, R; Ferris, S; Galasko, D; Jin, S; Kaye, J; Levey, A; Pfeiffer, E; Sano, M; van Dyck, CH; Thal, LJ; Alzheimer's Disease Cooperative Study Group. Vitamin E and donepezil for the treatment of mild cognitive impairment. *New England Journal of Medicine* 2005;352:2379-2388.

[324] Sano, M; Ernesto, C; Thomas, RG; Klauber, MR; Schafer, K; Grundman, M; Woodbury, P; Growdon, J; Cotman, CW; Pfeiffer, E; Schneider LS; Thal, LJ. A controlled trial of selegiline, alpha-tocopherol, or both as treatment for Alzheimer's disease. The Alzheimer's Disease Cooperative Study. *New England Journal of Medicine* 1997;336:1216-1222.

[325] Kang, JH; Cook, N; Manson, J; Buring, JE; Grodstein, F. A randomized trial of vitamin E supplementation and cognitive function in women. *Archives of Internal Medicine* 2006;166:2462-2468.

[326] Thomas, A; Iacono, D; Bonanni, L; D'Andreamatteo, G; Onofrj, M. Donepezil, rivastigmine, and vitamin E in Alzheimer disease: a combined P300 event-related potentials/neuropsychologic evaluation over 6 months. *Clinical Neuropharmacology* 2001;24:31-42.

[327] Onofrj, M; Thomas, A; Luciano, AL; Iacono, D; Di Rollo, A; D'Andreamatteo, G; Di Iorio, A. Donepezil versus vitamin E in Alzheimer's disease: Part 2: mild versus moderate-severe Alzheimer's disease. *Clinical Neuropharmacology* 2002;25:207-215.
[328] Jatoi, A; Kahanic, SP; Frytak, S; Schaefer, P; Foote, RL; Sloan, J; Petersen, RC. Donepezil and vitamin E for preventing cognitive dysfunction in small cell lung cancer patients: preliminary results and suggestions for future study designs. *Supportive Care in Cancer* 2005;13:66-69.
[329] Maurer, K; Ihl, R; Dierks, T; Frolich, L. Clinical efficacy of Ginkgo biloba special extract EGb 761 in dementia of the Alzheimer type. *Journal of Psychiatric Research* 1997;31:645-655.
[330] Francis, ST; Head, K; Morris, PG; Macdonald, IA. The effect of flavanol-rich cocoa on the fMRI response to a cognitive task in healthy young people. *Journal of Cardiovascular Pharmacology* 2006;47(Suppl 2):S215-220.
[331] Le Bars, PL; Katz, MM; Berman, N; Itil, TM; Freedman, AM; Schatzberg, AF. A placebo-controlled, double-blind, randomized trial of an extract of Ginkgo biloba for dementia. North American EGb Study Group. *Journal of the American Medical Association* 1997;278:1327-1332.
[332] [No authors listed] A randomized, double-blind, placebo-controlled trial of deprenyl and thioctic acid in human immunodeficiency virus-associated cognitive impairment. Dana Consortium on the Therapy of HIV Dementia and Related Cognitive Disorders. *Neurology* 1998;50:645-651.
[333] [No authors listed] Safety and tolerability of the free-radical scavenger OPC-14117 in Huntington's disease. The Huntington Study Group. *Neurology* 1998;50:1366-1373.
[334] [No authors listed] Safety and tolerability of the antioxidant OPC-14117 in HIV-associated cognitive impairment. The Dana Consortium on the Therapy of HIV Dementia and Related Cognitive Disorders. *Neurology* 1997;49:142-146.
[335] Duffy, R; Wiseman, H; File, SE. Improved cognitive function in postmenopausal women after 12 weeks of consumption of a soya extract containing isoflavones. *Pharmacology, Biochemistry, and Behaviour* 2003;75:721-729.
[336] Kritz-Silverstein, D; Von Muhlen, D; Barrett-Connor, E; Bressel, MA. Isoflavones and cognitive function in older women: the SOy and Postmenopausal Health In Aging (SOPHIA) Study. *Menopause* 2003;10:196-202.
[337] Kreijkamp-Kaspers, S; Kok, L; Grobbee, DE; de Haan, EH; Aleman, A; Lampe, JW; van der Schouw, YT. Effect of soy protein containing isoflavones on cognitive function, bone mineral density, and plasma lipids in postmenopausal women: a randomized controlled trial. *Journal of the American Medical Association* 2004;292:65-74.
[338] Kok, L; Kreijkamp-Kaspers, S; Grobbee, DE; Lampe, JW; van der Schouw, YT. A randomized, placebo-controlled trial on the effects of soy protein containing isoflavones on quality of life in postmenopausal women. *Menopause* 2005;12:56-62.
[339] Salas-Salvado, J; Torres, M; Planas, M; Altimir, S; Pagan, C; Gonzalez, ME; Johnston, S; Puiggros, C; Bonada, A; Garcia-Lorda, P. Effect of oral administration of a whole formula diet on nutritional and cognitive status in patients with Alzheimer's disease. *Clinical Nutrition* 2005;24:390-397.

[340] Young, KW; Greenwood, CE; van Reekum, R; Binns, MA. Providing nutrition supplements to institutionalized seniors with probable Alzheimer's disease is least beneficial to those with low body weight status. *Journal of the American Geriatrics Society* 2004;52:1305-1312.

[341] Lauque, S; Arnaud-Battandier, F; Gillette, S; Plaze, JM; Andrieu, S; Cantet, C; Vellas, B. Improvement of weight and fat-free mass with oral nutritional supplementation in patients with Alzheimer's disease at risk of malnutrition: a prospective randomized study. *Journal of the American Geriatrics Society* 2004;52:1702-1707.

[342] Riviere, S; Gillette-Guyonnet, S; Voisin, T; Reynish, E; Andrieu, S; Lauque, S; Salva, A; Frisoni, G; Nourhashemi, F; Micas, M; Vellas, B. A nutritional education program could prevent weight loss and slow cognitive decline in Alzheimer's disease. *Journal of Nutrition, Health and Aging* 2001;5:295-299.

[343] Serra-Majem, L; Roman, B; Estruch, R. Scientific evidence of interventions using the Mediterranean diet: a systematic review. *Nutrition Reviews* 2006;64(2 Pt 2):S27-47.

[344] Wolinsky, FD; Unverzagt, FW; Smith, DM; Jones, R; Stoddard, A; Tennstedt, SL. The ACTIVE cognitive training trial and health-related quality of life: protection that lasts for 5 years. *The Journal of Gerontology Series A: Biological Sciences and Medical Sciences* 2006;61:1324-1329.

[345] Ball, K; Berch, DB; Helmers, KF; Jobe, JB; Leveck, MD; Marsiske, M; Morris, JN; Rebok, GW; Smith, DM; Tennstedt, SL; Unverzagt, FW; Willis, SL; Advanced Cognitive Training for Independent and Vital Elderly Study Group. Effects of cognitive training interventions with older adults: a randomised controlled trial. *Journal of the American Medical Association* 2002;288:2271-2281.

[346] Kilonzo, MM; Vale, LD; Cook, JA; Milne, AC; Stephen, AI; Avenell, A; The MAVIS Trial Group. A cost-utility analysis of multivitamin and multimineral supplements in men and women aged 65 years and over. *Clinical Nutrition* 2007;26:364-370.

[347] White, PJ; Marette, A. Is omega-3 key to unlocking inflammation in obesity? *Diabetologia* 2006;49:1999-2001.

[348] Cereda, E; Malavazos, AE. Comment on: White PJ, Marette A (2006) is omega-3 key to unlocking inflammation in obesity? Diabetologia 49:1999-2001. *Diabetologia* 2006;49:2813-2814.

In: Nutrition for the Middle Aged and Elderly
Editors: N. E. Bernhardt, A. M. Kasko, pp. 107-156
ISBN: 978-1-60456-146-3

Chapter III

The Role of Diet and Nutrition in the Prevention of Cancer

Sa'eed Bawa
NND, Food Science and Technology; MSc, Food and Nutrition Sciences; PhD, Food and Nutrition Sciences
Department of Dietetics,
Faculty of Human Nutrition and Consumer Sciences,
Warsaw University of Life Sciences,
Nowoursynowska Street 159C, PL-02776 Warsaw, Poland

Abstract

The incidence of cancer in industrialized countries has increased since the early 1970s. It is estimated that more than one-third of cases are associated with factors related to a Western diet. Dietary factors are thought to account for about 30-40% of cancers in industrialized countries and therefore, diet is second only to tobacco as a potentially preventable cause of cancer. The contribution of diet to risk of cancer in developing countries is lower, perhaps around 20% or less. Obesity increases the risk of cancers in the esophagus, colorectum, breast, endometrium, and kidney. Alcohol causes cancers of the oral cavity, pharynx, larynx, esophagus, and liver, and causes a small increase in the risk of breast cancer. The consumption of nutrient sparse foods containing simple sugars brings about the impairment of glucose metabolism consequently leading to insulin resistance. Insulin resistance increases the risk of the development of cancer at many sites. Low intake of fiber, high consumption of red meat, and imbalance of omega-3 and omega-6 fats all increase significantly the risk of cancer. The inclusion to the diet of foods containing phytochemicals, such as flax seed, cruciferous vegetables, particularly broccoli sprouts can significantly decrease cancer risk. Antioxidant vitamins and minerals, such as the carotenoids (α-carotene, β-carotene, lycopene, lutein, and cryptoxanthin), vitamins C and E as well as selenium and zinc have been shown to protect against cancer. Recent scientific trials have shown the importance of pre-, pro- and synbiotics in decreasing the risk of the development of cancer, particularly of the gastrointestinal tract. Milk and dairy products are the good source of calcium and vitamin

D. Dairy products are a diverse food group comprising of various factors that could influence risk, e.g., relatively high saturated fat content, growth factors such as IGF-I, and chemical contaminants such as pesticide residues. However, the calcium, vitamin D, and CLA contents of dairy products have been hypothesized to reduce the cancer risk. Adherence to dietary food guidelines can help diminish the incidence of many types of cancers, including breast cancer, colorectal cancer, prostate cancer even by about 50-70%. The relationship between diet, nutrition and the development of cancer are presented in this review. Emphasis will be given to prospective epidemiologic studies because these are less subject to serious problems of confounding that can make cross-cultural comparisons completely misleading, and they avoid the problem of recall bias that can affect typical case-control studies of diet.

Introduction

Cancer is a multi-factorial disease that develops over a long period of time and progresses through different stages. Cancer is not a single disorder, because it covers a number of diseases that affect different sites in the body and have different causes. Whether we develop cancer depends on the environment we live in, how we live in that environment, and our family history (our genetic make-up). The development of cancer involves damage to the DNA of the cells making up the cancerous mass. This damage accumulates over time: cancerous cells replicate and escape the internal mechanisms that usually protect the person from the growth and spread of such cells.

All cancers are diseases of abnormal cell proliferation, development and death. During the earliest stages of human life all of the embryonic cells divide constantly, and differentiate to form the specialized tissues and organs. Throughout infancy and childhood cell proliferation continues at whatever rates are necessary to fulfill the requirements of growth, but as maturity is reached organs such as the central nervous system, muscles and skeletal tissues cease to grow, and cell division becomes minimal. However, certain tissues continue to proliferate throughout life. These include the blood-forming tissues, the epithelia which line the surfaces of the body exposed to the environment, the glandular tissues which produce secretions, and the sexual organs which produce new reproductive cells. Cancer can affect virtually any organ of the body but tissues such as those of the lungs and gut, which have characteristically high rates of cell division and chronic exposure to the external environment, are particularly vulnerable.

As mentioned earlier, carcinogenesis is a prolonged multi-stage process which usually occurs over many years. Because of its complexity there are, in principle, many critical steps at which food-related substances or metabolic processes may interact with the sequence of events so as to accelerate, delay or even reverse it. Diet-related anti-carcinogenesis can usefully be classified into blocking mechanisms, which operate during the initiation phase of carcinogenesis, and suppressing mechanisms, which delay or reverse tumor promotion at a later stage [1, 2].

The principal blocking mechanism through which dietary constituents are thought to act is modulation of the Phase I and Phase II biotransformation enzymes which are expressed strongly in the gastrointestinal mucosa and in the liver and act as a first line of defence against toxic substances in the environment [3]. Phase I enzymes such as the cytochrome P450 complex catalyze oxidation, reduction and hydrolytic reactions, thereby increasing the solubility of potentially toxic compounds. However, this phase may also create electrophilic intermediates and hence activate procarcinogens. Phase II enzymes such as glutathione *S*-transferase act on the products of Phase I metabolism to form conjugates, which generally reduces their reactivity and increases their excretion. Thus the biological activity of a carcinogen will often depend upon the relative activities of the Phase I and II enzymes involved in its metabolism. Pharmacological and dietary treatments can be used to block Phase I enzymes and enhance Phase II activity, so as to minimize the activation of carcinogens and increase their excretion. There is good evidence from experimental animal studies that this strategy can reduce DNA damage and tumor yield [4].

Experimental animal studies have also shown that some substances can inhibit the appearance of tumors, even when given days or weeks after exposure to a chemical carcinogen [5]. Hence the mechanism of action cannot involve protection against DNA damage, but can instead be due to some reduction in the rate at which initiated cells develop into tumors.

Suppression of carcinogenesis may involve inhibition of mitosis and increased expression of the differentiated phenotype, which serves to reduce the clonal expansion of initiated cells, or an increased susceptibility to undergo programmed cell death or apoptosis, which can eliminate precancerous cells from the tissue [6, 7].

The detoxifying/biotransformation enzymes play a vital role in deciding the final fate of carcinogens or procarcinogens and their subsequent influence on the process of carcinogenesis. As mentioned ealier, the purpose of physiological system is to increase the water solubility of carcinogenic substances in order to facilitate their excretion; this purpose is achieved in two phases. Phase I enzymes (cytochrome P450 and flavin-dependent monooxygenases) convert lipophilic compounds into more hydrophilic intermediates. In certain cases, this process can also give rise to carcinogens from biologically inactive compounds (procarcinogens) and, thus, inhibition of phase I enzymes may be protective. Subsequently, phase II enzymes (e.g., glutathione-*S*-transferases, UDP-glucuronosyltransferases, sulfotransferases, *N*-acetyl-transferases) catalyze conjugation reactions with molecules such as glutathione, glucuronic acid, or sulfate to render the toxic substances even more water soluble; and eventually, they are excreted through urine or bile.

Cancer is a disease strongly associated with age, as is evident from the very low occurrence of cancer in the first decade of life, which rises to an incidence of about 30% in the seventh decade. In this regard it may be considered a disease of the elderly, although from another viewpoint the multi-step nature of carcinogenesis suggests that the disease actually originates much earlier in life.

Diet is one of the most important lifestyle factors and has been estimated to account for up to 80% of cancers of the large bowel, breast, and prostate [8, 9]. Even lung cancer may have a dietary component, although cigarette smoking is the overwhelming cause of this and contributes also to oropharyngeal, esophageal, and bladder cancer. Physical activity, reproductive and sexual behavior, infection with hepatitis B and C viruses, infection with helicobacter, and exposure to sunlight, ionizing radiation, and environmental chemicals are also important at particular sites. Nevertheless, food and drink has a part to play in many if not all cancers, albeit to a variable extent.

Cancer Trends

Cancer is a major cause of mortality worldwide and, in the developed world, is generally exceeded only by cardiovascular diseases. An estimated 10 million new cases and over 6 million deaths from cancer occurred in 2000 [11]. As developing countries become urbanized, patterns of cancer, including those most strongly associated with diet, tend to shift towards those of economically developed countries. Cancer rates change as populations move between countries and adopt different dietary (and other) behaviors, further implicating dietary factors in the etiology of cancer.

Between 2000 and 2020, the total number of cases of cancer in the developing world is predicted to increase by 73% and, in the developed world, to increase by 29%, largely as a result of an increase in the number of old people [11].

Due to insufficient and lack of data on diet and cancer, it is quite difficult to define cancer trends in developing countries. Data are very limited from Africa, Asia and Latin America, yet these regions represent two-thirds or more of the world population. There is thus an urgent need for epidemiological research on diet and cancer in these regions. It is very important to address and evaluate the role of food processing methods, traditional and industrial in the development of cancer. Microbiological and chemical food contaminants may also contribute to carcinogenicity of diets. Nutrition transition is accompanied by changes in prevalence of specific cancers. For some cancers, such as stomach cancer, this may be beneficial while for others, such as colorectal and breast cancers, the changes are adverse. During nutrition transition and as developing countries become urbanized, people tend to adopt the Western lifestyle, including over-consumption of animal products. Excess consumption of meat can increase the risk of chronic diseases, including cancer (see Table 5 below).

Energy, Macronutrients and Cancer

Although prolonged energy as well as macro- and micronutrient malnutrition may increase an individual's risk of developing cancer, probably by decreasing the effectiveness of the immune system, life expectancy in societies with large malnourished populations is low, and infectious diseases are more likely to be the principal causes of illness and mortality. In prosperous Western societies, over-consumption of energy, coupled with inadequate exercise, appears to be a major risk factor for cancer.

For nearly a century, energy (caloric) restriction has been known to reduce the development of mammary tumors in animals. This effect has been observed in a variety of mammary tumor models and also for other tumors. The impact of energy restriction can be profound; for example, a 30-40% lower intake has reduced mammary tumors by 30-90% [14, 15, 16]. Mechanistically, the beneficial effect of this practice has been attributed largely to reduced oxidative stress on cellular structures, especially the mitochondrion, which results in less mitochondrial dysfunction arising from oxidatively induced mutations in mitochondrial DNA and consequent defects in the tricarboxylic acid cycle and the electron transport chain [16]. Also, although less definitive in outcome, high levels of antioxidant supplementation in several experimental animal studies have been reported to increase the average life span, which lends some further support to the notion of oxidative damage as a central mechanism in the aging process [16, 17].

It was estimated in a recent study, from a prospective cancer prevention cohort, that overweight and obesity accounted for 14 percent of all cancer deaths in men and 20 percent of those in women [18]. Significant positive associations were found between obesity and higher death rates for the following cancers: esophagus, colon and rectum, liver, gallbladder, pancreas, kidney, stomach (in men), prostate, breast, uterus, cervix, and ovary [18]. The authors estimated that over 90,000 cancer deaths per year could be avoided if the adult population maintained a normal weight (BMI < 25.0) [18].Taking into considerations the results of this study, it could be stated clearly that obesity is a major risk factor for cancer. It seems plausible to restrict energy intake to 70-80% of requirement to decrease cancer risk. This level of energy consumption does not comprise the delivery of vitamins and minerals that play important role in the prevention of cancer. Consumption of large amounts of energy and protein of animal origin can increase the risk of cancers at many sites, particularly breast via the elevation of insulin-like growth factors, especially IGF-1 concentration in the blood. Mechanisms, whereby IGF-1 increases cancer risk is presented in Figure 1 below.

Long-term positive energy balance increases the risk of overweight and obesity and there is now compelling evidence that excess body weight is a risk factor for many cancers. Cancers of the colon, breast, endometrium, kidney, and esophagus are convincingly associated with adiposity, but the link to prostate cancer is controversial. The strongest relationship observed for a nutrition-related factor and breast cancer is for relative body weight, generally indicated by body mass index (BMI: weight in kg divided by the square of height in m^2). The relationship of BMI with breast cancer risk differs by menopausal status. In premenopausal women, most studies have found either no association or a weak inverse relationship between BMI and breast cancer risk [20] although positive associations have sometimes been observed in countries with moderate or low rates of breast cancer [21].

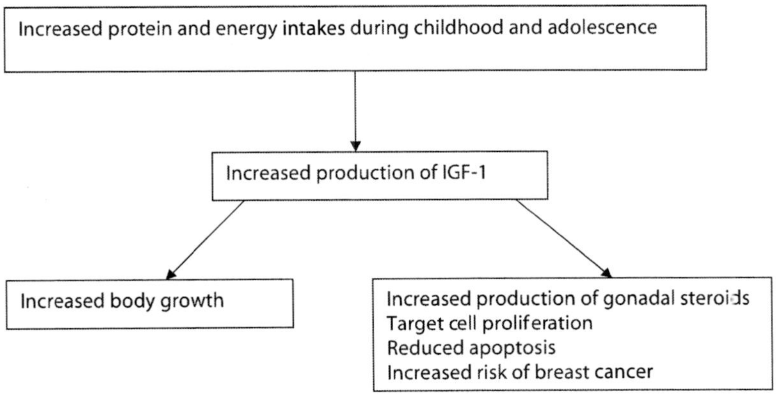

Figure 1. Cancer promoting actions of IGF-1 (19).

In postmenopausal women, however, the risk for breast cancer clearly increases with increasing BMI. A pooled analysis of seven prospective studies has shown that the risk of developing breast cancer is approximately 30% higher among postmenopausal women with a BMI of over 31 kg/m^2 compared with women with a BMI of about 20 kg/m^2 [22]. Due to the high and increasing prevalence of overweight and obesity this is an important potentially modifiable risk factor and there is a need to devise effective interventions at a population level.

The effect of BMI on breast cancer risk is probably due to the effects of BMI on endogenous estradiol levels. Women with a high BMI and more adipose tissue have more aromatase, which catalyses the conversion of androstenedione to estrone, which can then be converted to estradiol [23, 24]. This conversion occurs in women at all ages, but in premenopausal women estradiol production predominantly comes from the ovaries and is controlled by negative feedback, so there is little if any association between BMI and levels of free estradiol [25]. In postmenopausal women, the ovaries no longer produce estradiol, and most estradiol is derived from the conversion of androgens to estrogens in the adipose tissue; this estradiol production is not regulated by feedback, therefore obese postmenopausal women have up to about two-fold higher serum estradiol concentrations than thin postmenopausal women. Sex hormone-binding globulin levels fall with increasing body mass index, thus increasing the proportion of estradiol that is freely available to enter the cells. Thus, a high BMI is associated with an even greater increase in concentration of free estradiol than the two-fold increase in the concentration of total estradiol [25].

Fats and Cancer

Evidence suggests that dietary fats are associated with risk of cancer at many sites. The effects of fats depend not only on the quantity, but also on the composition of specific fatty acids. Moreover, fats particularly of the omega-6 family are peroxidizable, and peroxidation products as well as antioxidants play a role in the pathogenic process of cancer development. Essential fatty acids (EFAs) of the omega-6 family increase cancer risk, because the may induce COX-2 over-expression and augment PGE_2 production, which are features of cancer development and progression. Table 1 shows the properties and functions of different fatty acids.

Table 1. Major causes of cancer [8]

Factor	Estimated % of all cancer deaths
Diet	35
Tobacco	30
Infection	10
Reproductive and sexual behavior	7
Occupation	4
Alcohol	3
Geophysical factors	3
Pollution	2
Industrial products	1
Medicines and medical procedures	1
Food additives	<1

There are two categories of EFAs: omega-3 fatty acids (ω3FAs) and omega-6 fatty acids (ω6FAs); both groups originate from lipids ingested in the diet as the body is unable to synthesize them due to lack the enzymes Δ-15-desaturase and Δ-12-desaturase, respectively [26]. While ω6FAs are plentiful in foods such as cereal grains, processed foods, meat, milk, eggs and some vegetable oils, ω3FAs are found in significant quantity in only a few seeds and nuts, as well as in fish oil. Both families of fatty acids provide required substrate for the production of eicosanoids, which include important bioactive compounds such as prostaglandins, leukotrienes and thromboxanes (Figure 2).

Eicosanoids originating from ω6FAs act biochemically to promote cell proliferation, inflammation and blood clotting while eicosanoids originating from ω3FAs oppose these effects and facilitate anti-inflammatory action, inhibitory effects on cell growth, and blood thinning. Both groups of EFAs compete for the same limited supply of enzymes in the biochemical assembly of eicosanoids and diets with high ω6FAs:ω3FAs (ω6/3) ratios will diminish the effectiveness of ω3FAs-dependent processes, leading to an overabundance of omega-6 derived eicosanoids. The relative concentration of ω6FAs and ω3FAs consumed in the diet is a matter of major import to the biochemical and clinical functioning of many organs in the human body [26].

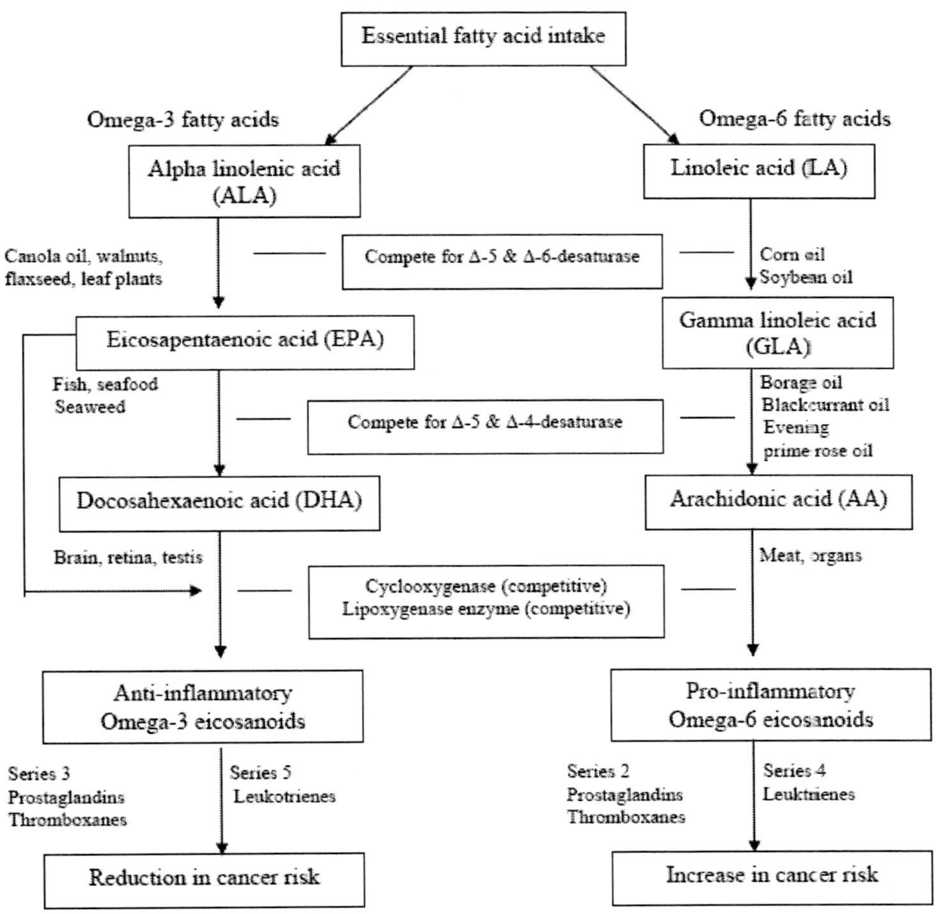

Figure 2. Metabolism of essential fatty acid and their sources.

Table 2. Summary of strength of evidence on lifestyle factors and the risk of developing cancer [10]

Evidence	Decreased risk	Increased risk
Convincing*	Physical activity (colon)	Overweight and obesity (esophagus, colorectum, breast in postmenopausal women, endometrium, kidney), alcohol (oral cavity, pharynx, larynx, esophagus, liver, breast), aflatoxin (liver), Chinese-style salted fish (nasopharynx)
Probable*	Fruits and vegetables (oral cavity, esophagus, stomach, colorectum**), physical activity (breast)	Preserved meat (colorectum) Salt-preserved foods and salt (stomach) Very hot (thermally) drinks and food (oral cavity, pharynx, esophagus)
Possible/ insufficient	Fiber, soy, fish, n-3 fatty acids, carotenoids, vitamins B_2, B_6, folate, B_{12}, C, D, E, calcium, zinc and selenium, non-nutrient plant constituents (e.g. allium compounds, flavonoids, isoflavones, lignans)	Animal fats, heterocyclic amines, polycyclic aromatic hydrocarbons, nitrosamines

* The ''convincing'' and ''probable'' categories correspond to the ''sufficient'' category of the IARC report on weight control and physical activity in terms of the public health and policy implications.

** For colorectal cancer, a protective effect of fruit and vegetable intake has been suggested by many case-control studies but this has not been supported by results of several large prospective studies, suggesting that if a benefit does exist it is likely to be modest.

Table 3. Dietary risk factors for major cancers [12, 13]

	Probable		Possible	
Site of cancer	Increases risk	Decreases risk	Increases risk	Decreases risk
Colorectum	Red meat, processed meat	Vegetables (non-starch polysaccharides (fiber)	Alcohol, fat	Folate
Breast	Alcohol, red meat, fried meat	Vegetables		Fruit, phytoestrogens
Lung			Alcohol, meat	Fruit and vegetables
Stomach	Salt, pickled and preserved foods	Fruit and vegetables, vitamin C		Carotenoids
Prostate		Vitamin E	Red meat, fat	Vegetables
Cervix		Fruit and vegetables, vitamin C		Folate, vitamin A
Pancreas			Red meat	Fruit and vegetables, vitamin C, non-starch polysaccharides (fiber)
Bladder		Fruit and vegetables		
Liver	Alcohol			

Table 4. Lifestyle and other factors affecting cancer risk [10, 11]

Type/site of cancer	Increased risk	Decreased risk
Colorectal	Adenomatous polyps, inflammatory bowel disease, obesity (men)	Physical activity
Breast	Early menarche, late menopause, older age at first pregnancy, height, obesity (after menopause)	Physical activity
Lung	Smoking, occupation	Physical activity
Stomach	*Helicobacter pylori* infection	
Prostate		
Cervix	Human papillomavirus, smoking	
Endometrium	Exposure to unopposed estrogen, obesity	
Esophagus	Smoking, Barrett's esophagus (gastro-esophageal reflux disease	
Pancreas	Smoking	
Bladder	Smoking, occupation, schistosoma infection	
Liver	Hepatitis B and C infection	
Ovary		Extended use of oral contraceptives

Table 5. A qualitative assessment of the relationships between the intakes of animal products and the of diet-related diseases

	Red meat (Beef, pork, lamb)	Poultry	Fish	Egg*	Dairy Products
Coronary heart diseases	Probably ↑	Possibly ↓	Probably ↓	Probably no increase in risk	Probably small ↑**
Hemorrhagic Stroke†	Possibly ↓	Possibly ↓	Uncertain §	Probably no increase in risk	Possibly ↓
Breast cancer	Possibly ↑	Probably no relation	Probably no relation	Probably no relation	Probably no relation
Colon cancer	Probably ↑	Possibly ↓	Possibly ↓	Probably no increase in risk	Probably no increase in risk
Prostate cancer	Probably ↑	Probably no relation	Probably no relation	Probably no relation	Probably ↑‡

↓ Increase in risk; ↑ decrease in risk

* Up to 1 egg per day

** It is possible that substitution of low-fat dairy (e.g., skim milk) for high-fat dairy products (e.g., whole milk) decreases risk of cardiovascular disease for individuals, but this is largely irrelevant for population disease rates because the dairy fat produced is almost inevitably consumed.

† The associations between animal products and risk of ischemic stroke, which is more common in the US, are probably similar to those for CHD.

‡ It is unclear whether it is due to fat or calcium.

§ Data are limited. It is possible that higher intake increases risk.

Table 6. Characteristics of different fatty acids

Fatty acid	Carbons: double bonds	Major dietary sources	Major functional roles
Butyric acid	4:0	Butter, cheese	Induction of apoptosis, gene regulation
Lauric acid	12:0	Coconut milk, baked sweets, chocolate	Protection of polyunsaturated fatty acids against peroxidation, inhibition of malignant cell lines growth
Myristic acid	14:0	Fish oil, coconut, meat	Protection of polyunsaturated fatty acids against peroxidation
Palmitic acid	16:0	Vegetable oil, salad dressing	Energy storage
Stearic acid	18:0	Shortening, butter	Phospholipid structure
Oleic	18:1	acid Beef, pork	Induction of fatty acid oxidation
Linoleic acid	18:2	Shortening, animal fat	Arachidonic acid precursor
α-Linolenic acid	18:3	Canola oil, mayonnaise	Eicosapentaenoic acid precursor
Arachidonic acid	20:4	Shitterlings, sardine oil	Substrate for 2-series prostaglandins
Eicosapentaenoic acid	20:5	Fish oil, fish	Substrate for 3-series prostaglandins
Docosahexaenoic acid	22:6	Fish oil, fish	Induction of apoptosis
Total *trans* fatty acids	–	Margarine, shortening	Disruption of eicosanoid synthesis and of the phospholipids cell membrane

Inflammation, which is the body's non-specific response to trauma and chemical or microbial aggression is associated with rubor, tumor, calor and dolor (redness, swelling, heat, and pain). These symptoms arise from the release of mediators derived mainly from the activation of leukocytes. They include prostaglandin E_2 and Leukotriene B_4 produced during the metabolism of arachidonate that belongs to the ω6FAs. EPA promotes the formation of prostaglandin E_3 and leukotriene B_5, which are less active proinflammatory compounds than the corresponding derivatives of omega-6 precursors. EPA and DHA can also inhibit the synthesis of other proinflammatory agents, such as interleukin-1, interleukin-6, and tumor necrosis factor. Under normal circumstances, the inflammatory response has a protective and beneficial function. However, when it becomes chronic or exaggerated, it can lead to generation of reactive oxygen species that can damage DNA, thereby increasing the risk of cancer.

Carbohydrates and Risk for the Development of Cancer

The consumption of complex carbohydrates, especially from whole grains has been reported to decrease cancer risk via many mechanisms. Complex carbohydrates ingested in the form of whole grains are rich sources of fermentable carbohydrates including dietary fiber, resistant starch and oligosaccharides. Undigested carbohydrate that reaches the colon is fermented by intestinal microflora to short chain fatty acids and gases. Short chain fatty acids include acetate, butyrate and propionate, with butyrate being a preferred fuel for the colonic mucosa cells. Undigested carbohydrates increase fecal wet and dry weight and speed intestinal transit.

SCFAs are the main end products of fermentation of dietary fibers in the human large bowel [27]. The principal SCFAs include acetic (C2:0), propionic (C3:0) and butyric acids (C4:0), which account for 85–95% of total fecal SCFAs [28]. Dietary sources of SCFAs are almost entirely dairy products. Recent data support the notion that endogenous colon production of SCFAs may decrease the risk of neoplasia in colonocytes through mechanisms that include the induction of apoptosis [29] as well as the regulation of histone acetylation, which is important in gene regulation [30]. Among the three major SCFAs, acetic and propionic acids have been scarcely investigated, particularly in relation to colorectal cancer risk. Butyric acid has attracted the most attention because it is considered a major candidate that could explain the hypothesized protective effect of dietary fibers against colorectal cancer.

Few epidemiologic studies collect biomarkers of gut function such as stool weight or transit time. Cummings et al. [31] collected data from 20 populations in 12 countries and found that average stool weight varied from 72 to 470 grams/day and was inversely related to colon cancer risk. It is known that different dietary fibers have different effects on stool weight. Wheat bran is most effective in increasing stool weight, with each gram of fiber fed as wheat bran increasing stool weight by 5.4 grams [32]. In contrast, soluble fibers like pectin only increase stool weight by 1.2 grams per gram of fiber fed.

Table 7. Dietary sources of soluble and insoluble fiber

<table>
<tr><td colspan="2">Sources of Fiber</td></tr>
<tr><td>Soluble Fiber</td><td>Insoluble Fiber</td></tr>
<tr><td>Oatmeal
Oat-bran
Nuts and seeds
Legumes
• Dried peas
• Beans
• Lentils
Apples
Pears
Strawberries
Blueberries</td><td>Whole grains
• Whole wheat breads
• Barley
• Couscous
• Brown rice
• Bulgur
Whole-grain breakfast cereals
• Wheat bran
• Seeds
• Carrots
• Cucumbers
• Zucchini
• Celery
• Tomatoes</td></tr>
</table>

Table 8. Sources of fiber in the American diet

Food Source	Serving Size	Grams of Dietary Fiber
Apple	1 medium	3.3
Banana	1 large (8-8 7/8 inches)	3.5
Baked Beans	½ cup, USDA recipe	4.2
Beans, Refried	½ cup, canned	6.7
Bread, Whole Wheat	Slice	Varies (read label)
Broccoli	½ cup, chopped, raw	1.2
Burrito, Beef	1, USDA recipe	2
Cantaloupe	½ cup, diced	0.7
Carrot	1 medium, raw	1.7
Celery	½ cup sticks	1.2
Cereal	1 oz	Varies (read label)
Chili Con Carne With Beans	½ cup, USDA recipe	2.5
Coleslaw	½ cup, USDA recipe	2
Corn	½ cup, frozen, cooked	2
Cucumber	½ cup, peeled	0.4
Grapes	½ cup	0.4
Kiwi Fruit	1 large without skin	2.7
Lentils	½ cup, cooked	7.8
Lettuce, Iceberg	1 cup, shredded	0.9
Mixed Vegetables, Frozen	½ cup, cooked	4
Oatmeal	½ cup, cooked	1.9
Peanuts	¼ cup, dry roasted	2.9
Peas, Split	½ cup, cooked	8.1
Potato, Baked with Skin	1 medium (2.25" x 3.25")	3.8
Potatoes, Mashed	½ cup, USDA commodity	0.8
Raisins	¼ cup	1.3
Rice, Brown, Medium Grain	½ cup, cooked	1.8
Rice, White, Long Grain	½ cup, cooked	0.4
Strawberries	½ cup, whole	1.4

Several mechanisms have been proposed for the protective action of dietary fiber against cancer. Increased fecal bulk and decreased transit time allow less opportunity for fecal mutagens to interact with the intestinal epithelium. Secondary bile acids are thought to promote cell proliferation, thus allowing increased opportunity for mutations to occur and increased replication of abnormal cells. The effect of fiber on the actions of bile acids may be attributable to the binding or diluting of bile acids. Fermentation of dietary fiber results in production of short chain fatty acids which lower intestinal pH; this inhibits the conversion of primary bile acids to secondary bile acids. At low pH, the solubility of free bile acids is reduced, diminishing their availability for cocarcinogenic activity. Fermentation of dietary fiber results in production of butyrate, a short-chain fatty acid that has been shown to be antineoplastic [33].

Not all starch is digested and absorbed during gut transit. Factors that determine whether starch is resistant to digestion include the physical form of grains or seeds in which starch is located, particularly if these are whole or partially disrupted, size and type of starch granules, associations between starch and other dietary components, and cooking and food processing, especially cooking and cooling [34]. Because the starch in whole grains is believed to be more resistant to digestion than refined starch, whole grains should improve the gut environment.

Besides dietary fiber and resistant starch, grains contain significant amounts of oligosaccharides. Oligosaccharides are defined as carbohydrates with low (2-20) degree of polymerization. Common oligosaccharides include oligofructose and inulin. Wheat flour contains from 1% to 4% fructan on a dry weight basis [35]. Fructans have also been found in rye and barley with very young barley kernels containing 22% fructan [35]. Van Loo has estimated that wheat provides 78% of the North American intake of oligosaccharides [35]. Oligosaccharides are thought to have similar effects as soluble dietary fibers in the human gut. Additionally, oligosaccharides have consistently been shown able to alter the human fecal flora. Many human studies [36, 37] find that consumption of fructooligosaccharides (FOS) increases bifidobacteria in the gut while decreasing concentrations of E. coli, clostridia and bacteroides.

Simple Sugars and Cancer Risk

Refined sugar is a high energy, low nutrient dense food. Refined wheat flour products do not contain the wheat germ and bran and have 78 percent less fiber, an average of 74 percent less of the B vitamins and vitamin E, and 69 percent less of the minerals. Concentrated sugars and refined flour products make up a large portion of the carbohydrate intake in the diet of the inhabitants of industrialized countries. One way to measure the impact of these foods on the development of chronic diseases is through the glycemic index. The glycemic index is an indication of the blood sugar response of the body to a standardized amount of carbohydrate in a food. The glycemic load takes into account the amount of food eaten. An international table of the glycemic index and glycemic load of a wide variety of foods has been published [38].

Case-control studies and prospective population studies have tested the hypothesis that there is an association between a diet with a high glycemic load and cancer. The case control studies have found consistent increased risk of a high glycemic load with gastric [39], upper aero digestive tract [40], endometrial [41], ovarian [42], colon or colorectal cancers [43, 44].

The results of prospective studies have been mixed. Some studies showed increased risk of cancer in the whole cohort with high glycemic load [45-47]; some studies found only increased risk among subgroups such as sedentary, overweight subjects [48-51]; other studies concluded that there was no increased risk for any of their cohort [52-55]. Even though there were no associations between glycemic load and colorectal, breast, or pancreatic cancer in the Nurses' Health Study there was still a strong link between diabetes and colorectal cancer [56].

Perhaps the dietary glycemic load is not consistently related to glucose disposal and insulin metabolism due to individual's different responses to the same glycemic load.

Glycated hemoglobin (HbA1c) is a time-integrated measurement of glucose control, and indirectly, of insulin levels. Increased risk in colorectal cancer was seen in the EPIC-Norfolk study with increasing HbA1c; subjects with known diabetes had a three-fold increased risk of colorectal cancer [57]. In a study of a cohort in Washington county, Maryland, increased risk of colorectal cancer was seen in subjects with elevated HbA1c, BMI > 30 kg/m2, or who used medications to control diabetes [58]. However, glycated hemoglobin was not found to be associated with increased risk of colorectal cancer in a small nested case-control study within the Nurses' Health Study [59]. Elevated fasting glucose, fasting insulin, 2 hour levels of glucose and insulin after an oral glucose challenge, and larger waist circumference were associated with a higher risk of colorectal cancer [60]. In multiple studies diabetes has been linked with increased risk of colorectal cancer [61-64], endometrial cancer [65], and pancreatic cancer [66, 67]. It is clear that severe dysregulation of glucose metabolism is a risk factor for cancer. Foods which contribute to hyperinsulinemia, such as refined sugar, foods containing refined sugar, and refined flour products should be avoided and eliminated from a cancer protective diet.

Low-Fiber, High-Sucrose Diet

Unrefined plant foods typically have an abundance of fiber. Dairy products, eggs, and meat all have this in common – they contain no fiber. Refined grain products also have most of the dietary fiber removed from them. So, a diet high in animal products and refined grains (a typical diet in the USA) is low in fiber. In prospective health studies low fiber was not found to be a risk for breast cancer [68]. It is possible that fiber measurements are just a surrogate measure for unrefined plant food intake. Slattery et al. [69] found an inverse correlation between vegetable, fruit and whole grain intake plant food intake and rectal cancer, while refined grains were associated with increased risk of rectal cancer. A threshold of about 5 daily servings of vegetables was needed to reduce cancer risk and the effect was stronger among older subjects [69].

High-sucrose products when heated at high temperatures may contain compounds that are genetoxic. Other harmful effects of high-sucrose diets include: (a) increase colon transit time, thereby increasing carcinogen contact time; (b) increase fecal concentration of total and secondary bile acids; (c) increase colorectal epithelial cell proliferation.

The Role of Selected Micronutrients in the Development of Cancer

Calcium, Vitamin D and the Prevention of Cancer

The calcium content of the human body is 25 to 30 g at birth (0.8% of the body weight) and between 900 and 1300 g in adult men (up to 1.7% of body weight) (Weaver et al, 1996). Over 99% of the total calcium of the body is located in the bones, where it accounts for 39% of the total body bone mineral content [70], and in the teeth, mostly as hydroxyapatite. Bone mineral provides structure and strength to the body and, very important, a reservoir of calcium that helps to maintain a constant concentration of blood calcium. Less than 1% of total body calcium is found in soft tissues (~7 g) and body fluids (~1 g). Calcium in the extracellular fluid and the blood are kept constant at 2.5 mmol/L (10 mg/dL) (between 2.25 and 2.75 mmol/L) via cell surface calcium-sensing receptors in parathyroid, kidney, intestine, lung, brain, skin, bone marrow, osteoblasts and other organs.

Calcium deficiency can result from low dietary intake, low absorption or excessive losses. A decrease in ionized calcium in the extracellular fluid stimulates the secretion of parathyroid hormone to mobilize calcium from bone and maintain the pre-set serum calcium level.

Calcium reduces the risk for the development of colon cancer by binding bile acids and fatty acids rendering them unavailable in this organ. Overall diets high in red meat and animal fat or calories may be associated with an increased risk of colorectal cancer [71]. These types of diets may increase the production of secondary bile acids, which may cause an increased proliferation of the colorectal epithelium [72]. Calcium binds to bile and fatty acids in the colon and may directly inhibit the growth of intestinal epithelial cells.

Table 9. Calcium content of selected foods

Foods	Calcium content (mg)
Collards	360
Orange juice (fortified)	350
Sardines	325
Oatmeal (instant)	325
Yogurt	300
Milk	300
Figs (dried)	270
Cheese	270
Spinach	244
Almonds	235
Brewer's yeast	210
Soybeans	175
Watercress	150
Beans (other)	50–100
Nuts (other)	50–100
Kale	95
Brussels sprouts	55
Orange	55
Raisins	50
Brown rice	50
Carrots	35

Table 10. Similarities and differences between some commercially available calcium supplements in the USA and Europe*

Calcium supplements	Brand name (examples)	Absorption directions
Calcium carbonate (contains 40% elemental calcium)	Caltrate, OsCal, Rolaids, TUMS, Viactiv (chewable calcium product (20 calories each)	Should be taken with food
Calcium citrate or calcium citrate malate (contains 21% elemental calcium)	Citracal	Can be taken with or without food probably the preferred form for those with a history or risk of oxalate kidney stones
Calcium phosphate (contains 39% elemental calcium)	Posture	Can be taken with or without food

Most of the epidemiologic data in humans demonstrate a reduction in the risk of colon cancer or colorectal adenoma with higher calcium intakes from diet or supplements, but only a limited number of these studies reached statistical significance [73, 74]. The major limitation of the epidemiologic data is the overall lack of specific assessment of calcium intake and the potential for confounding by other dietary compounds. A study of 930 patients with a history of colorectal adenomas were randomly assigned to receive either daily supplements consisting of 1200 mg of elemental calcium (3 g overall) or placebo daily for 4 years [75]. The analysis was limited to the 832 patients (409 in the calcium group and 423 in the placebo group) who completed both follow-up examinations (colonoscopies). A significant 15% lower rate of adenoma recurrence occurred in patients taking calcium dietary supplements. Interestingly, the effect of calcium was independent of baseline dietary fat and calcium intake. A recent 3-year randomized trial from Europe observed a similar result [76]. However, clinicians should keep in mind that the effect of calcium supplementation in patients without a history of polyps or as a cancer prevention supplement has not been evaluated. Regardless, some authors currently cite that the preliminary data on calcium supplements for colorectal cancer prevention is as promising as most other potential chemoprevention interventions [77]. Interestingly, cancers such as breast, colon, and prostate have preliminary evidence that higher intakes of vitamin D, and possibly calcium, may reduce the risk of these diseases and other carcinomas [78].

Milk and milk products are excellent sources of bioavailable calcium, but some vegetables, especially green leafy vegetables are also good sources of this mineral. Table 9 presents dietary sources of calcium, both of animal and plant origin.

Vitamin D

There are seven known forms of vitamin D, but only about two forms are well-known and heard by the general population. The most common form is D2 or egrocalciferol. This form of D is the most common commercial type, because it can be readily prepared from plant materials that contain the compound ergosterol. Vitamin D3, cholecalciferol, is the form that animals (including humans) synthesize from cholesterol.

Vitamin D is synthesized mainly from skin exposure to sunshine. The synthesis of vitamin D begins with cholesterol. When solar ultraviolet B radiation (UVB at 290-315 nm) penetrates the skin, 7-dehydrocholesterol in the plasma membrane of the skin cells absorbs it. This leads to the ring opening of 7-dehydrocholesterol to form previtamin D3 (cholecalciferol). Cholecalciferol, in turn, is metabolized first in the liver with the aid of 25α-hydroxylase enzyme to 25-hydroxycholecalciferol, then in the kidney, with the participation of 1α-hydroxylase to the active hormone 1,25-dihydroxycholecalciferol (see figure 3 below). This mechanism, should supply enough vitamin D such that dietary and supplemental forms are not needed in the presence of adequate sunlight exposure. It has been found that even sporadic contact of the face, hands, and arms with sunlight in the summer produces a large amount of vitamin D, but dark skinned individuals require 5 to 10 times this exposure. In fact, simulated sunshine, equivalent to standing on a sunny beach until a slight pinkness of the skin was detected, was equivalent to a 20,000 IU oral dose of vitamin D2 [79].

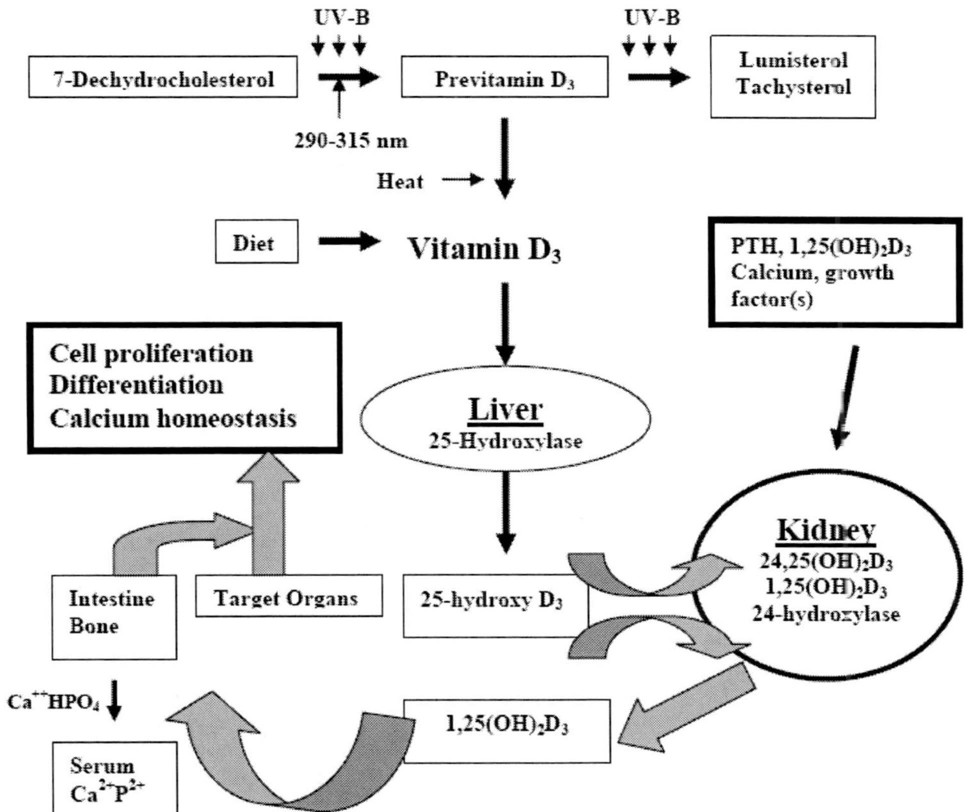

Figure 3. Metabolism of vitamin D with pathways for the conversion of 7-hydrocholesterol to previtamin D_3 by UV light and its subsequent processing to vitamin D_3 and active metabolite 1,25-dihydroxyvitamin D_3. Vitamin D metabolism by liver and its processing by kidney are also presented in this diagram.

It is worth stating that the RDA is 400 IU for most adults. It has been estimated that 1,000 IU per day is the minimal amount needed to maintain adequate levels of vitamin D in the absence of sunshine [79], and that up to 4,000 IU per day can be safely used with additional benefit [80].

Factors affecting the synthesis of vitamin D are: season, latitude, time of day, skin pigmentation, obesity, aging, sunscreen use and glass. During late autumn and early spring very little vitamin D is produced in the skin of people living above 37° latitude. In the absence of sunlight, 1000 IUs of vitamin D3 are necessary to maintain a physiological level of 25-hydroxyvitamin D above 75 nmol/l.

Table 11. Selected food sources of vitamin D

Food	International Units	%DV*
Cod Liver Oil, 1 Tbs.	1360 IU	340
Salmon, cooked, 3 1/2 oz	360 IU	90
Mackerel, cooked, 3 1/2 oz	345 IU	90
Sardines, canned in oil, drained,3 1/2 oz	270 IU	70
Eel, cooked, 3 1/2 oz	200 IU	50
Milk, nonfat, reduced fat, and whole, vitamin D fortified, 1 c	98 IU	25
Margarine, fortified, 1 Tbs.	60 IU	15
Cereal grain bars, fortified w/ 10% of the DV, 1 each	50 IU	10
Pudding, 1/2 c prepared from mix and made with vitamin D fortified milk	50 IU	10
Dry cereal, vitamin D fortified with 10%* of DV, 3/4 c * Other cereals may be fortified with more or less vitamin D	40-50 IU	10
Liver, beef, cooked, 3 1/2 oz	30 IU	8
Egg, 1 whole (vitamin D is present in the yolk)	25 IU	6

* DV = Daily Value. DVs are reference numbers based on the Recommended Dietary Allowance (RDA). They were developed to help consumers determine if a food contains very much of a specific nutrient. The DV for vitamin D is 400 IU. The percent DV (%DV) listed on the nutrition facts panel of food labels informs adults what percentage of the DV is provided by one serving. Percent DVs are based on a 2,000-calorie diet. Daily Values may be higher or lower depending on energy requirements. Foods that provide higher percentages of the DV will contribute to a healthful diet.

The concentration of the active hormonal form of vitamin D is tightly regulated in the blood by the kidneys. This active hormonal form of vitamin D has the potent anticancer properties. It has been discovered that various types of normal and cancerous tissues, including prostate cells [81], colon tissue [82], breast, ovarian and cervical tissue [83], pancreatic tissue [84] and a lung cancer cell line (85) all have the ability to convert the major circulating form of vitamin D, 25(OH)D, into the active hormonal form, 1,25(OH)2D. So, there is a local mechanism in many tissues of the body for converting the form of vitamin D in the body that is elevated by sunshine exposure into a hormone that has anticancer activity.

Indeed, 25(OH)D has been shown to inhibit the growth of colonic epithelial cells [86], primary prostatic epithelial cells [87], and pancreatic cells [84]. So, the laboratory work is confirming what had been seen some time ago in ecological studies of populations and sunshine exposure.

The mortality rates for colon, breast, and ovary cancer in the USA show a marked north-south gradient [88]. In ecological studies of populations and sunlight exposure (no individual data) sunlight has been found to have a protective effect for prostate cancer [89], ovarian cancer [90], and breast cancer [91]. Recently Grant found that sunlight was also protective for bladder, endometrial, renal cancer, multiple myeloma, and Non-Hodgkins lymphoma in Europe [92] and bladder, esophageal, kidney, lung, pancreatic, rectal, stomach, and corpus uteri cancer in the USA [93]. Several prospective studies of vitamin D and cancer have also shown a protective effect of vitamin D. It could be that sunshine and vitamin D are protective factors for cancers of many organs that can convert 25(OH)D into 1,25(OH)D_2.

Additionally, obtaining sufficient amounts of dietary vitamin D is not difficult. The human body produces adequate quantities when exposed to 10 to 15 min of sunlight several days a week and/or a cheap multivitamin generally contains a minimum of 400 International Units (IU) of vitamin D [94]. However, during fall and winter months in many geographic areas, it is difficult to obtain adequate amounts of sun exposure. Therefore, supplementing with vitamin D throughout the year, and especially during the colder months seems best.

Folic Acid

The vitamin that is most commonly deficient in the American diet is folate. Severe folate deficiency in humans is known to cause megaloblastic anemia and developmental defects, such as neural tube defects and is associated with an increased incidence of several forms of human cancer. Although the exact mechanisms by which this vitamin deficiency may cause these diseases are not known at the present time, recent work has shown that folate deficiency also causes genomic instability and programmed cell death (or apoptosis). Additionally, it is known that the DNA mismatch repair pathway mediates folate deficiency-induced apoptosis.

The importance of folate in cancer protection was first demonstrated in animal studies when folate deficiency was linked to enhanced chemically induced carcinogenesis and subsequently in humans in relation to cervical dysplasia and colon cancer. More recently, the importance of folate for the maintenance of genetic stability and for control of gene expression has further highlighted the potential importance of folate in cancer protection.

Folic acid is the dark green leafy vegetable vitamin. It has an integral role in DNA methylation and DNA synthesis. Folic acid works in conjunction with vitamin B-6 and vitamin B-12 in the single carbon methyl cycle. If insufficient folic acid is not available uracil is substituted for thymidine in DNA, which leads to DNA strand breakage. Mechanistically, folate deficiency may enhance carcinogenesis through the role of folate in maintaining the level of S-adenosyl methionine and consequently the production of deoxythymidine monophosphate for DNA synthesis, and because it is needed for the methylation of cytosine in cytosine-guanine sequences, which, if hypomethylated, may lead to enhanced expression of specific oncogenes. About 10% of the US population (and higher percentages among the poor) has low enough intakes of folic acid to make this a common problem [95]. Many studies have found a significant reduction in colon, rectal, and breast cancer with higher intakes of folic acid and their related nutrients (vitamin B-6 and B-12). Alcohol is an antagonist of folate, so that drinking alcoholic beverages greatly magnifies the cancer risk of a low-folate diet. Genetic polymorphisms (common single DNA base mutations resulting in a different amino acid encoded into a protein) in the methylenetetrahydrofolate reductase and the methionine synthase genes which increase the relative amount of folate available for DNA synthesis and repair also reduces the risk of colon cancer [96, 97, 98, 99]. Cravo et al. [100] used 5 mg of folic acid a day (a supraphysiological dose) in a prospective, controlled, cross-over study of 20 patients with colonic adenoma polyps. They found that the folic acid could reverse DNA hypomethylation in 7 of 12 patients who had only one polyp.

Folate may be more important for rapidly dividing tissue, like the colonic mucosa. Therefore, the cancer risk associated with low folate intake is probably higher for colon cancer than for breast cancer. Most of the breast cancer studies only found a protective effect of folate among women who consumed alcohol. However, among women residents of Shanghai who consumed no alcohol, no vitamin supplements and ate unprocessed, unfortified foods there was a 29% decreased risk of breast cancer among those with the highest intake of folate [101]. So, there may be a true protective effect that is masked in the western populations by so many other risk factors. Two studies showed that the risk of cancer due to family history can be modified by high folate intake, so a prudent anti-cancer diet would be high in dark green leafy vegetables.

Vitamin B_{12}

Vitamin B_{12} has not been proven to be an anti-cancer agent, but there is some evidence indicating that it could be beneficial. The form of administered vitamin B_{12} may be important. Some experimental cancer studies have been carried out with various forms of vitamin B-12. Methylcobalamin inhibited tumor growth of SC-3 injected into mice [102], and caused SC-3 mouse mammary tumor cells to undergo apoptosis, even when stimulated to grow by the presence of growth-inducing androgen [103]. Methylcobalamin, but not cyanocobalamin, increased the survival time of mice bearing implanted leukemia tumor cells [104]. 5'-deoxyadenosylcobalamin and methylcobalamin, but not cyanocobalamin, were shown to be effective cytotoxic agents [105]. Methylcobalamin also was able to increase survival time and reduce tumor growth in laboratory mice [106].

Laboratory mechanistic evidence for the effects of vitamin B_{12} was seen in a laboratory study with vitamin B_{12} deficient rats. Choi et al [107] found that the colonic DNA of the B_{12} deficient rats had a 35% decrease in genomic methylation and a 105% increase in uracil incorporation, both changes that could increase risk of carcinogenesis. In two prospective studies (one in Washington Country, Maryland and the Nurses' Health Study) a relation between lower vitamin B_{12} status (but not deficiency) and statistically significant higher risk of breast cancer was found [108, 109]. So, there is evidence from laboratory studies, prospective cohort studies, and mechanistic studies showing that vitamin B_{12} is an important nutrient for genetic stability, DNA repair, carcinogenesis, and cancer therapy.

Selenium

Selenium is an essential trace element, which on earth occurs in variable concentrations in the soil leading to very variable contents of selenium in food. There are natural selenium rich regions in some provinces in China and in the Americas (e.g. Venezuela) while in others (e.g. other provinces in China and Central Africa) selenium in food is very low, leading to deficiency symptoms. Central Europe generally has low selenium availability apart from the coastal areas.

The daily intake is especially low in the former region of East Germany. The recommended daily allowance for selenium according to the German Society for Nutrition is approx. 1 μg/kg/day. The real average intake in Germany is about 50 μg /day and thus some individuals are borderline deficient. The daily intake in the USA varies but usually is above 100 μg/day, the intake in Venezuela may be as high as >300 μg/day. Given this wide range of naturally occurring daily intake the probability that we do not know the optimal intake is very high. We do know that symptoms of deficiency occur below 20 μg/day and toxicity occurs above 800 μg/day. The main sources of selenium for nutrition are wheat, red meat and sea food. Some nuts contain huge amounts of selenium per kilogram but due to their low abundance in average daily food, they do not contribute very much to normal selenium supply [110].

Selenium is a mineral with anti-cancer properties. Many studies in the last several years have shown that selenium is a potent protective nutrient for some forms of cancer. The Arizona Cancer Center posted a selenium fact sheet listing the major functions of selenium in the body [111].

These functions are as follows:

1. Selenium is present in the active site of many enzymes, including thioredoxin reductase, which catalyze oxidation-reduction reactions. These reactions may encourage cancerous cells to under apoptosis.
2. Selenium is a component of the antioxidant enzyme glutathione peroxidase.
3. Selenium improved the immune systems' ability to respond to infections.
4. Selenium causes the formation of natural killer cells.
5. P450 enzymes in the liver may be induced by selenium, leading to detoxification of some carcinogenic molecules.
6. Selenium inhibits prostaglandins that cause inflammation.
7. Selenium enhances male fertility by increased sperm motility.
8. Selenium can decrease the rate of tumor growth.

A serendipitous randomized, double-blind, controlled trial of a 200 μg/day selenium supplement in the southeastern region of the USA (where soil selenium levels are low) found that the primary endpoints of skin cancer were not improved by the selenium supplement, but that other cancer incidence rates were decreased by selenium [112, 113]. There was a significant reduction in total cancer incidence (105 vs 137 cases, P = 0.03), prostate cancer (22 vs 42 cases, P = 0.005), a marginally significant reduction in colorectal cancer incidence (9 vs 19 cases, P = 0.057), and a reduction in cancer mortality, all cancer sites (40 vs 66 deaths, P = 0.008) (selenium versus control group cases reported, respectively) [112]. The selenium supplement was most effective in ex-smokers and for those who began the study with the lowest levels of serum selenium.

Several prospective studies have also examined the role of selenium in cancer prevention, particularly for prostate cancer and overall, it appears that poor selenium levels, especially for men, are a cancer risk. If a person has low selenium levels and other antioxidant defenses are also low the cancer risk is increased even further. Women do not appear to be as sensitive to selenium, as breast cancer has not been found to be influenced by selenium status in several studies [114, 115, 116, 117, 118], although both men and women were found to be protected by higher levels of selenium from colon cancer and lung cancer [119, 120].

Good vegetarian sources of selenium are whole grains and legumes grown in selenium-rich soil in the western United States, Brazil nuts (by far the densest source of selenium), nutritional yeast, brewers yeast, and sunflower seeds.

Selected Antioxidants and Cancer Prevention

Oxidative damage to DNA, lipids and proteins in the human body is generally considered to be an important factor in carcinogenesis. Reactive oxygen species such as superoxide, nitric oxide and hydroxyl radicals, formed continuously as a result of biochemical reactions, can cause significant oxidative damage. They can also be formed in response to excess pollution, too much UV sunlight and exposure to cigarette smoke. Evironmental carcinogens from various sources and industrial pollution as well as and food contaminants, such as heterocyclic aromatic amines (HAAs) contribute to an individual's total burden of oxidative stress [121]. Antioxidant defences, including enzymes that continually repair DNA damage, frequently cannot counteract all of the oxidative attack, and the resulting damage may lead to genetic mutations that could contribute to carcinogenesis. Dietary antioxidants, ubiquitous in plant foods where they have evolved to protect the plants against oxidative assault, may be protective to humans, in terms of reducing cancer risk.

Reactive oxygen species appear to be involved at all stages of cancer development; consequently, dietary antioxidants may have potential benefits throughout the carcinogenic process [122].

Epidemiologic data provide strong evidence of a cancer-protective effect for high intakes of vegetables, fruits and whole grains. Currently, the United States Department of Agriculture (USDA) and the National Cancer Institute (NCI) recommend the consumption of a minimum of five servings of fruits and vegetables per day to prevent cancer.

Table 12. Endogenous and dietary sources of antioxidants

Endogenous Antioxidants	Dietary antioxidants
Polyamines	Vitamin E
Melatonin	Vitamin C
estrogen	α-lipoate
Superoxide dismutase	Coenzyme Q10
Glutathione peroxidase	Carotenoids
Catalase	Polyphenols
Lipoic Acid	Phytates
Caeruloplasmin	Copper
Albumin	Zn
Lactoferrin	Se
Transferrin	Mn

Natural food derived components, such as antioxidative vitamins and Phenolic phytochemicals, have been receiving much attention, not only because they are safe and not perceived as "medicine," but also because some of them are known to function as chemopreventive agents. Many studies indicate that the risk of cancer incidence associated with lowest vegetable and fruit intakes is approximately twice that associated with highest intakes [123]. A review of more than 200 case–control and cohort studies found a probable protective effect for cancers of the breast, colon, endometrium, oral cavity and pharynx, pancreas and bladder, and convincing evidence for inverse associations with cancers of the stomach, oesophagus, and lung [124]. In 85% of the studies, raw vegetables appeared to be protective; highly protective categories included Allium vegetables, carrots, green vegetables, cruciferous vegetables, and tomatoes – all protective in 70% or more of the studies.

Total fruits and citrus fruit were protective in about 65% of the studies. The cancer-inhibitory effects reported for these plant foods may be attributed in part to various antioxidant constituents, including micronutrients (e.g. β-carotene (provitamin A), vitamins E and C, selenium) and certain phytochemicals (e.g. polyphenolics, carotenoids) [125]. It is likely that numerous constituents contribute to the overall protective effect. Lung cancer risk, for instance, consistently has been shown to be reduced by high vegetable and/or fruit consumption in both prospective and retrospective epidemiological studies, but the beneficial effect cannot be explained completely by either b-carotene or total provitamin A carotenoid intakes [126].

Protective Mechanisms of Antioxidants

Antioxidants are compounds that help to inhibit the many oxidation reactions caused by free radicals thereby preventing or delaying damage to the cells and tissues. Their mechanisms of action include: (a) scavenging reactive oxygen and nitrogen free radical species; (b) decreasing the localized oxygen concentration thereby reducing molecular oxygen's oxidation potential; (c) metabolizing lipid peroxides to non-radical products; (d) chelating transient metal ions to prevent the generation of free radicals.

By neutralizing reactive oxygen species, antioxidants can limit the processes of the development of chronic disease such as: (1) oxidation low density lipoprotein (LDL) cholesterol, which may increase the risk of atherosclerosis; (2) Promoting platelet adhesion, which can lead to thrombosis thereby increasing the risk of heart disease or stroke; (3) Damaging the cell's DNA, which may lead to cancer (4) Blocking the normal endothelial cell function and vasodilatation in response to nitric oxide, a potential mechanism for heart disease and cancer.

β-Carotene

ß-Carotene and carotenoids in general are isoprenoid compounds which are not synthesized in animals but biosynthesized by plants and micro-organisms. About 700 naturally occurring carotenoids have been identified so far. About 10% of them can be found in the human diet, and about 20 of these compounds have been found in plasma and tissues of the mammal. The predominant carotenoids observed in the plasma are ß-carotene, lycopene, lutein, ß-cryptoxanthin and α-carotene, accounting for more than 90% of the circulating carotenoids in humans.

Some dietary carotenoids, such as ß-carotene, serve as an important source of vitamin A, which is the major known function of carotenoids in humans. ß-Carotene is a hydrocarbon $C_{40}H_{56}$ that has a ß-ionone structure as the terminal ring system at each side of the poliene chain. Carotenoids containing at least one unsubstituted ß-ionone ring and a poliene chain are potential precursors of vitamin A. The preformed vitamin A is only present in animal products (e.g. liver, eggs, milk products), thus, in countries where the intake of animal products is low, carotenoids have to meet (i.e. by 80% or more in Asia and Africa) the vitamin A requirements. Even in developed countries carotenoids usually contribute to vitamin A supply by more than 40% [127].

Carotenoids can act as antioxidants and free radical/reactive species scavengers [128, 129]. *In vitro*, carotenoids efficiently quench excited molecules such as singlet oxygen and can scavenge peroxyl radicals; interactions with several other radicals have also been reported and a synergistic antioxidant protection by carotenoids with vitamins E and C has been shown [130]. The role *in vivo* and in humans is less clear [128]. The switch from antioxidant to pro-oxidant behavior can be, for example, a function of oxygen concentration [130]. The prooxidant activity of ß-carotene has been demonstrated at a high partial pressure of oxygen; because this is highest in the outermost cells of the lung, these cells might be particularly subject to the pro-oxidant effect of ß-carotene. Other effects of carotenoids, which can be related to cancer prevention, are the enhancement of the immune response observed in some experimental models, which may be due to production of tumor specific antigens [128]. In addition, carotenoids have been reported to modulate cytochrome P450 metabolism, inhibit arachidonic acid metabolism, inhibit chromosome instability and chromosome damage, influence apoptosis, and affect several other biological processes [128].

Clinical chemoprevention trials using β-carotene are based on extensive evidence from epidemiological studies. Weighing the evidence from studies conducted in the 1970s, which linked high vegetable and fruit intake - an index of β-carotene intake - with reduced cancer risk, Peto et al. [131] suggested that β-carotene might be the protective factor in these foods. Several possible mechanisms were proposed that supported the biological plausibility of β-carotene as a cancer-protective agent, including antioxidant protection and the differentiating action of vitamin A formed from β-carotene.

Clinical trials on oral cancer showed evidence of benefit from β-carotene. In Filipino betel nut chewers, who are at very high risk for oral cancer, the percentage of buccal mucosa cells with micronuclei - evidence of genotoxic damage – was significantly lower in people given β-carotene for 9 weeks than in those given canthaxanthin, a carotenoid with no vitamin A activity [132]. One study that examined the effect of β-carotene on leukoplakia, a precancerous oral lesion, reported that 17 of 24 patients showed significant reversal of lesions after 6 months of treatment [133]. In another study, however, low-dose 13-*cis*-retinoic acid was significantly more effective than β-carotene in maintaining the stability of leukoplakia reversed by high-dose 13-*cis*-retinoic acid [134].

β-carotene has been shown not to protect against colorectal polyps. Greenberg et al. [135] carried out a study in which 864 people, who previously had polyps removed, received either β-carotene, vitamins C and E, all three antioxidants, or placebo for 4 years, no reduction in polyp incidence and no evidence of harm was demonstrated for any of the interventions. Similarly, an Australian polyp prevention trial, in which approximately 400 patients with previous polyps received either β-carotene or placebo along with usual diet, low-fat diet, high-wheat bran diet or low-fat/high-wheat bran diet, found no significant polyp reduction [136]. The data suggested, however, that the low-fat/ high-wheat bran diet may inhibit the transition from smaller to larger polyps, which have greater malignant potential.

Numerous epidemiological studies investigating the possible association between β-carotene and the risk of various types of cancer have been conducted since the early 1980s, concurrent with clinical trials. A significant protective effect of dietary β-carotene for lung cancer is strongly supported by epidemiological data. A review by van Poppel and Goldbohm [137] of approximately 80 retrospective studies and 50 prospective studies reported that associations of either high intakes of β-carotene-rich vegetables and fruits or high blood concentrations of β-carotene with reduced cancer risk were most consistent for lung and stomach cancer. Esophageal cancer also showed a promising risk reduction, but the number of studies was limited.

Reported results for the effects of both b-carotene and vitamin A on prostate cancer have been equivocal, with studies being almost equally divided between inverse and positive associations [138]. For breast cancer, evidence from case–control studies has indicated a possible protective effect of β-carotene [139]. For colon cancer, some case–control studies have reported significantly reduced risk at high intakes, but the overall data have suggested only a modest risk reduction [137].

Controversies over β-Carotene Supplements

Existing evidence from human trials indicates that supplemental ß-carotene (20 mg/day or more) is contraindicated for use in current, heavy smokers [140]. However, there is insufficient scientific basis to set a precise figure for an upper limit of isolated ß-carotene as no dose-response relationship for ß-carotene effects is available either from the intervention trials in humans or from appropriate animal models. Moreover, it is not possible to be more specific in distinguishing different isomeric forms of ß-carotene or specific formulations.

There are 3 ß-carotene sources for humans: (a) natural food sources that may account for about 2-5 mg/day in the American and European diet; (b) food additives (1-2 mg/day); and (c) supplements. The contribution of (a) and (b) sources stands at about 3-7 mg/day (or up to 10 mg/day depending on seasonal and diet variations) of ß-carotene exposure. Thus, there may be a very small difference between the levels that may confer health benefits (up to 10 mg/d, mainly from natural sources) and those that may produce adverse effects in smokers in the general population (20 mg/day as shown in the ATBC study). In this situation it seems that the use of ß-carotene as a supplement should be regarded cautiously.

On one hand, human chemoprevention trials carried out in the last decade have shown that all-*trans* ß-carotene actually increases both lung-cancer incidence and mortality in human smokers and, more recently, mechanisms which offer likely explanations of these adverse effects have been derived from experimental studies in appropriate animal models.

On the other hand, a number of reviews have summarized the research on diet and lung cancer in humans during the preceding 30 year period. The consensus is that they consistently demonstrated reduced risk of lung cancer, with increased intake of vegetables and fruits rich in carotenoids. Further, high levels of ß-carotene in the blood were consistently associated with reduced incidence of lung cancer. However, these effects can not be attributed to α-carotene as the role of other carotenoids or other compounds from vegetables and fruits, and associated dietary or life style patterns, has not been adequately explored in the epidemiological studies.

Thus, the general assumption that individuals who eat more fruits and vegetables, rich in carotenoids, and/or have high levels of serum ß-carotene have a lower risk for cancer and cardiovascular diseases cannot be extended to specific formulations of ß-carotene.

Table 13. β-carotene phase III trials

Trial	Dosage (per day)	Results
PHS	25 mg BC	none
ATBC	30 mg BC	harm
CARET	30 mg BC + 25 mg retinoid	discontinued (potential harm)
Linxian	15 mg BC + Se + vitamin E	benefit

Note: PHS = Physician's Health Study (141); ATBC = Alpha-Tocopherol Beta-Carotene Study (140); CARET = Carotene and Retinoid Study (142); Linxian = Linxian Study (143); BC = beta-carotene, Se = selenium.

Vitamin C

Vitamin C, also known as ascorbic acid, is a water-soluble vitamin and is essential for normal functioning of the body. Unlike most mammals, humans do not have the ability to produce their own vitamin C and, therefore, must obtain it through the diet. Apart from its antioxidant capacity, vitamin C may also be able to reactivate other antioxidants, such as vitamin E, so that they can be reutilized. This vitamin is also involved in several enzyme systems for the synthesis of collagen (connective tissues, cartilage, teeth and skin), healing of wounds and conversion of nutrients into their functional forms. Furthermore, vitamin C is essential for immune system function, promotes resistance to infection, protects lung function, and enhances iron absorption from non-heme food sources, which is found primarily in fruits, vegetables, dried beans, nuts and grain products.

Table 14. Dietary Reference Intakes for Vitamin C

Gender	Age	EAR	RDA	AI	UL	NOAEL	LOAEL
	Years	mg/day	mg/day	mg/day	mg/day	mg/day	mg/day
Male/Female	0 – 0.5	-	-	40	-	-	-
	0.5 - 1	-	-	50	-	-	-
	1 – 3	13	15	-	400	-	-
	4 – 8	22	25	-	650	1000	3000
Male	9 – 13	39	45	-	1200	1000	3000
	14 – 18	63	75	-	1800	-	-
	19 – 30	75	90	-	2000	2000	3000
	31 – 50	75	90	-	2000	2000	3000
	51 – 70	75	90	-	2000	2000	3000
	> 70	75	90	-	2000	2000	3000
Female	9 – 13	39	45	-	1200	1000	3000
	14 – 18	56	65	-	1800	-	-
	19 – 30	60	75	-	2000	2000	3000
	31 – 50	60	75	-	2000	2000	3000
	51 – 70	60	75	-	2000	2000	3000
	> 70	60	75	-	2000	2000	3000
Pregnancy	≤ 18	66	80	-	1800	-	-
	19 – 30	70	85	-	2000	-	-
	31 – 50	70	85	-	2000	-	-
Lactation	≤ 18	96	115	-	1800	-	-
	19 – 30	100	120	-	2000	-	-
	31 – 50	100	120	-	2000	-	-

EAR = estimated average requirement, RDA = recommended daily allowance, AI = average intake, UL = tolerable upper intake level, NOAEL = no observed adverse effect level, LOAEL = the lowest intake at which an adverse effect has been demonstrated.

Vitamin C has the capacity to quench reactive oxygen metabolites in the stomach or duodenum and prevent the formation of N-nitroso compounds that are mutagenic. Nitrosamines have been linked to gastric cancer. Formation of nitrosamines in the gastrointestinal tract can be decreased by administration of vitamin C [144].

Table 15. Dietary sources of vitamin C [147]

Sources (Portion Size)	Vitamin C [mg]
Vegetables	
Pepper, red or green:	
Raw (1/2 Cup)	65
Cooked (1/2 Cup)	50
Cabbage:	
Red, raw, chopped (1/2 Cup)	20
Red, cooked (1/2 Cup)	25
Raw, chopped (1/2 Cup)	10
Cooked (1/2 Cup)	15
Kale, cooked (1 cup)	55
Mustard greens, cooked (1 cup)	35
Broccoli, cooked (1/2 Cup)	60
Brussels sprouts, cooked (1/2 Cup)	50
Cauliflower, raw or cooked (1/2 Cup)	25
Potato, baked (1 Medium)	25
Snow peas:	
Fresh, cooked (1/2 Cup)	40
Frozen, cooked (1/2 Cup)	20
Sweet potato:	
Baked (1 Medium)	30
Vacuum Can (1 Cup)	50
Canned, syrup-pack (1 Cup)	20
Plantains, sliced, cooked (1 Cup)	15
Tomato:	
Raw (1/2 Cup)	15
Canned (1/2 Cup)	35
Juice (6 fluid oz)	35
Fruit	
Cantaloupe (1/4 Medium)	60
Fresh grapefruit (1/2 fruit)	40
Honeydew Melon (1/8 Medium)	40
Kiwi (1 Medium)	75
Mango (1 Cup, sliced)	45
Orange (1 Medium)	70
Papaya (1 Cup, cubes)	85
Strawberries (1 Cup, sliced)	95
Tangerines or tangelos (1 Medium)	25
Watermelon (1 Cup)	15
Juice:	
Grapefruit (1/2 Cup)	35
Orange (1/2 Cup)	50
Fortified Juice:	
Apple (1/2 Cup)	50
Cranberry juice cocktail (1/2 Cup)	45
Grape (1/2 Cup)	120

High dietary vitamin C intake correlates with reduced gastric cancer risk [145]. Although high dietary vitamin C intake correlates with reduced gastric cancer risk [146], it is not certain what confers protection: vitamin C itself or other phytochemicals present in foods, particularly fruits and vegetables that also contain vitamin C.

Epidemiological evidence for a protective effect of diets high in vegetables and fruits that contain vitamin C is strong and consistent for cancers of the oral cavity, esophagus and stomach, but moderate and less consistent for colon and lung cancers. The data do not support an association with prostate cancer and the evidence for breast cancer has been conflicting [145, 146]. A review of more than 50 case – control and cohort studies that investigated intakes of vegetables and fruits, vitamin C, and vitamin E, reported that, across studies, individuals in the highest quartile or quintile of vegetable and fruit intake had approximately 40% less risk of gastrointestinal and respiratory tract cancers than those in the lowest intake levels [145]. Indices of vitamin C computed from vegetable and fruit intakes also were associated with lower risk.

Vitamin E

Vitamin E is the major lipid-soluble antioxidant in the cell antioxidant defence system and is exclusively obtained from the diet. The term "vitamin E" refers to a family of eight naturally occurring homologues that are synthesized by plants from homogentisic acid. All are derivatives of 6-chromanol and differ in the number and position of methyl groups on the ring structure. The four tocopherol homologues (*d*-α-, *d*-β-, *d*-γ-, and *d*-δ-) have a saturated 16- carbon phytyl side chain, whereas the tocotrienols (*d*-α-, *d*-β-, *d*-γ-, and *d*-δ-) have three double bonds on the side chain.

For dietary purposes, vitamin E activity is expressed as α-tocopherol equivalents (α-TEs). One α-TE is the activity of 1 mg *RRR*-α-tocopherol (*d*-α-tocopherol). To estimate the α-TE of mixed diet containing natural forms of vitamin E, the number of milligrams of β-tocopherol should be multiplied by 0.5, γ-tocopherol by 0.1, and α-tocotrienol by 0.3. Any of the synthetic all-*rac*-α-tocopherol (*dl*-α-tocopherol) should be multiplied by 0.74. One milligram of the latter compound in the acetate form is equivalent to 1 IU of vitamin E.

Because vitamin E is naturally present in plant-based diets and animal products and is often added by manufacturers to vegetable oils and processed foods, intakes are probably adequate to avoid explicit deficiency in most populations.

About half of the α-tocopherol in a typical northern European diet such as in the United Kingdom is derived from vegetable oils [148]. Animal fats, vegetables, and meats each contribute about 10 percent to the total per capita supply and fruit, nuts, cereals, and dairy products each contribute about 4 percent. Less than 2 percent is each obtained from eggs, fish and pulses.

Vitamin E is a typical example of a phenolic antioxidant. Such molecules readily donate the hydrogen from the hydroxyl (-OH) group on the ring structure to free radicals, which then become unreactive. On donating the hydrogen, the phenolic compound itself becomes a relatively unreactive free radical because the unpaired electron on the oxygen atom is usually delocalised into the aromatic ring structure thereby increasing its stability [149]

The major biologic role of vitamin E is to protect PUFAs and other components of cell membranes and low-density lipoprotein (LDL) from oxidation by free radicals. Vitamin E is located primarily within the phospholipid bilayer of cell membranes. It is particularly effective in preventing lipid peroxidation, a series of chemical reactions involving the oxidative deterioration of PUFAs. Elevated levels of lipid peroxidation products are associated with numerous diseases and clinical conditions [150]. Although vitamin E is primarily located in cell and organelle membranes where it can exert its maximum protective effect, its concentration may only be one molecule for every 2000 phospholipid molecules. This suggests that after its reaction with free radicals it is rapidly regenerated by other antioxidants, especially vitamin C and α-lipoic acid [151].

Epidemiological studies that have investigated associations of cancer risk at specific sites and diets high in vitamin E (a-tocopherol) are limited in number and data are inconsistent, possibly because estimation of vitamin E intake is difficult [124, 145]. A review that examined case–control and cohort studies of vitamin E intake and serum vitamin E levels in relation to breast cancer risk reported that the data were inconclusive [152]. One case-control study that investigated the association between micronutrient intake and colorectal adenomas reported that men in the highest quartile of vitamin E intake, compared with the lowest quartile, were about one-fifth as likely to develop adenomas (OR = 0.22 for men and 0.74 for women), after adjustment for possible confounding variables, including other micronutrients [153]. Similarly, another case–control study showed decreased risk of adenoma for the highest tertile of vitamin E intake (OR = 0.6, men and women combined, adjusted for total energy and physical activity) [154]. In the recently completed Alpha-Tocopherol Beta-Carotene (ATBC) Cancer Prevention Study [140] conducted in Finland in more than 29,000 male cigarette smokers at high risk for lung cancer, 34% fewer cases of prostate cancer and 16% fewer cases of colorectal cancer were diagnosed among men who received daily vitamin E supplements. Although these results suggest a protective effect of vitamin E, prostate and colon cancers were not primary study endpoints. Further research, targeted at these cancers, is needed before conclusions can be drawn about the potential of vitamin E for their prevention.

A recent review suggests that antioxidant effects of gamma-tocopherol may be superior to those of a-tocopherol, and that studies of vitamin E and colorectal cancer should consider all tocopherols [155].

Phytochemicals and Cancer Prevention

Table 16. Selected phytochemicals possessing anticancer properties, food sources and their mechanisms of action [156]

Phytochemical class	Typical compounds	Food sources	Cancer prevention-related activities
Carotenoids	α-Carotene, β-carotene, lycopene, β-cryptoxanthin, lutein, astaxanthin	Yellow–red and dark green vegetables and fruits	Antioxidant activity, modulation of carcinogen metabolism, inhibition of cell proliferation, inhibition of oncogene expression, beneficial effects on immune function, beneficial effects on cell transformation and differentiation, enhancement of cell-to-cell communication
Organosulphur compounds	Diallyl sulphide, diallyl disulphide, allyl methyl trisulphide, dithiolthiones	Sulphides, Allium vegetables (e.g. garlic, onion); dithiolthiones, cruciferous vegetables (e.g. broccoli, cabbage)	Increase phase II enzyme activity, inhibit cell proliferation, induce cell differentiation, alter steroid hormone metabolism, inhibit ornithine decarboxylase activity
Polyphenols	Phenolic acids (e.g. caffeic acid), hydroxycinnamic acids (e.g. curcumin), flavanols (e.g. quercetin, apigenin), flavanones (e.g. naringin, hesperidin), catechins (e.g. epigallocatechin gallate), theaflavins, resveratrol	Vegetables and fruits; catechins, green tea; theaflavins, black tea; resveratrol, red wine	Reduce carcinogen–DNA adduct formation, inhibit cell proliferation, induce cell cycle arrest and apoptosis, inhibit signal transduction pathways, enhance cell-to-cell communication, improve immune function
Phytoestrogens	Isoflavones (e.g. genistein, daidzein), lignans (e.g. matairesinol, secoisolariciresinol)	Isoflavones, soybeans, soy-based foods; lignans, vegetables, flaxseed, rye	Alter estrogen metabolism, decrease tyrosine kinase activity, induce cell cycle arrest and apoptosis, induce topoisomerase II-mediated DNA breakage
Glucosinolates, isothiocyanates, indoles	Glucobrassicin, sulphorophane, indole-3-carbinol	Cruciferous vegetables	Increase phase II enzyme activity, induce cell cycle arrest and apoptosis, inhibit cell adhesion and invasion
Terpenes	Monoterpenes (e.g. limonene, perillyl alcohol, geraniol), sesquiterpenes, e.g. farnesol)	Vegetables and fruits (e.g. citrus)	Increase phase II enzyme activity, influence cell cycle progression, induce apoptosis

Glucosinolates in Cruciferous Vegetables

Cruciferous vegetables play an important role against the risk of cancer [157, 158]. The Cruciferae (syn. Brassicaceae) are the family of plants that include a wide variety of familiar members of the species *Brassica oleracea* (e.g., broccoli, cabbage, cauliflower, parsnip, kale, kohlrabi, brussels sprouts, turnip, rutabaga) and many other plants which are commonly consumed in various parts of the world such as oriental cabbage, arugula, watercress, radish, daikon, wasabi, various mustards, horseradish, Chinese cabbage, etc. The role of cruciferous vegetables in protection against cancer is attributed to the presence of glucosinolates (β-thioglycoside-*N*-hydroxysulfates) in diet.

Glucosinolate content is about 1% of dry weight of the Brassica vegetables; and it plays important roles in plants such as in allelopathy (suppression of growth of neighboring plants), and in protection against predators including nematocidal, microbicidal, antifungal and insecticidal activities [159]. Glucosinolates are hydrolyzed by the plant enzyme myrosinase (β-thioglucosidase) when the cells in plants are damaged due to cutting or chewing in the presence of water, yielding the biologically active isothiocyanates which are basically organosulfur compounds. If myrosinase has been inactivated due to cooking, glucosinolates are broken down by intestinal bacterial myrosinase in the colon [160]. At least 120 different glucosinolates have been identified in the *Brassica oleracea* plant species [161] Glucobrassicin and glucoraphanin are generally found in high concentrations in broccoli. Chinese cabbage, radish and watercress contain high amount of gluconasturtiin; whereas, sinigrin is found in high concentrations in brussels sprouts, cabbage and cauliflower. As mentioned earlier, hydrolysis of glucosinolates by myrosinase produces various types of isothiocyanates.

Hydrolysis of glucoraphanin results in sulforaphane, hydrolysis of sinigrin results in allyl isothiocyanate, gluconasturtiin produces phenethyl isothiocyanate (PEITC) and glucobrassicin produces indole-3-carbinol [162]. The isothiocyanates formed from indole glucosinolates are unstable, and decompose spontaneously to indole-3-carbinol, indole-acetonitrile, thiocyanate and 3,3'-diindolylmethane. Indole-3-carbinol may then spontaneously condense under the acidic conditions of the stomach to form compounds that closely resemble 2, 3, 7, 8-tetrachlorodibenzo-*p*-dioxin (TCDD or dioxin), which is carcinogenic. In spite of this property, indole-3-carbinol has been investigated as a cancer chemopreventive agent [161]. A large amount of data demonstrate that isothiocyanates act as cancer chemopreventive agents by favorably modifying carcinogen metabolism via selective inhibition of cytochrome P450 enzymes involved in carcinogen metabolic activation and induction of phase II enzymes [163].

Interestingly, sulforaphane is an extremely potent inducer of phase II enzymes and effectively inhibits proliferation of cancer cells by causing caspase-9 and caspase-8 mediated apoptosis [157, 164].

Table 17. Sources of glucosinolates and their contents in selected foods of plant origin [161]

Product	Form of product	Mean content of glucosinolates (mg/100 g)
Broccoli	Raw	19-127
Broccoli	Cooked	20-37
Broccoli, frozen	Raw	50-70
Broccoli, frozen	Cooked	20·70
Brussels sprouts	Raw	50-445
Brussels sprouts	Cooked	00-148
Brussels sprouts, frozen	Raw	50-90
Brussels sprouts, frozen	Cooked	30-61
Cabbage, Chinese cabbage	Raw	19-84
Cabbage, Red	Raw	62-76
Cabbage, Red	Cooked	54-80
Kale	Raw	76-99
Cabbage, white	Raw	10-51
Cauliflower	Raw	23-43
Cauliflower	Cooked	00-42
Cauliflower, frozen	Raw	40-50
Cauliflower, frozen	Cooked	27-90
Coleslaw Salad	Raw	20-42
Horseradish	Raw	12-160
Kohlrabi	Raw	40-52
Kohlrabi	Cooked	40-73
Radish, red	Raw	64-67
Turnip	Raw	00-93

Cruciferous vegetables can modulate estrogen metabolism and it has been hypothesized that they might lower the risk of estrogen-dependent cancers like breast cancer [165]. 16-α-hydroxylation yields potent estrogen that may play a positive role in the development of breast cancer; whereas hydroxylation at the 2-position lowers the biosynthesis of 16-α-hydroxylation product of estrogen. Therefore, the ratio between the products of these two major pathways of estrogen metabolism may be important in the pathogenesis, e.g., 2-hydroxyestrone:16-α-hydroxyestrone, an increase in the ratio is thought to be protective. Several studies have observed that indole-3-carbinol increased the level of 2-hydroxyestrogen and simultaneously decreased the concentration of 16-α-hydroxyestrogen [166, 167]. Interestingly, cruciferous vegetables also contain other chemopreventive ingredients such as flavonoids and selenium [162, 168, 169].

Beneficial Effects of Phytoestrogens and Lignans

The higher soy intake in the Asian population compared to Europeans and Americans is believed to be an essential factor for the lower incidence of hormone-dependent tumors in Asia. It has already been shown that soybeans, with their ingredients genistein and daidzein from the isoflavonoid group, have protective effects on hormone-related diseases, such as breast and prostate cancer.

Phytoestrogens are naturally occurring plant-derived phytochemicals protect plants from stress and act as part of defense mechanism in plants. Although composed of a wide group of non-steroidal compounds of diverse structure, phytoestrogens have been shown to bind estrogen receptors and to behave as weak agonist/antagonist in both animals and humans. Phytoestrogens include mainly isoflavones, coumestans, and lignans. The structure of isoflavone molecule resembles those of many estrogenic and antiestrogenic compounds, including 17β-estradiol and the synthetic antiestrogen tamoxifen. Isoflavones have a common Phenolic structure that seems to be a prerequisite for binding to estrogen receptors (ERs). Isoflavones, particularly genistein have a more binding affinity for ER-β than for ER-α, therefore, taking into account different tissue distribution of the α and β receptors, there is clear potential that isoflavones could exhibit tissue-selective effects [170].

Many of the possible benefits of isoflavones and other phytoestrogens may be attributed to metabolic activities that involve systems other than ERs, including effects on enzymes, such as adenosine triphosphatase and inhibition of DNA topoisomerase. Isoflavones may also impart an influence on cell proliferation, angiogenesis, growth factor action, vascular smooth muscle cells, and cell differentiation [171].

The lignans, represented in the diet mainly by secoisolariciresinol and matairesinol, have been demonstrated to possess beneficial effects with cancer of the breast [172] prostate [173] and colon. Phytoestrogens, particularly genistein can act as an estrogen or antiestrogen, leading to both proliferatory and antiproliferatory effects. Genistein's anti-proliferatory effects that occur via estrogen-unrelated pathways are seen only at very high doses.

Phytoestrogens and lignans are present in fruits, vegetables, and whole grains commonly consumed by humans. Isoflavones are found in legumes, mainly soybeans, whereas flaxseed is a major source of lignans. Coumestans are present in significant amounts in clover, alfalfa and soybean sprouts. 8-Prenyl flavonoids are common in vegetables. Bioavailability of isoflavones requires an initial hydrolysis of the sugar moiety by intestinal enzymes - beta-glucosidases to allow the following uptake by enterocytes and the flow through the peripheral circulation. After absorption, isoflavones are reconjugated primarily to glucuronic acid and to a lesser extent to sulfuric acid. Gut metabolism seems key to the determination of the potency of action. In the colon, bacteria convert the botanical lignans into the mammalian lignans enterodiol and enterolactone. Evidence suggests that a healthy colon flora population may be necessary for humans to derive significant benefit from lignans.

Several epidemiological studies correlated high dose consumptions of soy isoflavones with multiple beneficial effects on breast and prostate cancers, menopausal symptoms, osteoporosis, atherosclerosis and stroke, and neurodegeneration. For cancer prevention the intakes of isoflavones at the level between 50 and 110 mg aglycones/day can reduce risks of breast, colon and prostate cancer [174].

It is worth mentioning that besides soybean, additional dietary factors present at high concentrations in the diet of Asians, such as fatty acids of the omega-3 family and a number of phytochemicals can inhibit cell proliferation via the same mechanisms as do soy isoflavones.

Table 18. Selected dietary sources of phytoestrogens and lignans (μg/100 g dry weight) [175]

Plant	Daidzein	Genistein	SEC*	MAT**
Legumes				
Soybean	10500-56 000	26800-84100	13-273	trace
Kidney bean	7-40	18-518	56-153	trace
Cowpea	21-30	12-56	195-196	0
Oil and nuts				
Flaxseed	0	0	369 900	1087
Sunflower seed	8	14	610	0
Peanut	58	64	298	trace
Grains and cereals				
Wheat (whole grain)	0	0	33	3
Wheat bran	4	7	110	0
Oat bran	0	0	24	155
Barley (whole grain)	14	8	58	0
Rye meal (whole grain)	0	0	47	65
Berries and fruits				
Lingonberry	0	0	1510	0
Strawberry	0	0	1205	5
Cranberry	0	0	1054	0
Apple	12	0	trace	0
Vegetables				
Pumpkin (peeled)	0	0	3870	4
Zuccinia (with peel)	0	0	817	trace
Broccoli	6	8	414	23
Carrot (with peel)	0	0	370	trace

*Secoisolariciresinol; **matairesinol.

Polyphenols and Cancer

The antioxidant characteristics of plant-derived materials can be attributed to their content of polyphenols. Until recently, most of the nutritional interest in polyphenols was in the deleterious effects caused by the ability of polyphenols to bind and precipitate macromolecules, such as dietary protein, carbohydrate, and digestive enzymes, and therefore reducing food digestibility. However, interest in food phenolics has increased, because of their antioxidant and free radical scavenging abilities. Polyphenols constitute one of the most numerous and widely distributed group of substances in the plant kingdom, with more than 8000 phenolic structures currently known [176]. Polyphenols are products of secondary metabolism of plants and ubiquitous in all plant organs. They arise biogenetically from two main synthetic pathways: the shikimate and the acetate pathway [176, 177].

Natural polyphenols can range from simple molecules, such as phenolic acids, to highly polymerised compounds, such as tannins. They occur primarily in conjugated form, with one or more sugar residues linked to hydroxyl groups, although direct linkages of the sugar unit to an aromatic carbon atom also exist. Polyphenols can be divided into at least 10 different classes depending on their basic chemical structure. Flavonoids, which constitute the most important single group, can be further subdivided into 13 classes, with more than 4000 compounds described until 1990 [176]. Flavonoids most widely occurred in the nature are flavonols, flavones, flavanols, isoflavones, flavanones, flavanols, anthocyanidines and proanthocyanidines [177]. The average intake of flavonoids by a human is in the range of 25–50 mg/day, including flavonols quercetin, myricetin and kaempferol, and the flavones luteolin and apigenin [178].

Acting as antioxidants, Polyphenols can decrease the risk of cancer. Many flavonoids and polyphenols can exhibit antioxidant activity as their extensive, conjugated π-electron systems allow ready donation of electrons, or hydrogen atoms, from the hydroxyl moieties to free radicals. Most polyphenols, especially flavonoids are very effective scavengers of hydroxyl and peroxyl radicals [180]. Flavonoids are chelators of metals and inhibit the Fenton and Haber-Weiss reactions, which are important sources of active oxygen radicals [181]. In addition, flavonoids retain their free radical scavenging capacity after forming complexes with metal ions.

Many studies in different cell lines, animal models and human epidemiological trials have shown the potential of dietary polyphenols as anticarcinogenic agents [182, 183]. These phenolic compounds may inhibit various stages in the carcinogenesis process by affecting molecular events in the initiation, promotion and progression stages.

Polyphenols have been shown to increase the expression of proapoptotic components in initiated proliferating cells and thereby prevent or delay tumor development. Although induction of apoptosis seems to be rather specific for cancer cells, it should be mentioned that certain human studies have shown no beneficial effects.

Table 19. Group of flavonoids and their dietary sources [179]

Group of flavonoids	Representative flavonoids	Dietary sources
Flavanols	EGCG, epigallocatechin, catechin, epicatechin	Chocolate, beans, tea, red wine apple, cherry, apricot
Flavones	Luteolin, apigenin, chrysin,	Capsicum pepper, thyme, celery, parsley
Flavanones	Naringenin, hesperidin, eriodictyol	Orange, grapefruit
Flavonols	Quercetin, myricetin, kaempherol, rutin	Onion, apple, cherry, broccoli, tomato, berries, tea, red wine, leek
Isoflavonoids	Genistein, daidzein	Soya beans, legumes
Anthocyanindins	Pelargonidin, cyanidin, malvidin	Rhubarb, cherry, strawberry, red wine

Tea, especially green tea and its polyphenols have been found to inhibit experimental tumorigenesis and tumor growth in animals. For instance, tea extracts inhibit most common cancers originating from skin, lung, esophagus, stomach, liver, duodenum, pancreas, colon, bladder, prostate and mammary gland [184]. The active anti-cancer compounds of tea are reported to be catechins, one of the main constituents in green tea. A typical tea beverage prepared with green tea contains 2.5-3.5 mg/ml tea solids, of which 30-42% are catechin compounds [185, 186]. The most abundant tea catechin compound is EGCG. In humans drinking green tea according to Chinese traditions, serum levels of EGCG are in the range of 0.1-0.3 μM [184]. Catechins are also found in most fresh fruits, some legumes and in chocolate.

In green tea-drinking populations, the lower incidence of esophageal and breast cancers has been attributed to flavonoids in tea, although epidemiological investigations on correlations of green tea consumptions and low risks of cancer incidences remain controversial [187].

EGCG is considered chemopreventive and has antitumor cell proliferative, invasive and metastasis effects, as well as anti-inflammatory characteristics [184]. Although the potential antitumor effects of green tea and its catechins had been investigated for a long time, little was known about their mechanisms. Several studies suggest that the antioxidative effect of catechins is involved in its antitumor activity.

Dietary Advice to Reduce Cancer Risk

- Eat plenty of fruit and vegetables (at least five portions a day). Evidence is strong that increasing consumption of fruits and vegetables to five servings a day will reduce risks of some cancers, including cancers of the lung and esophagus, and possibly breast and other cancers. Current U.S. guidelines include potatoes as a vegetable and these (as french fries) account for most of the recent increases in consumption; however, there is no good evidence that increasing potato consumption, or starch in general, will reduce cancer or cardiovascular disease risk;

- Eat plenty of cereal foods, mainly in an unprocessed form (as a source of non-starch polysaccharides);
- Limiting consumption of red meat to several times a month at most by replacement with chicken, fish, legumes, and nuts will probably reduce risk of colon cancer and possibly prostate cancer, although the evidence is not conclusive;
- Maintain ideal body weight (body mass index 20-25); avoid fatty foods;
- Eat red meat and processed meat in moderation (no more than 140 g/day);
- Supplements of folic acid may decrease risk of certain cancers in people who drink alcohol in excess. Substantial evidence indicates that consuming folic acid in the form of an RDA-level multiple vitamin (400 micrograms/day) will reduce risks of colon cancer and coronary heart disease. Alcohol antagonizes the bioavailability of folic acid, and epidemiologic studies suggest that the benefits of additional folate are greatest for those consuming alcohol on a daily basis. In principle, substantially increasing fruits and vegetables could also increase folic acid consumption, but folic acid from these foods has lower bioavailability than that from supplements;
- Avoid high doses of vitamin supplements;
- Alcohol in moderation (a maximum of two units a day for women and three units a day for men). The evidence is strong that high alcohol consumption increases risk of many cancers, and even intakes as low as one drink a day can increase risk of breast cancer. Personal decisions about alcohol consumption are complex and, in addition to the pleasures of consuming these beverages, should include consideration of benefits for coronary heart disease and risks of accidents and addiction;
- Avoid highly salted and moldy foods.

Advice on Lifestyle Factors to Reduce Cancer Risk

- Do not smoke;
- Take regular exercise. Physical activity is a primary method of weight control, and this goal is thus closely linked with weight control. However, evidence is strong that physical activity independently reduces risk of colon cancer, and higher levels of activity may reduce breast cancer risk, although the data are less consistent;
- Do not be sexually promiscuous;
- Avoid prolonged exposure to direct sunlight;
- Avoid hepatitis B and C risks.

Literature

[1] Johnson, IT; Williamson, GM; Musk, SRR. Anticarcinogenic factors in plant foods: a new class of nutrients? *Nutr. Res. Rev.*, 1994, 7, 175-204.

[2] Wattenberg, L. Inhibition of carcinogenesis by minor anutrient constituents of the diet. *Proc. Nutr. Soc.*, 1990, 49, 173-183.

[3] Greenwald, P; Nixon, DW; Malone, WF; Kelloff, GJ; Stern, HR; Witkin, KM. Concepts in cancer chemoprevention research. *Cancer*, 1990, 65, 1483-1490.

[4] Primiano, T; Egner, PA; Sutter, TR; Kelloff, GJ; Roebuck, BD; Kensler, TW. Intermittent dosing with oltipraz: relationship between chemoprevention of aflatoxin-induced tumorigenesis and induction of glutathione S-transferases. *Cancer Res.*, 1995, 55, 4319-4324.

[5] Wattenberg, LW. Inhibition of carcinogen-induced neoplasia by sodium cyanate, tert-butylisocyanate and benzyl isothiocyanate administered subsequent to carcinogen exposure. *Cancer Res.*, 1981, 41, 2991-2994.

[6] Chan, TA; Morin, PJ; Vogelstein, B; Kinzler, KW. Mechanisms underlying non-steroidal anti-inflammatory drug-mediated apoptosis. *Proc. Natl. Acad. Sci. USA*, 1998, 95, 681-686.

[7] Smith, TK; Lund, EK; Johnson, IT. Inhibition of dimethylhydrazineinduced aberrant crypt foci and induction of apoptosis in rat colon following oral administration of the glucosinolate sinigrin. *Carcinogenesis*, 1998, 19, 267-273.

[8] Doll, R; Peto R. The causes of cancer. *J. Natl. Cancer Inst.*, 1981, 66, 1191-308.

[9] Willett, WC. Diet, nutrition and avoidable cancer. *Environ Health Perspect*, 1995, 103(suppl 8), 165-70.

[10] Weight control and physical activity. Lyon, *International Agency for Research on Cancer*, 2002 (IARC Handbooks of Cancer Prevention, Vol. 6.

[11] Parkin, DM. Global cancer statistics in the year 2000. *Lancet Oncology*, 2001, 2:533-543.

[12] Department of Health: Chief Medical Officer's Committee on Medical Aspects of Food. *Nutritional aspects of the development of cancer*. London: Stationery Office, 1998. (Report on health and social subjects 48).

[13] World Cancer Research Fund. Food, nutrition and the prevention of cancer: a global perspective. Washington, DC: WCRF, American Institute for Cancer Research, 1997.

[14] Cargay, AB. Cancer-preventive foods and ingredients. *Food Technol.*, 1992, 46, 65-68.

[15] Luft, R. The development of mitochondrial medicine. *Proc. Natl. Acad. Sci. USA*, 1994, 91, 8731-8738.

[16] Harman, D. Free radical theory of aging: Consequences of mitochondrial aging. *Age*, 1983, 6, 86-94.

[17] Cutler, RG. Human longevity and aging: Possible role of reactive oxygen species. *In Annals of the New York Academy of Sciences*. W. Pierpaoli and N. Fabris, Eds.: 1991, 621, 1-28, New York Academy of Sciences, New York.

[18] Calle, EE; Rodriguez, C; Walker-Thurmond, K; Thun, MJ. Overweight, obesity, and mortality from cancer in a prospectively studied cohort of U.S. adults. *N. Engl. J. Med.*, 2003, 348, 1625-1638.

[19] Holly, J. Insulin-like growth factor-1 and new opportunities for cancer prevention. *Lancet*, 1998, 351, 1373-1375.

[20] Ursin, G; Longnecker, MP; Haile, RW; Greenland, S. A metaanalysis of body mass index and riskof premenopausal breast cancer. *Epidemiology*, 1995, 6, 137-141.

[21] Pathak, DR; Whittemore, AS. Combined effects of body size, parity, and menstrual events on breast cancer incidence in seven countries. *Am. J. Epidemiol.*, 1992, 135, 153-168.

[22] van den Brandt, PA; Spiegelman, D; Yaun, SS; et al. Pooled analysis of prospective cohort studies on height, weight, and breast cancer risk. *Am. J. Epidemiol.*, 2000, 152, 514-527.

[23] Siiteri, PK; MacDonald, PC. Role of extraglandular estrogen in human endocrinology. In: Geiger S R, Astwood E B, Greep R O, eds. *Handbookof Physiology*. Washington DC: American Physiological Society, 1973, 615-629.

[24] Judd, HL; Shamonki, IM; Frumar, AM; Lagasse, LD. Origin of serum estradiol in postmenopausal women. *Obstet. Gynecol.*, 1982, 59, 680-686.

[25] Key, TJ; Allen, NE; Verkasalo, PK; Banks E. Energy balance and cancer: the role of sex hormones. *Proc. Nutr. Soc.*, 2001, 60, 1-9.

[26] Simopoulos, AP. The importance of the ratio of omega-6/omega-3 essential fatty acids. *Biomed. Pharmacother*, 2002, 56:365-379.

[27] Cummings, JH; Englyst, HN. Fermentation in the human large intestine and the available substrates. *Am. J. Clin. Nutr.*, 1987, 45, 124-55.

[28] MacFarlane, GT; Cummings, JH. The colonic flora, fermentation, and large bowel digestive function. In: Philips, SF; Pemberton, JH; Shorter, RG, editors. *The large intestine: physiology, pathophysiology and disease*. New York: Raven Press; 1991. p. 51-92.

[29] Lipkin, M; Reddy, B; Newmark, H et al. Dietary factors in human colorectal cancer. *Annu. Rev. Nutr.*, 1999, 19, 545-86.

[30] D'Argenio, G; Mazzacca, G. Short-chain fatty acid in the human colon. Relation to inflammatory bowel diseases and colon cancer. In: Zappia, et al., editors. *Advances in nutrition and cancer.* vol. 2. New York: Plenum Press; 1999. p. 149-59.

[31] Cummings, JH; Bingham, SA; Heaton, KW; Eastwood, MA. Fecal weight, colon cancer risk and dietary intake of nonstarch polysaccharides (dietary fiber). *Gastroenterology*, 1992, 103, 1783-1789.

[32] Cummings, JH. The effect of dietary fiber on fecal weight and composition. In Spiller GA (ed): "*CRC Handbook of Dietary Fiber in Human Nutrition*." Boca Raton, FL: CRC Press, 1993, pp 263-333.

[33] Jenkins, DJA; Kendall, CWC; Vuksan, V; Augustin, LSA; Li, YM; Lee, B; Mehling, CC; Parker, T; Faulkner, D; Seyler, H; Vidgen, E; Fulgoni, V: The effect of wheat bran particle size on laxation and colonic fermentation. *J. Am. Coll. Nutr.*, 1999, 18, 339-345.

[34] Stephen, AM. Whole grains - Impact of consuming whole grains on physiological effects of dietary fiber and starch. *Crit. Rev. Food Sci. Nutr.*, 1994, 34, 499-511.

[35] Van Loo, J; Coussement, P; De Leenheer, L; Hoebregs, H; Smits, G. On the presence of inulin and oligofructose as natural ingredients in the western diet. *Crit. Rev. Food Sci. Nutr*, 1995, 35, 525-552

[36] Gibson, GR; Beatty, ER; Wang, X; Cummings, JH. Selective stimulation of bifidobacteria in the human colon by oligofructose and inulin. *Gastroenterology*, 1995, 108, 975-982.

[37] Buddington, RK; Williams, CH; Chen, S; Witherly, SA. Dietary supplement of neosugar alters the fecal flora and decreases activities of some reductive enzymes in human subjects. *Am. J. Clin. Nutr.*, 1996, 63, 709-716.

[38] Foster-Powell, K; Holt, SH; Brand-Miller, JC: International table of glycemic index and glycemic load values. *Am. J. Clin. Nutr.*, 2002, 76, 5-56.

[39] Augustin, LS; Gallus, S; Negri, E; La Vecchia C. Glycemic index, glycemic load and risk of gastric cancer. *Ann. Oncol.*, 2004, 15, 581-584.

[40] Augustin, LS; Gallus, S; Franceschi, S; Negri, E; Jenkins, DJ; Kendall, CW; Dal Maso, L; Talamini, R; La Vecchia, C. Glycemic index and load and risk of upper aero-digestive tract neoplasms (Italy). *Cancer Causes Control*, 2003, 14, 657-662.

[41] Augustin, LS; Gallus, S; Bosetti, C; Levi, F; Negri, E; Franceschi, S; Dal Maso, L; Jenkins, D;, Kendall, CW; La Vecchia, C. Glycemic index and glycemic load in endometrial cancer. *Int. J. Cancer*, 2003, 105, 404-407.

[42] Augustin, LS; Polesel, J; Bosetti, C; Kendall, CW; La Vecchia, C; Parpinel, M; Conti, E; Montella, M; Franceschi, S; Jenkins, DJ; Dal Maso, L. Dietary glycemic index, glycemic load and ovarian cancer risk: a case-control study in Italy. *Ann. Oncol.*, 2003, 14, 78-84.

[43] Franceschi, S; Dal Maso, L; Augustin, L; Negri, E; Parpinel, M; Boyle, P; Jenkins, DJ; La Vecchia, C. Dietary glycemic load and colorectal cancer risk. *Ann. Oncol.*, 2001, 12, 173-178.

[44] Slattery, ML; Boucher, KM; Caan, BJ; Potter, JD; Ma, KN. Eating patterns and risk of colon cancer. *Am. J. Epidemiol.*, 1998, 148, 4-16.

[45] Bostick, RM; Potter, JD; Kushi, LH; Sellers, TA; Steinmetz, KA; McKenzie, DR; Gapstur, SM; Folsom, AR. Sugar, meat, and fat intake, and non-dietary risk factors for colon cancer incidence in Iowa women (United States). *Cancer Causes Control*, 1994, 5, 38-52.

[46] Frazier, AL; Li, L; Cho, E; Willett, WC; Colditz, GA. Adolescent diet and risk of breast cancer. *Cancer Causes Control*, 2004, 15, 73-82.

[47] Higginbotham, S; Zhang, ZF; Lee, IM; Cook, NR; Giovannucci, E; Buring, JE; Liu, S. Dietary glycemic load and risk of colorectal cancer in the Women's Health Study. *J. Natl. Cancer Inst.*, 2004, 96, 229-233.

[48] Cho, E; Spiegelman, D; Hunter, DJ; Chen, WY; Colditz, GA; Willett, WC. Premenopausal dietary carbohydrate, glycemic index, glycemic load and fiber in relation to risk of breast cancer. *Cancer Epidemiol. Biomarkers Prev.*, 2003, 12, 1153-1158.

[49] Folsom, AR; Demissie, Z; Harnack, L. Glycemic index, glycemic load, and incidence of endometrial cancer: the Iowa women's health study. *Nutr. Cancer*, 2003, 46, 119-124.

[50] Higginbotham, S; Zhang, ZF; Lee, IM; Cook, NR; Buring, JE; Liu, S. Dietary glycemic load and breast cancer risk in the Women's Health Study. *Cancer Epidemiol. Biomarkers Prev.*, 2004, 13, 65-70.

[51] Michaud, DS; Liu, S; Giovannucci, E; Willett, WC; Colditz, GA; Fuchs, CS. Dietary sugar, glycemic load, and pancreatic cancer risk in a prospective study. *J. Natl. Cancer Inst.*, 2002, 94, 1293-1300.

[52] Holmes, MD; Liu, S; Hankinson, SE; Colditz, GA; Hunter, DJ; Willett, WC. Dietary carbohydrates, fiber, and breast cancer risk. *Am. J. Epidemiol.*, 2004, 159, 732-739.

[53] Jonas, CR; McCullough, ML; Teras, LR; Walker-Thurmond, KA; Thun, MJ; Calle, EE. Dietary glycemic index, glycemic load, and risk of incident breast cancer in postmenopausal women. *Cancer Epidemiol Biomarkers Prev.*, 2003, 12, 573-577.

[54] Oh, K; Willett, WC; Fuchs, CS; Giovannucci, EL. Glycemic index, glycemic load, and carbohydrate intake in relation to risk of distal colorectal adenoma in women. *Cancer Epidemiol. Biomarkers Prev.*, 2004, 13, 1192-1198.

[55] Terry, PD; Jain, M; Miller, AB; Howe, GR; Rohan, TE. Glycemic load, carbohydrate intake, and risk of colorectal cancer in women: a prospective cohort study. *J. Natl. Cancer Inst.*, 2003, 95, 914-916.

[56] Hu, FB; Manson, JE; Liu, S; Hunter, D; Colditz, GA; Michels, KB; Speizer, FE; Giovannucci, E. Prospective study of adult onset diabetes mellitus (type 2) and risk of colorectal cancer in women. *J. Natl. Cancer Inst.* 1999, 91:542-547.

[57] Khaw, KT; Wareham, N; Bingham, S; Luben, R; Welch, A; Day, N. Preliminary communication: glycated hemoglobin, diabetes, and incident colorectal cancer in men and women: a prospective analysis from the European prospective investigation into cancer-Norfolk study. *Cancer Epidemiol. Biomarkers Prev.*, 2004, 13, 915-919.

[58] Saydah, SH; Platz, EA; Rifai, N; Pollak, MN; Brancati, FL; Helzlsouer, KJ. Association of markers of insulin and glucose control with subsequent colorectal cancer risk. *Cancer Epidemiol. Biomarkers Prev.*, 2003, 12, 412-418.

[59] Platz, EA; Hankinson, SE; Rifai, N; Colditz, GA; Speizer, FE; Giovannucci, E. Glycosylated hemoglobin and risk of colorectal cancer and adenoma (United States). *Cancer Causes Control*, 1999, 10, 379-386.

[60] Schoen, RE; Tangen, CM; Kuller, LH; Burke, GL; Cushman, M; Tracy, RP; Dobs, A; Savage, PJ. Increased blood glucose and insulin, body size, and incident colorectal cancer. *J. Natl. Cancer Inst.*, 1999, 91, 1147-1154.

[61] Colangelo, LA; Gapstur, SM; Gann, PH; Dyer, AR; Liu, K. Colorectal cancer mortality and factors related to the insulin resistance syndrome. *Cancer Epidemiol. Biomarkers Prev.*, 2002, 11, 385-391.

[62] Coughlin, SS; Calle, EE; Teras, LR; Petrelli, J; Thun, MJ. Diabetes mellitus as a predictor of cancer mortality in a large cohort of US adults. *Am. J. Epidemiol.*, 2004, 159, 1160-1167.

[63] La Vecchia, C; Negri, E; Decarli, A; Franceschi, S. Diabetes mellitus and colorectal cancer risk. *Cancer Epidemiol. Biomarkers Prev.*, 1997, 6, 1007-1010.

[64] Sandhu, MS; Luben, R; Khaw, KT. Self reported non-insulin dependent diabetes, family history, and risk of prevalent colorectal cancer: population based, cross sectional study. *J. Epidemiol. Community Health*, 2001, 55, 804-805.

[65] Anderson, KE; Anderson, E; Mink, PJ; Hong, CP; Kushi, LH; Sellers, TA; Lazovich, D; Folsom, AR. Diabetes and endometrial cancer in the Iowa women's health study. *Cancer Epidemiol. Biomarkers Prev.*, 2001, 10, 611-616.

[66] Coughlin, SS; Calle, EE; Teras, LR; Petrelli, J; Thun, MJ. Diabetes mellitus as a predictor of cancer mortality in a large cohort of US adults. *Am. J. Epidemiol.*, 2004, 159, 1160-1167.

[67] Calle, EE; Murphy, TK; Rodriguez, C; Thun, MJ; Heath, CW Jr. Diabetes mellitus and pancreatic cancer mortality in a prospective cohort of United States adults. *Cancer Causes Control*, 1998, 9, 403-410.

[68] Holmes, MD; Liu, S; Hankinson, SE; Colditz, GA; Hunter, DJ; Willett, WC. Dietary carbohydrates, fiber, and breast cancer risk. *Am. J. Epidemiol.*, 2004, 159, 732-739.

[69] Slattery, ML; Curtin, KP; Edwards, SL; Schaffer, DM. Plant foods, fiber, and rectal cancer. *Am. J. Clin. Nutr.*, 2004, 79, 274-281.

[70] Weaver, CM. Calcium. In: *Present knowledge in nutrition*. Bowman BA and Russell RM (Eds.), ILSI Press, Washington, DC, 8th Edition, 2001, pp. 273-280.

[71] Giovannucci, E; Stampfer, MJ; Colditz, G; Rimm, EB; Willett, WC. Relationship of diet to risk of colorectal adenoma in men. *J. Natl. Cancer Inst*, 1992, 84, 91-8.

[72] Lipkin, M; Newmark, H. Effect of added dietary calcium on colonic epithelial-cell proliferation in subjects at high risk for familial colonic cancer. *N. Engl. J. Med.*, 1985, 313, 1381-4.

[73] Janne, PA; Mayer, RJ. Chemoprevention of colorectal cancer. *N. Engl. J. Med.*, 2000, 342, 1960-8.

[74] Burke, CA; Bauer, WM; Lashner, B. Chemoprevention of colorectal cancer: slow, steady progress. *Cleveland Clinic J. Med.*, 2003, 70, 346-50.

[75] Baron, JA; Beach, M; Mandel, JS, et al. Calcium supplements for the prevention of colorectal adenomas. *N Engl J Med*, 1999, 340, 101-7.

[76] Bonithon-Kopp, C; Kronborg, O; Giacosa, A; Rath, U; Faivre, J. Calcium and fibre supplementation in prevention of colorectal adenoma recurrence: a randomised intervention trial. European Cancer Prevention Organisation Study Group. *Lancet*, 2000, 356,1300-6.

[77] Pignone, M; Levin, B. Recent developments in colorectal cancer screening and prevention. *Am. Fam. Phys.*, 2002, 66, 297-302.

[78] Miller, GD; Anderson, JJB. The role of calcium in prevention chronic diseases. *J. Am. Coll. Nutr.*, 1999, 18, 371S-2S.

[79] Holick, MF. Vitamin D importance in the prevention of cancers, type 1 diabetes, heart disease, and osteoporosis. *Am. J. Clin. Nutr.*, 2004, 79, 362-371.

[80] Vieth, R; Kimball, S; Hu, A; Walfish, PG. Randomized comparison of the effects of the vitamin D3 adequate intake versus 100 mcg (4000 IU) per day on biochemical responses and the wellbeing of patients. *Nutr. J.*, 2004, 3, 8.

[81] Schwartz, GG; Whitlatch, LW; Chen,TC; Lokeshwar, BL; Holick, MF. Human prostate cells synthesize 1,25-dihydroxyvitamin D3 from 25-hydroxyvitamin D3. *Cancer Epidemiol. Biomarkers Prev.*, 1998, 7, 391-395.

[82] Tangpricha, V; Flanagan, JN; Whitlatch, LW; Tseng, CC; Chen, TC; Holt, PR; Lipkin, MS; Holick, MF. 25-hydroxyvitamin D-1alpha-hydroxylase in normal and malignant colon tissue. *Lancet*, 2001, 357, 1673-1674.

[83] Friedrich, M; Rafi, L; Mitschele, T; Tilgen, W; Schmidt, W; Reichrath, J. Analysis of the vitamin D system in cervical carcinomas, breast cancer and ovarian cancer. *Recent Results Cancer Res.*, 2003, 164, 239-246.

[84] Schwartz, GG; Eads, D; Rao, A; Cramer, SD; Willingham, MC; Chen, TC; Jamieson, DP; Wang, L; Burnstein, KL; Holick, MF; Koumenis, C. Pancreatic cancer cells

express 25-hydroxyvitamin D-1alphahydroxylase and their proliferation is inhibited by the prohormone 25-hydroxyvitamin D3. *Carcinogenesis*, 2004, 25, 1015-1026.

[85] Mawer, EB; Hayes, ME; Heys, SE; Davies, M; White, A; Stewart, MF; Smith, GN. Constitutive synthesis of 1,25-dihydroxyvitamin D3 by a human small cell lung cancer cell line. *J. Clin. Endocrinol. Metab.*, 1994, 79, 554-560.

[86] Holt, PR; Arber, N; Halmos, B; Forde, K Kissileff, H; McGlynn, KA; Moss, SF; Kurihara, N; Fan, K; Yang, K; Lipkin, M. Colonic epithelial cell proliferation decreases with increasing levels of serum 25-hydroxy vitamin D. *Cancer Epidemiol. Biomarkers Prev*, 2002, 11, 113-119.

[87] Barreto, AM; Schwartz, GG; Woodruff, R; Cramer, SD. 25-Hydroxyvitamin D3, the prohormone of 1,25-dihydroxyvitamin D3, inhibits the proliferation of primary prostatic epithelial cells. *Cancer Epidemiol Biomarkers Prev.*, 2000, 9, 265-270.

[88] Sunlight, Nutrition And Health Research Center [http://www.sunarc.org]

[89] Hanchette, CL; Schwartz, GG. Geographic patterns of prostate cancer mortality. Evidence for a protective effect of ultraviolet radiation. *Cancer*, 1992, 70, 2861-2869.

[90] Lefkowitz, ES; Garland, CF. Sunlight, vitamin D, and ovarian cancer mortality rates in US women. *Int. J. Epidemiol.*, 1994, 23, 1133-1136.

[91] Gorham, ED; Garland, FC; Garland, CF. Sunlight and breast cancer incidence in the USSR. *Int. J. Epidemiol.*, 1990, 19, 820-824.

[92] Grant, WB. Ecologic studies of solar UV-B radiation and cancer mortality rates. *Recent Results Cancer Res.*, 2003, 164, 371-377.

[93] Grant, WB. An estimate of premature cancer mortality in the U.S. due to inadequate doses of solar ultraviolet-B radiation. *Cancer*, 2002, 94, 1867-1875.

[94] Moyad, MA. *The ABCs of Nutrition and Supplements for Prostate Cancer*. Chelsea, MI: Sleeping Bear Press, 2000.

[95] Blount, BC; Mack, MM; Wehr, CM; MacGregor, JT; Hiatt, RA; Wang, G; Wickramasinghe, SN; Everson, RB; Ames, BN. Folate deficiency causes uracil misincorporation into human DNA and chromosome breakage: implications for cancer and neuronal damage. *Proc. Natl. Acad. Sci. USA*, 1997, 94, 3290-3295.

[96] Ma, J; Stampfer, MJ; Giovannucci, E; Artigas, C; Hunter, DJ; Fuchs, C; Willett, WC; Selhub, J; Hennekens, CH; Rozen, R. Methylenetetrahydrofolate reductase polymorphism, dietary interactions, and risk of colorectal cancer. *Cancer Res.*, 1997, 57, 1098-1102.

[97] Ma, J; Stampfe,r MJ; Christensen, B; Giovannucci, E; Hunter, DJ; Chen, J; Willett, WC; Selhub, J; Hennekens, CH; Gravel, R; Rozen, R. A polymorphism of the methionine synthase gene: association with plasma folate, vitamin B12, homocyst(e)ine, and colorectal cancer risk. *Cancer Epidemiol Biomarkers Prev.*, 1999, 8, 825-829.

[98] Giovannucci, E; Chen, J; Smith-Warner, SA; Rimm, EB; Fuchs, CS; Palomeque, C; Willett, WC; Hunter, DJ. Methylenetetrahydrofolate reductase, alcohol dehydrogenase, diet, and risk of colorectal adenomas. *Cancer Epidemiol Biomarkers Prev.*, 2003, 12, 970-979.

[99] Le Marchand, L; Donlon, T; Hankin, JH; Kolonel, LN; Wilkens, LR; Seifried, A. B-vitamin intake, metabolic genes, and colorectal cancer risk (United States). *Cancer Causes Control*, 2002, 13, 239-248.

[100] Cravo, ML; Pinto, AG; Chaves, P; Cruz, JA; Lage, P; Nobre Leitao, C; Costa Mira, F. Effect of folate supplementation on DNA methylation of rectal mucosa in patients with colonic adenomas: correlation with nutrient intake. *Clin. Nutr.*, 1998, 17, 45-49.

[101] Shrubsole, MJ; Jin, F; Dai, Q; Shu, XO; Potter, JD; Hebert, JR; Gao, YT; Zheng, W. Dietary folate intake and breast cancer risk: results from the Shanghai Breast Cancer Study. *Cancer Res.* 2001, 61, 7136-7141.

[102] Nishizawa, Y; Yamamoto, T; Terada, N; Fushiki, S; Matsumoto, K. Effects of methylcobalamin on the proliferation of androgensensitive or estrogen-sensitive malignant cells in culture and in vivo. *Int. J. Vitam Nutr. Res.*, 1997, 67:164-170.

[103] Nishizawa, Y; Goto, HG; Tanigaki, Y; Fushiki, S. Induction of apoptosis in an androgen-dependent mouse mammary carcinoma cell line by methylcobalamin. *Anticancer Res.*, 2001, 21, 1107-1110.

[104] Tsao, CS; Myashita, K. Influence of cobalamin on the survival of mice bearing ascites tumor. *Pathobiology*, 1993, 61:104-108.

[105] Tsao, CS; Miyashita, K; Young, M. Cytotoxic activity of cobalamin in cultured malignant and nonmalignant cells. *Pathobiology*, 1990, 58:292-296.

[106] Shimizu, N; Hamazoe, R; Kanayama, H; Maeta, M; Koga, S. Experimental study of antitumor effect of methyl-B12. *Oncology,* 1987, 44, 169-173.

[107] Choi, SW; Friso, S; Ghandour, H; Bagley, PJ; Selhub, J; Mason, JB. Vitamin B-12 deficiency induces anomalies of base substitution and methylation in the DNA of rat colonic epithelium. *J. Nutr.*, 2004, 134, 750-755.

[108] Wu, K; Helzlsouer, KJ; Comstock, GW; Hoffman, SC; Nadeau, MR; Selhub, J. A prospective study on folate, B12, and pyridoxal 5'-phosphate (B6) and breast cancer. *Cancer Epidemiol. Biomarkers Prev.*, 1999, 8, 209-217.

[109] Zhang, SM; Willett, WC; Selhub, J; Hunter, DJ; Giovannucci, EL; Holmes, MD; Colditz, GA; Hankinson, SE. Plasma folate, vitamin B6, vitamin B12, homocysteine, and risk of breast cancer. *J. Natl Cancer Inst.*, 2003, 95, 373-380.

[110] Thomson, CD. Assessment of requirements for selenium and adequacy of selenium status: a review. *Eur. J. Clin. Nutr.*, 2004, 58, 391-402.

[111] Selenium Information Sheet [http://www.selenium.arizona.edu/INFOse.htm]

[112] Duffield-Lillico, AJ; Reid, ME; Turnbull, BW; Combs, GF Jr; Slate, EH; Fischbach, LA; Marshall, JR; Clark, LC. Baseline characteristics and the effect of selenium supplementation on cancer incidence in a randomized clinical trial: a summary report of the Nutritional Prevention of Cancer Trial. *Cancer Epidemiol. Biomarkers Prev.*, 2002, 11:630-639.

[113] Clark, LC; Combs, GF Jr; Turnbull, BW; Slate, EH; Chalker, DK; Chow, J; Davis, LS; Glover, RA; Graham, GF; Gross, EG; Krongrad, A; Lesher, JL Jr; Park, HK; Sanders, BB Jr; Smith, CL; Taylor, JR. Effects of selenium supplementation for cancer prevention in patients with carcinoma of the skin. A randomized controlled trial. Nutritional Prevention of Cancer Study Group. *JAMA*, 1996, 276:1957-1963.

[114] Ghadirian, P; Maisonneuve, P; Perret, C; Kennedy, G; Boyle, P; Krewski, D; Lacroix, A. A case-control study of toenail selenium and cancer of the breast, colon, and prostate. *Cancer Detect Prev*, 2000, 24, 305-313.

[115] van den Brandt, PA; Goldbohm, RA; van't Veer, P; Bode, P; Dorant, E; Hermus, RJ; Sturmans, F. Toenail selenium levels and the risk of breast cancer. *Am. J. Epidemiol.*, 1994, 140:20-26.

[116] Hunter, DJ; Morris, JS; Stampfer, MJ; Colditz, GA; Speizer, FE; Willett, WC. A prospective study of selenium status and breast cancer risk. *JAMA*, 1990, 264, 1128-1131.

[117] van 't Veer, P van der Wielen, RP; Kok, FJ; Hermus, RJ; Sturmans, F. Selenium in diet, blood, and toenails in relation to breast cancer: a case-control study. *Am. J. Epidemiol.*, 1990, 131, 987-994.

[118] van Noord, PA; Collette, HJ; Maas, MJ; de Waard, F. Selenium levels in nails of premenopausal breast cancer patients assessed prediagnostically in a cohort-nested case-referent study among women screened in the DOM project. *Int J Epidemiol*, 1987, 16, 318-322.

[119] Reid, ME; Duffield-Lillico, AJ; Garland, L; Turnbull, BW; Clark, LC; Marshall, JR. Selenium supplementation and lung cancer incidence: an update of the nutritional prevention of cancer trial. *Cancer Epidemiol Biomarkers Prev.*, 2002, 11, 1285-1291.

[120] van den Brandt, PA; Goldbohm, RA; van 't Veer, P; Bode, P; Dorant, E; Hermus, RJ; Sturmans, F. A prospective cohort study on selenium status and the risk of lung cancer. *Cancer Res.*, 1993, 53, 4860-4865.

[121] Jacob, RA; Burri, BJ. Oxidative damage and defense. *Am J Clin Nutr*, 1996, 63, 985S-990S.

[122] 1222. Diplock, AT. Antioxidants and disease prevention. *Food Chem Toxicol*, 1996, 34, 1013-1023.

[123] Block, G; Patterson, BH; Subar, AF. Fruit, vegetables, and cancer prevention: a review of the epidemiological evidence. *Nutr. Cancer*, 1992, 18, 1-29.

[124] Steinmetz, KA; Potter, JD. Vegetables, fruit, and cancer prevention: a review. *JADA*, 1996, 96, 1027-1039.

[125] Wattenberg, LW. Inhibition of carcinogenesis by minor dietary constituents. *Cancer Res.*, 1992, 52, 2085S-2091S.

[126] Ziegler, RG; Mayne, ST; Swanson, CA. Nutrition and lung cancer. *Cancer Causes and Control*, 1996, 7, 157-177.

[127] Woutersen, RA; Wolterbeek, A; Appel, MJ; van den Berg, H. Safety evaluation of synthetic ß-carotene. (TNO report, V 97.221. TNO Nutrition and Food Research Institute). *Crit. Rev. Toxicol.*, 1999, 29, 515-542.

[128] IARC. International Agency for Research on Cancer Handbooks of Cancer Prevention. 1998, Vol 2, Carotenoids. IARC; Lyon, France.

[129] Omenn, GS. Chemoprevention of lung cancer: the rise and demise of beta-carotene. *Ann. Rev. Public Health*, 1998, 19, 73-99.

[130] Edge, R; Truscott, TG. Prooxidant and antioxidant reaction mechanisms of carotene and radical interactions with vitamins E and C. *Nutrition*, 1997, 13, 992-994.

[131] Peto, R; Doll, R; Buckley, JD; Sporn, MB. Can dietary beta-carotene materially reduce human cancer rates? *Nature*, 1981, 290, 201-208.

[132] Stich, HF; Stich, W; Rosin, MP; Vallejera, MO. Use of the micronucleus test to monitor the effect of vitamin A, beta-carotene and canthaxanthin on the buccal mucosa of betel nut/tobacco chewers. *Int. J. Cancer*, 1984, 34, 745-750.

[133] Garewal; HS; Meyskens, FL Jr; Killen, D; Reeves, D; Kiersch, TA; Elletson, H; Strosberg, A; King, D; Steinbronn, K. Response of oral leukoplakia to beta-carotene. *J. Clin. Oncol.*, 1990, 8, 1715-1720.

[134] Lippman, SM; Batsakis, JG; Toth, BB; Weber, RS; Lee, JJ; Martin, JW; Hays, GL; Goepfert, H; Hong, WK. Comparison of low-dose isotretinoin with beta carotene to prevent oral carcinogenesis. *NEJM*, 1993, 328, 15-20.

[135] Greenberg, ER; Baron, JA; Tosteson, TD; Freeman, DH Jr; Beck, GJ; Bond, JH; Colacchio, TA; Coller, JA; Frankl, HD; Haile, RW; Mandel, JS; Nierenberg, DW; Rothstein, R; Snover, DC; Stevens, MM; Summers, RW; van Stolk, RU. A clinical trial of antioxidant vitamins to prevent colorectal adenoma. *NEJM*, 1994, 331, 141-147.

[136] MacClennan, R; Macrae, F; Bain, C; Battistutta, D; Chapuis, P; Gratten, H; Lambert, J; Newland, RC; Ngu, M; Russell, A; Ward, M; Wahlqvist, ML. Randomized trial of intake of fat, fiber, and beta carotene to prevent colorectal adenomas. *JNCI*, 1995, 87, 1760-1766.

[137] van Poppel, G; Goldbohm, RA. Epidemiologic evidence for b-carotene and cancer prevention. *Am. J. Clin. Nutr.*, 1995, 62, 1393S-1402S.

[138] Kolonel, LN. Nutrition and prostate cancer. *Cancer Causes and Control*, 1996, 7, 83-94.

[139] Hunter, DJ; Willett, WC. Nutrition and breast cancer. *Cancer Causes and Control*, 1996, 7, 56-68.

[140] Alpha-Tocopherol Beta-Carotene Cancer Prevention Study Group. The effect of vitamin E and beta carotene on the incidence of lung cancer and other cancers in male smokers. *NEJM*, 1994, 330, 1029-1035.

[141] Hennekens, CH; Buring, JE; Manson, JE; Stampfer, M; Rosner, B; Cook, NR; Belanger, C; La Motte, F; Gaziano, JM; Ridker, PM; Willett, W; Peto, R. Lack of effect of long-term supplementation with beta-carotene on the incidence of malignant neoplasms and cardiovascular disease. *NEJM*, 1996, 334, 1145-1149.

[142] Omenn, GS; Goodman, GE; Thornquist, MD; Balmes, J; Cullen, MR; Glass, A; Keogh, JP; Meyskens, FL Jr; Valanis, B; Williams, JH Jr; Barnhardt, S; Cherniack, MG; Brodkin, CA; Hammar, S. Risk factors for lung cancer and for intervention effects in CARET, the Beta-Carotene and Retinol Efficacy Trial. *J. Natl. Cancer Ins.*, 1996, 88, 1550-1559.

[143] Blot, WJ; Li, J; Taylor, PR; Guo, W; Dawsey, SM; Li, B. The Lixian trials: mortality rates by vitamin-mineral intervention group. *Am. J. Clin. Nut.*, 1995, 62, 1424S-1426S.

[144] Helser, MA; Hotchkiss, JH; Roe, DA. Influence of fruit and vegetable juices on the endogenous formation of N-nitrosoproline and N-nitrosothiazolidine-4-carboxylic acid in humans on controlled diets. C*arcinogenesis*, 1992, 13, 2277-2280.

[145] Byers, T; Guerrero, N. Epidemiologic evidence for vitamin C and vitamin E in cancer prevention. *Am. J. Clin. Nutr.*, 1995, 562, 1385S-1392S.

[146] Block, G. Vitamin C and cancer prevention: the epidemiologic evidence. *Am. J. Clin. Nutr*, 1991, 53, 270S-282S.

[147] Padayatty, SJ; Katz, A; Wang, Y; Eck, P; Kwon, O; Je-Hyuk, L; Chen, S; Corpe, C; Dutta, A; Dutta, SK; Levine, M. Vitamin C as an Antioxidant: Evaluation of Its Role in Disease Prevention. *JACN*, 2003, 22, 18-35.

[148] Bellizzi, MC; Franklin, MF; Duthie, GG; James, WPT. Vitamin E and coronary heart disease: the European paradox. *Eur. J. Clin. Nutr.*, 1994, 48, 822-831.

[149] Scott, G. Antioxidants in science, technology, medicine and nutrition. Chichester, Albion Publishing, 1997.

[150] Duthie, GG. Lipid peroxidation. *Eur. J. Clin. Nutr.*, 1993, 47, 759-764.

[151] Kagan, VE; Recycling and redox cycling of phenolic antioxidants. *Ann. NY Acad. Sci.*, 1998, 854, 425-434.

[152] Kimmick, GG; Bell, RA; Bostick, RM. Vitamin E and breast cancer: a review. *Nutr Cancer*, 1997, 27, 109-117.

[153] Tseng, M; Murray, SC; Kupper, LL; Sandler, RS. Micronutrients and the risk of colorectal adenomas. *Amer. J. Epidemiol.*, 1996, 144, 1005-1014.

[154] Lubin, F; Rozen, P; Arieli, B; Farbstein, M; Knaani, Y; Bat, L; Farbstein, H. Nutritional and lifestyle habits and water–fiber interaction in colorectal adenoma etiology. *Cancer Epidemiol. Biomarkers Prevention*, 1997, 6, 79-85.

[155] Stone, WL; Papas, AM. Tocopherols and the etiology of colon cancer. *JNCI*, 1997, 89, 1006-1014.

[156] Greenwald, P; Clifford, CK; Milner, JA. Diet and cancer prevention. *Eur. J. Cancer*, 2001, 37, 948-965.

[157] Talalay, P; Fahey, JW. Phytochemicals from cruciferous plants protect against cancer by modulating carcinogen metabolism. *J. Nutr.*, 2001, 131, 3027S-33S.

[158] IARC Handbooks of Cancer Prevention. Cruciferous vegetables (Vol 9). *International Agency for Research on Cancer* (WHO), Lyon 2004.

[159] Rosa, EAS; Heaney, RK; Fenwick, GR; Portas, CAM. Glucosinolates in crop plants. *Hortic. Rev.*, 1997, 19, 99-215.

[160] Lampe, JW; Peterson, S. Brassica, biotransformation and cancer risk: Genetic polymorphisms alter the preventive effects of cruciferous vegetables. *J. Nutr.*, 2002, 132, 2991-2994.

[161] Fahey, JW; Zalcmann, AT; Talalay, P. The chemical diversity and distribution of glucosinolates and isothiocyanates among plants. *Phytochemistry*, 2001, 56, 5-51.

[162] Keck, AS; Finley, JW. Cruciferous vegetables: Cancer protective mechanisms of glucosinolate hydrolysis products and selenium. *Integr. Cancer Ther.*, 2004, 3, 5-12.

[163] Hecht, SS. Inhibition of carcinogenesis by isothiocyanates. *Drug Metab Rev.*, 2000, 32, 395-411.

[164] Singh, SV; Herman-Antosiewicz, A; Singh, AV; Lew, KL; Srivastava, SK; Kamath R, et al. Sulforaphane-induced G2/M phase cell cycle arrest involves checkpoint kinase 2 -mediated phophorylation of cell division cycle 25C. *J. Biol. Chem.*, 2004, 279, 25813-25822.

[165] Longcope, C. Relationships of estrogen to breast cancer, of diet to breast cancer, and of diet to estradiol metabolism. *J. Natl. Cancer Inst.*, 1990, 82, 96-97.

[166] Michnovicz, JJ; Adlercreutz, H; Bradlow, HL. Changes in levels of urinary estrogen metabolites after oral indole-3-carbinol treatment in humans. *J. Natl. Cancer Inst.*, 1997, 89, 718-723

[167] Brignall, MS. Prevention and treatment of cancer with indole-3-carbinol. *Altern. Med. Rev.*, 2001, 6, 580-589.

[168] Williamson, G; Plumb, GW; Uda, Y; Price, KR; Rhodes, MJ. Dietary quercetin glycosides: Antioxidant activity and induction of the anticarcinogenic phase II marker enzyme quinone reductase in Hepalclc7 cells. *Carcinogenesis*, 1996, 17, 2385-2387.

[169] Finley JW, Davis CD, Feng Y. Selenium from high selenium broccoli protects rats from colon cancer. *J. Nutr.* 2000;130:2384-9.

[170] Kuiper, GG; Carlsson, B; Grandien, K; Enmark, E; Häggblad, J; Nilsson, S; Gustafsson, J-Ă. Comparison of the ligand binding specificity and transcript distribution of estrogen receptors α and β. *Endocrinology*, 1997, 138, 863-870.

[171] Tham, DM; Gardner, CD; Haskell, WL. Potential health benefits of dietary phytoestrogens: a review of the clinical, epidemiological, and mechanistic evidence. *J. Clin. Endocrinol. Metab.*, 1998, 83, 2223-2235.

[172] Pietinen, P; Stumpf, K; Männistö, S; Kataja, V; Uusitupa, M; Adlercreutz, H. Serum enterolactone and risk of breast cancer: a case-control study in eastern Finland. *Cancer Epidemiol. Biomarkers Prev.*, 2001, 4, 339-344.

[173] Lin, X; Switzer, BR; Demark-Wahnefried, W. Effect of mammalian lignans on the growth of prostate cancer cell lines. *Anticancer Res.*, 2001, 21, 3995- 3999.

[174] Sung, MK; Lautens, M; Thompson, LU. Mammalian lignans inhibit the growth of estrogen-independent human colon tumor cells. *Anticancer Res.*, 1998, 18, 1405-1408.

[175] Mazur, W; Adlercreutz, H. Natural and ahthropogenic environmental oestrogens: the scientific basis for risk assessment. *Pure Appl. Chem.*, 1998, 70, 1759-1776.

[176] Harborne, JB. *The flavonoids: advances in research since 1986*. Chapman and Hall, London, UK, 1993.

[177] Bravo, L. Polyphenols: chemistry, dietary sources, metabolism, and nutritional significance. *Nutr. Rev.*, 1998, 56, 317-333.

[178] Hollman, PC; Katan, MB. Health effects and bioavailability of dietary flavonols. *Free Radic. Res.*, 1999, 31, S75-80.

[179] Ramos, S. Effects of dietary flavonoids on apoptotic pathways related to cancer chemoprevention. *J. Nutr. Biochem.*, 2007, 18, 427-442.

[180] Manach, C; Regerat, F; Texier, O; Agullo, G; Demigne, C; Remesy, C. Bioavailability, metabolism and physiological impact of 4-oxoflavonoids. *Nutr. Res.*, 1996, 16, 517-544.

[181] Shahidi, F; Wanasundara, PK. Phenolic antioxidants. *Crit. Rev. Food Sci. Nutr.*, 1992, 32,67-103.

[182] Watson, W; Cai, J; Jones, D. Diet and apoptosis. *Annu Rev Nutr*, 2000, 108, 153-64.

[183] Wenzel, U; Kuntz, S; Brendel, M; Daniel, H. Dietary flavone is a potent apoptosis inducer in human colon carcinoma cells. *Cancer Res.*, 2000, 60, 3823-31.

[184] Tosetti, F; Ferrari, N; De Flora, S; Albini, A. Angioprevention: angiogenesis is a common and key target for cancer chemopreventive agents. *FASEB J.*, 2002, 16, 2-14.

[185] Yang, CS; Chung, JY; Yang, G; Chhabra, SK; Lee, MJ. Tea and tea polyphenols in cancer prevention. *J. Nutr.*, 130, 472S-478S.
[186] Balentine, DA; Wiseman, SA; Bouwens, LC. The chemistry of tea flavonoids. *Crit. Rev. Food Sci. Nutr.*, 1997, 37, 693-704.
[187] Tsubono, Y; Nishino, Y; Komatsu, S; Hsieh, CC; Kanemura, S; Tsuji, I; Nakatsuka, H; Fukao, A; Satoh, H; Hisamichi, S. Green tea and the risk of gastric cancer in Japan. *N Engl. J. Med.*, 2001, 344, 632-636.

In: Nutrition for the Middle Aged and Elderly
Editors: N. E. Bernhardt, A. M. Kasko, pp. 157-194
ISBN: 978-1-60456-146-3

Chapter IV

The Significance of Diet and Nutrition in the Prevention and Management of Osteoporosis in the Elderly Population

Sa'eed Bawa
NND, Food Science and Technology; MSc, Food and Nutrition Sciences; PhD, Food and Nutrition Sciences
Department of Dietetics, Faculty of Human Nutrition and Consumer Sciences, Warsaw University of Life Sciences, Nowoursynowska Street 159C, PL-02776 Warsaw, Poland

Abstract

Osteoporosis is defined as a progressive systemic skeletal disease characterized by low bone mass and microarchitectural deterioration of bone tissue, with a consequent increase in bone fragility and susceptibility to fracture. More than one-third of the adult women will suffer one or more osteoporotic fractures in their lifetime. The lifetime risk in men is approximately one-half that in women. The decrease of the bone mineral density is the most important cause of risk fracture. Albeit bone mass and quality is mainly determined genetically, many other factors, including lifestyle (smoking, excess alcohol intake, physical inactivity) and nutrition also have an impact on bone health. Nutrition is the most significant modifiable factor that influences the development and maintenance of bone mass. Adequate intakes of macro- and micronutrients that modulate bone health can help in the prevention and management of osteoporosis. About 80-90% of mineral content in the bone is consisted of calcium and phosphorous. Among other factors, Ca^{2+} and vitamin D deficiencies are important risk factors for a decrease in bone mineral density, consequently inducing osteoporosis. The high prevalence of vitamin D deficiency in healthy elderly people living mainly in southern European countries increase the risk of osteoporotic fractures in these populations above those anticipated for the general elderly population of the European Community. In addition, the ageing of the world population, particularly the European population will double the number of osteoporotic fractures over the next 50 years, unless adequate preventative measures are undertaken. Apart from calcium, phosphorous and vitamin D, other nutrients, such as protein, magnesium, zinc, fluoride, sodium, copper, vitamins B_6, C, K, essential fatty acids from the omega-3 family, and antioxidants are also needed for normal bone turnover. In this paper, each of these nutrients is discussed separately. The efficacy and safety of Ca^{2+} and vitamin D supplements at preventing bone loss and reducing the risk of hip and other fractures are also discussed.

Introduction

Osteoporosis is a skeletal disorder characterized by compromised bone strength, a disorder that predisposes to fractures resulting from no identifiable injury or from minimal trauma insufficient to fracture normal bone. Bone strength is the result of two major determinants: bone mineral content and bone quality.

A person's bone mineral content is a function of the interaction of two key factors: the uppermost amount of bone achieved during youth (called the peak bone mass, PBM) in combination with the rate of subsequent bone loss. Growth in bone size and strength occurs during childhood, through adolescence and is usually completed in the 20s.

After peak bone mass is achieved during the third decade of life, bone architecture is maintained by a constant remodeling process. Osteoclasts attach to a specific area of bone, remove old bone (resorption pit), then osteoblasts move in and fill this pit with new bone. The balance between these processes shifts at menopause [1-4] and women typically undergo a rapid phase of bone loss that begins approximately 2 to 3 years before the cessation of menses and continues for up to 5 years postmenopause [5-7]. Although the decreased concentrations of circulating estrogen observed during menopause and the rapid phase of bone loss are chiefly responsible for the process [5], many other factors are associated with increased fracture risk [8]. These factors include prior fragility fracture, advanced age, a family history of osteoporotic fracture, and the use of certain medications [1, 3]. Additional predictors of bone loss and fracture risk in early postmenopause include prolonged low vitamin D and calcium intake and low body weight [1, 9-10]. Osteoporotic fractures are preventable (Brown and Josse, 2002); risk-factor assessment and methods to assess bone mass are available for the identification of women at risk, and management of osteoporosis is possible through pharmacologic and nonpharmacologic measures [11].

The quality of bone refers to the composition and structure of skeletal tissue and considers micro-architecture as well as existing damage (e.g., micro-fractures) (12). Dense bone is not necessarily strong bone as it is possible to have more quantity of poorer structural quality and less quantity of better structural integrity; geometric and structural differences in bone configuration can influence fracture potential.

Epidemiology of Osteoporosis

Osteoporosis is an established and well-defined disease that affects more than 75 million people in Europe, Japan and the USA, and causes more than 2.3 million fractures annually in

Europe and the USA alone. The lifetime risk for hip, vertebral and forearm (wrist) fractures has been estimated to be approximately 40%, similar to that for coronary heart disease.

Osteoporosis is three times more common in women than in men, partly because women have a lower peak bone mass and partly because of the hormonal changes that occur at the menopause. Estrogens have an important function in preserving bone mass during adulthood, and bone loss occurs as levels decline, usually from around the age of 50 years. In addition, women live longer than men [13] and therefore have greater reductions in bone mass.

Increasing life expectancy in many parts of the world means that women now live more than one-third of their lives after the menopause, and that the number of postmenopausal women is increasing. In Europe, for example, the number of women over 50 years of age is projected to increase by 30%-40% between 1990 and 2025 [13]. Among men over 50 years, the projected increase is expected to be even higher (50%). This trend is even more marked in other areas of the world. In North America, the proportion of the population over 50 years is expected nearly to double. The proportionate increases will be greatest in Africa, Asia and Latin America, but Asia will have the highest absolute increase because it has the largest population.

An estimated 1.3-1.7 million hip fractures occurred worldwide in 1990 [14, 15]. By 2025, this number is expected to increase to almost 3 million. This is probably an underestimate, since in many regions, hip fracture rates have increased even after age has been taken into consideration [15]. These projected estimates are relatively robust, since the group they apply to has already been born.

The prevalence of low bone density in the general population can be assessed by means of the WHO diagnostic criteria [16]. Osteoporosis is diagnosed based on the level of patient's BMD compared with the average peak BMD of young adult women [17] and expressed as T-score. The criteria are presented in Table 1.

Table 1. World Health Organization Criteria for the Diagnosis of Osteoporosis

Category	Criteria (expressed as T-score)
Normal	Patient BMD ≤ 1 SD of average peak young adult BMD (T-score, 0 to -1)
Osteopenia	Patient BMD between 1 SD and 2.5 SD below average peak young adult BMD (T-score, -1 to -2.5)
Osteoporosis	Patient BMD ≥ 2.5 SD below average peak young adult BMD (T-score, ≥ 2.5)
Severe osteoporosis	Patient BMD ≥ 2.5 SD below average peak young adult BMD with fragility fractures

BMD = Bone mineral density.

Factors Affecting Bone Health

Modifiable factors that promote bone health:

- Regular physical activity

- Healthy eating habits
- Adequate calcium consumption
- Adequate vitamin D status

Modifiable factors that increase risk for bone loss:

- Cigarette smoking and alcohol abuse
- Medications such as some types of anticonvulsants or glucocorticoids (corticosteroids, prednisone, dexamethasone)

Non-modifiable factors that increase risk for bone loss:

- Gender - women are at greater risk than men
- Age - bone loss increases with age
- Body size - small, thin women are more susceptible than larger women
- Ethnicity and heredity - Caucasian and Asian women are at greatest risk. African American and Hispanic women have a lower but significant risk
- Genetics - if a parent suffers from osteoporosis or an osteoporotic bone fracture, the children tend to have reduced bone mass and increased risk.

Macronutrients and Bone Health

Protein Intake and Osteoporosis

Negative Effects of Excess Protein on Bone Health

Increasing dietary protein increases urine calcium excretion such that for each 50 g increment of protein consumed and extra 60 mg of urinary calcium is excreted. It follows that the higher the protein intake, the more urine calcium is lost and the more negative calcium balance becomes.

Wachman and Bernstein [18] first hypothesized the alleged negative effect of dietary protein on bone calcium. The mechanism proposed by this hypothesis is that increased protein intake, especially of animal origin, because of the sulfur amino acid content and its acid-ash nature, leads to an increased glomerular filtration rate, reduced renal reabsorption of calcium, hypercalciuria and thus leaching of calcium out of the bone [19-23]. This gradual dissolution of bone mineral and its loss through the kidneys over time is often implicated in the etiology of osteoporosis [24-30].

In most individuals, the source of net acid load is from the metabolism of protein (when consumed in large amounts) and long-chain fatty acids (when they comprise more than 20 % of calories in the diet). A marker of net acid production is the extent of degradation of sulfur-containing amino aids: cysteine, cystine, and methionine. Moreover, the breakdown of any of the seven acidic amino acids (aspartate, glutamate, cysteine, cystine, proline/hydroxyproline, serine, and threonine), plus the keto-acids produced from amino acid metabolism, contribute to the body's fixed, organic acid load [31]. The metabolism of these amino acids produces H^+

without buffering partners. These H^+ accumulate and must be neutralized by matching buffering elements from the body. The buffering elements include the organize anions (usually as K^+ or other mineral salts) in fruits, vegetables, lentils/pulses, herbs, and spices. These also include metabolically alkaline forming citrate, malate, succinate, and fumarate. In addition, short- and medium-chain fatty acids reduce net acid burden by "scaking up" acetate and 2-carbon acidic units in the cells.

The major recognized sources of net acid load in the body are: a) large intakes of protein, especially of animal origin, b) dietary phosphate/phosphoric acid, c) dietary sulphate, d) excess consumption of long-chain fatty acids, e) distress (excess cortisol and adrenaline), f) delayed immune system reactions.

Many studies have shown that bone responds to an acid load by dissolving its basic buffering mineral salts. For background, the average adult skeleton contains a large but finite amount of Ca^{2+} (50-65,000 mEq, 99% of total body stores) and Mg^{2+} (1,060-1,600 mEq, 50% to 80% of body stores). Bone minerals serve as a sizeable reservoir of buffer, usable in the control of plasma pH [32, 33].

Diets of the citizens of industrialized nations commonly produce an excess load of fixed acids of 100 to 200 mEq per day [34, 35]. Remer and Manz [35] found that a diet containing 120 grams of protein yielded a net acid excretion of 135.5 mEq/day. Two "moderate" protein diets (95g/day protein) yielded net acid excess (NAE) of 69 to 112 mEq/day. A lactovegetarian "low" protein diet (49g/day) gave an NAE of 24 mEq/day. Therefore, the type of diet consumed influences net acid production. High-protein diets produce a six-fold (600%) increase in NAE. This results in low first-morning urine pH, indicating that buffering functional reserve is deficient, and that the risk of metabolic acidosis is correspondingly increased [35].

Barzel and Massey [32] demonstrated that the pH of colas with phosphoric acid is 2.8 to 3.2. However, the kidney cannot excrete urine with a pH much lower than 5, without significantly damaging the gentourinary tract. To achieve a urinary pH of 5, a 12 oz. (330mL) can of cola would have to be diluted 100-fold, requiring an additional 33 liters of urine. Otherwise, a corresponding amount of buffer must be drawn from the body to neutralize the excess acid. The body routinely buffers the acidic beverage with sodium and potassium if reserves permit, then with a corresponding loss of calcium, magnesium, and other minerals, as available.

Although several clinical trials [19, 21, 22, 36-41] have attempted to test the hypothesis proposed by Wachman and Bernstein [18], the effects of dietary protein on calcium retention and bone health remain unclear.

Positive Effects of Protein on Bone Health

Both underconsumption and excess intakes of protein can increase the risk of osteoporosis. The mechanism whereby a low protein intake has adverse effects on bone may be due to inadequate production of IGF-1, which exerts anabolic effects on bone mass, not only during growth, but also during adulthood [42]. Protein replenishment in patients with hip fracture can improve not only BMD, but also muscle mass and strength. These two variables are important determinants of the likelihood and consequences of falling and thus incidence of osteoporotic fractures. This observation underlines the importance of weight-bearing in the maintenance of bone mass [43]. At the tissue level, immobilization results in bone resorption being greater than bone formation. At the cellular level, immobilization increases bone reabsorption by osteoclasts associated with a decrease in osteoblastic formation (44). The molecular signal(s) perceiving the reduction in mechanical strain associated with immobility has not been identified.

While excess protein intake is common for the average American, consuming too little protein, especially from animal sources, can increase the risk for weakened bones and osteoporosis [45]. There is growing evidence that a low protein diet has a detrimental effect on bone. For example, Kerstetter et al. [46] reported that in healthy young women, acute intakes of a low-protein diet (0.7 g protein/kg) decreased urinary calcium excretion with accompanied secondary hyperparathyroidism. The etiology of the secondary hyperparathyroidism is due, in part, to a significant reduction in intestinal calcium absorption during a low protein diet.

In a recent short-term intervention trial, Kerstetter et al. [47] evaluated the effects of graded levels of dietary protein (0.7, 0.8, 0.9, and 1.0 g protein/kg) on calcium homeostasis. Secondary hyperparathyroidism developed by day 4 of the 0.7 and 0.8 g protein/kg diets (due to the decreased intestinal calcium absorption), but not during the 0.9 or 1.0 g protein/kg diets in eight young women. There were no significant differences in mean urinary calcium excretion over the relatively narrow range of dietary protein intakes studied, although the mean value with the 0.7-g/kg intake was lower than that with the 1.0 g/kg intake by 0.25 mmol (10 mg). According to authors of this study, the lack of change may be due to the small sample and the inherent variability in urinary calcium excretion. Similarly, when Giannini et al. [48] restricted dietary protein to 0.8 g protein/kg, they observed an acute rise in serum parathyroid hormone (PTH) in 18 middle-aged hypercalciuric adults. Taken together, both of studies suggest, at least in the short term, that the RDA for protein (0.8 g/kg) does not support normal calcium homeostasis.

Many other studies have shown that although excess protein intake is common for the average American and citizens of the European Union, consuming too little protein, especially from animal sources, can increase the risk for weakened bones and osteoporosis [45, 49-52]. In older adults, protein intake was found to be positively correlated with bone mineral density and inversely related to rates of bone loss [45, 49-52]. Bonjour et al. [49] carried out a 6-month, randomized, double-blind, placebo-controlled trial in 82 older adults who had suffered a hip fracture and found that increasing protein intake brought about a decrease in loss of leg bone density by 50% and an increase in blood levels of insulin-like growth factor, which promotes bone gain, and reduced the stay in the rehabilitation hospital by 10 days.

In the Iowa Women's Health Study of more than 32,000 women, higher intakes of protein, especially from animal sources, were associated with reduced risk of hip fractures in postmenopausal women [51]. Women with hip fractures consumed less red meat (beef, lamb, pork) than women who did not suffer hip fractures.

Dietary Calcium to Protein Ratio

The effect of protein intake on calcium balance is often interpreted as negative, especially in the consumer press. However, this is a classic case of a nutrient-nutrient interaction and should be viewed in terms of the calcium to protein intake ratio (Heaney, 1993). The calcium:protein ratio of the diet has been found to be more closely related (positively) to rate of bone gain than either calcium intake (positive) or protein intake (negative) alone [53].

The intakes of protein by Americans usually exceed recommended levels, but the consumption of calcium is well below recommended dietary intake levels [54-56]. Based on current dietary recommendations for calcium [57] and protein [58], a dietary calcium to protein ratio of 16:1 (mg:g) or higher likely provides adequate protection for the skeleton and can be considered optimal for adults (Table 2). However, nutrient intake data from USDA's 1994-96 Continuing Survey of Food Intakes by Individuals (CSFII) (54) reveal that calcium to protein ratio of about half the optimal ratio is achieved by adults (Table 2). Similar findings are observed from the Third National Health and Nutrition Examination Survey [55, 56]. Although protein intakes are somewhat higher than recommended, low calcium intake is the real problem [33].

Table 2. Optimal versus actual dietary calcium:protein ratio (mg:g) for adults (Institute of Medicine, 1997; National Research Council, 1989; USDA, 1997)

Sex/age group	Optimal calcium: protein ratio* (mg:g)	Calcium intake (mg)	Protein intake (g)	Dietary calcium: protein ratio (mg:g)
Males				
30-39	16	951	102.7	9.3
40-49	16	876	95.3	9.2
50-59	19	791	90.3	8.8
60-69	19	796	83.5	9.5
70+	19	746	72.9	10.2
Females				
30-39	20	661	65.3	10.1
40-49	20	634	63.5	10.0
50-59	24	630	64.1	9.8
60-69	24	604	60.4	10.0
70+	24	584	56.6	10.3

*Based on DRI for calcium [57] and RDA for protein [58].

Essential Fatty Acids (EFAs)

Fatty acids act in several ways to modulate bone health. First and foremost, dietary fats can influence bone health by affecting intestinal calcium absorption, and possibly renal calcium excretion. Individual fatty acids have been shown in several studies to influence enterocyte membrane dynamics, Vitamin D_3 activity, and prostaglandin formation, which can have important effects on intestinal calcium absorption as well as urinary calcium excretion; this has been reviewed comprehensively by [59]. Calcium absorption is increased and excretion decreased not only when essential fatty acid deficiencies are corrected, but also when standard diets are supplemented with specific oils. Supplementation of diet with evening primrose oil or fish oil increased the unsaturation index of intestinal brush border membrane vesicles and significantly enhanced calcium transport [60]. Supplementation with these oils also reduced urinary calcium excretion [61, 62].

While small quantities of dietary fat may have benefits, large amounts, especially saturated fat can increase intestinal and urinary calcium excretion. For instance, a high-fat diet increased urinary calcium losses induced by ovariectomy in rats [63]. Earlier work indicated that high-fat diets can also cause the formation of insoluble calcium soaps in the intestines, resulting in increased fecal calcium excretion [64]. The effects of fats on intestinal calcium excretion were exacerbated with age, and were strongest when saturated fatty acids were consumed [65-67]. Since intestinal calcium absorption normally decreases with age, consumption of high-fat diets, particularly those rich in saturated fatty acids may put the elderly at risk for increased calcium excretion and associated bone disorders [65, 68, 69].

Recent research confirms that adequate and balanced levels of EFAs in the diet positively impact bone health and that EFA deficiency may be a major contributor to osteoporosis.

Although the complex mechanisms of bone physiology are not fully understood, many molecular factors which are inextricably linked to bone formation and resorption are controlled or influenced by the availability and action of EFAs [70-73]. The finding that animals deficient in EFAs develop severe osteoporosis [74] has prompted further study of the role of these essential nutrients in bone health.

There are two categories of EFAs: omega-3 fatty acids (ω3FAs) and omega-6 fatty acids (ω6FAs); both groups originate from lipids ingested in the diet as the body is unable to synthesize them due to lack the enzymes Δ-15-desaturase and Δ-12-desaturase, respectively [75]. While ω6FAs are plentiful in foods such as cereal grains, processed foods, meat, milk, eggs and some vegetable oils, ω3FAs are found in significant quantity in only a few seeds and nuts, as well as in fish oil. Both families of fatty acids provide required substrate for the production of eicosanoids, which include important bioactive compounds such as prostaglandins, leukotrienes and thromboxanes (Figure 1).

Eicosanoids originating from ω6FAs act biochemically to promote cell proliferation, inflammation and blood clotting while eicosanoids originating from ω3FAs oppose these effects and facilitate anti-inflammatory action, inhibitory effects on cell growth, and blood thinning. Both groups of EFAs compete for the same limited supply of enzymes in the biochemical assembly of eicosanoids and diets with high ω6FAs:o3FAs (ω6/3) ratios will diminish the effectiveness of ω3FAs-dependent processes, leading to an overabundance of omega-6 derived eicosanoids. The relative concentration of ω6FAs and ω3FAs consumed in the diet is a matter of major import to the biochemical and clinical functioning of the individual [76], including skeletal tissue function [73].

The ω6/3 dietary ratio affects calcium metabolism [73] as bone formation and bone resorption are influenced locally by prostaglandins and cytokines which in turn are regulated by EFAs. High intake of ω6FAs results in elevated prostaglandin E2 and other cytokines, which are pro-inflammatory [77] and which activate osteoclasts and bone resorption. As a result, excess 6FAs in the diet has been associated with increased periodontal disease and bone resorption as well as lower bone density at the hip in both men and women [70].

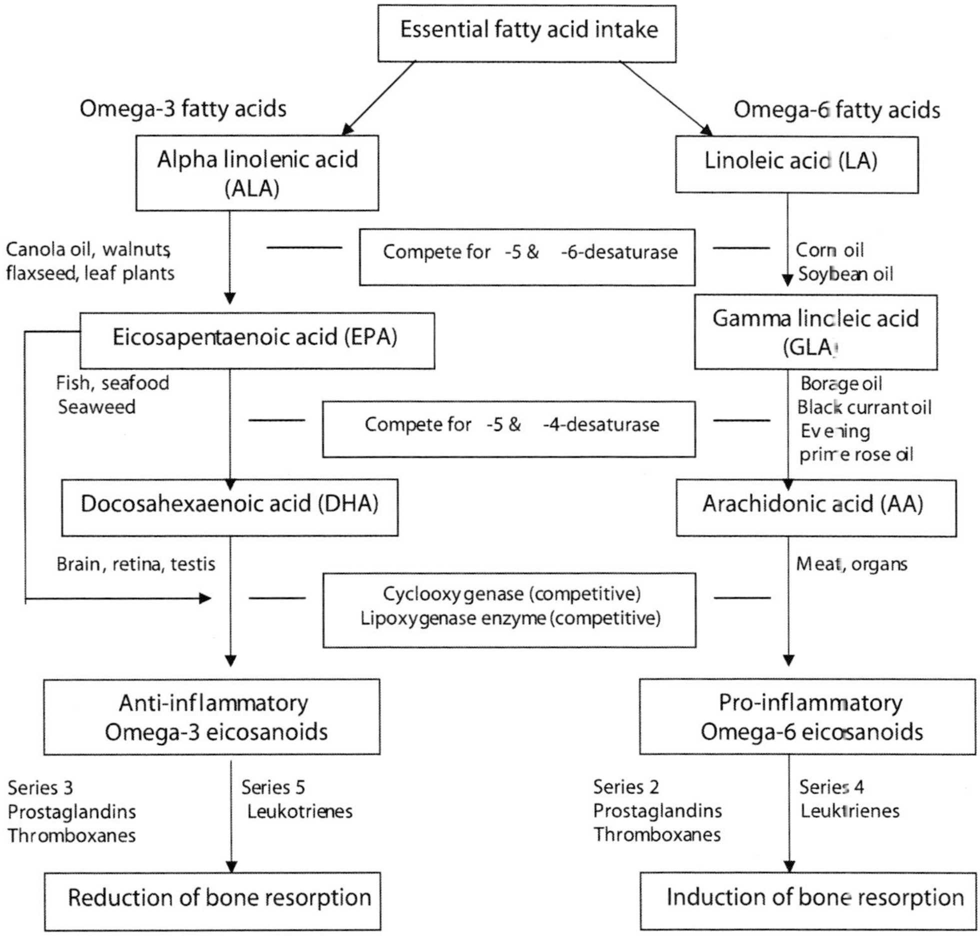

Figure 1. Metabolism of essential fatty acid and their sources.

On the other hand, ω3FAs downregulate inflammatory cytokines; bone resorption is reduced when ω3FAs levels are high [78]. Adequate dietary ω3FAs facilitate absorption of calcium in the gut, reduce excretion of calcium in the urine, increase calcium deposition in bone and enhance bone collagen synthesis. Significant reductions in cytokine production can be achieved by dietary supplementation with foods containing abundant ω3FAs such as fish oil [79], flaxseeds, and flaxseed oil [80] resulting in increased calcium absorption, bone calcium and BMD. Abundant volumes of recent literature confirm that a low ω6/3 ratio ‘‘may be necessary for optimal health, normal development, and prevention of chronic disease [70].

The relatively high ω6/3 ratio in the typical North American diet may have a significant impact on osteoporosis and other degenerative diseases; while the ω6/3 ratio was about 1–2:1 as recent as 200 years ago, it is now estimated at 16:1 (Simopoulos, 2002). By way of contrast, osteoporotic hip fractures are much less prevalent in Japan [81] a country where the dietary ratio of ω6/3 is 4:1 [82].

In conclusion, a low nutritional ratio of ω6/3 appears to enhance calcium absorption, reduce excretion, and increase calcium deposition in bone, which in turn decreases the risk of osteoporosis and resultant fragility fractures. Furthermore, by improving bone quality and BMD [73], in addition to reducing inflammatory cytokines, ω3FA supplementation has been shown to slow the rapid rate of postmenopausal bone loss (Kettler, 2001). Accordingly, it may be prudent in clinical medicine to discuss EFA intake with patients and to supplement ω3FAs as a routine aspect of care for individuals with compromised bone health.

Micronutrients and Bone Health

The Impact of Major Minerals on Bone Status

Calcium

Calcium is the fifth most abundant element in the human body. The amount of calcium the human body is about 25 to 30 g at birth (constituting 0.8% of the body weight) and between 900 and 1300 g in adult men (which is about 1.7% of body weight) [84]. Over 99% of the total calcium of the body is located in the bones, where it accounts for 39% of the total body bone mineral content [85], and in the teeth, mostly as hydroxyapatite.

Bone mineral provides structure and strength to the body and, very important, a reservoir of calcium that helps to maintain a constant concentration of blood calcium. Less than 1% of total body calcium is found in soft tissues (~7 g) and body fluids (~1 g). Calcium in the extracellular fluid and the blood are kept constant at 2.5 mmol/L (10 mg/dL) (between 2.25 and 2.75 mmol/L) via cell surface calcium-sensing receptors in parathyroid, kidney, intestine, lung, brain, skin, bone marrow, osteoblasts and other organs. Calcium is present in blood in three different forms: as free Ca^{2+} ions, bound to protein (about 45%), and complexed to citrate, phosphate, sulphate and carbonate (about 10%).

Ionised calcium is kept within narrow limits [86] by the action of three hormones, parathyroid hormone, 1,25-dihydroxycholecalciferol, and calcitonin. Extracellular calcium serves as a source for the skeleton and participates in blood clotting and intercellular adhesion. Intracellular calcium varies widely between tissues and is predominantly bound to intracellular membrane structures of the nucleus, mitochondria, endoplasmatic reticulum or contained in special storage vesicles. Free Ca^{2+} is only 0.1 μmol/L in the cytosol, which is 10,000 times lower than in the extracellular fluid (1 mmol/L).

Intracellular calcium rises in response to stimuli interacting with the cell surface receptor. The increase of intracellular calcium comes from influx of extracellular calcium or from release of intracellular calcium stores. This activates specific responses like hormone or neurotransmitter release, muscle contraction, cellular differentiation and many others.

Calcium must be ingested with the diet in sufficient amounts to allow for calcium deposition during bone growth and modeling and to compensate for obligatory intestinal, fecal and dermal losses during the life-time.

In the elderly, several factors contribute to negative calcium balance. With ageing, calcium intake decreases because of reduced consumption of dairy products, and the absorptive capacity of the intestinal epithelium to adapt to low calcium intake is impaired. Exposure to sunlight and the capacity of the skin to produce vitamin D are also reduced. The capacity of the renal tubule to reabsorb calcium and its responsiveness to PTH are impaired. Finally, the decease in glomerular filtration rate observed in the elderly may contribute to chronic hyperparathyroidism, favouring a negative bone mineral balance and thus osteoporosis. Increasing calcium intake is certainly an important strategy which is relatively easier to implement than other possible preventive measures. Older people have a higher calcium requirement than young adults. Table 3 shows the current reference intakes of calcium in selected countries.

Table 3. Reference intakes for calcium in selected countries [87]

Country	Children age 4-6	Adults	Pregnancy	Lactation
Australia	700	800	1100	1300
France	700	800	1000	1200
Germany	700	700F, 800M	1200	1200
India	450	450	1000	1000
Mexico	500	500	1000	100
Netherlands	400-600	700-900	800-1000	900-1100
Scandinavia	600	600	1000	1000
UK	450	700	700	1250
US*	800	1000*	1000	1000

*The US dietary reference intakes for adults over age 50 is 1200 mg/day.

Foods vary widely in calcium content. The best sources are milk (120 mg/100 g) and milk products (up to 1100 mg/100 g), from which about 32% is absorbable [85]. Tables 4 to 7 show the calcium content of various foods.

Table 4. Approximate calcium contents of one serving of some common foods (From references [88-93])

Food	Serving size	Calcium (mg)
Milk (whole)	1 cup	290-300
Milk skim	1 cup	300-310
Swiss cheese	1.5 oz	400
Yogurt, low fat	8 oz	300-415*
Calcium-fortified orange juice	1 cup	300
Tofu, raw, firm (calcium added)	½ cup	200-434
Calcium enriched bread	3 oz	290
Instant oatmeal	1 package	150
Salmon, canned, with bones	3 oz	150
Sardines, canned, with bones	6 oz	250

Table 4. (Continued)

Food	Serving size	Calcium (mg)
Sweet potatoes, mashed	½ cup	44
Soybean, boiled	1 cup	175
Soybean, boiled	1 cup	175
Refried beans	1 cup	188
Baked beans, canned	1 cup	128
Black beans, boiled	1 cup	47
Kidney beans, boiled	1 cup	50

*Varies by brand.

Table 5. Approximate calcium contents of one serving of variety of vegetables and greens [89, 91, 94]

Vegetable	Serving size	Calcium (mg)
Acorn squash	½ cup	45
Butternut squash	½ cup	42
Beet greens	½ cup	82
Blackeyed peas	1 cup	42
Broccoli raw	½ cup	82
Cabbage, green, boiled	½ cup	25
Cabbage, red, boiled	½ cup	28
Cardoon, boiled	3.5 oz	72
Carrots, raw	1 medium	19
Carrots	½ cup	24
Cabbage, Chinese, boiled	½ cup	79
Chickpeas	1 cup	80
Chicory, greens, raw	½ cup	90
Collard greens	1 cup	148-350
Dandelion greens	½ cup	73
Fuki (butterbur), boiled	3.5 oz	79
Garlic, raw	3 cloves	16
Kale, boiled	½ cup	47
Mustard greens, boiled	½ cup	52
Parsley, raw	½ cup	39
Pigeon peas	1 cup	72
Spinach, raw	½ cup	122
Turnip greens, raw	1 cup	165-200

Table 6. Approximate calcium contents of one serving of nuts and seeds [89, 91]

Food	Serving size	Calcium (mg)
Almonds	24 (dried)	75
Brazil nuts	8 (dried)	50
Carob flour	1 cup	359
Pistachios	38 (dried)	38
Sesame seeds	1 tablespoon	10
Sunflower seeds	1 oz (dried)	33
Soybean nuts (roasted)	½ oz	20

Table 7. Some calcium-fortified foods commonly available in the US [95] as well as based on an informal 1996 FDA market survey conducted in the Washington, DC metropolitan area, except for fruit punch. Some data on fruit punch were derived from the 1989-1991 CSFII

Food	Amount of calcium (mg)
Frozen yogurt, fat free, calcium added (1/2 cup)	450
Soy milk, calcium added (1 cup)	250-300
Tofu made with calcium (1/2 cup)	200-434
Calcium fortified orange juice (6 fluid oz)	300
Milk (100 g)	160-200
Meal replacements, milk-based (100 g)	150-360
Meal replacements, fruit-based (100 g)	70
Cottage cheese (100 g)	170
Breakfast cereals, ready to eat (100 g)	220-710
Bread, light (100 g)	330
Sweet bakery products (100 g)	160-230
Cereal bars (100 g)	540-870
Weight loss candy/bars	460-910
Apple sauce (100 g)	160
Fruit juice (100 g)	80-130
Fruit punch	60-130

The Significance of Calcium Supplements in Increasing BMD in the Elderly Population

There is some evidence that calcium supplementation in young women before the menopause is beneficial, but most research on the effects of calcium intake on bone has been in postmenopausal subjects. The considerable, but often contradictory observational data can now be replaced by the increasing amount of data from more than 20 randomized controlled trials, most of which have recently been reviewed and tabulated [96]. Almost all of these studies show a small increase in BMD (~1%) in calcium-treated subjects. In the great majority of these studies, this increase is statistically significant at one or more skeletal sites (e.g. the forearm, spine, proximal femur or total body). The benefits appear to be more marked in late postmenopausal life than at the perimenopause [97], although some studies have found beneficial effects in this latter group also [98]. The greater variation in rates of bone loss in perimenopausal women may obscure the relatively small effect of calcium supplementation. Some studies have reported that such effects are greater in those on lower calcium intakes [97].

A number of studies have suggested that the beneficial effect of calcium supplements is most marked in the first year of treatment, particularly at the sites where cancellous bone predominates [99]. This effect is probably the result of a fall in circulating PTH concentrations, which decreases the number of bone remodelling units on the surface of cancellous bone. However, there is also a smaller residual positive effect on BMD of about 0.25% per year after the first year [99]. If this were to continue over 30 years of postmenopausal life, a cumulative benefit of 7.5% would be expected, which would reduce fracture risk by about one-third. Furthermore, three studies have found a significant effect of calcium monotherapy on fracture incidence despite observed between-group differences in bone density of <2% [99-101]. However, when all randomized clinical trials reporting fractures are meta-analysed, calcium supplementation is associated with a relative risk (RR) of vertebral fracture of 0.77 (95% confidence interval [CI] 0.54–1.09) and a relative risk of non-vertebral fracture of 0.86 (95% CI 0.43–1.72) [102]. A large, international case-control study found that hip fractures were less frequent in those receiving calcium supplements (RR 0.75, 95% CI 0.60–0.94) [103].

Based on this evidence, a number of agencies have adopted recommendations for dietary calcium intake throughout life. These vary widely from country to country, reflecting some of the scientific uncertainties [104]. The fractional absorption of calcium from dairy products is higher than that from vegetables, and cheese may be marginally superior to milk in this respect [105].

Calcium supplements are generally well tolerated and reports of significant side-effects are rare (106), but some individuals complain of constipation when taking them. The possibility that high calcium intakes might lead to urinary calculi in susceptible subjects was a cause for concern, and it was found in an observational study that whereas dietary calcium intake was inversely related to the risk of stone formation, the use of calcium supplements increased this risk by 20% [107]. This apparent inconsistency may arise from the reduction in intestinal oxalate absorption that occurs when calcium is taken with meals. It has been suggested that high calcium intakes are associated with a reduced risk of colorectal cancer [108], reduced blood pressure [109] and reduced serum lipid concentrations [110], but these associations require further investigation.

Table 8. Elemental calcium content of calcium salts [111]

Calcium salt	Elemental calcium (mg/g)	mEq/g	Approx. equivalent dose mg of salt
Calcium acetate	250	12.7	354
Calcium carbonate	400	20	225
Calcium chloride	270	13.5	330
Calcium citrate	211	10.6	425
Calcium glucobionate	64	3.2	1400
Calcium gluconate	90	4.5	1000
Calcium lactate	130	6.5	700
Calcium phosphate, tribasic	390	19.3	233

Phosphorous

The phosphorus content of the adult human body is about 700 g (as elemental phosphorus). About 85% of total phosphorus is present in the skeleton, the remainder in the soft tissues and in the extracellular fluids (≈ 1%) [112]. Total body phosphorus content increases from 0.5% on a body weight basis in infancy up to 0.65-1.1% in adults [113]. Total phosphorus concentration in whole blood is approximately 13 mmol/L (40 mg/dL). Approximately 70% is present as organic phosphates, such as in the phospholipids of red blood cells and in the plasma lipoproteins. The other 30% is present as inorganic phosphate, of which 15% is protein bound. About 50% of the inorganic phosphate is in the soluble divalent cation form (HPO_4^{2-}), the remaining as the monovalent anion (H_2PO_{4-}, 10%) and the trivalent cation (PO_4^{3-}, <0.01%), or as HPO_4^{2-} complexed with sodium, calcium and magnesium salts. These anion forms are interconvertible and effective buffers of blood pH and involved in regulation of the whole body acid-base balance.

Effects of Phosphorous on Calcium Regulating Hormones, Calcium Balance and Skeletal Mass

An increase in phosphorus intake can induce an increase in serum PTH, as part of the normal homeostatic control to maintain serum calcium levels. This effect depends on the actual increase in serum Pi, and the subsequent (small) decrease in the serum ionized calcium level. PTH adjusts renal clearance of Pi and through this mechanism the phosphate balance is maintained. It is not clear at what dietary intake level of phosphorus PTH secretion is stimulated. Only in the first days of life a (linear) relationship exists between serum PTH and phosphorus intake in the normal nutritional range. After the renal excretion capacity has fully developed and remains intact, the excess absorbed phosphate is excreted and serum Pi levels are kept within the normal range, i.e. no hyperphosphatemia develops.

Acute oral phosphorus loading with dosages of 1.0-1.5 g phosphorus did not result in an increase in serum PTH in young adults [114]. Also in an earlier study in osteoporotic postmenopausal women a supplemental phosphorus dosage of 1000 mg (total intake up to 2740 mg/day) for 12 months did not affect fasting serum PTH [115]. Also in more recent chronic supplementation studies in young healthy men [116], and women [117], with total intakes up to 3000 mg phosphorus/day, no significant effect on changes in serum PTH could be demonstrated. However in a study with a similar group of postmenopausal women supplemental dosages >1500 mg phosphorus/day resulted in an increase in PTH levels (+35%) [118]. A normal phosphorus intake (1700 mg/day) in combination with a low calcium diet (400 mg/day) also resulted in a persistent increase in PTH, but is likely due to the low calcium content, rather than the relatively higher phosphorus content [119].

The skeletal effects of carbonated beverage consumption, if any, as reported in a relatively small study in children [120] might be due to milk displacement, i.e. a low calcium intake rather than an effect of phosphoric acid. Such a trend in the consumption of milk and soft drinks, i.e. a decrease in milk consumption with a concurrent increase in soft drink consumption, resulting in a lower calcium, but higher phosphorus intake, has been reported for the US [121].

A comparative study in adult women showed no effect of phosphoric acid compared to citric acid as the acidulant in carbonated beverages on urinary calcium excretion [122].

Ectopic calcification (e.g. nephrocalcinosis) and skeletal deformations and bone loss, as observed in animal studies with high phosphorus loads, have not been reported to occur in humans as long as the renal excretion capacity is not seriously compromised, such as in end-stage renal disease. It should also be noted that standard diets for laboratory animals generally have a relatively high phosphorus and low calcium content [123]. It cannot be excluded therefore that the observed effects in some of the animal studies were associated with the relatively low calcium intakes, rather than the high phosphorus intake as such. Besides the sensitivity of the PTH-vitamin D axis to variations in calcium and phosphorus intake might be different between animals and humans.

The suppression of the renal 1,25-(OH)2D synthesis by an increase in the serum Pi level [124] contributes to the already decreased intestinal phosphate absorption, and increased renal phosphate excretion. This effect may be mediated by phosphatonins, under conditions of high phosphorus intake, due to down-regulation of the NTP2 co-transporters [125]. Decreased absorption and increased renal excretion therefore protect the human body against the development of chronic hyperphosphatemia under conditions of high phosphorus intake. The observed decrease in responsiveness of osteoclasts to PTH with increasing serum Pi levels likely explain why a (temporary) increase in serum PTH, if any, induced by a high phosphorus load does not result in an increased rate of bone resorption (remodelling), as compared to a low calcium intake which induces both an increased PTH and 1,25-(OH)2D synthesis. The role of the phosphatonins in these processes remains to be established [125].

The phosphorus-induced nephrocalcinosis as observed in rats [123], and the upper boundary of the normal distribution curve for serum Pi in infants [126] have been used as critical endpoints to set a maximum tolerable daily intake level. Both approaches have their limitations however. The phosphorus-induced nephrocalcinosis in rats seems less relevant for humans. Also derivation of a hypothetical NOAEL (no adverse effect level) based upon serum Pi distribution curves is doubtful as no actual adverse effects on bone mineralization have been observed. The Panel decides therefore not to use these endpoints to derive an upper level.

Potassium and the Prevention of Hypercalciuria and Osteoporosis

Potassium is an essential nutrient involved in fluid, acid and electrolyte balance and is required for normal cellular function. Dietary deficiency of potassium is very uncommon due to the widespread occurrence of potassium in foods. Important potassium sources include potatoes, fruit and berries, vegetables, milk products (excluding cheese) and nuts. Potassium occurs in foods mainly associated with weak organic acids. Potassium is also found in mineral, spring, and table waters, but the content varies considerably. Some mineral waters available on the market can, when consumed in large quantities, contribute significantly to the daily intake.

Increasing potassium intake reduces urinary calcium excretion and causes a positive calcium balance [127, 128]. Increasing potassium intake may therefore help manage hypercalciuria. Eleven children with idiopathic hypercalciuria who were treated with potassium in the form of potassium citrate (two patients), potassium gluconate (one patient), potassium chloride (seven patients), or a high potassium diet (one patient) all had a significant reduction in their urinary calcium:creatinine ratio after two weeks [127]. By reducing calcium excretion, a high potassium intake may also reduce the risk of kidney stones [129]. If increasing potassium intake reduces calcium excretion and causes a positive calcium balance, it may be associated in the longer term with a higher bone mass. In a cross sectional study of 994 healthy premenopausal women aged 45 to 49 years, bone mineral density in the lumbar spine and femoral neck increased with increasing potassium intake [130]. A study of 62 healthy women aged 45 to 55 years found that a higher potassium intake was associated not only with a higher bone mass but also with lower excretion of pyridinoline and deoxypyridinoline [131]. Administration of potassium bicarbonate to 18 postmenopausal women for 18 days reduced urinary calcium and hydroxyproline excretion and increased serum osteocalcin concentration, indicating a reduction in reabsorption of bone and an increase in the rate of bone formation [132].

Urinary calcium excretion is also associated directly with sodium intake and affected by acid-base homeostasis. To try to clarify the separate effects of potassium, sodium, and the accompanying anions Lemann et al. [128] compared the effects of administering potassium chloride potassium chloride, potassium bicarbonate, sodium chloride, and sodium bicarbonate (90 mmol/day) in 10 healthy adults on fixed metabolic diets. Each supplement was given for four days in random order. They also studied the effects of a reduction in potassium chloride and potassium bicarbonate in eight people. Giving potassium bicarbonate had the greatest effect on reducing calcium excretion, but potassium chloride also reduced the fasting urinary calcium:creatinine ratio significantly. Sodium bicarbonate did not affect calcium excretion, whereas sodium chloride increased calcium excretion.

Sodium and Bone Health

Sodium is found widely in nature and as a normal constituent of foods. It is added to foods, most frequently as sodium chloride (NaCl), common known as salt (1 mmol is equivalent to 23 mg sodium and approximates 58 mg sodium chloride), but also as other salts, e.g. nitrate, nitrite, phosphates, glutamate. In the European Community, in drinking water, the guide level of sodium is 20 mg/L (Council Directive 80/778/EEC). Sodium is an essential nutrient and a dietary inadequacy may lead to serious consequences. Sodium is present in biological systems as the main cation in the extracellular space, acting to maintain extracellular volume and plasma osmolality.

The sodium content of natural foods varies from around 0.1 to 3 mmol/100g, with fruit containing 0.1 mmol/100g, vegetables 0.3 mmol/100g, and meat, fish or eggs 3.0 mmol/100g. The content of sodium as sodium chloride in processed foods may be much higher; bread 20 mmol/100g; cheese, 30 mmol/ 100g; salted butter, 40 mmol/100g; and lean raw bacon, 80 mmol/100g. It is difficult to obtain reliable information on the sodium chloride content of foods as consumed, because of variable practices in terms of processing, food preparation and personal preferences.

In surveys of free living individuals and in physiological studies where dietary loads of sodium chloride have been administered, there is consistent evidence that increased sodium ingestion induces a substantial increase in the urinary excretion of calcium [133-135]. On this basis, it has been hypothesised that higher levels of sodium ingestion might compromise bone health. The available evidence suggests that sodium-induced increase in urinary calcium excretion leads to an increased calcium absorption by the gastrointestinal tract, mediated via parathyroid hormone [136]. However, this adaptive mechanism may be insufficient to prevent an increase in bone resorption in some individuals, e.g. postmenopausal women with a particular vitamin D receptor genotype [137]. Whether this increase in bone resorption leads to net bone loss is unclear and thus the evidence for a direct effect of sodium ingestion on bone health is not conclusive.

Magnesium

The adult healthy body contains approximately 21-28 g (about 1 mole) of Mg. 60% of the body's magnesium are in the skeleton and the rest in the soft tissue. It is the fourth most abundant cation in the mammalian body and the second most abundant cation in intracellular fluid.

Depending on the degree of the deficiency, symptoms are latent, moderate or even life threatening because Mg is a cofactor in hundreds of enzymatic reactions, many of which involve energy metabolism. It also plays an important role in protein and nucleic acid synthesis and has a stabilizing and protecting effect on membranes. Mg is also considered essential in maintaining Ca, K and Na homeostasis [138]. Magnesium deficiency interferes with calcium metabolism, leading to hypocalcemia and vitamin D abnormalities.

Only a small amount of the magnesium in the bone can be freely exchangeable with extracellular magnesium. In a kinetic model of magnesium metabolism in healthy men based on investigations with the stable isotopes ^{25}Mg and ^{26}Mg it has been determined that 24% of the human total magnesium exchanges rapidly; of this 79% turns over in 115 h, representing probably the bone surface pool and the remaining part - which may represent serum and easily accessible extracellular space - in less than 9 h [139]. In growing animals magnesium deficiency induced a loss of bone magnesium with few days [140]. Bone magnesium, therefore, represents a magnesium reservoir that buffers extracellular magnesium concentration. In humans this magnesium buffering capacity is reduced with increasing age as over lifetime nearly half of the magnesium content of bone is lost [141]. This might be explained by slight changes in acid–base balance at increasing age. Due to a reduced ability to excrete acid together with an increased nutritional acid load a general loss of minerals from the skeleton occurs with increasing age [142]. The usual amount of magnesium in the diet seems not to be high enough to avoid this magnesium loss from the bones that are also accompanied by calcium losses and reduced bone mineral density. This might be of importance for the development of osteoporosis. Animal experiments and human studies [143, 144] showed a positive effect of supplementing magnesium on bone density and bone absorption parameters.

Vitamin D

Vitamin D_3, or cholecalciferol, is produced in the skin as a result of the action of ultraviolet light on 7-dehydrocholesterol. The efficiency of this conversion is reduced with age, skin pigmentation, and potentially with the extensive use of sunscreens applied on the skin. Where foods are not fortified, the diet is relatively unimportant in determining vitamin D status, the principal dietary source being fatty fish and the oils derived from them. Severe and marked vitamin D deficiency still occurs in many regions of the world, causing rickets in childhood and osteomalacia in adults. Recently it has been increasingly recognized that vitamin D insufficiency is common in the elderly, and particularly those who are no longer fully independent and therefore less exposed to sunlight. This problem is greater at higher latitudes. In addition, vitamin D insufficiency leads to secondary hyperparathyroidism and consequently to greater bone loss. It also impairs muscle metabolism and may increase the likelihood of falls.

The most critical role of 1,25(OH)2D in mineral homeostasis is to enhance the efficiency of the small intestine to absorb dietary calcium. This was clearly demonstrated in the VDR null mouse [145]. Calcium absorption from the intestine is dependent on the amount of calcium in the diet and on physiological requirements, and is adaptable. When dietary calcium concentrations are low, almost all calcium is absorbed. The same happens in pregnancy and during lactation. 1,25$(OH)_2$D also promotes the intestinal absorption of phosphate. However a significant phosphate absorption also occurs in 1,25(OH)2D-deficient states [146].

1,25(OH)2D is essential for development and maintenance of a mineralised skeleton. Deficiency results in rickets during growth and osteomalacia in adults. 1,25(OH)2D induces bone formation by regulation of matrix proteins important for bone formation, such as osteocalcin, osteopontine, alkaline phosphatase, matrix-gla- protein and collagen, as well as mineral apposition. The bone forming osteoblasts express VDR and it appears that 1,25(OH)2D inhibits osteoblast proliferation through VDR-dependent signal pathway, and promotes their differentiation [147]. Vitamin D does not appear to be absolutely essential for the ossification process, but enhances this through increasing serum levels of calcium and phosphate. It has been suggested that not only 1,25$(OH)_2$D is involved in bone mineralisation, but also 24,25(OH)2D may be required (146).

1,25(OH)2D enhances the mobilisation of calcium and phosphorus stores from bone at times of calcium deprivation. 1,25(OH)2D induces stem cell monocytes to become mature osteoclasts. It appears though that this effect is not direct, but is mediated via osteoblasts that secrete a factor promoting osteoclast differentiation (147). 1,25(OH)2D regulate calcium homeostasis in close co-operation with PTH, which is the principal hormone regulating extracellular ionised calcium from minute to minute. PTH stimulates 1,25(OH)2D synthesis and 1,25(OH)2D suppresses the synthesis and secretion of PTH and controls parathyroid growth through negative gene regulation. Studies in the VDR null mouse suggest that VDR is not essential, but works in co-operation with calcium and phosphate [146].

The most important effects of 1,25(OH)2D in the kidney is suppression of 1α-hydroxylase activity and induction of 24-hydroxylase activity. 1,25(OH)2D increases renal calcium reabsorption and calbinding expression, and it accelerates PTH dependent calcium transport in the distal tubule, which has the highest level of VDR. The enhancing effect of 1,25(OH)2D on renal phosphate absorption might be an indirect action via PTH suppression [146].

The Benefits of Vitamin D Supplementation

Suboptimal vitamin D status is very common in the elderly, mainly because of reduced exposure to sunlight. A daily intake of 400-800 IU of vitamin D can help in the prevention of osteoporosis and fractures.

Malabanan et al. [148] have shown that vitamin D supplementation suppressed levels of PTH only in subjects whose baseline serum 25- hydroxycholecalciferol was less than 50 nmol/l (20mg/l). This suggests that 50 nmol/l is an appropriate threshold concentration for serum 25-hydroxycholecalciferol, below which individuals are at risk. However, some cross-sectional studies suggest that this threshold may be as high as 100 nmol/l (40mg/l) [149].

Physiological supplements of calciferol (e.g. 400-800IU/day) reduce PTH concentrations in elderly subjects and increase bone density, particularly at the femoral neck [150-153]. Similar changes in biochemical end-points have been reported with regular exposure to sunlight for 15–30 minutes daily (Reid et al., 1986). The effect of calciferol supplementation alone on fracture rates has been assessed in two large studies. In the first [153], no difference in fracture incidence was found in 2578 Dutch men and women over the age of 70 years randomized to calciferol 400 IU/day or placebo. In the second [154], however, 150000 IU of vitamin D annually reduced symptomatic fracture rates by 25% in a cohort of 800 elderly subjects in Finland. In another study, in which calcium was co-administered with calciferol to elderly subjects [155], a reduction of more than one-quarter in all non-vertebral and hip fracture rates was reported in a cohort of 3000 elderly women given 800 IU of vitamin D and 1200 mg of calcium daily over a period of 3 years. A further randomized study comparing calcium (500 mg/d) plus vitamin D (700 IU/d) to placebo in 400 older men and women showed a reduction in non-vertebral fracture rates of more than one-half [156].

Whether the calcium, the vitamin D or both together were responsible for reducing fracture rates is impossible to determine, though the most consistent results are in the two studies that used calcium plus vitamin D in the elderly [155, 156] (RRs of 0.45 and 0.75 in the respective studies, $P < 0.05$ for each). These studies show that it may be possible to markedly reduce morbidity in the elderly by means of a safe and inexpensive intervention.

Vitamin D supplements appear to produce no benefit in early postmenopausal women who are vitamin D replete [157]. Their use as a physiological supplement is fundamentally different from the use of high doses of calciferol or 1a-hydroxylated derivatives of vitamin D to manipulate intestinal calcium absorption pharmacologically. These agents bypass the normal homeostatic control of vitamin D metabolism and therefore incur a significant risk of hypercalcaemia and hypercalciuria. The use of pharmacological doses of calciferol has not been demonstrated to confer any beneficial effects on bone density [158].

Vitamin K

Vitamin K (VTK) is a fat-soluble molecule that naturally occurs in two forms: (a) VTK-1 (phylloquinone) is synthesized by plants and is abundantly found in green leafy vegetables and some vegetable oils (soybean, canola, and olive); (b) VTK-2 (menaquinones) refers collectively to a group of compounds that are commonly synthesized from bacteria that normally colonize the colon as well as from enteric metabolism of VTK-1. The "K" component of VTK is derived from the German word "Koagulation" as this essential molecule is a required coenzyme involved in blood coagulation, but recent work has also recognized VTK as a cofactor in many biochemical pathways associated with cell growth, brain development [159] and bone health [160].

Increasing epidemiological research has demonstrated that healthy bone mineralization and adequate bone integrity is dependent on adequate levels of VTK. Various VTK-dependent proteins have been isolated in bone, the deficiencies of which may be associated with diminished BMD and other adverse sequelae [161, 162]. The Nurses Health Study, for example, confirmed that women with low VTK consumption had dramatically higher rates of hip fracture [163] and the Framingham Heart study found that both men and women with higher VTK intakes sustained about a 35% relative risk of hip fracture compared to those with low intake [164]. Furthermore, a 3-year, double-blind, controlled study recently concluded that 1mg of VTK-1 daily may substantially contribute to reducing postmenopausal bone loss at the site of the femoral neck [165].

More recently, there has been increased focus on the VTK-2 form of this micro-nutrient. VTK-2 is involved in the induction of bone mineralization in human osteoblasts [166, 167] and in vitro studies suggest that this molecule also inhibits osteoclast formation [168] as well as diminishing bone resorption by inhibiting prostaglandin E2 synthesis [169]. A form of VTK-2, menatetrenone (MK-4), is well tolerated with oral intake and is under extensive study in Japan for the management of osteoporosis and the prevention of fractures [170-173]. A number of human clinical trials have been undertaken and prove VTK-2 to be an effective agent in maintaining BMD and diminishing the risk of fracture. In a recent randomized control trial, for example, osteoporotic women receiving VTK-2 and calcium were significantly less likely to sustain clinical fractures and lose BMD than controls who received calcium alone [171].

Furthermore, another recent trial on patients with Alzheimer's disease confirmed that supplemental VTK-2 preserved BMD and significantly decreased the risk of non-vertebral fractures including hip fractures in these high risk patients [174]. Various authors report that no adverse effects are usually associated with this intervention (175), but caution has been expressed that VTK-2 may counteract the effects of anticoagulant therapy and may be contraindicated in individuals who have sustained thrombotic illness previously.

In a recent review paper on the effects of VTK on osteoporosis, the authors conclude that deficiency may contribute to osteoporotic fractures and that use of VTK-2 may stimulate bone formation and suppress bone resorption, thus contributing to the prevention of osteoporotic fractures [160]. Deficiency of this nutrient typically occurs with insufficient intake or with depletion of bacterial flora in the intestine potentially from antibiotic usage [176]. Accordingly, it appears prudent to ensure that dietary requirements for VTK are being met [177], to incorporate laboratory testing for functional measures of VTK status if indicated [178], and to consider VTK-2 supplementation for patients with compromised bone health [179]. It is uncertain whether probiotic usage to enhance bacterial flora is associated with improved VTK-2 production.

Vitamin C

One important function of vitamin C is in the formation and maintenance of collagens, the basis of connective tissues, which are found in skin, ligaments, cartilages, vertebral discs, joint linings, capillary walls and the bones and teethes. Collagen protein requires vitamin C for hydroxylation, a process that allows the molecule to achieve the best configuration and prevent collagen from becoming weak and susceptible to damage. It has been shown that vitamin C increases the level of procollagen messenger RNA [180].

Collagen subunits are formed with in fibroblasts as procollagen, which are excreted into extra cellular spaces. Vitamin C is required to export the procollagen molecules out of the cell. The final structure of the collagen is formed after pieces of the procollagen are enzymatically cleaved [180]. Collagen and thus vitamin C is needed to give support and shape to the body to help wounds heal and to maintain healthy blood vessels. Specifically ascorbic acid works as a coenzyme to convert proline and lysine to hydroxyproline and hydroxylysine both important to the collagen structure. Deficiency of vitamin C leads to secretion of premature collagen fibers into the bone.

Vitamin C is important for collagen formation and strong collagens are necessary for strong bones. Both the densities of bones and level of vitamin C begin to decrease with age. While a number of factors contribute to osteoporosis, studies show that a person's vitamin C status is also related to the maintenance of healthy bones. In fact, vitamin C may directly affect the growth of bone cells, above and beyond its call of duty in forming collagen. Ascorbic acid intake at moderate doses is important and safe for bone maintenance and therefore a factor in mitigating or delaying osteoporosis [180].

Fluoride

Fluoride (F) is an essential ultratrace element that is required for skeletal and dental development. F is present in very small amounts in food and water. The concentration of fluoride in the soil, water, and many foods varies by geographic region. Major dietary sources include drinking water, tea, coffee, rice, soybeans, spinach, onions, and lettuce. It is well known that water fluoridation at the level of 1 mg/L can help prevent dental caries, but is unlclear if this process can affect bone mass. Incorporation of F into bone increases its size and decreases the solubility of apatite crystals [181]. Fluoride action on bones include stimulation of osteoblast replication and sensitizing skeletal growth factors through the inhibition of osteoblastic acid phosphatase [182]. The adequate daily adult intake is 4 mg for males and 3 mg for females. Excess fluoride ingestion causes fluorosis, a painful condition associated with extra-osseous calcification and brittle bones and for that reason in some endemic high fluoride areas, higher hip fracture rates have been seen. High doses of fluoride can stimulate osteoblasts; however, the quality of bone that is formed may be abnormal and the effect on fracture rates is unclear [183].

Boron

Boron occurs in foods as borate and boric acid. Boron has not been established to be an essential nutrient for humans and no specific biochemical function for boron has been identified in higher animals or man. There is some evidence that, in humans, boron intake within the usual dietary range may influence the metabolism and utilisation of other nutrients, particularly calcium, and may have a beneficial effect on bone calcification and maintenance. Recommended intakes for boron have not been established.

The first findings demonstrating the significance of boron in human nutrition came from two studies in which male subjects over the age of 45, postmenopausal women, and postmenopausal women on estrogen therapy consumed a low boron diet (about 0.25 mg/2000 kcal) for 63 days and later ingested daily the same diet supplemented with 3.0 mg of this ultratrace element for the period of 49 days [184]. The major differences between the two investigations were the levels of copper and magnesium in the diets; in one experiment they were marginal (1.6 mg Cu/2000 kcal) or inadequate (115 mg Mg/2000 kcal), in the other, they were adequate (2.4 mg Cu and 300 mg Mg/2000 kcal). Results from these researches showed that boron has an impact on the metabolism of macrominerals, energy, nitrogen, and reactive oxygen in humans; they also demonstrated that boron affects brain function, psychomotor performance and the response to estrogen ingestion.

Mechanisms, whereby boron affects bone health include the metabolism of minerals and changes in hormones that are involved in their turnover. Serum 25-hydroxycholecalciferol concentration was found to be lower during boron depletion than during the period of its repletion [185, 186]. It was also reported that when dietary copper was marginal and magnesium was inadequate, calcitonin values were much higher than when these two elements were adequate. The results of these studies suggest that, because the calcitonin values obtained with adequate copper and magnesium were close to those reported by others as being normal, the combined magnesium-low, copper-marginal diet caused elevated serum calcitonin indicative of an abnormal calcium metabolism. [185]. Similar findings were obtained with serum osteocalcin. Further evidence that boron affects the metabolism of major minerals is that plasma ionised calcium and serum magnesium concentrations were lower during born depletion than repletion in the studies where dietary copper and magnesium were marginal or inadequate.

Copper

It is well established that the trace element copper is essential for life. Copper in living organisms, including humans, forms an essential component of many enzymes (cuproenzymes) and proteins. The biochemical role for copper is primarily catalytic, with many copper metalloenzymes acting as oxidases to achieve the reduction of molecular oxygen, for example cytochrome-C-oxidase and superoxide dismutase. Studies have also shown that copper is required for infant growth, host defence mechanisms, bone strength, red and white cell maturation, iron transport, cholesterol and glucose metabolism [187].

Copper influences bone formation, skeletal mineralization, and the integrity of the connective tissue. Lysyl oxidase, a copper-containing enzyme, is essential for cross-linking of collagen fibrils, thereby increasing the mechanical strength of the protein and forming strong, flexible connective tissue. Copper deficiency has been shown to decrease bone strength in animal studies [188]. In humans, copper supplementation for 2 years was associated with a reduction in bone loss in perimenopausal [189] and postmenopausal women [190]. A variety of indicators were used to establish the recommended levels for copper, including plasma copper concentration, serum ceruloplasmin activity, superoxide dismutase activity, and platelet copper concentration [190]. The RDA for copper reflects the results of depletion-repletion studies and was based on the prevention of deficiency (900 mg/d for adults). However, higher levels (2.5-3 mg/d) have been associated with greater BMD and lower bone loss in pre and post-menopausal women [189, 190].

Oxidative Stress as a Risk Factor for the Development of Osteoporosis

Oxidative stress and antioxidants may contribute to the pathogenesis of the skeletal system including osteoporosis, the most prevalent metabolic bone disease [191]. Oxidative stress control the functions of both osteoclasts [192, 193] and osteoblasts [194]. Endogenous [193, 195] and synthetic [196] antioxidants counteract the effects of oxidative stress in these cells. Recent studies reported that antioxidants from natural sources, such as the lycopene from tomatoes, can also counteract the damaging effects of oxidative stress. The findings that lycopene has a stimulatory effect on the cell proliferation [197] and the differentiation marker alkaline phosphatase of osteoblasts [197, 198], as well as its inhibitory effects on osteoclasts formation and resorption [199, 200] are evidence of the involvement of lycopene in bone health and warranted further investigation in clinical studies.

Epidemiological studies have shown that oxidative stress is associated with osteoporosis and that antioxidants may counteract this effect. Certain antioxidants including vitamin C, E and beta-carotene may reduce the risk of osteoporosis [201-204] and counteract the adverse effects of oxidative stress on bone that are produced during strenuous exercise [203] and among smokers [201]. Osteoporotic women have been shown to have reduced levels of antioxidant vitamins and enzymes indicating a decrease in their antioxidant defences [205].

A recently published clinical study showed a direct correlation between serum lycopene and decrease in the risk of osteoporosis among postmenopausal women for the first time [206]. The relationship between serum lycopene, oxidative stress parameters and bone turnover markers in postmenopausal women were investigated. Study participants were asked to complete a seven-day food intake record prior to giving fasting blood samples. Oxidative stress parameters, total antioxidant capacity, serum lycopene and the bone turnover markers including bone alkaline phosphatase (bone formation) and cross-linked N-telopeptides of type I collagen (NTx) (bone resorption) were measured in the serum samples. Results showed a direct correlation between lycopene intake and serum lycopene levels. Increase in serum lycopene levels resulted in significant decreases in protein oxidation and NT*x* values [206]. Based on these results an important role for lycopene mediated via its antioxidant property in reducing the risk of osteoporosis is suggested. Dietary intervention studies with varying levels of lycopene are currently being conducted with the objective of demonstrating the beneficial effects of lycopene in the prevention and management of osteoporosis.

Conclusion

Bone is strongly influenced by the intake of several nutrients. Not only the traditional nutrients related to bone, e.g. calcium, protein, phosphorus, magnesium, vitamin D, and fluoride, are important in bone health, but also several other vitamins, minerals and phytochemicals. The intakes of many of these nutrients by the general population and in particular by the elderly population are inadequate for bone health. Several recent epidemiological studies and clinical trials have shown that higher intakes of some of these nutrients through supplementation may help in building bone mass, preventing bone loss and fractures, and decreasing bone resorption and/or increasing bone formation. These dietary nutrients include zinc, copper, manganese, vitamin K, and vitamin C. Other nutrients that have been shown to maintain bone health include boron and antioxidants.

These nutrients are found in a variety of foods. Dairy products provide ample calcium, as well as protein, vitamin D, phosphorus, potassium, magnesium, and zinc Calcium is also found in green leafy vegetables, such as bok choy, broccoli, collard, and kale, which also provide magnesium, potassium, boron, vitamins K, A, and C. Fruits and vegetables provide magnesium, boron, vitamins K, A, and C. In addition, they promote an alkaline environment, thereby reducing the demand for skeletal salts to balance the acid generated from meats. Legumes and whole-grain products provide phosphorus, potassium, magnesium, manganese, zinc, copper, and vitamin K. In addition, beef, fish, or poultry, and nuts and seeds are good sources of protein, zinc, magnesium, copper, phosphorus, manganese, and iron.

References

[1] National Osteoporosis Foundation. Physician's guide to prevention and treatment of osteoporosis. Washington (DC): National Osteoporosis Foundation; 2003. p. 1-37.

[2] North American Menopause Society. Management of postmenopausal osteoporosis: position statement of the North American Menopause Society. *Menopause,* 2002, 9, 84-101.

[3] Brown, JP; Josse, RG. 2002 clinical practice guidelines for the diagnosis and management of osteoporosis in Canada. For the Scientific Advisory Council of the Osteoporosis Society of Canada. *CMAJ*, 2002, 167(Suppl 10), S1-34.

[4] US Preventive Services Task Force. Screening for osteoporosis in postmenopausal women: recommendations and rationale. *Ann. Intern. Med.*, 2002, 137, 526-528.

[5] Eastell, R. Pathogenesis of postmenopausal osteoporosis. In: Favus MJ, editor. *Primer on the metabolic bone diseases and disorders of mineral metabolism. 5th ed.* Washington (DC): American Society for Bone and Mineral Research; 2003. p. 314-316.

[6] Recker, R; Lappe, J; Davies, K; Heaney, R. Characterization of perimenopausal bone loss: a prospective study. *J. Bone Miner Res.*, 2000, 15, 1965-1973.

[7] Abrahamsen, B; Nissen, N; Hermann, AP; Hansen, B; Barenholdt, O; Vestergaard, P; Tofteng, CL; Pors-Nielsen, S. When should densitometry be repeated in healthy peri- and postmenopausal women?: The Danish Osteoporosis Prevention Study. *J. Bone Miner Res.*, 2002, 17, 2061-2067.

[8] Marshall, D; Johnell, O; Wedel, H. Meta-analysis of how well measures of bone mineral density predict occurrence of osteoporotic fractures. *BMJ*, 1996, 312, 1254-1259.

[9] Picard, D; Imbach, A; Couturier, M ; Lepage, R ; Ste Marie, L-G. Longitudinal study of bone density and its determinants in women in peri- or early menopause. *Calcif Tissue Int.*, 2000, 67, 356-3560.

[10] Ravn, P; Cizza, G; Bjarnason, NH; Thompson, D; Daley, M; Wasnich, RD; McClung, M; Hosking, D; Yates, AJ; Christiansen, C. Low body mass index is an important risk factor for low bone mass and increased bone loss in early postmenopausal women. Early Postmenopausal Intervention Cohort (EPIC) study group. *J. Bone Miner Res.*, 1999, 14, 1622-1627.

[11] Genant, HK; Cooper, C; Poor, G; Reid, I; Ehrlich, G; Kanis J; et al. Interim report and recommendations of the World Health Organization task-force for osteoporosis. *Osteoporosis Int. 1999*, 10, 259-264.

[12] Cooper, C. The epidemiology of fragility fractures: is there a role for bone quality? *Calcif Tissue Int.*, 1993, 53(Suppl 1), S23-26.

[13] United Nations: The sex and age distributions of population. The 1994 revision of the United Nations global population estimates and projections. New York, NY, United Nations, 1995.

[14] Cooper, C; Campion, G; Melton, LJ III. Hip fractures in the elderly: a worldwide projection. *Osteoporosis Int.*, 1992, 2, 285-289.

[15] Gullberg, B; Johnell, O; Kanis, JA. Worldwide projections for hip fracture. *Osteoporosis Int.*, 1997, 7, 407-413.

[16] Jonston, Jr CC. Development of clinical practice guidelines for prevention and treatment of osteoporosis. *Calcif Tissue Int.*, 1996, 59 Suppl 1, S30-S-33

[17] Kanis, JA; Melton 3rd, LJ; Christiansen, C; Johnston Jr, CC; Khaltaev, N. The diagnosis of osteoporosis. *J. Bone Miner Res.*, 1994, 9, 1137-1141.

[18] Wachman, A; Bernstein DB. Diet and osteoporosis. *Lancet*, 1968, 1, 958-959.

[19] Allen, LH; Oddoye, EA; Margen, S. Protein-induced hypercalciuria: a longer term *study. Am. J. Clin. Nutr.*, 1979, 32, 741–749.

[20] Kim, Y; Linkswiler, H M. Effect of level of protein intake on calcium metabolism and on parathyroid and renal function in the adult human male. *J. Nutr.*, 1979; 109, 1399-1404.

[21] Schuette, SA; Zemel, MB; Linkswiler, HM. Studies on the mechanism of protein-induced hypercalciuria in older men and women. *J. Nutr.*, 1980, 110, 305-315.

[22] Hegsted, M; Schuette, SA; Zemel, MB; Linkswiler, HM. Dietary calcium and calcium balance in young men as affected by level of protein and phosphorus intake. *J. Nutr.*, 1981, 111, 553-562.

[23] Hegsted, M; Linkswiler, HM. Long-term effects of level of protein intake on calcium metabolism in young adult women. *J. Nutr.*, 1981, 111, 244-251.

[24] Heaney, RP. Nutritional factors in osteoporosis. *Annu. Rev. Nutr.*, 1993, 13, 287-316.

[25] Bunker, VW. The role of nutrition in osteoporosis. *Br. J. Biomed. Sci.*, 1994, 51, 228-240.

[26] Feskanich, D; Willett, WC; Stampfer, MJ; Colditz, GA. Protein consumption and bone fractures in women. *Am. J. Epidemiol.*, 1996, 143, 472-479.

[27] Cohen, A J; Roe, FJ. Review of risk factors for osteoporosis with particular reference to a possible aetiological role of dietary salt. *Food Chem. Toxicol.*, 2000, 38, 237-253.

[28] Hegsted, DM; Fractures, calcium, and the modern diet. *Am. J. Clin Nutr.*, 2001, 74, 571-573.

[29] Hegsted, DM. Calcium and osteoporosis. *J. Nutr.*, 1986, 116, 2316-2319.

[30] Sellmeyer, DE; Stone, KL; Sebastian, A; Cummings, SR. A high ratio of dietary animal to vegetable protein increases the rate of bone loss and the risk of fracture in postmenopausal women. *Am. J. Clin. Nutr.*, 2001, 73, 118-122.

[31] Halperin, ML; Goldstein, MB. Fluid, Electrolyte, and Acid-Base Physiology: A Problem-Based Approach, 3rd Edition. Philadelphia: WB Saunders Company, 1999.

[32] Barzel, US; Massey, LK. Excess dietary protein can adversely affect bone. *J. Nutr.,* 1998, 128, 1051-1053.

[33] Heaney, RP. Excess dietary protein may not adversely affect bone. *J. Nutr.*, 1998, 128, 1054-1057.

[34] Frassetto, L; Morris, R; Sebastian, A. Potassium bicarbonate reduces urinary nitrogen excretion in postmenopausal women. *J. Clin. Endocrinol. Metab.*, 1997, 82, 254-259.

[35] Remer, T; Manz, F. Estimation of the renal net acid excretion by adults consuming diets containing variable amounts of protein. *Am. J. Clin. Nutr.*, 1994, 59, 1356-1361.

[36] Walker, RM; Linkswiler, HM. Calcium retention in the adult human male as affected by protein intake. *J. Nutr.*, 1972, 102, 1297-1302.

[37] Johnson, NE; Alcantara, EN; Linkswiler, H. Effect of level of protein intake on urinary and fecal calcium and calcium retention of young adult males. *J. Nutr.*, 1970, 100, 1425-1430.

[38] Spencer, H; Kramer, L; Osis, D; Norris, C. Effect of phosphorus on the absorption of calcium and on the calcium balance in man. *J. Nutr.*, 1978; 108, 447-457.

[39] Hunt, JR; Gallagher, SK; Johnson, LK; Lykken, GI. High- versus low-meat diets: effects on zinc absorption, iron status, and calcium, copper, iron, magnesium, manganese, nitrogen, phosphorus, and zinc balance in postmenopausal women. *Am. J. Clin. Nutr.*, 1995, 62, 621-632.

[40] Spencer, H; Kramer, L; Osis, D; Norris, C. Effect of a high protein (meat) intake on calcium metabolism in man. *Am. J. Clin. Nutr.*, 1978b, 31, 2167-2180.

[41] Spencer, H; Kramer, L; Osis, D. Do protein and phosphorus cause calcium loss? *J. Nutr.*, 1988, 118, 657-660.

[42] Bonjour, J-P; Schurch, MA; Chevalley, T; Ammann, P; Rizzoli, R. Protein intake, IGF-1 and osteoporosis. *Osteoporosis Int.*, 1997, 7(suppl. 3), S36-S42.

[43] Marcus, R. Mechanisms of exercise effects on bone. In: Bilezikian JP, Raisz LG, Rodan GA, eds. *Principles of bone biology*. San Diego, CA, Academic Press, 1996:1135-1146.

[44] Rodan, GA. Coupling of bone resorption and formation during bone remodeling. In: Marcus R., Feldman D, Kelsey J, eds. *Osteoporosis*. San Diego, CA, Academic Press, 1996, 289-299.

[45] Heaney, RP; Abrams, S; Dawson-Hughes, B; Looker, A; Marcus, R; Matkovic, V; Weaver, C. Peak bone mass. *Osteoporosis Int.*, 2000, 11, 985-1009.

[46] Kerstetter, JE; O´Brien, KO; Insogna, KL. Dietary protein affects intestinal calcium absorption. *Am. J. Clin. Nutr.*, 1998, 68, 859-865.

[47] Kerstetter, JE; Svastislee, C; Caseria, D; Mitnick, MAE; Insogna, K.L. A threshold for low-protein-diet-induced elevations in parathyroid hormone. *Am. J. Clin. Nutr.*, 2000, 72, 168-173.

[48] Giannini, S; Nobile, M; Sartori, L; Carbonare, LD; Ciuffreda, M; Corro, P; D'Angelo, A; Calo, L; Crepaldi, G. Acute effects of moderate dietary protein restriction in patients with idiopathic hypercalciuria and calcium nephrolithiasis. *Am. J. Clin. Nutr.*, 1999, 69, 267-271.

[49] Bonjour, J-P; Schurch, M-A; Rizzoli, R. Nutritional aspects of hip fractures. *Bone*, 1996; 18: 139S-144S.

[50] Schurch, M-A; Rizzoli, R; Slosman, D; Vadas, L; Vergnaud, P; Bonjour J-P. Protein supplements increase serum insulin-like growth factor-I levels and attenuate proximal femur bone loss in patients with recent hip fracture. *Ann. Intern. Med.*, 1998, 128, 801-809.

[51] Munger, RG; Cerhan, JR; Chiu, BC-H. Prospective study of dietary protein intake and risk of hip fracture in postmenopausal women. *Am. J. Clin. Nutr.*, 1999, 69, 147-152.

[52] Hannan, MT; Tucker, KL; Dawson-Hughes, B; Cuppler, LA; Felson, DT; Kiel, D.P. Effect of dietary protein on bone loss in elderly men and women: the Framingham Osteoporosis Study. *J. Bone Miner Res.*, 2000, 15, 2504-2512.

[53] Recker, RR; Davies, KM; Hinders, SM; Heaney, RP; Stegman, MR; Kimmel, DB. Bone gain in young adult women. *JAMA*, 1992, 268, 2403-2408.

[54] USDA. Agricultural Research Service. 1997. Data tables: Results from USDA's 1994-96 Continuing Survey of Food Intakes by Individuals and 1994-96 Diet and Health Knowledge Survey. February 1999. http://www.barc.usda.gov/bhnrc/foodsurvey /home.htm

[55] McDowell, MA; Briefel, RR; Alaimo, K; Bischof, AM; Caughman, CR; Carroll, MD; Loria, CM; Johnson, CL. Energy and macronutrient intakes of persons ages 2 months and over in the United States: Third National Health and Nutrition Examination Survey, Phase I, 1988-91. Advance data from Vital and Health Statistics No. 255. Hyattsville, MD: National Center for Health Statistics; 1994.

[56] Alaimo, K; McDowell, MA; Briefel, RR; Bischof, AM; Caughman, CR; Loria, CM; Johnson, CL. Dietary intake of vitamins, minerals, and fiber of persons ages 2 months and over in the United States: Third National Health and Nutrition Examination Survey, Phase 1, 1988-91. Advance Data from Vital and Health Statistics No. 258. Hyattsville, MD: National Center for Health Statistics; 1994.

[57] Institute of Medicine, Food and Nutrition Board. Standing Committee on the Scientific Evaluation of Dietary Reference Intakes. Dietary Reference Intakes for Calcium, Phosphorus, Magnesium, Vitamin D, and Fluoride. Washington, D.C.: National Academy Press; 1997.

[58] National Research Council, Subcommittee on the Tenth Edition of the RDAs, Food and Nutrition Board, Commission on Life Sciences. Recommended Dietary Allowances. 10th ed. Washington, D.C.: National Academy Press; 1989.

[59] Kruger, MC; Horrobin, DF. Calcium metabolism, osteoporosis and essential fatty acids: a review. *Prog. Lipid Res.*, 1997, 36, 131-151.

[60] Coetzer, H; Claassen, N; van-Papendorp, DH; Kruger, MC. Calcium transport by isolated brush border and basolateral membrane vesicles: role ofessential fatty acid supplementation. *Prostaglandin Leukot Essent Fatty Acids*, 1994, 50, 257-266.

[61] Buck, AC; Davies, RL; Harrison, T. The protective role of eicosapentaenoic acid [EPA] in the pathogenesis of nephrolithiasis *J. Urol.*, 1991, 146, 188-194.

[62] Tulloch, I; Smellie, WS; Buck, AC. Evening primrose oil reduces urinary calcium excretion in both normal and hypercalciuric rats. *Urol. Res.*, 1994, 22, 227-230.

[63] Chanda, S; Islam, MN; Pramanik, P; Mitra, C. High lipid diet intake is a possible predisposing factor in the development of hypogonadal osteoporosis. *Jpn. J. Physiol.*, 1996, 46, 383-388.

[64] Beadles, JR; Mitchell, HH; Hamilton, TS. The utilization of dietary calcium by growing albino rats fed diets containing lard or cocoa butter. *J. Nutr*, 1951, 45, 399-405.

[65] Kane, GG; Lovelace, FE; McCay, CM. Dietary fat and calcium wastage in old age. *J. Gerontol.*, 1949, 4, 185-192.

[66] Kaup, SM; Behling, AR; Chodquitte, L; Greger, JL. Calcium and magnesium utilization in rats: effect of dietary butterfat and calcium and of age. *J. Nutr.*, 1990, 120, 266-273.

[67] Atteh, JO; Leeson, S. Effects of dietary saturated or unsaturated fatty acids and calcium levels on performance and mineral metabolism of broiler chicks. *Poult Sci.,* 1984, 673, 2252-2260.

[68] Bullamore, JR; Wilkinson, R; Gallagher, JC; Nordin, BE. Effect of age on calcium absorption *Lancet*, 1970, 2, 535-537.

[69] Gallagher, JC; Riggs, BL; Eisman, J; Hamstra, A; Arnaud, SB, DeLuca, HF. Intestinal calcium absorption and serum vitamin D metabolites in normal subjects and osteoporotic patients: effect of age and dietary calcium. *J. Clin. Invest.*, 1979, 64, 729-736.

[70] Weiss, LA; Barrett-Connor, E; von Muhlen, D. Ratio of n-6 to n-3 fatty acids and bone mineral density in older adults: the Rancho Bernardo Study. *Am. J. Clin. Nutr.*, 2005, 81, 934-938.

[71] Watkins, BA; Li, Y; Lippman, HE; Seifert, MF. Omega-3 polyunsaturated fatty acids and skeletal health. *Exp. Biol. Med. (Maywood)*, 2001, 226, 485-97.

[72] Watkins, BA; Li, Y; Lippman, HE; Feng, S. Modulatory effect of omega-3 polyunsaturated fatty acids on osteoblast function and bone metabolism. *Prostaglandins Leukot Essent Fatty Acids*, 2003, 68, 387-98.

[73] Albertazzi, P; Coupland, K. Polyunsaturated fatty acids. Is there a role in postmenopausal osteoporosis prevention? *Maturitas*, 2002, 42, 13-22.

[74] Kruger, MC; Horrobin, DF. Calcium metabolism, osteoporosis and essential fatty acids: a review. *Prog. Lipid Res.*, 1997, 36, 131-151.

[75] Genuis, SJ; Schwalfenberg, G. Time for an oil check: the role of essential omega 3 fatty acids in maternal and pediatric health. *J. Perinatol.*, 2006, 26, 359-365.

[76] Simopoulos, AP. The importance of the ratio of omega-6/omega-3 essential fatty acids. *Biomed Pharmacother*, 2002, 56:365-379.

[77] Masi, L; Brandi, ML. Physiopathological basis of bone turnover. *Q. J. Nucl. Med.*, 2001, 45, 2-6.

[78] Fernandes, G; Lawrence, R; Sun, D. Protective role of n-3 lipids and soy protein in osteoporosis. *Prostaglandins Leukot Essent Fatty Acids*, 2003, 68, 361-372.

[79] Corey, EJ; Shih, C; Cashman, JR. Docosahexaenoic acid is a strong inhibitor of prostaglandin but not leukotriene biosynthesis. *Proc. Natl. Acad. Sci. USA*, 1983, 80, 3581-3584.

[80] Meydani, SN; Lichtenstein, AH; Cornwall, S. Immunologic effects of national cholesterol education panel step-2 diets with and without fish-derived n-3 fatty acid enrichment. *J. Clin. Invest.*, 1993, 92, 105-113.

[81] Caughey, GE; Mantzioris, E; Gibson, RA; Cleland, LG; James, MJ. The effect on human tumor necrosis factor alpha and interleukin 1 beta production of diets enriched in n-3 fatty acids from vegetable oil or fish oil. *Am. J. Clin. Nutr.,* 1996, 63, 116-122.

[82] Fujita T. Osteoporosis in Japan: factors contributing to the low incidence of hip fracture. *Adv. Nutr. Res.*, 1994, 9, 89-99.

[83] Sugano M, Hirahara F. Polyunsaturated fatty acids in the food chain in Japan. *Am. J. Clin. Nutr.*, 2000, 71, 189S-196S.

[84] Kettler, DB. Can manipulation of the ratios of essential fatty acids slow the rapid rate of postmenopausal bone loss? *Altern. Med. Rev.*, 2001, 6, 61-77.

[85] Weaver, CM; Peacock, M; Martin, BR; Plawecki, KL; McCabe, GP. Calcium retention estimated from indicators of skeletal status in adolescent girls and young women. *Am. J. Clin. Nutr.*, 1996, 64, 67-70.

[86] Weaver, CM. Calcium. In: Present knowledge in nutrition. Bowman BA and Russell RM (Eds.). ILSI Press, Washington, DC, 8th Edition, 2001; pp. 273-280.

[87] Worth, GK; Retallack, RW; Devlin, RD; Jefferies, M; Gutteridge, DH. Ionized calcium: aspects of techniques and some factors affecting results. *Clin. Chim. Acta*, 1981, 114, 283-286.

[88] Fishbein, L. Multiple sources of calcium – some aspects of its essentiality. Regulatory *Toxicol. Pharmacol.*, 2004, 39, 67-80.

[89] American Academy of Pediatrics. Calcium requirements of infants, children and adolescents. *Pediatrics,* 1999, 104, 1152-1157.

[90] Harvard University Health Services, 2003. Calcium content of common foods in common portions. Available from: http://www.uhs.harvard.edu/CWHC/CWHC WellnessInformationCalciumContent.htm

[91] Johns Hopkins Student Health and Wellness Center, 2003. Calcium concepts - what are good sources of calcium? Available from: http://www.jhu.edu/-shcenter/calcium.html

[92] Medical Network, Inc, 2002. Health A to Z. Available from: http://www.Healthatoz.com/atoz/osteo/osmilk.asp.

[93] McKinley Health Center, University of Illinois, 2002. Calcium. Available from: http://www.mckinley.uiuc.edu/handouts/calcium/html.

[94] USDA, 2001. Nutrient Value of Food. Publ. HG-7. US Department of Agriculture, Washington, DC. Available from: http://www.nal.usda.gov/fnicfoodcomp.

[95] Baylor College of Medicine, 1999. USDA/ARS Children's Nutrition Center. What are good non-dairy sources of calcium? Available from: http://www.bcm.tmc.edu/cnrc/consumer/archives/nondairy.htm.

[96] National Institute of Child Health and Human Development, 2000. Why calcium? National Institutes of Health, Bethesda, MD. Available from: http://www.nlm.nih.gov/milk/whycal/foods.afm.

[97] Nordin, BEC. Calcium and osteoporosis. *Nutrition*, 1997, 13, 664-686.

[98] Dawson-Hughes, B; Dallal, GE; Krall, EA; Sadowski, L; Sahyoun, N; Tannenbaum S. A controlled trial of the effect of calcium supplementation on bone density in postmenopausal women. *NEJM*, 1990, 323, 878-883.

[99] Elders, PJ; Netelenbos, JC; Lips, P; van Ginkel, FC; Khoe, E; Leeuwenkamp, OR; Hackeng, WH; van der Stelt, PF. Calcium supplementation reduces vertebral bone loss in perimenopausal women: a controlled trial in 248 women between 45 and 55 years of age. *J. Clin. Endocrinol. Metab.*, 1991, 73, 533-540.

[100] Reid, IR; Ames, R; Evans, MC; Gamble, GD; Sharpe, SJ. Long-term effects of calcium supplementation on bone loss and fractures in postmenopausal women - a randomized controlled trial. *Am. J. Med.*, 1995, 98, 331-335.

[101] Chevalley, T; Rizzoli, R; Nydegger, V; Slosman, D; Rapin, C-H; Michel, J-P; Vasey, H; Bonjour J-P. Effects of calcium supplements on femoral bone mineral density and vertebral fracture rate in vitamin-D-replete elderly patients. *Osteoporosis Int.*, 1994, 4, 245-252.

[102] Recker, RR; Hinders, S; Davies, KM; Heaney, RP; Stegman, MR; Lappe, JM; Kimmel, DB. Correcting calcium nutritional deficiency prevents spine fractures in elderly women. *J. Bone Min. Res*. 1996, 11, 1961-1966.

[103] Cranney, A; Guyatt, G; Griffith, L; Wells, G; Tugwell, P; Rosen C. The Osteoporosis Methodology Group and the Osteoporosis Research Advisory Group. Summary of meta-analyses of therapies for postmenopausal osteoporosis. *Endocrine Rev.*, 2002, 23, 570-578.

[104] Kanis, JA. Calcium nutrition and its implications for osteoporosis. Part II. After menopause. *Eur. J. Clin. Nutr.*, 1994, 48, 835-841.

[105] Report on osteoporosis in the European Community. Strasbourg, European Community, 1998.

[106] Karkkainen, MUM; Wiersma, JW; Lambergallardt, CJE. Postprandial parathyroid hormone response to four calcium-rich foodstuffs. *Am. J. Clin. Nutr.*, 1997, 65, 1726-1730.

[107] Whiting, SJ; Wood, RJ. Adverse effects of high-calcium diets in humans. *Nutr. Rev.*, 1997, 55, 1-9.

[108] Curhan, GC; Willett, WC; Speizer, FE; Spiegelman, D; Stampfer, MJ. Comparison of dietary calcium with supplemental calcium and other nutrients as factors affecting the risk for kidney stones in women. *Ann. Internal. Med.* 1997, 126, 497-504.

[109] Baron, JA; Beach, M; Mandel, JS; van Stolk, RU; Haile, RW; Sandler, RS; Rothstein, R; Summers, RW; Snover, DC; Beck, GJ; Bond, JH; Greenberg, ER; Frankl, H; Pearson, L; Calcium supplements for the prevention of colorectal adenomas. *NEJM,* 1999, 340, 101-107.

[110] Griffith, LE; Guyatt, GH; Cook, RJ; Bucher, HC; Cook, D.J. The influence of dietary and nondietary calcium supplementation on blood pressure - An updated metaanalysis of randomized controlled trials. *Am. J. Hyperten.*, 1999, 12, 84-92.

[111] Reid, IR; Mason, B; Horne, A; Ames, R; Clearwater, J; Bava, U;, Orr-Walker, B; Wu, F; Evans, MC; Gamble, GD. Effects of calcium supplementation on serum lipid concentrations in normal older women: a randomized controlled trial. *Am. J. Med.*, 2002, 112, 343-347.

[112] Taketomo, CKL; Hodding, JH; Kraus, DM. In: Pediatric Dosage Handbook. Lexi-Comp, Inc, Cleveland, OH, 2001; pp. 167-170.

[113] Lloyd, CW; Johnson, CE. Management of hypophosphatemia. *Clinic Pharmacy*, 1988, 7, 123-128.

[114] Fomon, SJ; Nelson, SE. Calcium, phosphorus, magnesium, and sulfur. In: Fomon S.J. ed. *Nutrition of normal infants*. St. Louis: Mopsby-Year book, 1993, 192-216.

[115] Calvo, MS; Heath H. 3rd. Acute effects of oral phosphate-salt ingestion on serum phosphorus, serum ionized calcium, and parathyroid hormone in young adults. *Am. J. Clin. Nutr.*, 1988, 47, 1025-1029.

[116] Goldsmith, RS; Jowsey, J; Dube, WJ; Riggs, BL; Arnaud, CD; Kelly, PJ. Effects of phosphorus supplementation on serum parathyroid hormone and bone morphology in osteoporosis. *J. Clin. Endocrin. Metab.*, 1976, 43, 523-532.

[117] Whybro, A; Jagger, H; Barker, M; Eastell, R. Phosphate supplementation in young men: lack of effect on calcium homeostasis and bone turnover. *Eur. J. Clin. Nutr.*, 1998, 52, 29-33.

[118] Grimm, M; Muller, A; Hein, G; Funfstuck, R; Jahreis, G. High phosphorus intake only slightly affects serum minerals, urinary pyridinium crosslinks and renal function in young women. *Eur. J. Clin. Nutr.*, 2001, 155, 153-161.

[119] Brixen, K; Nielsen, HK; Charles, P; Mosekilde, L. Effect of a short course of oral phosphate treatment on serum parathyroid hormone (I-84) and biochemical markers of bone turnover: a dose-response study. *Calcif Tissues Int.*, 1992, 51, 276-281.

[120] Calvo, MS; Heath H 3rd. Persistently elevated parathyroid hormone secretion and action in young women after four weeks of ingesting high phosphorus, low calcium diets. *J. Clin. Endocrinol. Metab.*, 1990, 70, 1334-1340.

[121] Mazarlegos-Ramos, E; Guerrero-Romero, F; Rodriguez-Moran, M; Lazcano-Burciaga, G; Paniagua, R; Amato, D. Consumption of soft drinks with phosphoric acid as a risk factor for the development of hypocalcemia in children: a case-control study. *J. Pediatr.*, 1995, 126, 940-942.

[122] Anderson, JJB; Sell, ML; Garner SC; Calvo, MS. Phosphorus. In: *Present Knowledge in Nutrition*. 8th Ed. BA Bowman and Russell RM (eds). ILSI Press, Washington DC, 2001.

[123] Heaney, RP; Rafferty, K. Carbonated beverages and urinary calcium excretion. *Am. J. Clin. Nutr.*, 2001, 74, 343-347.

[124] JECFA (Joint FAO/WHO Expert Committee on Food Additives) (1982). Toxicological evaluations of certain food additives. Twenty-sixth report of the joint FAO/WHO Expert Committee on Food Additives. WHO Food Additives Series No 17.

[125] Portale, AA; Halloran, BP; Mutphy, MM; Morris, RC. Oral intake of phosphorus can determine the serum concentration of 1,25-dihydroxyvitamin D by determining its production rate in humans. *J. Clin. Invest.*, 1986, 77, 7-12.

[126] Blumsohn, A. What have we learnt about the regulation of phosphate metabolism? *Curr. Opin. Nephrol. Hypertens,* 2004, 13, 397-401.

[127] FNB (Food and Nutrition Board). Dietary Reference Intakes for calcium, phosphorus, magnesium, vitamin D and fluoride. Institute of Medicine National Academy Press, Washington DC, 1997.

[128] Osorio, AV; Alon, US. The relationship between urinary calcium, sodium, and potassium excretion and the role of potassium in treating idiopathic hypercalciuria. *Pediatrics*, 1997, 100, 675-681.

[129] Lemann, J; Pleuss, JA; Gray, RW; Hoffmenn RG. Potassium administration reduces and potassium deprivation increases urinary calcium excretion in healthy adults. *Kidney Int.*, 1991, 39, 973-83.

[130] Gurhan, GC; Willett, WC; Rimm, EB; Stampfer, MJ. A prospective study of dietary calcium and other nutrients and the risk of symptomatic kidney stones. *N. Engl. J. Med.*, 1993, 328, 833-838.

[131] New, SA; Bolton-Smith, C; Crubb, DA; Reid, DM. Nutritional influences on bone mineral density: a cross-sectional study in premenopausal women. *Am. J. Clin. Nutr.*, 1997, 65, 183-189.

[132] New, SA; Robins, SP; Campbell, MK; Martin, JC; Garton, MK; Bolton-Smith, C; Grubb, DA; Lee, SJ; Reid, DM. Dietary influences on bone mass and bone metabolism: further evidence of a positive link between fruit and vegetable consumption and bone health. *Am. J. Clin. Nutr.*, 2000, 71, 142-151.

[133] Sebastian, A; Harris, ST; Ottaway, JH; Todd, KM; Morris, RC. Improved mineral balance and skeletal metabolism in postmenopausal women treated with potassium bicarbonate. *N. Engl. J. Med.*, 1994, 330, 1776-81.

[134] SACN (Scientific Advisory Committee on Nutrition). Salt and Health. London, The Stationery Office, 2003.

[135] FNB (Food and Nutrition Board) (2004). Dietary Reference Intakes for water, potassium, sodium, chloride and sulfate. Institute of Medicine. National Academy of Sciences. Food and Nutrition Board. Standing Committee on the Scientific Evaluation of Dietary Reference Intake, Institute of Medicine, Dietary Reference Intakes for Vitamin A, Vitamin K, Arsenic, Boron, Chromium, Copper, Iodine, Iron, Manganese, Molybdenum, Nickel, Silicon, Vanadium, and Zinc. Washington, D.C.: National Academy Press 2002.

[136] New, SA, Bonjour, J-P. Nutritional Aspects of Bone Health. London, The Royal Society of Chemists, 2003.

[137] Cashman, KD; Flynn A. Sodium effects on bone and calcium metabolism. In: New SA, Bonjour J-P. *Nutritional Aspects of Bone Health*. London, The Royal Society of Chemists, 2003, pp267-289.

[138] Harrington, M; Bennett, T; Jakobsen, J; Brot, C; Ovesen, L; Flynn, A; Cashman, K.D. The effect of a high-protein, high-salt diet on calcium and bone metabolism in

postmenopausal women and its interaction with vitamin D receptor genotype. *Br. J. Nutr.*, 2004, 91, 41-51.

[139] Seelig, MS. Cardiovascular consequences of magnesium deficiency and loss: pathogenesis, prevalence and manifestations - magnesium and chloride loss in refractory potassium repletion. *Am. J. Cardiol.*, 1989, 63, 46-216.

[140] Sabatier, M; Pont, F; Keyes, WR; Arnaud, M; Turnlund, JR. A kinetic model of magnesium metabolism in healthy men based on two stable isotope tracers. *Trace Elem. Man. Animal* 11, 2002, abstracts.

[141] Vormann, J; Forster, C; Zippel, U; Lozo, E; Gunther, T; Merker, H; Stahlmann, R. Effects of magnesium deficiency on magnesium and calcium content in bone and cartilage in developing rats in correlation to chondrotoxicity. *Calcif Tissue Int.*, 1997, 61, 230-238.

[142] Vormann, J; Anke, M. Dietary magnesium: supply, requirements and recommendations - results from duplicate and balance studies in man. *J. Clin. Basic Cardiol.*, 2002, 5, 49-53.

[143] Frassetto, LA; Morris, Jr. RC; Sebastian, A. Effect of age on blood acid-base composition in adult humans: role of age-related renal functional decline. *Am. J. Physiol.*, 1996; 271:F1114-F1122.

[144] Stendig-Lindberg, G; Tepper, R; Leichter, I. Trabecular bone density in a two year controlled trial of peroral magnesium in osteoporosis. *Magnes. Res.*, 1993, 6, 155-163.

[145] Dimai, HP; Porta, S; Wirnsberger, G; Lindschinger, M; Pamperl, I; Dobnig, H; Wilders-Truschnig, M; Lau, KH. Daily oral magnesium supplementation suppresses bone turnover in young adult males. *J. Clin. Endocrinol. Metab.*, 1998, 83, 2742-2748.

[146] Yoshizawa, T; Handa, Y; Uematsu, Y; Takeda, S; Sekine, K; Yoshihara, Y; Kawakami, T; Arioka, K; Sato, H; Uchiyama, Y; Masushige, S; Fukamizu, A; Matsumoto, T; Kato, S. Mice lacking the vitamin D receptor exhibit impaired bone formation, uterine hypoplasia and growth retardation after weaning. *Nat. Genet.*, 1997, 16, 391-396.

[147] Brown, AJ; Dusso, A; Slatopolsky, S. Vitamin D. Invited Review. *Am. J. Physiol.*, 1999, 277 (Renal Physiol 46), F157-175.

[148] Kveiborg, M; Mosekilde, L; Eriksen, EF; Kassem, MS. Calcitriols biologiske virkningsmekanismer og effekter. *Ugeskr Laeger*, 1999, 161, 5669-5674.

[149] Malabanan, A; Veronikis, IE; Holick, MF. Redefining vitamin D insufficiency. *Lancet*, 1998, 351, 805-806.

[150] Dawson-Hughes, B; Harris, SS; Dallal, GE. Plasma calcidiol, season, and serum parathyroid hormone concentrations in healthy elderly men and women. *Am. J. Clin. Nutr.*, 1997, 65:67-71.

[151] Ooms, ME; Roos, JC; Bezemer, PD; van der Vijgh, WJ; Bouter, LM; Lips, P. Prevention of bone loss by vitamin D supplementation in elderly women: A randomized double-blind trial. *J. Clin. Endocrinoal. Metab.*, 1995, 80, 1052-1058.

[152] Dawson-Hughes, B; Harris, SS; Krall, EA; Dallal, GE; Falconer, G; Green, CL. Rates of bone loss in postmenopausal women randomly assigned to one of two dosages of vitamin D. *Am. J. Clin. Nutr.*, 1995, 61, 1140-1145.

[153] Reid, IR; Gallagher, DJA; Bosworth, J. Prophylaxis against vitamin D deficiency in the elderly by regular sunlight exposure. *Age and Ageing*, 1986, 15, 35-40.

[154] Lips, P; Graafmans, WC; Ooms, ME; Bezemer, D; Bouter, LM. Vitamin D supplementation and fracture incidence in elderly persons - a randomized, placebo-controlled clinical trial. *Ann. Internal. Med.*, 1996; 124; 400-406.

[155] Heikinheimo, RJ; Inkovaara, JA; Harju, EJ; Haavisto, MV; Kaarela, RH; Kataja, JM; Kokko, AM-L; Kolho, LA; Rajala, S.A. Annual injection of vitamin D and fractures of aged bones. *Calcif Tissue Int.*, 1992; 51:105-110.

[156] Chapuy, MC; Arlot, ME; Delmans, PD; Meunier, PJ. Effect of calcium and cholecalciferol treatment for three years on hip fractures in elderly women. *BMJ*, 1994, 308, 1081-1082.

[157] Dawson-Hughes, B; Harris, SS; Krall, EA; Dallal, GE. Effect of calcium and vitamin D supplementation on bone, density in men and women 65 years of age or older. *NEJM*, 1997b, 337, 670-676.

[158] Komulainen, M; Tuppurainen, MT; Kroger, H; Heikkinen, AM; Alhava, PE; Honkanen, R; Saarikoski, S. Vitamin D and HRT - no benefit additional to that of HRT alone in prevention of bone loss in early postmenopausal women - a 2.5-year randomized placebo-controlled study. *Osteoporosis Int.*, 1997, 7, 126-132.

[159] Nordin, BEC; Horsman, A; Crilly, RG; Marshall, DH; Simpson, M.. Treatment of spinal osteoporosis in postmenopausal women. *BMJ*, 1980, 1, 451-454.

[160] Tsaioun, KI. Vitamin K-dependent proteins in the developing and aging nervous system. *Nutr. Rev.*, 1999, 57, 231-240.

[161] Iwamoto, J; Takeda, T; Sato, Y. Effects of vitamin K2 on osteoporosis. *Curr. Pharm. Des*, 2004, 10, 2557-2576.

[162] Shearer, MJ. The roles of vitamins D and K in bone health and osteoporosis prevention. *Proc. Nutr. Soc.*, 1997, 56, 915-937.

[163] Booth, SL; Skeletal functions of vitamin K-dependent proteins: not just for clotting anymore. *Nutr. Rev.*, 1997, 55, 282-284.

[164] Feskanich, D; Weber, P; Willett, WC; Rockett, H; Booth, SL; Colditz, GA. Vitamin K intake and hip fractures in women: a prospective study. *Am. J. Clin. Nutr.*, 1999, 69, 74-79.

[165] Booth, SL; Tucker, KL; Chen, H; Hannan, MT; Gagnon, DR; Cupples, LA; Wilson, PWF; Ordovas, J; Schaefer, EJ; Dawson-Hughes, B; Kiel, DP. Dietary vitamin K intakes are associated with hip fracture but not with bone mineral density in elderly men and women. *Am. J. Clin. Nutr.*, 2000, 71, 1201-1208.

[166] Braam, LAJL; Knapen, MH; Geusens, P; Brouns, F; Hamulyak, K; Gerichhausen, MJW; Vermeer, C. Vitamin K1 supplementation retards bone loss in postmenopausal women between 50 and 60 years of age. *Calcif Tissue Int.*, 2003, 73, 21-26.

[167] Koshihara, Y; Hoshi, K; Ishibashi, H; Shiraki, M. Vitamin K2 promotes 1α,25(OH)2 vitamin D3-induced mineralization in human periosteal osteoblasts. *Calcif Tissue Int.*, 1996, 59, 466-473.

[168] Yamaguchi, M; Taguchi, H; Gao, YH; Igarashi, A; Tsukamoto, Y. Effect of vitamin K2 (menaquinone-7) in fermented soybean (natto) on bone loss in ovariectomized rats. *J. Bone Miner Metab.*, 1999, 17, 23-29.

[169] Koshihara, Y; Hoshi, K; Okawara, R; Ishibashi, H; Yamamoto, S. Vitamin K stimulates osteoblastogenesis and inhibits osteoclastogenesis in human bone marrow cell culture. *J. Endocrinol.*, 2003, 176, 339-348.

[170] Hiruma, Y; Nakahama, K; Fujita, H; Morita, I. Vitamin K2 and geranylgeraniol, its side chain component, inhibited osteoclast formation in a different manner. *Biochem. Biophys. Res. Commun.*, 2004, 314, 24-30.

[171] Asakura, H; Myou, S; Ontachi, Y; Mizutani, T; Kato, M; Saito, M; Morishita, E; Yamazaki, M; Nakao, S. Vitamin K administration to elderly patients with osteoporosis induces no hemostatic activation, even in those with suspected vitamin K deficiency. *Osteoporosis Int.,* 2001, 12, 996-1000.

[172] Shiraki, M; Shiraki, Y; Aoki, C; Miura, M. Vitamin K2 (menatetrenone) effectively prevents fractures and sustains lumbar bone mineral density in osteoporosis. *J. Bone Miner Res.*, 2000, 15, 515-521.

[173] Akiyama, Y; Hara, K; Tajima, T; Murota, S; Morita, I. Effect of vitamin K2 (menatetrenone) on osteoclast-like cell formation in mouse bone marrow cultures. *Eur. J. Pharmacol.,* 1994, 263:181-185.

[174] Hara, K; Akiyama, Y; Tajima, T; Shiraki, M. Menatetrenone inhibits bone resorption partly through inhibition of PGE2 synthesis in vitro. *J. Bone Miner Res.*, 1993, 8, 535-542.

[175] Sato, Y; Kanoko, T; Satoh, K; Iwamoto, J. Menatetrenone and vitamin D2 with calcium supplements prevent nonvertebral fracture in elderly women with Alzheimer's disease. *Bone*, 2005, 36, 61-68.

[176] Tanaka, Y; Shibata, R. Effects of vitamin K2 administration in the patients with severely motor and intellectual disabilities: assessment of bone metabolic marker and bone mineral density. *No To Hattatsu*, 2000, 32, 491-496.

[177] Conly, J; Stein, K. Reduction of vitamin K2 concentrations in human liver associated with the use of broad spectrum antimicrobials. *Clin. Invest. Med.*, 1994, 17, 531-539.

[178] Ryan-Harshman, M; Aldoori, W. Bone health. New role for vitamin K? *Can. Fam. Physician*, 2004, 50, 993-997.

[179] Sokoll, LJ; Booth, SL; O'Brien, ME; Davidson, KW; Tsaioun, KI; Sadowski, JA. Changes in serum osteocalcin, plasma phylloquinone, and urinary gamma-carboxyglutamic acid in response to altered intakes of dietary phylloquinone in human subjects. *Am. J. Clin. Nutr.*, 1997, 65, 779-784.

[180] Vermeer, C; Shearer, MJ; Zittermann, A; Bolton-Smith, C; Szulc, P; Hodges, S; Walter, P; Rambeck, W; Stocklin, E; Weber, P. Beyond deficiency: potential benefits of increased intakes of vitamin K for bone and vascular health. *Eur. J. Nutr.*, 2004, 43, 325-335.

[181] Gaby, SK; Singh, VN. "Vitamin C," – Vitamin intake and health: A Scientific Review, Gaby, S.K., Bendich, A., Singh, V. and Machlin, L. (eds.). Marcel Dedder, N.Y., 1991.

[182] Grynpas, MD. Fluoride effects on bone crystals. *J. Bone Miner Res.*, 1990, Suppl. 1, S169-S175.

[183] Caverzasio, J; Imal, T; Ammann, P; Burgener, D; Bonjour J-P. Aluminium potentiates the effect of fluoride on tyrosine phosphorylation and osteoblast replication in vitro and bone mass in vivo. *J. Bone Miner Res.*, 1996, 11, 46-55.

[184] Riggs, BL. Treatment of osteoporosis with sodium fluoride or parathyroid hormone. *Am. J. Med.*, 1993, 95, 625-665.

[185] Nielsen F. H. Biochemical and physiologic consequences of boron deprivation in humans. *Environ. Health Perspect.* 1994; 102 (Suppl 7): 59-63.

[186] Nielsen, FH; Mullen, LM; Gallagher, SK. Effect of boron depletion and repletion on blood indicators of calcium status in humans fed a magnesium-low diet. *J. Trace Elem. Exp. Med.*, 1990, 3, 45-54.

[187] Nielsen F. H., Gallagher S. K., Johnson L. K., Nielsen E. J. Boron enhances and mimics some effects of estrogen therapy in postmenopausal women. *J. Trace Elem. Exp. Med.* 1992; 5: 237-246.

[188] Uauy, R; Olivares, M; Gonzalez, M. Essentiality of copper in humans. *Am. J. Clin. Nutr.*, 1998, 67, S952-S959.

[189] Jonas, J; Burns, J; Abel, EW; Cresswell, MJ; Strain, JJ; Paterson, CR. Impaired mechanical strength of bone in experimental copper deficiency. *Ann. Nutr. Metab.*, 1993, 37, 245-252.

[190] Eaton-Evans, J; Mcllrath, EM; Jackson, WE; McCartney, H; Strain, JJ. Copper supplementation and the maintenance of bone mineral density in middle-aged women. *J. Trace Elem. Exp. Med.*, 2003, 9, 87-94.

[191] Strause, L; Saltman, P; Smith, KT; Bracker, M; Andon, MB. Spinal bone loss in postmenopausal women supplemented with calcium and trace minerals. *J. Nutr.*, 1994, 124, 1060-1064.

[192] Rao, LG. Tomato lycopene and bone health: Preventing osteoporosis. In: Rao AV, editor, *Tomatoes, lycopene and human health.* Scotland: Caledonian Science Press; 2006. p. 153-68.

[193] Silverton, S. Osteoclast radicals. *J. Cell Biochem.*, 1994, 56(3), 367-373.

[194] Suda, N; Morita, I; Kuroda, T; Murota, S. Participation of oxidative stress in the process of osteoclast differentiation. *Biochim. Biophys. Acta*, 1993, 1157, 318-323.

[195] Liu, H-C; Cheng, R-M; Lin, F-H; Fang, H-W. Sintered beta-dicalcium phosphate particles induce intracellular reactive oxygen species in rat osteoblasts. *Biomed. Eng. Appl. Basis Commun.*, 1999, 11, 259-264.

[196] Key, LL; Ries, WL; Taylor RG; Hays, BD; Pitzer, BL. Oxygen derived free radicals in osteoclasts: the specificity and location of the nitroblue tetrazolium reaction. *Bone*, 1990, 11, 115-119.

[197] Hall, TJ; Schaeublin, M; Fuller, K; Chambers, TJ. The role of oxygen intermediates in osteoclastic bone resorption. *Biochem. Biophys. Res. Commun.*, 1995, 207, 280-287.

[198] Kim, L; Rao, AV; Rao, LG. Lycopene II - effect on osteoblasts: the carotenoid lycopene stimulates cell proliferation and alkaline phosphatase activity of SaOS-2 cells. *J. Med. Food*, 2003, 6(2), 79-86.

[199] Park, CK; Ishimi, Y; Ohmura, M; Yamaguchi, M; Ikegami, S. Vitamin A and carotenoids stimulate differentiation of mouse osteoblastic cells. *J. Nutr. Sci. Vitaminol.*, 1997, 43, 281-296.

[200] Rao, LG; Krishnadev, N; Banasikowska, K; Rao, AV. Lycopene I - Effect on osteoclasts: Lycopene inhibits basal and parathyroid hormone-stimulated osteoclast

formation and mineral resorption mediated by reactive oxygen species in rat bone marrow cultures. *J. Med. Food*, 2003, 6(2), 69-78.

[201] Ishimi, Y; Ohmura, M; Wang, X; Yamaguchi, M; Ikegami, S. Inhibition by carotenoids and retinoic acid of osteoclast-like cell formation induced by bone-resorbing agents in vitro. *J. Clin. Biochem. Nutr.*, 1999, 27, 113-122.

[202] Melhus, H; Michaelsson, K; Holmberg, L; Wolk, A; Ljunghall, S. Smoking, antioxidant vitamins, and the risk of hip fracture. *J. Bone Miner Res.*, 1999, 14, 129-135.

[203] Morton, DJ; Barrett-Connor, EL; Schneider, DL. Vitamin C supplement and bone mineral density in postmenopausal women. *J. Bone Miner Res.*, 2001, 16, 135-140.

[204] Singh, VN. A current perspective on nutrition and exercise. *J. Nutr.*, 1992, 122, 760-765.

[205] Leveille, SG; LaCroix, AZ; Koepsell, TD; Beresford, SA; VanBelle, G; Buchner, DM. Dietary vitamin C and bone mineral density in postmenopausal women in Washington State, USA. *J. Epidemiol. Community Health*, 1997, 51, 479-485.

[206] Maggio, D; Barabani, M; Pierandrei, M; Polidori, MC; Catani, M; Mecocci, P; Senin, U; Pacifici, R; Cherubini, A. Marked decrease in plasma antioxidants in aged osteoporotic women: results of a cross-sectional study. *J. Clin. Endocrinol. Metab.*, 2003, 88(4), 1523-1527.

[207] Rao, LG; Mackinnon, ES; Josse, RG; Murray, TM; Strauss, A; Rao, AV. Lycopene consumption decreases oxidative stress and bone resorption markers in postmenopausal women. *Osteoporosis Int.*, 2007, 18(1), 109-115.

In: Nutrition for the Middle Aged and Elderly
Editors: N. E. Bernhardt, A. M. Kasko, pp. 195-212
ISBN: 978-1-60456-146-3

Chapter V

The Impact of Transtheoretical Model-Based Multiple Behavior Interventions on Nutrition

Sara Johnson, Carol Cummins and Kerry Evers
Pro-Change Behavior Systems, Inc., West Kingston, RI, USA

Abstract

The Transtheoretical Model (TTM), an overview of which will be provided in this chapter, offers a promising intervention framework for nutrition interventions. Several recent applications of the TTM (e.g., Rossi et al., 2005; Prochaska et al., 2005; Prochaska et al., 2004; Campbell et al., 2004; Johnson et al., under review) have included interventions targeting multiple health behaviors such as healthy eating or fruit and vegetable consumption. These interventions will be reviewed, with particular emphasis on how the interventions are effective across the lifespan, including middle-aged and senior populations. Preliminary evidence supporting the notion that co-variation of behavior change can be produced by tailored interventions will be presented. Johnson et al. (under review), for example, reported that a tailored intervention for healthy eating that targeted calorie and fat intake in the context of a weight management intervention had significant effects on an untreated nutrition behavior (i.e., fruit and vegetable intake).

Advantages of multiple behavior approaches will be highlighted and alternative delivery channels for these interventions will be presented. The chapter will conclude with recommendations for maximizing the potential of multiple behavior change interventions that include nutrition targets.

Introduction

Because of the essential role dietary behaviors play in preventable diseases and premature death, Healthy People 2010 includes unhealthy diet as a key indicator of the health of the US (USDHHS, 2000). Despite the extensive public health messaging surrounding healthy eating, adults in the US are not adopting nutrition practices recommended by experts. Based on Behavioral Risk Factor Surveillance data from more than 150,000 participants in 2000, Reeves and Rafferty (2005) reported that only 23.3% of adults are consuming 5 fruits and vegetables per day. According to Healthy People 2010 reports, among individuals two years of age or older, fewer than 30% consumed at least two servings of fruit per day; 3% consumed at least three daily servings of vegetables; 36% consumed less than 10 percent of daily calories from saturated fat; and 33% consumed no more than 30 percent of daily calories from total fat (USDHHS, 2000). Americans also eat on average 300 more calories per day now than they did in 1985 (Putnam, Allshouse, and Kantor, 2002). Poor nutritional practices are likely contributing to the alarming obesity epidemic in the US: Wang and Beydoun (2007) recently estimated that the prevalence of overweight and obesity will increase to 75% by 2015. There is, therefore, an urgent need for effective and easily disseminable interventions to address healthy eating behaviors.

After conducting an extensive review of behavioral interventions intended to change nutrition behaviors, Ammerman et al. (2001) reported that, with regard to interventions designed to increase fruit and vegetable intake, studies utilizing a theoretical framework were more likely to report significant treatment effects than studies not employing a theory. A variety of theoretical frameworks have been employed to intervene upon nutrition behaviors among adults and seniors, including Social Cognitive Theory (e.g., Emmons et al., 2005; Toobert et al., 2007); the Transtheoretical Model (TTM) (e.g., Clark et al., 2005 Greene and Rossi, 1998); social support theory (e.g., Campbell et al., 2002); and social ecological theory (e.g., Toobert et al., 2007). According to Glanz, Rimer, and Lewis (2002), the TTM is one of the most dominant models of health behavior change. Clark et al. (2002) report that the TTM has provided the theoretical foundation for a number of effective health behavior change studies, including several addressing nutrition. In a recent meta-analysis regarding the effect of tailored print communications, Noar et al. (2007) reported that the constructs of the TTM (i.e., pros and cons, self-efficacy, stage of change, and processes of change, as outlined below) are the theoretical constructs most likely to produce behavior change. The inclusion of each of these TTM constructs produced higher effect sizes. Other constructs, such as perceived susceptibility, produced lower effect sizes, while social norms and behavioral intentions made no difference (Noar et al., 2007).

The Transtheoretical Model of Behavior Change

The TTM (Prochaska and DiClemente, 1983; Prochaska, Johnson, and Lee, 1998) is an integrative and comprehensive model of behavior change that incorporates process oriented variables to explain and predict how and when individuals change behaviors.

Stage of change is the central organizing construct of the TTM. As people make a behavior change, they progress through a series of five stages. Each stage represents an interval of time and a group of tasks that must be completed before progression to the next stage takes place (Prochaska and DiClemente, 1992). The length of time individuals spend in each stage is variable, but the tasks required are the same for most individuals (Prochaska and

DiClemente, 1992). *Precontemplation* is the stage in which individuals have no intention of taking action in the forseeable future, typically defined as the next six months. *Contemplation* is the stage in which individuals intend to take action in the next six months. This stage is characterized by ambivalence and doubt. In the *Preparation* stage, individuals intend to take action in the next 30 days and may have already taken some small behavioral steps toward Action (e.g., adding a serving of vegetables each day). Individuals in Preparation typically represent only a small proportion of the population. *Action* is the stage in which successful behavior change has been achieved for a period of less than six months. In the *Maintenance* stage, change has been maintained for more than six months (Prochaska et al., 1998). Rather than involving a linear movement through the stages, behavior change is cyclical. Most people relapse—or recycle—to previous stages several times before complete behavior change is achieved (Prochaska, DiClemente, and Norcross, 1992). Stage is a powerful predictor of behavior. Smokers in Preparation, for example, are twice as likely to be abstinent at one and six month post-treatment than Contemplation, who in turn are twice as likely as Precontemplation to be abstinent (Prochaska et al., 1993). An intervention that helps individuals progress one stage doubles their chances of taking action in the next six months (Prochaska et al., 1992).

Another central aspect of the TTM is an individual's decisional balance, or relative weighting of the pros and cons of making a health behavior change (Prochaska, et al., 1994; Velicer, Prochaska, DiClemente, and Brandenburg, 1985). The decisional balance measure, originally based on Janis and Mann's (1977) model of decision making, has been empirically reduced to two well-defined, orthogonal components: pros and cons (Velicer et al., 1985). Meta-analyses (Prochaska et al., 1994; Hall and Rossi, 2004; Hall, 2004) revealed a consistent pattern of the pros and cons across stages for 55 behaviors. The cons of changing outweighed the pros in the Precontemplation stage while the pros outweighed the cons in the Action stage (Prochaska, 1994). For all behaviors, the cross-over occurred prior to Action (Hall and Rossi, 2004; Hall 2004).

The processes of change represent both the covert and overt activities that individuals perform to make a behavior change (i.e., how a person changes). Each of the 10 common processes can be operationalized by a wide range of techniques and strategies (Prochaska, Velicer, DiClemente, and Fava, 1988; Prochaska and DiClemente, 1992). The processes are integrally related with stages of change (Prochaska et al., 1992). Research demonstrates that experiential—or cognitive, affective, and evaluative processes—are emphasized by individuals in the earlier stages (Prochaska et al., 1992; Hall and Rossi, 2005). Although prior research indicated that individuals in later stages rely more on the behavioral processes—social support, commitments, and behavior management techniques (Prochaska et al., 1988), Hall and Rossi (2005) report that the behavioral processes may be important in earlier stages as well.

Self-efficacy, another central construct of the TTM (Velicer, DiClemente, Rossi, and Prochaska, 1990), represents the degree to which an individual believes s/he has the ability to attain a goal. Self-efficacy is operationalized as confidence to make and sustain changes and temptation to relapse (Prochaska and DiClemente, 1992). Assessment of this dimension often involves asking individuals to rate how tempted they would be to engage in a problem behavior in a variety of situations and/or how confident they are that they could avoid engaging in a behavior in a variety of situations (Prochaska and DiClemente, 1986;1992a). Temptation and confidence scores are inversely related and highly correlated (-.60) and vary with stage of change. Individuals in Precontemplation report the most temptation, while those in later stages report decreasing levels. The converse occurs for confidence (DiClemente et al., 1991).

Importance of Tailoring

Tailoring is now recognized as a crucial strategy for delivering effective behavior change interventions (Skinner et al., 1999). Kreuter, Strecher, and Glassman (1999) define tailoring as delivering a combination of messaging and strategies about a particular outcome to a specific individual based on that individual's responses to an assessment. Dynamic tailoring is a similar term that can be defined as tailoring on multiple occasions to deliver unique feedback based on a new assessment on each occasion. In addition to providing a framework through which behavior change can be better understood, the TTM provides a guiding theoretical framework for tailoring interventions. After conducting a meta-analysis of 57 studies of tailored print communications, Noar et al. (2007) reported that interventions tailored on behavior only had the weakest effects (r=.026) among tailored communications. In comparison, interventions tailored on theoretical constructs and behavior had an effect of r=.092. From a usability perspective, Brug et al. (1998) reported that computer-tailored print reports were rated very favorably by participants: Tailored materials are more likely to have been read (Campbell et al., 1994; Brug, 1998; Skinner, Campbell, Rimer, Curry, and Prochaska 1999); remembered (Campbell et al., 1994; Skinner et al., 1999); discussed with others (Brug et al., 1998); and considered personally relevant, interesting, and credible (Brug et al., 1998; Skinner et al., 1999; Kreuter et al., 1999). Participants receiving computer-tailored letters reported that the letters were more likely to change their behavior and/or increase their intention to change (Brug et al., 1998; Skinner et al., 1999; Kreuter et al., 1999). Consistent with the Elaboration Likelihood Model (Petty and Cacioppo, 1986), greater interest, perceived personal relevance and individualization may account, in part, for the greater effect tailored materials appear to have on nutrition and other health behaviors as they may increase motivation for central route processing. In fact, in a recent study of the short-term effect of a web-based tailored nutrition intervention, Oenema, Tan, and Brug (2005) reported that perceived personal relevance, individualization, and interstingness were mediators of the tailoring effects on fat and vegetable intake. The authors hypothesized that tailoring on stage may contribute to the effects of tailoring by reducing resistance and reactance to the tailored materials.

The Application of the TTM to Tailored Nutrition Interventions

The effectiveness of TTM-based interventions on nutrition behaviors (e.g., reducing dietary fat, increasing fruit and vegetable intake) has been demonstrated in a number of studies in the past decade. Greene and Rossi (1998), for example, reported that a single TTM-based individually tailored report regarding dietary fat consumption could accelerate stage progression over 18 months relative to a control group. Brug, Glanz, Van Assema, Kok, and van Breukelen (1998) reported that computer tailored feedback reports that provided individualized feedback on the constructs of the TTM (i.e., intention to change, current behavior, attitudes, and self-efficacy) had more of an effect on dietary intake (i.e., decreasing fat reduction and increasing fruit and vegetable consumption) than general information letters about nutrition in a sample of 762 Dutch adults recruited via newspaper and radio ads (mean age = 44 years, SD = 14 years). Furthermore, an additional tailored report enhanced the effect. Individuals randomized to the group receiving two computer tailored reports scored significantly lower on fat intake at the final assessment than those receiving a single tailored report, who in turn had a significantly lower fat intake than those receiving general information. Participants randomized to computer tailored reports also had higher vegetable intakes than those receiving general information at the first follow-up, whereas at the second follow-up only those receiving two computer-tailored reports differed significantly on vegetable intake from those receiving general information. Across both post-tests, the group receiving two tailored reports significantly increased their fruit intake as compared to those receiving a single report or general information.

In a similar study, Campbell et al. (1994) delivered a single computer tailored report to the homes of patients randomized to receive tailored materials in a study of 558 adult primary care patients. The remainder of participants were randomized to groups receiving either a non-tailored report regarding diet of equivalent length and style or no nutrition information (control group). All participants then completed a 4-month follow-up survey. The tailored reports provided feedback on stage of change, as well as several other constructs of the TTM (e.g., motivators and barriers, self-efficacy). Participants receiving the reports were more likely than the control group to report a decrease in fat and saturated fat intake. There was, however, no treatment effect for fruit and vegetable intake.

In a study of nearly 2025 economically disadvantaged young adults recruited from community settings in ten states, Nitzke et al. (2007) reported that a combination of monthly stage-matched newsletters, two tailored reports addressing each of the constructs of the TTM, and two educational phone calls designed to reinforce the reports over a 6-month period had a significant effect on intake of fruit and vegetables, as well as on forward stage progression. At the 12-month follow-up, a significantly higher proportion of the treatment group was in Maintenance and a significantly lower proportion was in Precontemplation relative to the control group, despite the absence of baseline differences in the stage distributions of the two groups.

In summary, tailored interventions providing feedback on multiple constructs of the TTM have been demonstrated effective in facilitating stage progress and progression to Action and Maintenance for dietary fat and fruit and vegetable intake in adults recruited from community and primary care settings. It appears that additional tailored materials increased the effects on nutritional targets (e.g., Brug et al., 1998).

The Potential of Multiple Behavior Interventions

A promising recent innovation in health behavior change is multiple behavior interventions (Prochaska and Prochaska, in press). Interventions targeting more than one behavior are logical, particularly for adults who are likely to have more than one behavioral risk (Fine et al., 2004). In fact, Pronk and colleagues (2004) reported that only 10.8% of adults and 12.8% of seniors met public health guidelines for five healthy lifestyle behaviors (i.e., physical activity, healthy diet, non-smoking, healthy weight, and moderate alcohol consumption). Increasingly dismal estimates have been reported more recently: Some studies estimate that only 3% of American adults have four key lifestyle factors, including not smoking, consuming 5 fruits and vegetables per day, having a BMI between 18.5-25, and engaging in at least 30 minutes of physical activity at least 5 times a week (Reeves and Rafferty, 2005). The World Health Organization (WHO) has estimated that by 2015, world deaths from lifestyle diseases attributable to three major lifestyle factors will double unless major efforts are taken to change lifestyle behaviors, namely unhealthy diet, physical inactivity, and smoking (WHO, 2007).

Multiple behavior interventions also have the potential to be more efficient by creating synergy, as many of the processes and principles of behavior change apply to multiple behaviors (Atkins and Clancy, 2004; Prochaska and and Prochaska, in press). This hypothesis was supported by the findings of Hyman et al. (2007), who reported that individuals receiving simultaneous interventions for multiple risks fared better than participants receiving sequential interventions for individual behaviors. In addition to contributing to disease outcomes, having multiple risks contributes to decreased productivity (Burton et al., 2005), increased health care costs (Edington, 2001), and increased pharmaceutical claims (Burton et al., 2003). Because of the potential effects on multiple behavioral risks, multiple behavior interventions offer an increased likelihood of greater impact, improved quality of life, and reductions in health care utilization (Nigg, Allegrante, and Ory, 2002).

Innovators in the area of multiple behavior change have begun to examine the effects of interventions targeting several behavioral risks. Prochaska, Velicer, Prochaska, Delucchi, and Hall (2006), for example, compared the outcomes of smokers treated for a single behavior versus those treated for multiple behaviors (including high-fat diets) in three population-based trials involving more than 2300 smokers. The outcomes for smoking cessation were comparable to previous population-based trials for single behaviors. Equally important, the interventions for other behaviors were effective. The stability of 24-month point prevalence cessation rates at approximately 25% indicates that treating up to three risk factors does not decrease the effectiveness of tailored interventions on treating any of the single behaviors, underscoring the promise of multiple behavior interventions.

Multiple Behavior Interventions Including Nutrition Targets

Many multiple behavior interventions that include nutrition have been successful to date. In one study of over 5400 primary care patients randomized to receive either usual care or three individualized, dynamically tailored feedback reports based on the TTM over a 12-month period, significant treatment effects were found for four behaviors related to cancer prevention or detection (Prochaska et al., 2005). Generalized Estimating Equations (GEE) revealed that 28.8% of those assigned to fully dynamically tailored TTM-based interventions for reducing dietary fat progressed to Action or Maintenance at 24 months as compared to 19.8% of the comparison group. Approximately 25% of smokers assigned to the treatment group progressed to Action or Maintenance for smoking cessation versus 18.5% of the usual care comparison group. A significantly greater proportion of the treatment group also reached Action or Maintenance for sun protection (23.4% versus 12.5%). Finally, a significantly higher proportion of those in the treatment group remained in Action or Maintenance for mammography at 24 months (93.8% versus 89.7%). These significant treatment effects at long-term follow-up are particularly compelling because the treatment protocol included tailored interventions for 12 months. These differences therefore represent the treatment effects at one year post-treatment. Furthermore, the recruitment rate for the study, which included those at risk (i.e., in a pre-action stage) for at least one of the risk behaviors, was nearly 70%, indicating that this is not a highly select sample. This study clearly demonstrates that TTM-based stage-matched interventions for multiple behaviors have a significant effect on multiple risks, including dietary fat reduction on a population basis.

Similar results were obtained in a randomized effectiveness trial of dynamically tailored interventions for three behaviors (i.e., dietary fat reduction, smoking cessation, and sun protection) in a population of 2460 parents of adolescents (Prochaska et al., 2004). The large sample is the result of a recruitment rate of 84%, indicating a highly representative sample of this population. Treatment consisted of three series of tailored reports that addressed each of the TTM constructs for each of the behaviors for which an individual was at risk mailed over a 12-month period (0, 6, and 12 months). Among those in a pre-action stage for dietary fat reduction at baseline, significantly more of those assigned to the treatment group (34%) reached Action or Maintenance at 24 months versus 26% of those assigned to usual care. GEE also indicated that the treatment had significant effects on smoking cessation rates and sun protection with 22% versus 16% and 30 % versus 18% progressing to Action or Maintenance at 24 months, respectively.

A more recent effectiveness trial (i.e., Johnson et al., in press) further underscores the population impact of tailored multiple behavior interventions delivered to participants' homes. Twelve hundred seventy-seven overweight or moderately obese adults (BMI 25-39.9) were recruited nationally, primarily from large employers. Those randomly assigned to the treatment group received a stage-matched multiple behavior change guide and a series of dynamically tailored, individualized interventions for three health behaviors that are crucial to effective weight management: healthy eating (i.e., reducing calorie and dietary fat intake), moderate exercise, and managing emotional distress without eating. Up to three tailored reports (one per behavior) were delivered based on assessments conducted at four time points: baseline, 3, 6, and 9 months. All participants were followed up at 6, 12, and 24 months. GEE indicated that at 24 months, those who were in a pre-Action stage for healthy eating at baseline and received treatment were significantly more likely to have reached Action or Maintenance than the comparison group (47.5% vs. 34.3%). Individuals in the treatment group who were in a pre-Action stage for exercise at baseline were also significantly more likely to reach Action or Maintenance (44.9% versus 38.1%). The treatment also had a significant effect on managing emotional distress without eating, with 49.7% of those in a pre-Action stage at baseline moving to Action or Maintenance versus 30.3% of the comparison group. The intervention also impacted a related, but untreated behavior: fruit and vegetable consumption. Over 48% of those in the treatment group in a pre-Action stage at baseline progressed to Action or Maintenance for eating at least 5 servings a day of fruit and vegetables as opposed to 39% of the comparison group. The groups differed on weight lost at 24 months with the treatment group losing significantly more than the comparison group. Among those in a pre-Action stage for both healthy eating and exercise at baseline, 30.0% of those randomized to the treatment group lost 5% or more of their body weight versus 18.6% in the comparison group. Co-variation of behavior change occurred and was much more pronounced in the treatment group. Within the treatment group, individuals progressing to Action/Maintenance for a single behavior were 2.5-5 times more likely to make progress on another behavior. This study demonstrates the ability of TTM-based tailored feedback to improve healthy eating, exercise, managing emotional distress, and weight on a population basis. Furthermore, the results highlight the potential for multiple behavior interventions to leverage synergy of health behavior change. The treatment also produced the highest population impact to date on multiple health risk behaviors: The impact of the intervention was more than three times that of typical single behavior interventions (Johnson et al., under review).

Multiple behavior TTM-based weight management interventions have also been disseminated in group-based clinic settings (Riebe et al., 2003). One hundred and forty-four primarily middle-aged overweight or moderately obese participants received a multi-disciplinary, multiple behavior intervention targeting lifestyle changes related to physical activity and nutrition. In addition to structured, supervised hour long bi-weekly exercise sessions (during which actual exercise time was gradually increased from 15-45 minutes), participants participated in an hour long bi-weekly behavior change group that focused on the processes and principles of change (i.e., the TTM). Participants also submitted weekly food diaries that were reviewed by a registered dietitian. After the first three months of the program, participants attended a three month tapering phase, beginning with four weekly hourly meetings. The subsequent eight weeks included meetings every other week. During the course of the program, participants also received three individualized, dynamically tailored expert system reports for both exercise and dietary fat reduction. Depending on randomization, participants also received one of two additional mailings at 9 and 12 months: action-oriented materials or dynamically tailored expert system reports. At the final 24-month follow-up, data were available from 104 participants. Though the effects of the intervention diminished over time, the intervention had significant effects on weight, BMI, percent body fat, calorie and saturated fat intake, and self-reported exercise. There were, however, no differences on percent of calories from fat, and fruit and vegetable intake had declined from baseline. Receiving additional tailored reports versus action-oriented materials did not have a differential effect on Maintenance, which is likely due to the fact that the majority of participants were in Action or Maintenance at the end of the 6-month program. In addition to effects on weight and important behavioral outcomes, the intervention also had a positive effect on several factors on health related quality of life (HRQOL) as measured by the SF-36. Improvements in HRQOL were independent of maintaining a clinically significant (i.e., more than 5%) weight loss (Blissmer et al., 2006).

Kim et al. (2006) delivered multiple behavior weight management group-based interventions in churches in a rural African-American community. The 8-week faith-based program, which was delivered by lay people in the community who completed a 10-hour training, was theory-based, drawing heavily upon the TTM, social support models, and social cognitive theory. Group meetings included self-assessment of stage of change, as well as discussions about how to overcome cons of changing and how to seek social support. Participants in intervention churches lost a mean of 3.0 pounds more than the control group and had larger reductions in hip and waist circumference. The treatment effect remained significant after controlling for baseline body mass index (BMI), education, and age. Other studies have also underscored the potential for theoretically-based, tailored multiple behavior interventions to be effectively disseminated in church settings. Campbell et al. (2004) developed and examined the effectiveness of a multiple behavior intervention for colorectal cancer prevention that addressed fruit and vegetable intake, physical activity, and colon cancer screening in a sample of 587 members of 12 rural African American churches (mean age=52 years). Participants were randomly assigned to receive 1) a series of four dynamically tailored newsletters intervening on stage of change, barriers, motivators, knowledge, social support, and other psychosocial variables and four targeted videos; 2) interventions from lay health advisors who operated within the social networks of the church community; 3) both tailored materials and lay health advisors; or 4) generic health education sessions on unrelated topics. The tailored materials had a significant effect on fruit and vegetable consumption (0.6 servings per day increase), recreational physical activity, and colon cancer screening rates. The addition of the lay health advisors did not significantly affect the outcome behaviors measured, alone or in combination with the tailored materials.

Trials of multiple behavior interventions have also been conducted at worksites. Campbell et al. (2002), for example, examined the effectiveness of a multiple behavior change intervention for fruit and vegetable intake, physical activity, smoking cessation, and cancer screening over an 18-month period. The intervention, which was delivered to 859 rural female blue collar workers in nine worksites, included a combination of trained natural helpers and individually computer-tailored women's magazines that addressed stage of change, barriers, and social support, as well as other psychosocial variables. Control participants received a single tailored magazine after the first 6 months of the study. A total of 538 women completed all three timepoints (baseline, 6 month, and 18 month). Among those randomized to treatment, there was a significant increase in fruit and vegetable intake (0.7 servings) at 18 months relative to controls. There was a significant difference on fat intake at 6 months, but the difference between groups did not remain significantly different at 18 months. The intervention group demonstrated significant increases in strength and flexibility exercise at 6 months. Differences on flexibility remained significant at 18 months. There was no significant treatment effect on rates of smoking or cancer screening.

The efficacy of TTM-based multiple behavior change interventions (i.e., fruit and vegetable intake and physical activity) on seniors has also been examined (Clark et al., 2005). The Study of Exercise and Nutrition in Older Rhode Islanders (SENIOR) was conducted with a sample of 1277 seniors in an urban, culturally diverse community in Northern Rhode Island. The 12-month intervention consisted of dynamically tailored reports mailed to participants' homes once every four months, a stage-based manual for each behavior, stage-matched newsletters, and three coaching calls that relied on motivational interviewing to deliver stage appropriate messages (Clark et al., 2002; Clark et al., 2005). At the 24-month follow-up, those randomly assigned to the treatment group reported a significant increase in number of servings of fruit and vegetables despite the absence of difference in proportion progressing to Action or Maintenance (Rossi et al., 2005). In fact, those assigned to the treatment group increased their consumption by 1/2-1 servings per day (Greene et al., in press). Greene et al. (in press) reported that there was no effect of age, gender, income, or marital status on stage progression for fruit and vegetable intake. This is an important finding given that 25% of the sample was over 80 years old. Significantly more of the treatment group progressed to Action/Maintenance for physical activity (44% versus 26%) (Rossi et al., 2005).

Multiple behavior interventions for disease management based on the TTM have also been successful. Jones et al. (2003) examined the effectiveness of a multiple behavior diabetes self-management intervention that targeted self-monitoring of blood glucose (SMBG), healthy eating, and smoking cessation in a sample of 1029 individuals with diabetes. Participants randomized to the treatment group received dynamically tailored, TTM-based expert system reports once per quarter, newsletters, and telephone coaching calls over the course of 12 months. At the end of the study, 30.5% of those randomized to the treatment group progressed to Action or Maintenance for SMBG as compared to only 18.4% of the usual care group. Similarly, 32.5% versus 25.8% of those receiving tailored treatment materials progressed to Action or Maintenance for healthy eating. Those receiving the healthy eating intervention significantly decreased fat intake and increased servings of fruit and vegetables. The smoking cessation intervention was also effective, with 23.3% versus 11.6% of the treatment group reaching Action or Maintenance. Furthermore, sub-group analyses indicated that among participants progressing to Action for both SMBG and healthy eating, there were significant reductions in glycosolated hemoglobin. Thus, multiple behavior change interventions can have important implications for physiologic outcomes as well as behavioral outcomes.

Other studies have examined the potential impact of optimal tailoring. Optimal tailoring in this case means providing dynamically tailored feedback on all of the constucts of the TTM for one behavior and providing brief feedback on a limited set of TTM constructs (e.g., stage and decisional balance) for the remaining target behaviors. Johnson et al. (2005) examined the effectiveness of a population-based, individualized TTM-based expert system intervention to improve adherence and increase exercise and diet in a randomized 18-month trial involving 404 adults who had received a prescription for a lipid-lowering drug. Individuals randomized to the treatment group received a fully tailored report for medication adherence that addressed each of the TTM constructs. The report also provided feedback on stage of change for diet and physical activity, two behaviors essential for the management of hypercholesterolemia. The stage-matched manual for adherence also included one example per stage of how the processes and principles of behavior change could be applied to these other important lifestyle behaviors. More than half of the intervention group (56%) who were previously in a pre-Action stage for adherence were adhering to their prescribed medication regimen at the 18-month follow-up. Additionally, a vast majority (85%) of those in the intervention group who were in Action or Maintenance at baseline remained in Action or Maintenance at 18 months as opposed to 55.6% of the usual care group. Those receiving treatment were significantly more likely to progress to Action or Maintenance for exercise 43.3% versus 24.7%) and dietary fat reduction (24.7% versus 12.5% for diet) at 24 months. The results for dietary fat and exercise suggest co-variation of treatment effects, indicating that when paired with fully tailored interventions, minimal stage-matched interventions have the potential to have significant impacts on behavior change.

Future Opportunities and Directions for Multiple Behavior Interventions

The field of multiple behavior change research is in its infancy. While it is clear that we must avail ourselves of this innovative intervention approach, many questions remain about how to maximize its effectiveness. One such question is how many contacts are optimal. Taken together, the findings above suggest that multiple, dynamically tailored contacts may be superior to single tailored communications. Glodstein et al. (2004) underscored the need for multiple follow-up contacts for successful multiple behavior change interventions, emphasizing that assessments were crucial to tailor to patients' needs. Noar et al. (2007) also emphasized that interventions offering multiple contacts in which messages are dynamically tailored over time are more effective.

Another question is whether tailored TTM-based multiple-behavior interventions can be as effective in vulnerable populations. Evidence available to date indicates that there is a high probability that they will be. In a review of five population-based smoking cessation studies, Velicer, Redding, Sun, and Prochaska (2007) reported that there were no significant differences in the effectiveness of tailored interventions across gender, race, and ethnic subgroups. Although that type of programmatic research is not yet available for tailored nutrition interventions, the recent meta-analysis conducted by Noar et al. (2007) also indicated that the effect sizes of tailored interventions were generally unrelated to participant characteristics (e.g., race, education level), suggesting that tailored communication are indeed a promising approach in low-income groups. As is reported above, Nitzke et al. (2007) demonstrated that a TTM-based fruit and vegetable intervention was effective in a racially diverse sample reporting limited income (60% of their sample earned less than $800/month). Future larger studies including socioeconomically disadvantaged participants are needed, however.

Additional questions relate to the relative effectiveness of various delivery channels. Many of the interventions reviewed above were provided via print. Increasingly, Inter- and intra-nets are being explored as alternative, potentially more cost-effective delivery channels. Glasgow, Bull, Piette, and Steiner (2004) report that interactive behavior change technologies are a promising approach to multiple behavior change interventions. Oenema, Brug, and Lechner (2001) reported that participants exposed to a single session of a tailored web-based intervention provided ratings similar to those seen when tailored print communications are compared to non-tailored materials: Specifically, participants perceived the tailored web-based intervention as more personally relevant, novel, and specifically designed for them. This tailored intervention also had an impact on intention to eat less fat and more fruit and vegetables (Oenema et al., 2001). It is not yet clear, however, if tailored interventions delivered electronically will have equivalent effectiveness. Oenema et al. (2005), for example, reported that they did not observe effects of the same magnitude of tailoring on fat intake as they had in studies of print-based tailored materials. Issues with recruitment and retention may also pose problems for evaluation. In a recent study of the effectiveness of a web-based weight management program, Rothbert et al. (2006) reported retention rates of only 20% at the 6 month follow-up. Web-based multiple behavior change programs will likely require innovative recruitment and retention techniques. Systematic research on the effectiveness of such techniques is needed.

The practical limitations of multiple behavior change interventions also need to be explored. Given the response burden of the assessments for each behavior, it is not clear how many behaviors can be realistically intervened upon. Prochaska et al. (2005) and Johnson et al. (under review) demonstrated that up to three-four behaviors can be effectively treated simultaneously. The weight management intervention (Johnson et al., under review), which intervened on three behaviors including healthy eating (i.e., calorie and dietary fat reduction), also had a significant effect on fruit and vegetable consumption. This is an important finding that highlights the potential synergy of multiple behavior change interventions because fruit and vegetable intake was not a target behavior. Individuals received no specific tailored feedback on it. The differential co-variation in the treatment group reported by Johnson et al. (under review) coupled with the findings from Johnson et al. (2006) suggest that optimally tailored interventions may be a promising, and potentially more cost-effective approach for multiple behavior change interventions.

Measurement of the outcomes of multiple behavior change interventions also presents some challenges. In addition to measuring the effect of the intervention on each of the targeted behaviors and related behaviors, it will be important to include global measures that can be used for comparison across studies (Prochaska and Prochaska, in press). Measures of Health Related Quality of Life, for example, could be an important common metric (e.g., Blissmer et al., 2006). If properly quantified, the impact of multiple behavior change interventions could also serve as a benchmark. In single behavior interventions, impact is the product of participation rates multiplied by the effectiveness of the intervention. In multiple behavior interventions, measures for assessing impact must take into account the number of behaviors treated effectively and the participation rates in each of those behavioral interventions (Prochaska and Prochaska, in press). The following impact equation (Prochaska and Prochaska, in press) can be employed: $I = \Sigma_{\text{\# of behaviors(n)}} (E_n \text{ x } P_n)$, where E is the efficacy for each behavior and P is the proportion of at risk individuals participating in the intervention for each behavior.

Finally, more studies with longer follow-up are needed to demonstrate sustained effects of multiple behavior change interventions (Ammerman et al., 2001). Riebe et al. (2005) reported that the effects of the clinic-based intervention declined slightly during the follow-up period. This finding differs from that of Johnson et al. (under review), who reported increasing treatment effects of a home-based intervention through the 24-month follow-up timepoint on behavioral and weight outcomes. Multiple behavior change interventions also need to include strategies to sustain maintenance of health behavior change (Ammerman et al., 2001). Historically, individuals in Maintenance were considered not at risk for relapse, but Johnson et al. (2007) report that among individuals in Maintenance at baseline for health eating, only 58.9% remained in Maintenance at 24 months. Dynamically tailored TTM-based interventions that address each participant's particular risk factors for relapse have the potential to increase long-term maintenance of behavior change. Therefore, the effectiveness of such enhanced interventions for individuals in Maintenance needs to be systemically evaluated.

Conclusion

Based on the literature summarized in this chapter, it is evident that TTM-based, tailored, multiple behavior change interventions which include nutrition targets are effective across a variety of dissemination channels with adults and seniors. TTM-based tailored interventions appear to be effective with adults from the community, primary care patients, adults with chronic health conditions, and adults recruited into clinic-based weight management programs. Additional research is needed to determine the optimal dissemination techniques and channels, as well as to provide guidance on how these interventions can be delivered most cost-effectively.

References

Ammerman, A., Lindquist, C., Hersey, J., Jackman, A., Gavin, N., Garces, C., Lohr, K., Cary, T., and Whitener, B.L. (2001). *The Efficacy of Interventions to Modify Dietary Behavior Related to Cancer Risk.* AHRQ Publication Number 01-E029: AHRQ.

Atkins, D. and Clancy, C. (2004). Multiple behavior interventions: Are we up to the challenge? *American Journal of Preventive Medicine*, *27(2S)*, 102-103.

Blissmer, B., Riebe, D., Dye, G., Ruggiero, L., Greene, G., and Caldwell, M. (2006). Health-related quality of life following a clinical weight loss intervention among overweight and obese adults: Intervention and 24 month follow-up effects. *Health and Quality of Life Outcomes*, *4*, 43-51.

Brug, Glanz, Van Assema, Kok, G., Van Breukelen, G.J. (1998). The impact of computer-tailored feedback and iterative feedback on fat, fruit, and vegetable intake. *Health Education and Behavior*, *25(4)*, 517-531.

Burton, W., Chen, C., Conti, D., Schultz, A., and Edington, D. (2003). Measuring the relationship between employees' health risk factors and corporate pharmaceutical expenditures. *Journal of Occupational and Environmental Medicine*, *45(8)*, 793-802.

Burton, W., Chen, C., Conti, D., Schultz, A., Pransky, G., and Edington, D. (2005). The association of health risk factors with on-the-job productivity. *Journal of Occupational and Environmental Medicine*, *47*, 769-777.

Campbell, M., DeVellis, B., Strecher, V., Ammerman, A., DeVellis, R., and Sandler, R. (1994). Improving dietary behavior: The effectiveness of tailored messages in primary care settings. *American Journal of Public Health*, *84(5)*,783-7.

Campbell, M.K., James, A., Hudson, M.A., Carr, C., Jackson, E., Oates, V., Demissie, S., Farrell, D. and Tessaro, I. (2004). Improving multiple behaviors for colorectal cancer prevention among African American church members. *Health Psychology*, *23(5)*, 492-502.

Campbell, M.K., Tessaro, I., DeVellis, B., Benedict, S., Kelsey, K., Belton, L., and Sanhueza, A. (2002). Effects of a tailored health promotion program for female blue collar workers: Health works for women. *Preventive Medicine*, *34*, 313-323.

Clark, P., Nigg, C., Greene, G., Riebe, D., Saunders, S., et al. (2002). The study of exercise and nutrition in older Rhode Islanders (SENIOR): Translating theory into research. *Health Education Research*, *17(5)*, 552-561.

Clark, P., Rossi, J.S., Greaney, M., Riebe, D., Greene, G., Saunders, S., Lees, F., Nigg, C. (2005). Intervening on Exercise and Nutrition in Older Adults: The Rhode Island Senior Project. *Journal of Aging and Health*, *17*, 753.

DiClemente, C., Prochaska, J., Fairhurst, S., et al. (1991). The process of smoking cessation: An analysis of precontemplation, contemplation, and preparation stages of change. *Journal of Consulting and Clinical Psychology*, *59(2)*, 295-304.

Edington, D.W. (2001). Emerging research: A view from one research center. *American Journal of Health Promotion*, *15(5)*, 341-349.

Emmons, K.M., McBride, C.N., Puleo, E., Pollak, K., Clipp, E., Kuntz, K., Marcus, B.H., Napolitano, M., Onken, J., Farraye, F., and Fletcher, R. (2005). Project PREVENT: A randomized trial to reduce multiple behavioral risk factors for colon cancer. *Cancer Epidemiologic Biomarkers Prevention, 14(6)*, 1453-1459.

Fine, L.J., Philogene, G., Gramling, R., Coups, E.J., and Sinha, S.. (2004). Prevalence of multiple chronic disease risks factors: 2001 National Health Interview Survey. *American Journal of Preventive Medicine*, *27(2)*, 18-24.

Glanz, K, Rimer, B., Lewis, F.M. (2002). Theory, Research, and Practice in Health Behavior and Health Education. In K. Glanz, B. Rimer, and M.L. Lewis (Eds.*) Health Behavior and Health Education: Theory, Research, and Practice*, Third Edition, pp 22-40. Jossey-Bass: San Francisco.

Glasgow, R.E., Bull, S., Piette, J., and Steiner, J.F. (2004). Interactive behavior change technology: A partial solution to the competing demands of primary care. *American Journal of Preventive Medicine, 27(2S),* 80-87.

Goldstein, M.G., Whitlock, E.P., DePue, J. (2004). Multiple behavioral risk factor interventions in primary care: Summary of research evidence. *American Journal of Preventive Medicine*, *27(2 Suppl)*, 61-79.

Greene, G. W., Fey-Yensan, N., Padula, C., Rossi, S. R., Rossi, J. S., Clark, P. (in press) Change in Fruit and Vegetable Intake over 24 Months in Older Adults: Results of the SENIOR Project Intervention. *The Gerontologist.*

Greene, G.W. and Rossi, S.R. (1998). Stages of change for reducing dietary fat intake over 18 months. *Journal of the American Dietetic Association*, *98*, 529-534.

Hall, K. (2004). A Meta-Analytic Examination of Decisional Balance Across Stage Transitions: A Cross-Sectional Analysis and Longitudinal Cross-Validation. Unpublished doctoral dissertation. University of Rhode Island.

Hall, K.L., and Rossi, J.S. (2004). Examining the Transtheoretical Model using meta-analytic procedures and integrative analyses. In S. Keller and W.F. Velicer (Eds.), Research on the Transtheoretical Model: Where are we now, where are we going? (pp. 56-58). Lengerich, Germany: Pabst Science Publishers.

Hall, K. and Rossi, J.S. (2005). A meta-analysis of the processes of change across 20 health behaviors: Testing theory and informing interventions. *Annals of Behavioral Medicine*, *29*, S162.

Hyman, D.J., Pavlik, V., Taylor, W.C., Goodrick, G.K., and Moye, L. (2007). Simultaneous vs. sequential counseling for multiple behavior change. *Archives of Internal Medicine*, *167*, 1152-1158.

Janis, I.L. and Mann, L. (1977). *Decision Making: A psychological analysis of conflict, choice, and commitment.* New York: Free Press.

Johnson, S.S., Driskell, MM., Johnson, J.L, Dyment, S., Prochaska, J.O., Prochaska, J.M., Bourne, l. (2006). Transtheoretical model intervention for adherence to lipid-lowering drugs. *Disease Management*, *9(2)*, 102-114.

Johnson, S.S, Paiva, A.L. Cummins, C., Johnson, J.L. Dyment, S., Wright, J.A., Prochaska, J.O., Prochaska, JM., Sherman, K. (2007, September). *Effectiveness and Dissemination of Transtheoretical Model-based Individualized Weight Management Interventions.* Paper presented at the 8th Annual Disease Management Leadership Forum. Las Vegas.

Johnson, S.S, Paiva, A.L. Cummins, C., Johnson, J.L. Dyment, S., Wright, J.A., Prochaska, J.O., Prochaska, JM., Sherman, K. (under review). Evidence-based Multiple Behavior Intervention for Weight Management: Effectiveness on a Population Basis. *Preventive Medicine*.

Jones, H., Edwards, L., Ruggiero, L., Rossi, S., Rossi, J., Greene, G., Prochaska, J., and Zinman, B. (2003). Changes in diabetes self-care behaviors make a difference in glycemic control. *Diabetes Care*, *26*, 732-737.

Kim, K.H., Linnan, L., Campbell, M., Brooks, C., Koenig, H., and Wiesen, C. (2006). The WORD (Wholeness, Oneness, Righteousness, and Deliverance): A faith-based weight loss program utilizing a community-based participatory research approach. *Health Education and Behavior*, 1-17.

Kreuter, M.W., Strecher,V., Glassman, B. (1999). One size does not fit all: The case for tailoring print materials. *Annals of Behavioral Medicine, 21(4)*, 276-283.

Nigg, C., Allegrante, J. and Ory, M. (2002). Theory comparison and multiple behavior research: Common themes advancing health behavior research. *Health Education Research*, *17(5)*, 670-679.

Nitze, S., Kritsch, K., Boeckner, L., Greene, G., Hoerr, S., Horacek, T., Kattelmann, K., Lohse, B., Oakland, M.J., Phillips, B., and White, A. (2007). A stage-tailored multi-modal intervention increases fruit and vegetable intakes of low-income young adults. *American Journal of Public Health, 21(4)*, 1-9.

Noar, S., Benac, C. N., Harris, M.S. (2007). Does tailoring matter? Meta-analytic review of tailored print health behavior change interventions. *Psychological Bulletin, 133(4),* 673-693.

Oenema, A., Brug, J. and Lechner, L. (2001). Web-based tailored nutrition education: Results of a randomized controlled trial. *Health Education Research, 16(6)*, 647-660.

Oenema, A., Tan, F., and Brug, J. (2005). Short-term efficacy of a web-based computer-tailored intervention: Main effects and mediators. *Annals of Behavior Medicine, 29(1)*, 54-63.

Petty, R.E., Cacioppo, J.T., (1986). Communication and Persuasion: Central and Peripheral Routes to Attitude Change. New York: Springer.

Prochaska, J.J. and Prochaska, J.M. (in press). Multiple risk behavior change: What most individuals need. Handbook of Health Behavior Change, Third Edition. Springer Publishing.

Prochaska, J.J., Velicer, W.F., Prochaska, J.O., Delucchi, K., and Hall, S. (2006). Comparing intervention outcomes in smokers treated for single versus multiple behavioral risks. *Health Psychology, 25(3)*, 380-388.

Prochaska, J.O. (1994). Strong and weak principles for progressing from precontemplation to action on the basis of twelve problem behaviors. *Health Psychology*, 13(1), 1-5.

Prochaska, J.O. and DiClemente, C.C. (1983). Stages and processes of self-change of smoking: Toward an integrative model of change. *Journal of Consulting and Clinical Psychology, 51*, 390-395.

Prochaska, J.O. and DiClemente, C.C. (1986). Toward a comprehensive model of change. In W.R. Miller and N. Heather (Eds.), *Treating Addictive Behaviors* (pp. 4-27). New York: Plenum Publishing.

Prochaska, J.O. and DiClemente, C.C. (1992). Stages of change in the modification of problem behaviors. In M. Herson, R. Eisler, and P. Miller (Eds.), *Progress in Behavior Modification* (pp. 3-60). Sycamore, IL: Sycamore.

Prochaska, J.O., DiClemente, C.C., and Norcross, J.C. (1992). In search of how people change: Applications to addictive behaviors. *American Psychologist, 47(9)*, 1102-1114.

Prochaska, J.O., DiClemente, et al. (1993). Standardized, individualized, interactive, and personalized self-help programs for smoking cessation. *Health Psychology, 12(5)*, 399-405.

Prochaska, J.O., Johnson, S.S., and Lee, P. (1998). The Transtheoretical Model of Behavior Change. In S.A. Shumaker, E.B. Schron, J.K. Ockene, W.L. McBee (Eds.) *The Handbook of Health Behavior Change, 2nd Edition* (pp. 59-87). New York: Springer Publishing.

Prochaska, J.O., Velicer, W.F., DiClemente, C.C., and Fava, J. (1988). Measuring processes of change: Applications to the cessation of smoking. *Journal of Consulting and Clinical Psychology, 56(4)*, 520-528.

Prochaska, J.O., Velicer, W.F., Redding, C., Rossi, J.S., et al. (2005). Stage-based expert systems to guide a population of primary care patients to quit smoking, eat healthier, prevent skin cancer, and receive regular mammograms. *Preventive Medicine*, *41*, 406-416.

Prochaska, J.O., Velicer, W.F., Rossi, J.S., Goldstein, M.G., et al., (1994). Stages of change and decisional balance for 12 problem behaviors. *Health Psychology*, *13(1)*, 39-46.

Prochaska, J.O., Velicer, W.F., Rossi, J.S., Redding, C.A., et al. (2004). Multiple Risk Expert Systems Interventions: Impact of simultaneous stage-matched expert system interventions for smoking, high fat diet, and sun exposure on a population of parents. *Health Psychology*, *23(5)*, 503-516.

Pronk, N.P., Anderson, L.H., Crain, L., Martinson, B.C., O'Connor, P.J., Sherwood, N.E., and Whitebird, R.R. (2004). Meeting recommendations for multiple healthy lifestyle factors: Prevalence, clustering, and predictors among adolescent, adult, and senior health plan members. *American Journal of Preventive Medicine*, *27(2S)*, 25-33.

Putnam, J., Allshouse, J., Kantor, L.S. (2002). U. S. per capita food supply trends: more calories, refined carbohydrates, and fats. *Food Review, 25*, 2-15.

Reeves, M.J., and Rafferty, A.P. (2005). Healthy lifestyle characteristics among adults in the United States, 2000. *Archives of Internal Medicine*, *165*, 854-857.

Riebe, D., Blissmer, B., Greene, G., Caldwell, M., Ruggiero, L., Stillwell, K., and Nigg, C. R., (2005). Long-term Maintenance of Exercise and Healthy Eating Behaviors in Overweight Adults. *Preventive Medicine*, *40*, 769-778.

Riebe, D., Greene, G. W., Ruggiero, L., Stillwell, K. M. Blissmer, B., Nigg, C. R., and Caldwell, M. (2003). Evaluation of a Healthy-Lifestyle Approach to Weight Management. *Preventive Medicine*, *36*, 45-54.

Rossi, J.S., Clark, P., Greaney, M., Riebe, D., Greene, G., Saunders, S., Lees, F., and Nigg, C. (2005). Effectiveness of transtheoretical model-based interventions on exercise and fruit and vegetable consumption in older adults. *Annals of Behavioral Medicine*, *29 (Suppl)*, S134.

Rothbert, K., Strecher, V., Doyle, L., Caplan, W., Joyce, J., Jimison, H., Karm, L., Mims, A., and Roth, M. (2006). Web-based weight management programs in an integrated care setting: A randomized controlled trial. *Obesity*, *14(2)*, 266-272.

Skinner, C.S., Campbell, M.K., Rimer, B., Curry, S., and Prochaska, J.O. (1999). How effective is tailored print communication? *Annals of Behavioral Medicine*, *21(4)*, 290-298.

Toobert, D., Glasgow, R.E., Strycker, L.A., Barrera, M., Ritzwoller, D., and Weidner, G. (2007). Long term effects of the Mediterranean lifestyle program: A randomized clinical trial for postmenopausal women with type 2 diabetes. *International Journal of Behavioral Nutrition and Physical Activity*, *4,* 1-12.

USDHHS. (2000). Healthy People 2010. Washington, DC. US Government Printing Office.

Velicer, W.F., DiClemente, C.C., Rossi, J.S., and Prochaska, J.O. (1990). Relapse situations and self efficacy: An intergrative model. *Addictive Behaviors, 15*, 271-283.

Velicer, W.F., Prochaska, J.O., DiClemente, C.C., and Brandenburg, N. (1985). Decisional balance measure for assessing and predicting smoking status. *J Personality and Social Psychology*, *48(5)*, 1279-1289.

Velicer, W.F., Redding, C.A., Sun, X., and Prochaska, J.O. (2007). Demographic variables, smoking variables, and outcome across five studies. *Health Psychology, 26(3)*, 278-287.

Wang, Y. and Beydoun, M.A. (2007). The obesity epidemic in the United States: Gender, age, socioeconomic, racial/ethnic, and geographic characteristics: A systematic review and meta-regression analysis. *Epidemiologic Reviews, 29(1),*6-28.

In: Nutrition for the Middle Aged and Elderly
Editors: N. E. Bernhardt, A. M. Kasko, pp. 213-233
ISBN: 978-1-60456-146-3

Chapter VI

The Assessment of Protein-Energy Malnutrition in Elderly People

Roberto Buffa[1], Giovanni Floris[1], Paolo Francesco Putzu[2] and Elisabetta Marini[1*]

[1]Department of Experimental Biology, Anthropological Science Section, University of Cagliari, Italy
[2]Geriatric Division, SS Trinità Hospital, ASL 8, Cagliari, Italy

Abstract

Protein-energy malnutrition (PEM) refers to an inadequate supply of nutrients and energy with respect to the body's demand. This condition, caused by organic disturbances or by psychological, social and cultural factors, is highly prevalent in the elderly and can lead to a significant increase of morbidity and mortality.

Early detection of individuals at risk for malnutrition is important to prevent a large proportion of chronic diseases.

However, the objective evaluation of malnutrition in the elderly is difficult because of the lack of reference data for comparisons and of the poor standardization of methods and threshold values.

The aim of this chapter is to discuss the different properties of various methods to diagnosis PEM and the concordance among their results.

The techniques differ in portability, expense and invasiveness, and reflect different aspects of PEM. They are: anthropometry (Body Mass Index, BMI); body composition analysis (phase angle and Bioelectrical Impedance Vector Analysis, BIVA); multi-dimensional techniques (Mini Nutritional Assessment, MNA); biochemical markers (albumin).

* Correspondence address: prof. Elisabetta Marini, Department of Experimental Biology, Anthropological Science Section, University of Cagliari, Cittadella Universitaria, 09042 Monserrato (Cagliari), Italy. Tel 0039-070-6754156; fax 0039-070-6754032; e-mail: emarini@unica.it

We used literature data and unpublished results for healthy (548 individuals) and pathological (50 individuals with Alzheimer disease) elderly samples from Sardinia (Italy).

The MNA is a valid and suitable method for the global evaluation of the nutritional status, and distinguishes malnourished, at risk of malnutrition, and well nourished individuals.

BMI is an indicator of size, but does not distinguish between changes of body components. Is inexpensive and easy to perform. Clear agreement between MNA and BMI has been shown in many studies and in the healthy and pathological samples from Sardinia. The cut-off of 24 kg/m^2 showed the greater accuracy (73.5%) in the diagnosis of under-nourishment based on the MNA.

Several authors have reported a significant correlation between MNA and albumin; however, this was not found in Alzheimer disease.

The phase angle, a bioelectrical parameter, is considered an applicable indicator of nutritional status. It decreases as the nutritional state worsens. In the Sardinian sample it showed different means between MNA groups, but a weak correlation with MNA.

The application of BIVA demonstrated that the bioelectric characteristics of malnourished individuals or subjects at risk of malnutrition are significantly different from those of people with normal nutrition (MNA≥24). BIVA appears a suitable and promising alternative technique for the nutritional assessment in the elderly.

Keywords: *methodological comparison, Mini Nutritional Assessment, anthropometry, bioimpedance, albumin.*

Introduction

Aging is characterized by changes in body mass and composition which generally occur even in the absence of diseases. So-called "physiological aging" implies a reduction of body mass due to the loss of bone mass (Abrams, 2003; Arking, 1998; Kanis and Adami, 1994), the decrease of lean soft tissue mass, that starts at around 30-40 years (Arking, 1998; Baumgartner et al., 1995; Buffa et al., 2002; Forbes and Reina, 1970; Kyle et al., 2001a, 2001b; Novak, 1972), and the decrease of fat mass (FM), that starts at about 75 years of age (Baumgartner et al., 1995; Buffa et al., 2002; Hughes et al., 2002; Silver et al., 1993). Dehydration is a common condition in the elderly (Sheehy et al., 1999). The loss of muscle mass, a component of fat free mass (FFM), is termed sarcopenia and is a common process in healthy individuals, particularly men, who may not manifest weight loss (Gallagher et al., 2000). Fat accumulation in the trunk increases (Buffa et al., 2002; Cronck and Roche, 1982; Hughes et al., 2004; Kuk et al., 2005), leading to a fat pattern associated with increased risks of metabolic and cardiovascular diseases (Després, 2006). Moreover, the loss of height due to compression of the intervertebral disks and osteoporosis may lead to a reduction of stature, which has been quantified in 1 cm per decade (Sorkin et al., 1999).

These morphological variations are related to significant changes in bioelectrical parameters (especially a decrease of the phase angle) (Bosy-Westphal et al., 2005, 2006; Buffa et al., 2003; Guida et al., 2007; Kyle et al., 2004; Piccoli et al., 2002).

Aging is also characterized by a high risk of protein-energy malnutrition (PEM), i.e. an inadequate supply of nutrients and energy with respect to the body's demand. The prevalence of PEM is quite low in independently living individuals (0-6%), higher in institutionalized individuals (10-30%) and patients receiving public home assistance (up to 50%), and epidemic among individuals with acute diseases (Finch et al., 1998; Guigoz et al., 2002; Ruiz-Lopez et al., 2003; Saletti et al., 2005).

The high prevalence of PEM depends on a multi-factorial process involving both central and peripheral mechanisms. It is characterized by the interaction of physiological ("anorexia of aging") and non-physiological (psychological, social and medical) causes.

Anorexia of aging, i.e. the reduction of appetite and food intake, is frequent in the healthy elderly (Morley, 1997). The reduction of hunger and increased satiation are related to delayed gastric emptying in older individuals, due to both anatomical-functional modifications of the stomach and variations in the concentration of hormones regulating food intake (Morley, 1997). Several hormones play a role in the regulation of appetite and their concentrations vary with age. Wilson and Morley (2003) discuss the role of increased levels of cholecystokinin and, in men, the decline in testosterone that leads to an increase in leptin. Other authors report that leptin, ghrelin and insulin alter the control of hunger and satiety in the elderly (Di Francesco et al., 2006).

Poor appetite can also be due to the progressive decline of taste and, more particularly, olfactory sensitivity which reduces the enjoyment of food. Taste and smell dysfunctions are common in the elderly and can be amplified by diseases (especially Alzheimer disease) or drugs (Doty et al., 1984; Hetherington, 1998; Schiffman, 1997, 2000; Stevens et al., 1995).

Finally, age-related declines of visual performance and functional ability can reduce the aptitude to prepare meals and limit the type and quantity of food eaten (Payette et al., 1995).

The social and psychological difficulties that often affect the senile population, together with the high prevalence of diseases, are important etiological factors in malnutrition (Hickson, 2006; Morley, 1997).

Poverty, isolation, and loneliness are important social causes (Finch et al., 1998), while lifestyle factors, such as cooking abilities or food beliefs, have less influence on the development of malnutrition (Payette et al., 1995). Other social causes of weight loss (monotony or poor choice of food, limited and established meal times, dislike of communal eating) may occur in institutionalized individuals.

Depression is the most frequent psychological cause of malnutrition (Blaum et al., 1995; Blazer et al., 1987; Thompson and Morris, 1991) but other psychological disorders (anxiety, stress) are also associated with changes in food intake (Morley, 1997).

Common diseases in the elderly, such as gastrointestinal, respiratory, endocrine, neurological disorders, dementia, cancer, acute and chronic infections, oral and dental diseases, are associated with high rates of malnutrition (Donini et al., 2003; Morley, 1997). Many illnesses can result in cachexia which causes changes in body composition and weight loss (Morley et al., 2006b). In addition, various drugs can cause malabsorption of nutrients and loss of appetite.

PEM can lead to a significant increase of morbidity and mortality (Kagansky et al., 2005; Van Nes et al., 2001). The clinical consequences of this condition have a strong impact on the quality of life and have high social costs (Stechmiller, 2003). In fact, malnutrition is an important predictor of frailty syndrome in the elderly (Morley et al., 2006a).

Old people are also less able to reverse weight loss and restore FFM than young people (Hebuterne et al., 1995). For these reasons, prevention and treatment of malnutrition in the elderly are primary aims of geriatric medicine. The correct and timely diagnosis of PEM, followed by adequate therapeutic and nutritional interventions, results in a significant improvement of the general condition of the patient (Hudgens et al., 2004).

However, malnutrition in the elderly is often underdiagnosed (Nursal et al., 2005; Wells and Drumbell, 2006). The objective evaluation of malnutrition in elderly subjects is difficult because of the lack of methodological standardization and reference data for comparisons. Moreover, there is not a general agreement on the appropriate cut-offs for the diagnosis of under-nutrition and malnutrition. The use of too low values, such as those adopted for adults, underestimate the prevalence of malnourished individuals and does not allow the recognition of individuals at risk of malnutrition.

This chapter discusses the different properties of the principal methods to assess nutritional status in the elderly (multi-dimensional techniques, anthropometry, body composition analysis, biochemical markers) and their concordance in the classification of under-nourishment.

For this purpose, we used literature data and unpublished results for healthy and pathological (Alzheimer disease) elderly samples from Sardinia (Italy). Alzheimer disease was considered because of the changes in nutritional status and the related weight loss characterizing this pathology (Buffa et al., 2007a; Gillette-Guyonnet et al., 2000; Vellas et al., 2005; White et al., 1997, 1998a, 1998b).

Methods for the Assessment of Malnutrition in the Elderly

Methods to assess the nutritional status in elderly subjects must be simple and practical so as to allow a wide range of applications, the detection of subclinical cases and timely interventions.

In this research, we considered various types of methods: anthropometry, body composition analysis, multi-dimensional techniques and biochemical markers. The techniques differ in portability, expense and invasiveness and they reflect different aspects of malnutrition.

Anthropometry

Anthropometry is the most portable, applicable, inexpensive and non-invasive technique to assess nutritional status. It also has an important advantage over other nutritional indicators, in that body measurements are sensitive over the full spectrum of malnutrition. The main disadvantage of anthropometry is its lack of specificity, as changes in body measurements are influenced by several factors, especially the genetic background.

Descriptions of standard anthropometric measurements can be found in Lohman et al. (1988). Individual anthropometric variables can be analyzed in relation to their longitudinal changes or to a set of reference values that determine the limits of normality.

The problem with reference standards is that they are population-, age- and sex-specific and should be periodically updated to take account of diachronic changes in body size and proportions, i.e. the secular trend. Nevertheless, since sample data for population-specific standards are inadequate, international reference values are generally utilized. The cut-off points for the elderly population are usually those determined for adults in general.

The most common anthropometric indicators of nutritional status are: weight, subcutaneous skinfolds, mid-arm circumference and body mass index. Anthropometric measurements can also be used to predict body density and to calculate body fatness and fat free mass but these applications are obsolete.

Body weight is a size dimension and it has an important role in the assessment of nutritional status: historical weight loss is a cardinal measure of nutritional depletion in the elderly. There are no defined cut-off points but most authors consider a loss of 10% of body weight (with respect to habitual weight) indicative of risk of malnutrition (ANAES, 2003). Beck and Ovesen (1998) suggested that a clinically significant weight loss for the elderly is less (around 5% annually) than in younger age groups (around 5% in 1-6 months). Weight can also be compared with an ideal measure (for example, the formula by Lorentz; Spyckerelle et al., 1984), where a variation of 75-85% indicates malnutrition. The limitation of this indicator is that changes in body weight do not reveal alterations of body composition and they can be confounded by changes in hydration.

Triceps skinfold and upper arm circumference have been used to assess nutritional status in field studies. Their combination appears to be a more precise indicator of nutritional status than either of the individual variables alone. Although proper training and quality control can render the method acceptable, these measurements are generally considered of low precision.

Body mass index (BMI) refers to relative weight for height (weight / height^2, kg/m^2) (WHO, 1995, 2000). The index was devised to consider body mass independently of height; in fact, the correlation between BMI and height is generally low (Shetty and James, 1994). BMI is considered the most suitable objective anthropometric indicator of nutritional status in adults (Bailey and Ferro-Luzzi, 1995; WHO, 1995, 2000). However, like weight, BMI does not indicate body composition changes.

The WHO defines the normal range of BMI for adults (over 20 years) as 18.5-24.9 kg/m^2 (WHO, 2000). The need for population-specific BMI standards seems to be less critical than for other anthropometric variables since differences among ethnic groups are considered the result of environmental rather than genetic influences. However, most authors agree that the cut-off points should increase in relation to age. This seems appropriate in view of the changes in body composition during aging and the decrease in height. The shorter height of elderly individuals, due to the combined effects of aging and secular trend, might result in higher BMI values with respect to younger adults. Moreover, the higher cut-offs would allow the identification of subclinical malnutrition and the earlier prevention of associated complications. Beck and Ovesen (1998) suggest a cut-off of 24 kg/m^2 for the classification of individuals at risk of malnutrition in the elderly. The diagnostic cut-off for malnutrition proposed for persons over 65 years varies from 18.5 kg/m^2 (WHO, 2000) to 22 kg/m^2

(Nutrition Screening Initiative, American Academy of Family Physicians, American Dietetic Association, 2002). However, 20 kg/m² is the most common value in the literature and it is considered very sensitive for the diagnosis of malnutrition in the elderly (ANAES, 2003).

Body Composition Analysis

The most common way to describe body composition is in terms of a 2-component model of fat mass and fat free mass. Human body composition can be assessed with direct, indirect and doubly indirect methods. Direct measurement techniques - anatomical dissection and chemical analysis - are most accurate but unsuitable in most cases. Indirect methods, e.g. densitometry, dual energy X-ray absorptiometry (DXA), magnetic resonance imaging (MRI) and computed tomography (CT), are based on the direct techniques and involve assumptions on the tissues characteristics. These techniques are accurate and technologically advanced but time-consuming and expensive, so they are impractical in large-scale studies and field applications. Doubly indirect methods are calibrated against indirect methods. They are the most widely used methods and include anthropometry and bioelectrical impedance analysis (BIA).

BIA is based on the conductive and dielectric properties of biological tissues. It is a simple and non-invasive technique for the determination of body composition, which has gained wide acceptance as a field and bedside body composition technique. The procedure to measure the bioelectrical parameters, resistance (R, Ω) and reactance (Xc, Ω), is indicated by the National Institutes of Health Technology Assessment Conference Statement (N.I.H., 1996). The derived variables, phase angle (Φ, degrees) and impedance (Z, Ω), are calculated as $\Phi = \arctan(Xc/R)$ and $Z = (R^2 + Xc^2)^{0.5}$.

In the conventional BIA procedure, regression equations are used to estimate the body compartments. However, these equations are significantly influenced by age, sex, population, pathological condition and validation method. Moreover, they are not sensitive to individual variability in the density of mineral mass, hydration and protein content of fat free mass. For these reasons, the predictive accuracy of the BIA equations is inadequate and their application could lead to substantial estimation errors, especially in the elderly.

Piccoli et al. (1994) proposed the direct use of resistance (R) and reactance (Xc) normalized for height (H). Bioelectrical impedance vector analysis (BIVA) allows the semiquantitative examination of body composition and provides an evaluation of nutritional and hydration status without the need for predictive equations or models of the electrical properties of human tissues. The R and Xc values are standardized by height (R/H, Ω /m; Xc/H, Ω /m) to eliminate the effect of conductor length on the bioelectrical parameters. Individual impedance vectors can be plotted within the tolerance ellipses (R-Xc graph), where the major axis refers to hydration status and the minor axis to the body cell mass (BCM). In particular, the upper pole of the ellipse refers to dehydration, the lower pole to edema, the left side to obesity or athletic condition, the right side to cachexia or anorexia. Comparison of the individual vectors with the reference standards of the healthy population (tolerance ellipses) allows us to assess the affinity between their bioelectrical characteristics and to make a clinical evaluation (De Palo et al., 2000; Piccoli et al., 1995, 2002).

The mean impedance vectors from groups of individuals can be compared graphically by means of confidence ellipses and statistically by the Hotelling T^2 test (Piccoli and Pastori, 2002).

Because of its characteristics, BIVA is an appropriate method to study the quantitative and qualitative changes of body composition in normal and pathological aging. It combines the BIA characteristic of suitability with improved accuracy.

Biochemical Markers

Nutritional status can also be assessed with biochemical indicators, although they are generally useful only at the extremes of malnutrition. The most commonly used biomarkers are: serum albumin, pre-albumin, retinol-binding protein, transferrin and insulin-like growth factor-1 (IGF-I) levels, lymphocyte count, creatinine height index, urinary creatinine and urinary 3-methylhistidine.

Serum albumin is the most widely used indicator of malnutrition (ANAES, 2003). It has a long half-life of about 20 days and provides information about the degree of protein-visceral malnutrition (Heymsfield and Williams, 1988). However, the utility of serum albumin in older people has been questioned because of its poor specificity. Pathological factors, especially inflammation processes but also impaired physical functions, can influence albumin concentrations in older people. Moreover, age-related variations of albumin levels are present (ca. 0.5 g/l per decade) (International Federation of Clinical Chemistry, 1996; Kuzuya et al., 2007; Thérond, 1994).

In spite of these limitations, serum albumin remains a good prognostic indicator and its use is justified by the significant association with morbidity and mortality rates (ANAES, 2003). A serum level of 35 g/l is generally adopted as a cut-off for moderate malnutrition and 30 g/l for severe malnutrition (ANAES, 2003).

Multi-Dimensional Techniques

Various multi-dimensional methods to assess nutritional status in the elderly are reported in the literature. They are characterized by non-invasiveness, ease of use and low costs. These methods consider a heterogeneous set of variables, mainly: clinical variables (medical history data, gastrointestinal symptoms), anthropometric variables (changes in body weight and in subcutaneous and muscle mass), nutritional variables (alimentary habits), biochemical variables (cholesterolemia and albuminemia), and psychological and socio-behavioral variables. The diagnosis leads to classification of individuals into groups with different nutritional status. The most common methods are (for an extensive review, see Buffa et al., 2007b): Subjective Global Assessment (SGA), Sadness, Cholesterol, Albumin, Loss of weight, Eating problems, Shopping problems or inability to prepare a meal, SCALES, Geriatric Nutritional Risk Index (GNRI), Nutrition Risk Score (NRS), Nutrition Screening Initiative (NSI) (DETERMINE), Nutritional Risk Assessment Scale (NuRAS), Prognostic Nutritional Index (PNI), Mini Nutritional Assessment (MNA).

The MNA protocol (Guigoz et al., 1994; Rubenstein, 1998) is recommended by the European Society of Parenteral and Enteral Nutrition (Kondrup et al., 2003) and is considered the gold standard technique by some authors (Morley, 1997). Therefore, we used this method in the present research.

The sensitivity and specificity of MNA in detecting states of malnutrition are 96% and 98% respectively (Vellas et al., 1999). The level of reliability (R) is 0.89 (Bleda et al., 2002).

The method is useful to evaluate the effects of therapeutic interventions on nutritional status (Barone et al., 2003; Gil Gregorio et al., 2003). It is also a valid predictor of short- and long-term morbidity and mortality in hospitalized patients (Persson et al., 2002).

The versatility of the technique has been documented in different populations and in different acute pathological conditions (see details and bibliography in Buffa et al., 2007b).

The MNA test involves the compilation of a questionnaire consisting of 18 items divided into three sections: anthropometry; alimentation; cognitive and disability status. A score lower than 17 indicates malnutrition, 17-23.5 indicates a risk of malnutrition, and 24 or higher indicates normal nutrition.

The Sardinian Sample and the Applied Methods

The sample consisted of 548 healthy individuals and 50 individuals with Alzheimer disease from Sardinia (Italy) (table 1). The Sardinian origin of the sample was verified to the first parental generation. All individuals were over 70 years old.

The subjects agreed to participate in the study after being informed about the objectives and methods of the research.

Measurements of healthy volunteers were carried out at various cultural and recreational meeting places habitually frequented by older people. Individuals who were admitted to the hospital in the 3 months before the survey or were under medical treatment were excluded from the sample.

Alzheimer patients were chosen from the Geriatrics Division, SS. Trinità Hospital, ASL 8 of Cagliari. The diagnosis of AD was made on admission to the center based on the DSM IV and NINDS-ADRDA (National Institute of Neurological Disorders and Stroke – Alzheimer's Disease and Related Disorders Association) criteria. The Clinical Dementia Rating (CDR) scale was used to identify the stage of AD and patients in the mild-moderate stage (CDR 1 and 2) were selected for the study.

Table 1. Sardinian sample composition

	N	Age mean±s.d. range	
Healthy men	265	79.3±7.1	70.0 - 99.8
Healthy women	283	81.4±7.0	70.0-101.4
Alzheimer men	13	80.1±5.1	71.4-93.4
Alzheimer women	37	82.3±6.0	70.1-95.4

All anthropometric measurements were taken by an experienced operator according to standard procedures (Lohman et al., 1988). Height was measured with a portable anthropometer with an accuracy of 1 mm. Body weight was measured to 0.1 kg with a portable spring scale. The Body Mass Index (BMI, kg/m^2) was calculated and the individuals were categorized into five groups (<18.5 kg/m^2, 18.5-19.9 kg/m^2, 20.0-23.9 kg/m^2, 24.0-28.9 kg/m^2, ≥29 kg/m^2).

The bioelectrical parameters, R (Ω) and Xc (Ω), were measured with a single-frequency impedance analyzer (BIA 101, Akern, Florence, Italy), using an operating frequency of 50 kHz at 800 μA. The instrumental accuracy was checked with a calibration circuit of known impedance (R = 380 Ω, Xc = 47 Ω, 1% error).

Bioelectrical impedance vector analysis (BIVA) was performed (Piccoli et al., 1994).

Serum albumin was determined in the Alzheimer group.

The MNA method was applied to a sub-group of 219 individuals adopting the full questionnaire and standard cut-off values.

Using MNA as the gold standard and a cut-off of MNA<24 (at risk of malnutrition), we calculated the sensitivity (proportion of individuals correctly assigned to the under-nourished category), the specificity (proportion of individuals correctly diagnosed as well-nourished), and the accuracy of the nutritional indicators. Different BMI values (20 - 25 Kg/m^2) were tested to identify the best cut-off for classification of nutritional status. The standard serum albumin cut-off for moderate malnutrition (< 35 g/l) was applied. The evaluation was performed with the sexes combined but with the healthy and Alzheimer individuals separated. Confidence intervals (95% CI) for sensitivity, specificity, and accuracy were also calculated.

The statistical comparison between mean values in the groups of well- and under-nourished individuals was performed applying the Student's t test for independent samples. The association among nutritional indicators and the relationship with age were evaluated by correlation analysis.

Results

Nutritional Assessment

Table 2 shows the frequencies of nutritional assessment using BMI, albumin, and MNA.

In the healthy sub-sample, the prevalence of individuals identified as malnourished by means of MNA was 1.1% in the men and 1.3% in the women. The prevalence of individuals classified as under-nourished ("at risk of malnutrition" plus malnourished, i.e. with a MNA < 24) was 26.9% in the men and 49.4% in the women.

The nutritional classification using the BMI threshold of 20 kg/m^2 identified a frequency of malnourished individuals equal to 0.4% in the men and 5.7% in the women. The percentage of individuals with a BMI<24 kg/m^2 was 15.1% in the men and 26.5% in the women.

In the Alzheimer group, the MNA recognized 5.6% of the women as malnourished, 38.5% of the men and 50.0% of the women as under-nourished. The percentage of patients with a BMI under the value of 20 kg/m^2 was 7.7% in the men and 10.8% in the women. The frequency of individuals with a BMI<24 kg/m^2 was 46.2% in the men and 40.5% in the women. The classification based on albumin levels identified a prevalence of Alzheimer individuals with severe malnutrition (albumin level < 30 g/l) equal to 9.1% in the men and 28.6% in the women. The cumulative frequency of patients moderately malnourished (albumin < 35 g/l) was 27.3% in the men and 48.6% in the women.

Table 2. Nutritional assessment

		Healthy men		Healthy women		Alzheimer men		Alzheimer women	
		N	%	N	%	N	%	N	%
BMI (kg/m^2)	BMI≥29	72	27.2	121	42.8	1	7.7	11	29.7
	24≤BMI<29	153	57.7	87	30.7	6	46.1	11	29.7
	20≤BMI<24	39	14.7	59	20.8	5	38.5	11	29.7
	18.5≤BMI<20	1	0.4	11	3.9	1	7.7	1	2.7
	16≤BMI<18.5	0	0.0	5	1.8	0	0.0	3	8.2
Albumin (g/l)	alb≥35	-	-	-	-	8	72.7	18	51.4
	30≤alb<35	-	-	-	-	2	18.2	7	20.0
	25≤alb<30	-	-	-	-	1	9.1	10	28.6
MNA	MNA≥24	68	73.1	39	50.6	8	61.6	18	50.0
	17≤MNA<24	24	25.8	37	48.1	5	38.5	16	44.4
	MNA<17	1	1.1	1	1.3	0	0.0	2	5.6

BMI: Body Mass Index; alb: Albumin; MNA: Mini Nutritional Assessment. N: absolute frequency; %: relative frequency.

Both in the healthy and Alzheimer samples, few individuals were diagnosed as malnourished by means of MNA (1.2% and 4.1%, respectively). A greater proportion was found for at risk of malnutrion individuals (healthy: 35.9%; Alzheimer: 42.9%). Similar results were found in the literature. Data on free-living and healthy institutionalized elderly people show a low prevalence (0-6%) of malnutrition (Davidson and Getz, 2004; Delacorte et al., 2004; Guigoz et al., 2002), and a greater proportion (20-61%) of at risk condition, especially in institutionalized individuals (Ruiz-Lopez et al., 2003; Saava and Kisper-Hint, 2002).

The prevalence of under-nourished individuals was greater in women than in men. A similar gender discrepancy was found by other authors (Castel et al., 2006). This pattern seem counter-intuitive, as women represent the larger proportion of the elderly population and have an average longer life span. However, selective mechanisms related to the sex differences in mortality could play a role. The underlying mechanisms are poorly understood and they will require *ad hoc* investigations.

The greater frequency of under-nourished Alzheimer patients with respect to the healthy individuals is in agreement with the theoretical expectations and experimental observations from the literature. Weight reduction is an important aspect of the complex clinical picture of Alzheimer's disease: it represents a typical manifestation of the pathology and is an indicator of its progression (Gillette-Guyonnet et al., 2000; White et al., 1997, 1998a, Wolf-Klein and

Silverstone, 1994). Malnutrition appears in the sub-clinical phase and initial onset of dementia (Barrett-Connor et al., 1996, Buchman et al., 2005, Knittweis, 1998), accelerates by the time of diagnosis (Stewart, 2005), and reaches very high proportions in the advanced stages (Gillette-Guyonnet et al., 2000; White et al., 1998b).

Agreement between Methods

The Mini Nutritional Assessment was used as the reference method, since it is the most appropriate and best validated instrument for the nutritional screening in the elderly (Vellas et al., 1999; Morley, 1997).

Descriptive and comparative statistics for the nutritional indicators in the under nourished (MNA<24) and well nourished (MNA≥24) sub groups are shown in table 3. The association among nutritional indicators, evaluated by means of correlation analysis, is shown in table 4 (a: healthy individuals, b: Alzheimer individuals).

Body mass shows a reduction with the worsening of nutritional status. In the healthy sub sample, the mean BMI values were significantly lower in the under-nourished with respect to the normo-nourished individuals, both in men ($p<0.05$) and in women ($p<0.001$) (table 3). A similar pattern was observed in the Alzheimer subgroup, but the difference was not statistically significant. Mean BMI values range from 22.69 (Alzheimer men) to 28.65 (healthy women). On the basis of the classification adopted for adults by the World Health Organization (2000), such values indicate normal or overweight conditions. This result confirms the inadequacy of the cut-off points for adults, and the need for the use of higher values in the elderly (Beck and Ovesen, 1998). In the healthy and Alzheimer individuals of both sexes, the MNA scores were significantly related to the BMI values (table 4). A clear association between MNA and BMI has been already shown in many studies (Kucukerdonmez et al., 2006; Magri et al., 2003; Saletti et al., 2000; Vellas et al., 2000).

The better classification of nutritional status in the healthy sample was reached using the cut-off of BMI = 24 Kg/m^2, which showed an accuracy of 73.5% ± 6.6, a sensitivity 50.1% ± 12.1, and a specificity 86.9% ± 8.2. The cut-off of 20 Kg/m^2 furnished the worse results (accuracy = 67.6% ± 7.0; sensitivity = 12.7 % ± 6.0; specificity = 100 % ± 4.0). In the Alzheimer sample, accuracy, sensitivity and specificity of the cut-off of 24 Kg/m^2 were 63.3% ± 13,5, 56.5% ± 21,6, and 69.2% ± 21,1, respectively.

The mean albumin levels were slightly lower in the under-nourished with respect to the normo-nourished subgroups (table 3), especially in men, but the difference was not significant. Mean values were above the cut-off for normal nutrition (35 g/l). Similarly, Vellas et al. (1999), found normal levels of albumin in patients with a MNA score between 17 and 23.5. MNA scores were not significantly related to albumin levels (Alzheimer sample) (table 4). Some authors reported a significant correlation between MNA and albumin (Saletti et al., 2000; Vellas et al., 1999, 2000), but a lack of significant correlation was already found in Alzheimer disease (Nourhashemi et al., 1999). The accuracy, sensitivity and specificity of albumin classification of under-nutrition (<35 g/l) were 62.2% ± 14.1, 57.1% ± 22.7, and 66.7% ± 26.6, respectively. The quite low accuracy of albumin as indicator of nutritional status could be due to its poor sensitivity for detecting mild degrees of malnutrition, but also to the presence of inflammatory conditions in Alzheimer individuals.

Table 3. Descriptive statistics and Student's t test in groups with different nutritional status

	Well nourished (MNA<24)		Under nourished (MNA≥24)		Statistical comparison	
	Mean	s.d.	Mean	s.d.	*t*	*p*
Healty men						
Age	78.46	4.83	86.02	8.96	-5.22	0.000
MNA	25.68	1.26	21.84	1.72	11.75	0.000
BMI (kg/m^2)	27.11	2.97	25.30	3.77	2.41	0.018
Phase angle (°)	6.20	0.91	5.67	1.11	2.27	0.026
Healty women						
Age	77.52	5.14	84.87	7.64	-4.97	0.000
MNA	25.31	0.98	21.53	2.00	10.57	0.000
BMI (kg/m^2)	28.65	4.72	23.26	3.84	5.50	0.000
Phase angle (°)	6.04	0.87	5.37	0.95	3.09	0.003
Alzheimer men						
Age	79.70	6.46	80.62	1.92	-0.31	0.766
MNA	26.88	0.95	19.70	2.05	8.67	0.000
BMI (kg/m^2)	25.38	2.28	22.69	2.81	1.90	0.084
Phase angle (°)	5.34	0.78	4.85	0.42	1.27	0.231
Albumin (g/l)	40.76	3.58	37.60	2.16	1.41	0.193
Alzheimer women						
Age	83.49	5.20	80.87	6.69	1.31	0.199
MNA	26.72	1.57	20.11	2.71	8.94	0.000
BMI (kg/m^2)	28.15	5.02	24.64	5.78	1.94	0.060
Phase angle (°)	5.20	0.91	4.78	0.54	1.68	0.102
Albumin (g/l)	38.74	5.14	38.48	5.40	0.15	0.884

s.d.: standard deviation, *t*: Student's t test.

Table 4. Correlation among nutritional indicators and relation with age

a. Healthy individuals

	Age	Phase angle	BMI	MNA
Age	-	-0.30*	-0.22*	-0.55*
Phase angle	-0.32*	-	0.15*	0.27*
BMI	-0.28*	0.04	-	0.61*
MNA	-0.45*	0.20	0.31*	-

b. Alzheimer individuals

	Age	Phase angle	BMI	MNA	Albumin
Age	-	-0.35*	0.24	0.04	0.01
Phase angle	-0.68*	-	0.05	0.34*	0.12
BMI	-0.32	0.42	-	0.31*	-0.15
MNA	-0.21	0.33	0.59*	-	0.09
Albumin	-0.42	0.23	0.22	0.36	-

Men are shown below the diagonal and women are shown above the diagonal. BMI: Body mass Index; MNA: Mini Nutritional Assessment. *: $p<0.05$.

The mean phase angle was lower in the under-nourished with respect to the normo-nourished subgroups, but the difference is significant only in the healthy sample (table 3). The relation between MNA and phase angle was positive and significant in the healthy women and the Alzheimer men (table 4).

Literature data show that the phase angle decreases as the nutritional state worsens (Barbosa-Silva et al., 2005; Nagano et al., 2000; Norman et al., 2007; Selberg and Selberg, 2002; Wirth and Miklis, 2005). Moreover, phase angle has demonstrated to be a good prognostic indicator, in some case superior to other serum or anthropometric nutritional markers (Gupta et al., 2004; Ott et al., 1995; Schwenk et al., 2000). However some authors criticized the univariate approach to body composition assessment by means of the phase angle (Toso et al., 2000). In fact, changes in phase angle may be due either to variations in body cell mass or to modifications in fluid volume.

Figure 1 shows the R-Xc graph with the mean bioelectrical vectors from healthy individuals grouped by sex and MNA classes (under-nourished, MNA<24; well-nourished, MNA≥ 24). In both sexes, the 95% confidence ellipses were significantly separated between MNA classes (men: T^2=9.4, p<0.01; women: T^2=11.9, p<0.01). The mean vector of under-nourished individuals showed a clear shift to the down, thus reflecting a reduction of the body cell mass. The only other study on the relation between BIVA and MNA detected a similar significant displacement of the mean vector in under-nourished individuals (Norman et al., 2007). Alzheimer individuals showed similar results (Buffa et al in prep.).

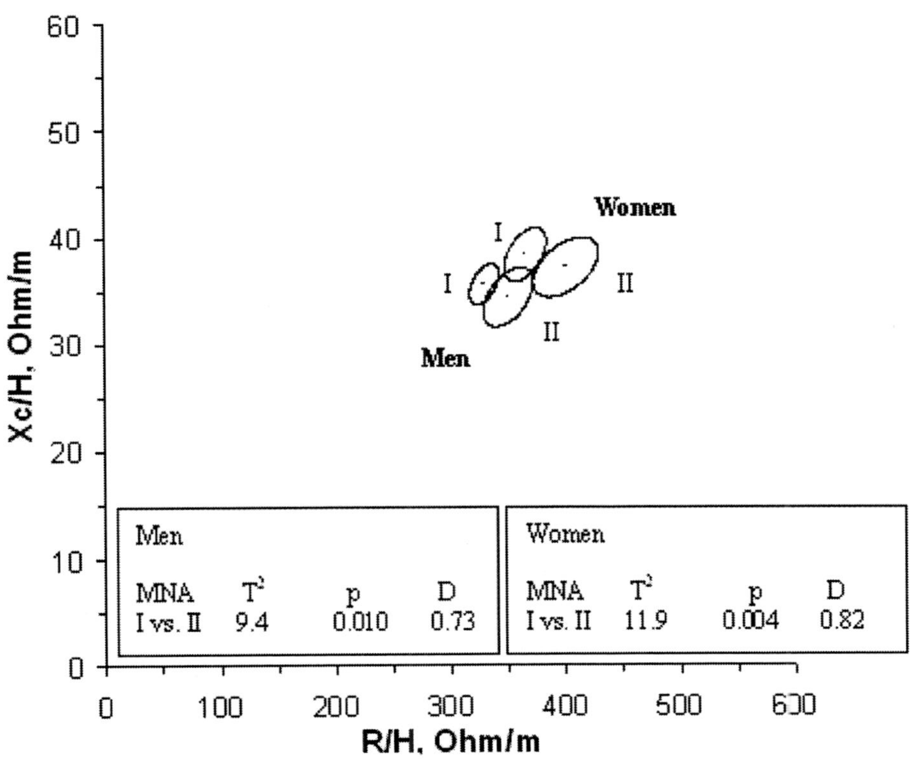

Figure 1. Bioelectrical mean vector with 95% confidence ellipses form subjects grouped by sex and MNA classes (healthy individuals). I= MNA≥ 24; II= MNA<24; T^2= Hotelling's T^2 statistic; p= probability level; D= Mahalanobis distance.

Under nourished healthy individuals had significantly higher mean ages than well nourished individuals. Moreover, all nutritional indicators showed a significant association with age, indicating a progressive decline of the nutritional status in the healthy aging. There is evidence for the age related changes of BMI (Sanchez-Garcia et al., 2007; Zamboni et al., 2003), bioelectrical parameters (Bosy-Westphal et al., 2005, 2006; Buffa et al., 2003; Guida et al., 2007; Kyle et al., 2004; Piccoli et al., 2002), albumin (ANAES, 2003), and MNA (Delacorte et al., 2004; Kuzuya et al., 2005; Saletti et al., 2000). These trends indicate that physiological changes of aging are associated with the decline of nutritional status and place the elderly at increased risk for malnutrition.

The weaker association between nutritional indicators and age in the Alzheimer sample could be due to a greater influence on nutritional status of pathological factors than of physiological aging.

Conclusion

Older persons experience physiological changes of body mass and composition, which progressively place them at increased risk for developing protein energy malnutrition. Moreover, the ability to reverse weight loss is reduced in the elderly.

As a matter of fact, malnutrition is a prevalent condition in the elderly, especially in institutionalized individuals and when a pathological condition is present. Women seem to be at markedly increased risk. This gender discrepancy should be analyzed in detail to understand the underlying mechanisms.

The impact of malnutrition on the quality of life can be considerable and its relation with increased morbidity and mortality has been well documented. Early detection of individuals at risk for malnutrition is crucial. It should allow a timely nutritional interventions, so preventing a large proportion of chronic diseases, with considerable health and economic benefits. In spite of the above, malnutrition in the elderly is often under diagnosed and under treated. This is mainly due to the lack of consensus on methods and on the appropriate cut-off for the diagnosis of under-nutrition and malnutrition. At this purpose, more data on older healthy people should be useful.

The more used methods for the assessment of nutritional status in the elderly are multi-dimensional techniques, anthropometry, body composition analysis, biochemical markers.

The Mini Nutritional Assessment (MNA) is a multi-dimensional technique. MNA furnishes a global evaluation of the nutritional status, considering a heterogeneous set of variables, and distinguishes malnourished, at risk of malnutrition, and well nourished individuals. It is considered a valid and suitable method.

Body Mass Index (BMI) is an anthropometric indicator of size. It is considered an effective proxy indicator of undernutrition, useful as a screening tool because it is inexpensive and easy to perform. However, it is unable to distinguish between changes of fat mass and fat free mass. Moreover, there is no agreement on the cut-off values for the diagnosis of under-nutrition and malnutrition in the elderly. The standard cut-off for adults seem too low in the aged population. The cut-off 24 kg/m^2 showed the greater accuracy (73.5%) in the diagnosis of under-nourishment based on the MNA.

Even if frequently used, the ability of serum albumin to predict nutritional status in the elderly is questionable, especially in case of associated diseases. In fact, albumin is dependent from physiological and pathological factors. Moreover, as other biochemical markers, it is sensitive only to the extremes of malnutrition. The relation with MNA, the sensitivity, the specificity, and the accuracy resulted quite low in the Sardinan Alzheimer sample.

Bioimpedance techniques for the study of body composition are simple, inexpensive and non invasive. However, the conventional use of BIA is susceptible of equation-inherent errors. The direct use of bioelectrical parameters (phase angle, BIVA) is more accurate.

The phase angle, which is considered an applicable indicator of nutritional status, showed different means between MNA groups, but a weak correlation with MNA. However, some authors criticized this univariate approach to body composition assessment.

Bioelectrical impedance vector analysis well agreed with the MNA classification, as shown by this research and by a recent similar investigation. Further, it provides meaningful information on body cell mass and hydration, i.e. two cardinal variables of aging. BIVA appears a suitable and promising alternative technique for the nutritional assessment in the elderly. The definition of specific cut-off values for the evaluation of malnutrition and risk of malnutrition would improve the usefulness for screening programs and clinical practice.

Acknowledgments

We acknowledge the support of the Sardinian individuals that participated in the study.

We thank A. Piccoli and G. Pastori (Department of Medical and Surgical Sciences, University of Padova, Italy) for providing the BIVA software (Piccoli and Pastori, 2002).

This research was financially supported by the MIUR contributions.

References

Abrams, SA. Normal Acquisition and Loss of Bone Mass. *Horm. Res,* 2003 60 (Suppl.3), 71-76.

ANAES, Agence Nationale d'Accréditation et d'Évaluation en Santé. Évaluation diagnostique de la dénutrition protéino-énergétique des adultes hospitalisés. Service des recommandations professionnelles. Available from: septembre 2003. URL: http://www.has-sante.fr/portail/display.jsp?id=c_432199.

Arking, R. Biology of aging. Sunderland: Sinauer Associates; 1998.

Bailey, KV; Ferro-Luzzi A. Use of body mass index of adults in assessing individual and community nutritional status. *Bull. World Health Org.,* 1995 73(5), 673-680.

Barbosa-Silva, MC; Barros, AJ; Wang, J; Heymsfield, SB; Pierson, RN Jr. Bioelectrical impedance analysis: population reference values for phase angle by age and sex. *Am. J. Clin. Nutr.,* 2005 82(1), 49-52.

Barone, L; Milosavljevic, M; Gazibarich, B. Assessing the older person: is the MNA a more appropriate nutritional assessment tool than the SGA? *J. Nutr. Health Aging,* 2003 7, 13-17.

Barrett-Connor, E; Edelstein, SL; Corey-Bloom, J; Wiederholt, WC. Weight loss precedes dementia in community-dwelling older adults. *J. Am. Geriatr. Soc.*, 1996 44, 1147-1152.

Baumgartner, RN; Stauber, PM; McHugh, D; Koehler, KM; Garry, PJ. Cross-sectional age differences in body composition in persons 60 +years of age. *J. Gerontol. A Biol. Sci. Med. Sci.*, 1995 50, 307 –316.

Beck, AM; Ovesen, L. At which body mass index and degree of weight loss should hospitalized elderly patients be considered at nutritional risk? *Clin. Nutr.*, 1998 17(5), 195-198.

Blaum, CS; Fries, BE; Fiatarone, MA. Factors associated with low body mass index and weight loss in nursing home residents. *J. Gerontol. A Biol. Sci. Med. Sci*, 1995 50, 162–168.

Blazer, D; Bachas, JR; Hughes, DC. Major depression with melanchoha: a comparison of middle-aged and elderly adults. *J. Am. Geriatr. Soc.*, 1987 35, 927-932.

Bleda, MJ; Bolibar, I; Pares, R; Salva, A. Reliability of the mini nutritional assessment (MNA) in institutionalised elderly people. *J. Nutr. Health Aging,* 2002 6, 134-137.

Bosy-Westphal, A; Danielzik, S; Dörhöfer, RP; Later, W; Wiese, S; Müller, MJ. Phase angle from bioelectrical impedance analysis: population reference values by age, sex, and body mass index. *JPEN J. Parenter. Enteral. Nutr.*, 2006 30(4), 309-316.

Bosy-Westphal, A; Danielzik, S; Dörhöfer, RP; Piccoli, A; Muller, MJ. Patterns of bioelectrical impedance vector distribution by body mass index and age: implications for body-composition analysis. *Am. J. Clin. Nutr.*, 2005 82(1), 60-68.

Buchman, AS; Wilson, RS; Bienias, JL; Shah, RC; Evans, DA; Bennett, DA. Change in body mass index and risk of incident Alzheimer disease. *Neurology*, 2005 65, 892–897.

Buffa, R; Floris, G; Marini, E. Migration of bioelectrical vector in healthy elderly subjects. *Nutrition,* 2003 19(11-12), 917-921.

Buffa, R; Floris, G; Marini, E; Porcu, A. Caratteristiche antropometriche di un campione di popolazione senile della Sardegna. In: Guerci A, Consigliere S editors. *Curare la vecchiaia.* Genova: Erga Edizioni; 2002; 51-61.

Buffa, R; Lodde, M; Floris, GU; Zaru, C; Putzu, PF; Marini, E. Somatotype in Alzheimer disease. *Gerontology,* 2007a 53 (4), 200-204.

Buffa, R; Marini, E; Putzu, PF; Floris, G. La malnutrizione proteico-energetica nell'anziano: tecniche di analisi e applicazioni. *Antropo*, 2007b 14, 19-27.

Castel, H; Shahar, D; Harman-Boehm, I. Gender differences in factors associated with nutritional status of older medical patients. *J. Am. Coll. Nutr.*, 2006 25(2),128-134.

Cronck, CE; Roche, AF. Race and sex specific reference data for triceps and subscapular skinfolds and weight/stature. *Am. J. Clin. Nutr.,* 1982 35, 347–354.

Davidson, J; Getz, M. Nutritional risk and body composition in free-living elderly participating in congregate meal-site programs. *J. Nutr. Elder.*, 2004 24(1), 53-68.

De Palo, T; Messina, G; Edefonti, A; Perfumo, F; Pisanello, L; Peruzzi, L; Di Iorio, B; Mignozzi, M; Vienna, A; Conti, G; Penza, R; Piccoli, A. Normal values of the bioelectrical impedance vector in childhood and puberty. *Nutrition*, 2000 16, 417.

Delacorte, RR; Moriguti, JC; Matos, FD; Pfrimer, K; Marchinil, JS; Ferriolli, E. Mini-nutritional assessment score and the risk for undernutrition in free-living older persons. *J. Nutr. Health Aging,* 2004 8(6), 531-534.

Després, J-P. Abdominal obesity: the most prevalent cause of the metabolic syndrome and related cardiometabolic risk. *Eur. Heart J. Suppl.,* 2006 8, 4–12.

Di Francesco, V; Zamboni, M; Zoico, E; Mazzali, G; Dioli, A; Omizzolo, F; Bissoli, L; Fantin, F; Rizzotti, P; Solerte, SB; Micciolo, R; Bosello, O. Unbalanced serum leptin and ghrelin dynamics prolong postprandial satiety and inhibit hunger in healthy elderly: another reason for the "anorexia of aging". *Am. J. Clin. Nutr.*, 2006 83(5), 1149-1152.

Donini, LM; Savina, C; Cannella, C. Eating habits and appetite control in the elderly: the anorexia of aging. *Int. Psychogeriatr.,* 2003 15(1), 73-87.

Doty, RI; Shaman, P; Applebaum, SL; Giberson, R; Siksorski, L; Rosenberg, L. Smell identification ability: changes with age. *Science,* 1984 226, 1441-1443.

Finch, S; Doyle, W; Lowe, C; Bates, CJ; Prentice, A. Smithers, G; Clarke, PC. *National Diet and Nutrition Survey: People Aged 65 Years and Over. Report of the Diet and Nutrition Survey*. London: The Stationery Office; 1998.

Forbes, GB; Reina, JC. Adult lean body mass declines with age: some longitudinal observations. *Metabolism,* 1970 19, 653 –663.

Gallagher, D; Ruts, E; Visser, M; Heshka, S; Baumgartner, RN; Wang, J; Pierson, RN; Pi-Sunyer, FX; Heymsfield, SB. Weight stability masks sarcopenia in elderly men and women. *Am. J. Physiol. Endocrinol. Metab.*, 2000 279(2), 366-375.

Gil Gregorio, P; Ramirez Diaz, SP; Ribera Casado, JM. Dementia and Nutrition. Intervention study in institutionalized patients with Alzheimer disease. *J. Nutr. Health Aging,* 2003 7, 304-308.

Gillette-Guyonnet, S; Nourhashemi, F; Andrieu, S; de Glisezinski, I; Ousset, PJ; Riviere, D; Albarede, JL; Vellas, B. Weight loss in Alzheimer disease. *Am. J. Clin. Nutr.*, 2000 71, 637–642.

Guida, B; Laccetti, R; Gerardi, C; Trio, R; Perrino, NR; Strazzullo, P; Siani, A; Farinaro, E; Colantuoni, A. Bioelectrical impedance analysis and age-related differences of body composition in the elderly. *Nutr. Metab. Cardiovasc. Dis.,* 2007 17(3), 175-80.

Guigoz, Y; Lauque, S; Vellas, BJ. Identifying the elderly at risk for malnutrition. The Mini Nutritional Assessment. *Clin. Geriatr. Med.*, 2002 18(4), 737-757.

Guigoz, Y; Vellas, B; Garry, PJ. Mini Nutritional Assessment: A practical assessment tool for grading the nutritional state of elderly patients. *Facts Res. Gerontol.*, 1994 2, 15-59.

Gupta, D; Lammersfeld, CA; Burrows, JL; Dahlk, SL; Vashi, PG; Grutsch, JF; Hoffman, S; Lis CG. Bioelectrical impedance phase angle in clinical practice: implications for prognosis in advanced colorectal cancer. *Am. J. Clin. Nutr.,* 2004 80(6), 1634-1638.

Hebuterne, X; Broussard, JF; Rampal, P. Acute renutrition by cyclic enteral nutrition in elderly and younger patients. *JAMA*, 1995 273, 638–643.

Hetherington, MM. Taste and appetite regulation in the elderly. *Proc. Nutr. Soc*, 1998 57, 625–631.

Heymsfield, SB; Williams, PJ. Nutritional assessment by clinical and biochemical methods. In: *Shils ME, Young VR editors. Modern nutrition in health and disease*. Philadelphia: Lea and Febiger; 1988, 817-860.

Hickson, M. Malnutrition and ageing. *Postgrad. Med. J.*, 2006 82, 2-8.

Hudgens, J; Langkamp-Henken, B. The Mini Nutritional Assessment as an assessment tool in elders in long-term care. *Nutr. Clin. Pract.,* 2004 19, 463-470.

Hughes, VA; Frontera, WR; Roubenoff, R; Evans, WJ; Singh, MA. Longitudinal changes in body composition in older men and women: role of body weight change and physical activity. *Am. J. Clin. Nutr.,* 2002 76(2), 473-81.

Hughes, VA; Roubenoff, R; Wood, M; Frontera, WR; Evans, WJ; Fiatarone Singh, MA. Anthropometric assessment of 10-y changes in body composition in the elderly. *Am. J. Clin. Nutr.,* 2004 80(2), 475-82.

International Federation of Clinical Chemistry; Shenkin, A; Cederblad, G; Elia, M; Isaksson, B. Laboratory assessment of protein-energy status. *Clin. Chim. Acta*, 1996 253, 5-59.

Kagansky, N; Berner, Y; Koren-Morag, N; Perelman, L; Knobler, HH; Levy, S. Poor nutritional habits are predictors of poor outcome in very old hospitalized patients. *Am. J. Clin. Nutr.,* 2005 82, 784-791.

Kanis, JA; Adami S. Bone loss in the elderly. *Osteoporos. Int.,* 1994 4, 59-65.

Knittweis, J. Weight loss precedes Alzheimer's disease symptoms: a case study. *J. Am. Geriatr. Soc.*, 1998 46, 540–541.

Kondrup, J; Allison, SP; Elia, M; Vellas, B; Plauth, M. ESPEN guidelines for nutrition screening 2002. *Clin. Nutr.,* 2003 22, 415-421.

Kucukerdonmez, O; Koksal, E; Rakicioglu, N; Pekcan, G. Assessment and evaluation of the nutritional status of the elderly using 2 different instruments. *Saudi Med. J.,* 2005 26(10), 1611-1616.

Kuk, JL; Lee, S; Heymsfield, SB; Ross, R. Waist circumference and abdominal adipose tissue distribution: influence of age and sex. *Am. J. Clin. Nutr.*. 2005 81(6), 1330-4.

Kuzuya, M; Izawa, S; Enoki, H; Okada, K; Iguchi, A. Is serum albumin a good marker for malnutrition in the physically impaired elderly? *Clin. Nutr.*, 2007 26(1), 84-90.

Kuzuya, M; Kanda, S; Koike, T; Suzuki, Y; Satake, S; Iguchi, A. Evaluation of Mini-Nutritional Assessment for Japanese frail elderly. *Nutrition*, 2005 21(4), 498-503.

Kyle, UG; Bosaeus, I; De Lorenzo, AD; Deurenberg, P; Elia, M; Manuel Gómez, J; Lilienthal Heitmann, B; Kent-Smith, L; Melchior, JC; Pirlich, M; Scharfetter, H; M W J Schols, A; Pichard, C; ESPEN. Bioelectrical impedance analysis-part II: utilization in clinical practice. *Clin. Nutr.,* 2004 23(6), 1430-53.

Kyle, UG; Genton, L; Hans, D; Karsegard, VL; Michel, JP; Slosman, DO; Pichard, C. Total body mass, fat mass, fat-free mass, and skeletal muscle in older people: cross-sectional differences in 60-year-old persons. *J. Am. Geriatr. Soc.,* 2001a 49, 1633 –1640.

Kyle, UG; Genton, L; Slosman, DO; Pichard, C. Fat-free and fat mass percentiles in 5225 healthy subjects aged 15 to 98 years. *Nutrition*, 2001b 17(7-8), 534-41.

Lohman, TG; Roche, AF; Martorell, R. Anthropometric Standardization Reference Manual. Champaign IL: Human Kinetics; 1988.

Magri, F; Borza, A; del Vecchio, S; Chytiris, S; Cuzzoni, G; Busconi, L; Rebesco, A; Ferrari, E. Nutritional assessment of demented patients: a descriptive study. *Aging Clin. Exp. Res.,* 2003 15(2), 148-153.

Morley, JE. Anorexia of aging: physiologic and pathologic. *Am. J. Clin. Nutr.*, 1997 66, 760–773.

Morley, JE; Haren, MT; Rolland, Y; Kim, MJ. Frailty. *Med. Clin. North Am.*, 2006a 90(5), 837-847.

Morley, JE; Thomas, DR; Wilson, MM. Cachexia: pathophysiology and clinical relevance. *Am. J. Clin. Nutr.*, 2006b 83(4), 735-743.

N.I.H. Bioelectrical impedance analysis in body composition measurement: National Institutes of Health Technology Assessment Conference Statement. *Am. J. Clin. Nutr.*, 1996 64(3 Suppl), 524S-532S.

Nagano, M; Suita, S; Fukuoka, TY. The validity of bioelectrical impedance phase angle for nutritional assessment in children. *J. Pediatr. Surg.* 2000 35, 1035–1039.

Norman, K; Smoliner, C; Valentini, L; Lochs, H; Pirlich, M. Is bioelectrical impedance vector analysis of value in the elderly with malnutrition and impaired functionality? *Nutrition*, 2007 23(7-8), 564-569.

Nourhashemi, F; Guyonnet, S; Ousset, PJ; Kostek, V; Lauque, S; Chumlea, WC; Vellas, B; Albarede, JL. Mini Nutritional Assessment and Alzheimer patients In: *Mini Nutritional Assessment (MNA): Research and practice in elderly.* Nestlé Clinical and performance Nutrition Workshop series. Philadelphia: Lippincott-Raven: edited by Vellas, B; Garry, PJ; Guigoz, Y, 1999; 87-91.

Novak, LP. Ageing, total body potassium, fat-free mass, and cell mass in males and females between ages 18 and 85 years. *J. Gerontol.*, 1972 27, 438 –443.

Nursal, TZ; Noyan, T; Atalay, BG; Koz, N; Karakayali, H. Simple two-part tool for screening of malnutrition. *Nutrition,* 2005 21, 659-665.

Nutrition Screening Initiative, American Academy of Family Physicians, American Dietetic Association. A physician's guide to nutrition in chronic disease management for older adults. Leawood (KS): NSI; 2002.

Ott, M; Fischer, H; Polat, H; Helm, EB; Frenz, M; Caspary, WF; Lembcke, B. Bioelectrical impedance analysis as a predictor of survival in patients with human immunodeficiency virus infection. *J. Acquir. Immune Defic. Syndr. Hum. Retrovirol.,* 1995 9, 20–25.

Payette, H; Gray-Donald, K; Cyr, R; Boutier, V. Predictors of dietary intake in a functionally dependent elderly population in the community. *Am. J. Public Health*, 1995 85, 677–683.

Persson, MD; Brismar, KE, Katzarski, KS, Nordenstrom, J; Cederholm, TE. Nutritional status using mini nutritional assessment and subjective global assessment predict mortality in geriatric patients. *J. Am. Geriatr. Soc.,* 2002 50, 1996-2002.

Piccoli, A; Nigrelli, S; Caberlotto, A; Bottazzo, S; Rossi, B; Pillon, L; Maggiore, Q. Bivariate normal values of the bioelectrical impedance vector in adult and elderly populations. *Am J. Clin. Nutr.*, 1995 61(2), 269.

Piccoli, A; Pastori, G. BIVA software. Padova: *Department of Medical and Surgical Sciences*, University of Padova; 2002.

Piccoli, A; Pillon, L; Dumler, F. Impedance vector distribution by sex, race, body mass index, and age in the United States: standard reference intervals as bivariate Z scores. *Nutrition*, 2002 18, 153-167.

Piccoli, A; Rossi, B; Pillon, L; Bucciante, G. A new method for monitoring body fluid variation by bioimpedance analysis: the RXc graph. *Kidney Int,* 1994, 46(2), 534.

Rubenstein, LZ. Development of a short version of the Mini Nutritional Assessment. In: Vellas B, Garry PJ, Guigoz Y. *Mini Nutritional Assessment (MNA): Research and practice in elderly. Nestlé Clinical and performance Nutrition Workshop series.* Philadelphia: Lippincott-Raven; 1998; 101-111.

Ruiz-Lopez, MD; Artacho, R; Oliva, P; Moreno-Torres, R; Bolanos, J; de Teresa, C; Lopez, MC. Nutritional risk in institutionalized older women determined by the Mini Nutritional Assessment test: what are the main factors? *Nutrition*, 2003 19(9), 767-771.

Saava, M; Kisper-Hint, IR. Nutritional assessment of elderly people in nursing house and at home in Tallinn. *J. Nutr. Health Aging*, 2002 6(1), 93-95.

Saletti, A; Johansson, L; Yifter-Lindgren, E, Wissing, U; Osterberg, K; Cederholm, T. Nutritional status and a 3-year follow-up in elderly receiving support at home. *Gerontology*, 2005 51, 192-198.

Saletti, A; Lindgren, EY; Johansson, L; Cederholm, T. Nutritional status according to mini nutritional assessment in an institutionalized elderly population in Sweden. *Gerontology*, 2000 46(3), 139-145.

Sanchez-Garcia, S; Garcia-Pena, C; Duque-Lopez, MX; Juarez-Cedillo, T; Cortes-Nunez, AR; Reyes-Beaman, S. Anthropometric measures and nutritional status in a healthy elderly population. *BMC Public Health*, 2007 3(7), 2.

Schiffman, SS. Taste and smell losses in normal aging and disease. *JAMA*, 1997 278(16), 1357-1362.

Schiffman, SS; Graham, BG. Taste and smell perception affect appetite and immunity in the elderly. *Eur. J. Clin. Nutr.*, 2000 54(3), 54-63.

Schwenk, A; Beisenherz, A; Römer, K; Kremer, G; Salzberger, B; Elia, M. Phase angle from bioelectrical impedance analysis remains an independent predictive marker in HIV-infected patients in the era of highly active antiretroviral treatment. *Am. J. Clin. Nutr.*, 2000 72, 496–501.

Selberg, O; Selberg, D. Norms and correlates of bioimpedance phase angle in healthy human subjects, hospitalized patients, and patients with liver cirrhosis. *Eur. J. Appl. Physiol.*, 2002 86, 509–516.

Sheehy, CM; Perry, PA; Cromwell, SL. Dehydration: biological considerations, age-related changes, and risk factors in older adults. *Biol. Res. Nurs.*, 1999 1(1), 30-37.

Shetty, PS; James, WPT. Body mass index. A measure of chronic energy deficiency in adults. *FAO Food Nutr. Pap.*, 1994 56, 1-57.

Silver, AJ; Guillen, CP; Kahl, MJ; Morley, JE. Effect of ageing on body fat. *J. Am. Geriatr. Soc.*, 1993 41, 211 –213.

Sorkin, JD; Muller, DC; Andres, R. Longitudinal change in height of men and women: implications for interpretation of the body mass index: the Baltimore Longitudinal Study of Aging. *Am. J. Epidemiol.*, 1999 150 (9), 969-977.

Spyckerelle, Y; Garillot, S; Deschamps, JP. Histoire du "poids idéal" de Lorentz. *Cah. Nutr. Diét.*, 1984, 19(6), 365-366.

Stechmiller, JK. Early nutritional screening of older adults: review of nutritional support. *J. Infus. Nurs.*, 26 2003, 170-177.

Stevens, JC; Cruz, LA; Hoffman, JM; Patterson, MQ. Taste sensitivity and aging: high incidence of decline revealed by repeated threshold measures. *Chem. Senses*, 1995, 20, 451-459.

Stewart, R; Masaki, K; Xue, QL; Peila, R; Petrovitch, H; White, LR; Launer, LJ. A 32-year prospective study of change in body weight and incident dementia: the Honolulu-Asia Aging Study. *Arch. Neurol.*, 2005 62, 55–60.

Thérond, P. Albumine. In: Vassault A. *Société Française de Biologie Clinique. Cahier de formation biochimie. Assurance qualité. Tome II.* Paris: SFBC; 1994; 61-67.

Thompson, MP; Morris, LK. Unexplained weight loss in the ambulatory elderly. *J. Am. Geriatr. Soc.,* 1991 39, 497-500.

Toso, S; Piccoli, A; Gusella, M; Menon, D; Bodoni, A; Crepaldi, G; Terrazzi, E. Altered tissue electric properties in lung cancer patients as detected by bioelectric impedance vector analysis. *Nutrition,* 2000 16(2), 120-124.

Van Nes, MC; Herrmann, FR; Gold, G; Michel, JP; Rizzoli, R. Does the mini nutritional assessment predict hospitalization outcomes in older people? *Age Ageing,* 2001 30, 221-226.

Vellas, B; Guigoz, Y; Baumgartner, M; Garry, PJ; Lauque, S; Albarede, JL. Relationships between nutritional markers and the mini-nutritional assessment in 155 older persons. *J. Am. Geriatr. Soc.*, 2000 48(10), 1300-1309.

Vellas, B; Guigoz, Y; Garry, PJ; Nourhashemi, F; Bennahum, D; Lauque, S; Albarede, JL. The Mini Nutritional Assessment (MNA) and its use in grading the nutritional state of elderly patients. *Nutrition*, 1999 15(2), 116-122.

Vellas, B; Lauque, S; Gillette-Guyonnet, S; Andrieu, S; Cortes, F; Nourhashemi, F; Cantet, C; Ousset, PJ; Grandjean, H; REAL.FR Group. Impact of nutritional status on the evolution of Alzheimer's disease and on response to acetylcholinesterase inhibitor treatment. *J. Nutr. Health Aging*, 2005 9(2), 75-80.

Wells, JL; Dumbrell, AC. Nutrition and aging: assessment and treatment of compromised nutritional status in frail elderly patients. *Clin. Int. Aging, 2006 1(1), 67-79.*

White, H; Pieper, C; Schmader, K. The association of weight change in Alzheimer's disease with severity of disease and mortality: a longitudinal analysis. *J. Am. Geriatr. Soc.*, 1998b 46, 1223–1227.

White, H; Pieper, C; Schmader, K; Fillenbaum, G. A longitudinal analysis of weight change in Alzheimer's disease. *J. Am. Geriatr Soc.*, 1997 45, 531–532.

White, H; Pieper, C; Schmader, K; Fillenbaum, GJ. Weight change in Alzheimer's disease. *J. Am. Geriatr. Soc.*, 1998a 46, 540–541.

Wilson, MM; Morley, JE. Invited review: Aging and energy balance. *J. Appl. Physiol.,* 2003 95(4), 1728-1736.

Wirth, R; Miklis, P. Bioelectric impedance analysis in the diagnosis of malnutrition. *Z. Gerontol. Geriatr.*, 2005 8(5), 315-21.

Wolf-Klein, GP; Silverstone, FA. Weight loss in Alzheimer's disease: an international review of the literature. *Int. Psychogeriatr.*, 1994 6, 135–142.

World Health Organization. Obesity: preventing and managing the global epidemic. Report on a WHO consultation. *Geneva: WHO Tech. Rep. Ser.*, No. 894; 2000.

World Health Organization. Physical status: the use and interpretation of anthropometry. Report of a WHO Expert Committee. *Geneva: WHO Tech. Rep. Ser.*, No. 854; 1995.

Zamboni, M; Zoico, E; Scartezzini, T; Mazzali, G; Tosoni, P; Zivelonghi, A; Gallagher, D; De Pergola, G; Di Francesco, V; Bosello, O. Body composition changes in stable-weight elderly subjects: the effect of sex. *Aging Clin. Exp. Res.*, 2003 15(4), 321-7.

In: Nutrition for the Middle Aged and Elderly ISBN: 978-1-60456-146-3
Editors: N. E. Bernhardt, A. M. Kasko, pp. 235-252

Chapter VII

Rationale to Integrate Nutritional Aspect in the Comprehensive Geriatric Assessment

Thierry Pepersack*
Geriatrics, Hópital Erasme, Université Libre de Bruxelles, Belgium

Abstract

We first propose a definition of the "geriatric patient" and a holistic management of his multiple dimensions using a "comprehensive geriatric assessment". Then the nutritional status of the geriatric patient was described. We review data from the literature which showed that malnutrition represents a cardinal symptom of frailty in older persons. We underscored the importance of an early detection of malnutrition and we stressed on the fact that geriatricians should increase their vigilance to detect early weight loss and institute-appropriate preventive and health promotion measures. In view of this preoccupant malnutrition, a quality programs are proposed to improve nutritional status of the geriatric patients. A comprehensive screening tool for assessment of nutritional status is needed that is clinically relevant and cost-effective to perform. If malnutrition is suggested by such screening tests, then they should be supplemented by conventional nutritional assessment before treatment is planned.

Introduction

This paper gives an overview of the recently published literature concerning the concept of comprehensive geriatric assessment. The rationale to integrate nutritional assessment in the comprehensive geriatric assessment is pointed out.

* Corresponding author : Thierry PEPERSACK, Geriatrics, Hôpital Erasme, Université Libre de Bruxelles, 808 route de Lennik, 1070 Bruxelles, Belgium. Tel: +32.2.5553806. Fax: +32.2.5553211. E-mail : tpepersa@alb.ac.be

The «Geriatric Patient»: A Proposition of Definition

The increase of the average human lifespan due to the improvement of the social, and sanitary conditions, as well as the development of the medical sciences, has led to the apparition of a growing cohort of « very old » subjects (Mayence et al. 2000).

The majority of these very old people has gone through an aging process without major problems (Pepersack 2000a, Pepersack 2004). Others who reach a very old age, however, are more vulnerable and present a so called « geriatric » profile. How can this "geriatric" profile be defined? In Table 1 some of the characteristics of the typical geriatric patient are presented.

Decreased homeostasis represents the low defense margins of the somatic functions. The example of the decreased awareness of thirst is well known and is associated with an increased mortality during heat waves.

The *atypical presentation* of the diseases confers a risk of delayed recognition of the disease leading to increased risk of complication and mortality. Beside the age-related altered physiological mechanisms, the attitudes of the caregivers may also be dangerous: symptoms are often attributed to age itself. This complex phenomenon is probably due to a different perception of old adults or to their fear to be hospitalized; this may lead to symptoms being minimized or even concealed.

« *Polypathology* » is another characteristic of the geriatric patient. Many of these diseases may be chronic in nature. Cardiovascular diseases are common but also degenerative osteo-articular (osteoporosis and osteoarthrosis) and cerebral diseases (dementia, Parkinson, etc.) commonly occur.

Polypathology leads to another characteristic of the geriatric patient which is his *functional dependence* for the instrumental and/or basic activities of daily living (Pepersack 1997, Pepersack et al. 1998a, Pepersack et al. 1998b, Duez et al. 2003). We observed that less than 30 percent of the patients of our unit were able to eat without any help (Pepersack et al. 1998b).

The *psychosocial* evaluation should be a cornerstone of the geriatric patient's assessment. Indeed, the geriatric patient is often confronted to major events in his life (bereavement, moving house, institutionalization, etc.). Depression and anxiety disorders are common and may be a cause of increasing dependence (Pepersack and Bastan 2000, Pepersack et al. 2005).

Table 1. Characteristics of the « geriatric» patient

1.	Decreased homeostasis
2.	Atypical presentations of the diseases
3.	Multiple pathologies and functional dependencies
4.	Combination of somatic, psychological and social factors
5.	Altered pharmacokinetics

Polypharmacy is the rule. However, few data are available for the use of drugs for the geriatric patient. All the geriatric characteristics are often to be found among the exclusion criteria for enrolment into a randomized controlled trial. Therefore, very few data are available to guide a geriatrician about the best way to manage e.g. an 85 year old patient presenting a combination of e.g. diabetes, osteoporosis, hypertension, renal failure, visual disorders, urinary incontinence, and depression associated with social retirement... Nevertheless, this situation is common in the geriatric units. Moreover, any prescription of medication should take into account: polymedication, age-related altered body composition, low serum albumin level, decreased renal and/or liver metabolisation and/or excretion, and drugs interactions. The problem of polypharmacy (both iatrogenous and self-medication) is complex and results from multiple actors (relatives, family, pharmacist, practitioners, etc.…). Interventional programmes in order to reduce polypharmacy (Kelly 1986) stress on the usefullness of a systematic monthly review of therapeutics for all old institutionalized subjects. Polypharmacy is also a risk factor for malnutrition.

Finally, the geriatric patient either is at high *risk of malnutrition* or presents severe malnutrition (Gazzotti et al. 2000). The recognition and the correction of malnutrition is an important step to help the patient to recover health (Pepersack et al. 2002, Pepersack 2002, Pepersack 2005, Pepersack 2007).

The Concept of "Comprehensive Geriatric Assessment"

In view of these multiples dimensions of the geriatric patient, an holistic approach seems to be useful: it is the concept of the « comprehensive geriatric assessment ».

For vulnerable elderly patients, hospitalization can be hazardous (Becker et al. 1987, Hirsh et al. 1990, Creditor 2003). Too often their treatment is complicated by delirium (Pepersack 2005b), depression, adverse drug reactions, poor nutrition (Pepersack 2005a), and loss of physical strength. Often e.g. their pneumonia is cured or their hip fractures repaired, but they never regain the independence they had previously to the acute event. Over the past 15 years, programs in geriatrics have been developed at most American medical centres with the prime clinical mission to achieve better results for hospitalized, high-risk elderly patients. There are two main strategies. One is to admit older patients at risk to a specialized unit for acute or post-acute care (Rubenstein et al. 1984, Appelgate et al. 1990). The other is to provide an out patient assessment, usually by an interdisciplinary team. Geriatric assessments have been evaluated in many controlled trials. Landefeld et al. (1995) showed that there are benefits from having a specially designed acute care unit, but Reuben et al. (1995) found little benefit from comprehensive geriatric consultation. The interpretation of these two studies is complicated and sometimes contradictory.

More than twenty years ago, Rubenstein reported on the astonishing effectiveness of a geriatric evaluation and management unit (Rubenstein 1984). In that randomized trial, conducted in the Sepulveda Veterans Administration Medical Centre, the patients assigned to the geriatric unit had improved functional status, fewer discharges to nursing homes, and much lower mortality at one year (24 percent, as compared with 48 percent for the controls). These results raised high expectations and have affected the interpretation of all subsequent trials of clinical geriatric programs in the USA. It must be remembered however that in this study screening selected only one patient out of twelve, that the intervention group stayed on average 36 days longer in the hospital, and that the geriatric team later directed much of the outpatient management. Most of the differences in mortality emerged after the initial hospital stay. As the authors of this often-cited study said of the marked reduction in mortality, "There seems to be no simple explanation for this outcome" (Rubenstein 1984). It remains possible that the large differences were partly due to chance or even to management errors in the relatively small control group (only 60 patients). Nonetheless, there is reason to believe that any geriatric intervention that improves strength and functional independence may reduce mortality (Appelgate et al 1990, Guralnik et al 1995).

As in other geriatric interventions, use of the specialized acute care unit in the study by Landefeld et al (1995) emphasized rehabilitation, independence in self-care, detailed planning for home discharge, and avoidance of iatrogenic illness. Few patients were excluded from this study, so the results should apply widely. Even though care in the separate, specialized unit began from the day of admission, there was no difference in mortality either while the patients were in the hospital or three months later. The extra efforts did produce some improvements in function. At discharge, 34 percent of the intervention group had improved, and only 16 percent were worse in performing the basic activities of daily living; in the usual-care group, 24 percent improved and 21 percent got worse. In the intervention group, 14 percent were discharged to nursing homes or other institutions, as compared with 22 percent in the usual-care group. It has to be noted that in demonstration studies there is great pressure to avoid discharges to nursing homes, and clinicians may take extra risks in sending home some patients who are quite impaired. Hence, it is reassuring that the subsequent rates of nursing home admission were comparable for the two groups during the three-month follow-up. In the intervention group the greatest improvements were in the patients' ability to bathe and dress themselves, and the scores for global health status were significantly higher. At three months, however, there were no differences between the two groups. If the geriatrics team had directed the patients' care longitudinally, greater differences might have emerged over time.

Although none of the outcomes from the special care unit are dramatic, the gains are admirable and clinically valuable, particularly the reduction in discharges to nursing homes. Some would argue that patients should be screened so that this intervention could be directed to those who are most vulnerable, which might make the outcomes more impressive. However, screening and selection are tricky tasks. The most impaired are easy to identify, but they also generally have less potential for improvement. Since the costs were no greater for the special unit, it would be wise to apply this model widely. Moreover, there should be some benefits to all patients that do not show up in the outcome measures: improved safety, greater motivation, better compliance, and the reassurance that comes from close attention to the details of how to return home after an acute illness. Clearly, the patients themselves felt they were in better health after this short, one-week program. Improvement in the well-being of patients and their satisfaction is of value in itself.

Many geriatric programs offer a consultation assessment service, although the details of this intervention vary from one program to the other. Such services follow in the tradition of medical consultation and are relatively easy to set up, since there are no struggles over the control of hospital beds. The hope has been that a geriatric consultation team could deliver some of the benefits seen with the inpatient evaluation units. Some even expressed the hope that such assessments might have the impact and power of a new technological advance

(Epstein et al. 1987). The study by Reuben et al (1995) involved four hospitals and 2353 at-risk patients in a health maintenance organization, of whom 1337 were assigned randomly to undergo a comprehensive assessment by a social worker, nurse practitioner, and geriatrician. These consultants often recommended rehabilitation programs, adjustments in medications, and additional diagnostic tests, and most of the recommendations were implemented. Nonetheless, over the follow-up period of one year there were no differences in survival between the groups and no consistent or convincing improvement in the functional status of those who received the geriatric consultation. This was a large study, carefully performed experienced geriatrics. Several earlier studies also could not demonstrate any major difference in outcomes after geriatric consultations (Campion et al. 1983, McVey et al. 1989, Fretwell et al. 1990, Winograd et al. 1993).

Do these negative results mean that geriatric consultations are ineffective and should be discouraged and not paid for? In the study by Reuben et al., with so many consultations being conducted, physicians may have become quite familiar with the geriatricians' advice and applied it to the benefit of all their patients, including those in the control group. In research design this problem is known as contamination. In addition, some benefits of consultation are difficult to measure, particularly in a large, heterogeneous population. More important, it is unrealistic to expect major differences in outcomes from a single consultation, especially when the geriatric team does not control the care that will have to follow (Cohen et al. 1989).

Geriatric assessment is a diagnostic, not a therapeutic, intervention, and by itself cannot cure chronic disease or reverse disability (Solomon 1988). The data do show that geriatric consultations should not be mandatory or expected to produce remarkable improvements. These bedside consultations are not a form of technology, and we should not be as severe in judging them as we are in evaluating e.g. a surgical procedure or the use of a monoclonal antibody. The appropriate measure of the value of a consultation is the opinion of those who request it and those who receive it. The physicians, nurses, family, and patient may well see value in the way an experienced geriatrics team helps with complicated problems such as incontinence, confusion, immobility, and complex drug interactions.

These studies concern geriatric interventions that are safe, cheap, and sensible and that can help vulnerable elderly patients. Moreover, both approaches have additional value for education and quality assurance, and as prerequisites to future discoveries that will protect functional independence better (Pepersack 2005, Pepersack et al. 2007a, 2007b). A further value of both studies is that they encourage physicians to look beyond the laboratory results to see how people live and cope with the hazards of disease.

The aim this papers is to stress on the importance to detect malnutrition and to propose intervention to improve the nutritional care among geriatric patients. Unintentional weight loss and malnutrition represent a cardinal symptom of frailty in older persons (Fried et al. 2001, Gillick et al. 2001, Zuliani et al. 2001, Newman et al 2001, Bortz 2002, Morley et al 2002). Even a small decline in body mass in older persons is associated with mortality (Reynish W et al. 2001, Newman et al 2001). Protein energy malnutrition is associated with anemia, pressure ulcers, sarcopenia, bone loss and hip fractures, declining immune function, impaired immune response to vaccinations, infections, cognitive impairment, functional decline, and poor quality of life (MacIntosh et al. 2000, Chao et al. 2002, Amarantos et al. 2001, Drewnowski et al. 2001, Thomas 2001a, Thomas 2001b, Coleman et al. 2002,

McElhaney et al. 2002, Wouters-Wesseling et al. 2002). Weight loss is a sentinel event in long-term care facilities and associated with particularly poor outcomes (Morley et al. 1995, Thomas et al. 2002). Despite this, aggressive nutritional management when weight loss is well established is often not associated with improved outcomes (Borum et al. 2000, Callahan et al. 2000, Gessert et al. 2000, Mitchell et al. 2000, Ahronhein et al. 2001). For this reason, it is important that geriatricians increase their understanding of the pathophysiological processes that underlie weight loss in older persons (Morley 2001) and increase their vigilance to detect early weight loss and institute-appropriate preventive and health promotion measures (Morley et al. 2000, Chernoff 2001).

Nutritional Status of the Geriatric Patient

What Does It Mean to Be "At Nutritional Risk"?

Most clinical nutritionists would agree that in the care of sick or frail elderly patients, nutrition and hydration often rank far too low on the list of evaluation and treatment priorities. In hospitals, nursing homes (McWhirter et al. 1994, Morley et al. 1995) and in the community, elderly patients may receive a variety of costly and complex medical interventions, eg, extensive drug therapy (Flaherty et al. 2000) and mechanical ventilatory support (Montuclard et al. 2000), while the routine availability of adequate food and fluids is neglected.

The following tables resume the prevalence of malnutrition in hospital, in geriatric wards and in institutions:

Hospitalized patients

	year	N=	%
Kyle	**2005**	**1707**	**51**
Pichard	**2004**	**996**	**46**
Wyszynski	**2003**	**1000**	**48**
Waitzberg	**2001**	**4000**	**48**
Kyle	**2001**	**995**	**38**
McWhirter	**1994**	**300**	**45**
McWhirter	**1994**	**300**	**45**
Coats	**1993**	**228**	**38**
Larsson	**1993**	**382**	**29**
Reilly	**1988**	**365**	**59**
Robinson	**1987**	**100**	**56**
Bistrian	**1980**	**251**	**44**
Σ		***10858***	***46***

Geriatric Hospitalized patients			
Pepersack	2005	1139	30-60*
Wyszynski	2003	466	50-76**
Kyle	2002	172	61
Σ		*1177*	

*60% at risk and 30% presenting overt malnutrition. ** >60 y: 50; > 70 y: 53, > 80 y: 77 %.

Institutions

	Year	**N=**	**%**
Shaver	**1980**	**115**	**85%**
Pinchocofsky-Devin	**1987**	**227**	**52%**
Silver	**1988**	**130**	**23%**
Thomas	**1991**	**61**	**54%**
Larson	**1991**	**501**	**29%**
Nelson	**1993**	**100**	**39%**
Wright	**1993**	**309**	**51%**
Abbasi	**1993**	**2811**	**28%**
Morley	**1994**	**185**	**15%**
Blaum	**1995**	**6832**	**10%**
Σ		***11971***	

Why is nutrition not more clearly recognized as a priority for the elderly by health professionals other than nutritionists? The need for nutritional assessment and intervention is particularly crucial in this age group, in whom the incidence of chronic illness is high and a myriad of socioeconomic factors enhance the likelihood of malnutrition (Barrocas et al. 1995). In the search for an answer to this question, let us consider the terminology used to express the findings of nutritional status studies of the elderly (and other age groups, for that matter). The findings of these studies often indicate that the elderly subjects are "at nutritional risk" or "at risk of malnutrition." As nutritionists, we all have an idea of what being at nutritional risk means. But, as evidenced in the literature, although we agree that this is an important issue, we do not always agree about its exact interpretation (Sahyoun et al. 1997) or implications. For some, being at risk of malnutrition is different from actually being malnourished: being malnourished certainly sounds worse than being at risk of it. Others think that these two terms are one and the same. It is not too surprising, then, that our counterparts in the clinic sometimes pay too little attention to nutrition. When compared with the many serious diseases already established and diagnosed in elderly patients, being at risk of malnutrition sounds less than urgent.

The terminology of nutritional risk can also cause difficulties in certain research situations, especially when nutritionists collaborate with clinical investigators from other disciplines. That a particular demographic or physiologic factor might increase or decrease the risk of being at nutritional risk can be a difficult concept to convey, and the selection of statistical methods can be hampered by the seemingly circular logic.

In addition, there is sometimes a lack of consistency in the interpretation of results from different tools used for nutritional screening and assessment in the published literature. For example, although some groups have used the DETERMINE checklist from the Nutrition Screening Initiative to assess nutritional risk (MacLellan et al. 1998), it is generally not considered to be a clinical diagnostic tool (Posner et al. 1993). The checklist is intended mainly to provide education and to increase awareness of nutritional problems in the elderly and thus may not be a particularly good predictor of health outcomes related to nutritional status (Sahyoun et al. 1997). In fact, several different instruments have been developed for the assessment of nutritional risk [eg, the Mini Nutritional Assessment (Vellas et al. 1999), and the Nutritional Risk Assessment Scale (Nikolaus T et al. 1995)], and all are used more or less interchangeably in the literature to detect risk, although they obviously differ in the data collected.

Jensen et al. (2001) reported the results of a study of nutritional risk in the elderly, noting the importance of using nutrition assessment instruments according to their intended purpose and the need for validation testing of these screening tools. They commented that screening tools "are being used in capacities that far exceed those for which they were originally intended" and recommended that the ability of these tools to predict health and nutrition outcomes should be more thoroughly tested. Their study was designed to determine whether elderly subjects found to be at nutritional risk were likely to have poor health outcomes within the subsequent year. They compared the ability of the Level II Nutrition Screen and that of the Probability of Repeated Admission (P_{ra}) questionnaire to predict a recognized marker of poor health outcomes—repeated hospital admissions—in 386 enrollees in a Medicare managed-risk health plan. The Level II Nutrition Screen, from the Nutrition Screening Initiative, was developed to compliment the DETERMINE checklist by providing a more comprehensive nutritional assessment for use in medical settings. The P_{ra} was developed especially to assess the likelihood of hospitalization in older persons and was previously tested for reliability and validity.

The results of the study by Jensen et al showed that the Level II Nutrition Screen predicted future hospitalization with an effectiveness comparable with that of the P_{ra}. Moreover, subjects with a high P_{ra} score were more likely to have lost weight and to report consuming special diets. The authors concluded that regardless of the screening approach selected, answers to questions about eating problems, weight loss, and special diets help to predict future hospital admissions in the elderly and should be included in health screenings. In addition, these results underscore the clinical importance of being at nutritional risk and thus help to establish a clearer meaning of the term. The findings provide supporting evidence that nutritional risk should also be considered to be a serious health risk. Certainly, more work of this type, in different and larger populations, is needed to help define the implications of a high nutritional risk and to ensure that the term is recognized as a valid predictor of health outcomes.

We should not necessarily discourage the application of any particular screening tool or abandon the use of the term *nutritional risk*. The term is embedded in the nutrition and aging literature and is unlikely to be given up. We need to establish a clear and widely held understanding of the descriptive terms commonly used to indicate nutritional status and then to use these terms as specifically as possible. Moreover, studies like the one by Jensen et al.

can help to explain and confirm the extent of health endangerment that the condition of nutritional risk may contribute and thus, it is hoped, increase recognition of this problem in the elderly.

Nutritional Intervention Studies in Elderly People: Importance of a Comprehensive Geriatric Assessment

Malnutrition is a major risk factor for mortality in elderly people (Sullivan et al. 1991, Lipski et al. 1993, Morley et al. 1995, Wallace 1995). It may also worsen the progression of several age-related diseases. Data from the different surveys recently conducted in Europe reveal that over 25% of the non-institutionalized population has a lower-than-recommended intake, corresponding to 1700 kcal/day for women and 2100 kcal/day for men. When Mini Nutritional Assessment (MNA) is used, low percentages of malnutrition (1%, range 0%–2% with MNA < 17) are found among the general population, but 29% (range 15%–44%) present nutritional risk criteria (23.5 > MNA > 17) (Vellas et al. 1999, Moreiras et al. 1991, Wallace 1995, Christensson et al. 2002, Thomas et al. 2002, Margetts et al. 2003). In hospitals or nursing homes, such nutritional risk may affect 20% to 60% of the population; and 25% (range 10%–32%) are considered as undernourished (MNA < 17). Comparable conclusions were reached using the criteria of the Malnutrition Advisory Group in the United Kingdom (Margetts et al. 2003). We found 30% of hospitalized geriatric patients presenting a MNA < 17 (Pepersack et al. 2002, Pepersack 2005)

Such protein-energy malnutrition should be detected as soon as possible to initiate interventions to prevent any further decrease in weight (Posner et al 1993, Morley et al. 1995, Payette et al. 1995). Once established, this malnutrition state must be corrected by appropriate diet, supplementation, artificial nutrition, or therapeutic treatment. If carried out well, these interventions should reduce the risk of mortality and, for some diseases such as degenerative diseases, may postpone morbidity and dependence (Delmi et al. 1990, Akner et al. 2001)

The efficiency of nutritional interventions has already been evaluated by different means including measurement of anthropometric and laboratory parameters. However, in the absence of any consensus on the use of these parameters, comparison between studies and even effectiveness of the proposed treatment are frequently unconvincing. It may be that an apparent absence of effect in some studies was merely linked to an inappropriate choice of parameters—with confusing results.

To overcome this lack of standardization in protocols and outcomes in nutritional interventions in elderly people, a minimum data set should be proposed. This was the goal of a Task Force of international experts from Europe, the United States, and Japan, joined by the International Association of Gerontology and International Academy of Nutrition and Aging. Analysis of the literature was performed to identify the most common markers used in epidemiologic studies on malnutrition and nutritional interventions in elderly persons. The relevance of these parameters for establishing a minimum data set was detailed during three consecutive meetings with experts over a period of 3 months to reach a consensus (Salva et al. 2004).

Minimum Data Set

A majority of experts in nutrition stated that parameters for a minimum data set have to fulfil a number of criteria taking into account the feasibility of measurements under most conditions, low time-consuming or resource-consuming, and a high probability of being affected by nutritional intervention. In addition, the population of patients at the beginning of the intervention must be carefully described to allow further comparisons between studies and allow meta-analysis.

- Birth date and gender.
- Education level, characterized by the number of years at school or university.
- Social status (live alone or with family) as well as income are relevant to describe the initial population. These parameters are likely to interfere with nutritional habits and compliance with interventions.
- *Anthropometry.* The body measurement protocol must be standardized using accepted World Health Organization criteria measurements. Equipment accuracy and sensitivity have to be recorded. Baseline body weight should be recorded before starting the intervention to allow stratification of further evolution including stable body weight, weight loss, or weight gain. Weight has to be measured at timely intervals during the study to determine the trends.
- *Body Mass Index (BMI).* The body mass index (weight/height squared) suffers from the same difficulties as the measurements previously mentioned for body weight assessment (Chumlea et al. 1992, Chumlea et al. 1998). Height measurements may be difficult in elderly people but can be calculated from the height from the heel to the knee. Knee–heel length (knee-height) has been suggested as a surrogate measurement by using the equation of Chumlea and Guo (Chumlea et al. 1992) to calculate standing height. However, these equations were derived from healthy North American people. Attention will be paid to the variability of BMI standards according to ethnic and social subset of populations.
- *Mini Nutritional Assessment (MNA) and its Short Form (MNA-SF).* The MNA was developed to assess the nutritional status of the at-risk elderly population (Guigoz et al. 1996, Chumlea et al. 1998, Beck et al. 1998, Vellas et al. 2000, Guigoz et al. 2002,). This scale includes 18 items covering anthropometric measurements, risk situation, dietary survey, and self-perception of health. The maximum score is 30, and the threshold for normality is 23.5. A score below 17 is indicative of malnutrition, and intermediate values between 17 and 23.5 are indicative of nutritional risk. It is a relatively simple and quick test that is not time consuming. Over the past few years, several studies with different levels of care and clinical conditions have included the MNA and have validated its reliability by comparison with other nutritional markers. The results of the shortened version with 6 of the 18 initial items were highly correlated with those of the full MNA (Rubenstein et al. 2001). A score of 12 or more on the MNA-SF reflects a satisfactory nutritional status. A score of 11 or less suggests a risk of malnutrition and calls for full assessment. If

not all of the anthropometric parameters are available, at least the MNA-SF is recommended.

- *Functional Status.* Different available scales have to be used to define the population under study and to test possible changes in functional status due to nutritional interventions: Instrumental and basic Activities of Daily Living (IADL and ADL, respectively) measure the ability to perform daily life activities such as feeding, washing, dressing, walking, and determining mobility and the occurrence of incontinence (Katz et al. 1962, Katz et al. 1970, Pepersack et al. 1998a, Pepersack et al. 1998b).
- Geriatric Depression Scale (GDS), a 15-item version test for screening depressive symptoms and their severity in elderly persons (Yesavage et al. 1983, Neal et al. 1994, Van Marwijk et al. 1995, Pepersack et al. 2001).
- Folstein's Mini-Mental State Examination (MMSE) is used to evaluate cognitive function and to identify dementia and Alzheimer's disease (Folstein et al. 1975). Impaired cognitive function, which is quite frequent in elderly people, is a clear risk for malnutrition.
- Gait and balance are additional parameters. Within a study, investigators have to choose to use consistently either "the timed chair stand" or a "timed 4-meter walk" (Tinetti et al. 1986, Bischoff et al. 2003). They should use standardized measurements from a written protocol, whichever measurement they choose, and should plan to do periodic quality controls during the study.
- R*elevant Current Medical Conditions (Comorbidity).* Every acute and chronic disease that constitutes a malnutrition risk in elderly people or that would impair the effectiveness of any nutritional intervention have to be recorded.
- *Care and Medication.* Different levels of care may be defined. It is recommended to stratify patients on the basis of their health status and their residence at the initiation of the study. Any medical cotreatment will be recorded, with the number and kinds of major prescribed drugs. This also applies to over-the-counter or enriched foods, which could interfere with nutritional assessment, such as vitamin or other self-administered oral supplements.

A limited number of items are proposed to be used in every study on nutritional intervention in elderly people. They concern tools from the comprehensive geriatric assessment (Pepersack 2007).

Conclusion

Malnutrition among geriatric patient could be an important part of his frailty. Screening for malnutrition and his causes should be systematically integrate in comprehensive geriatric assessment. Quality programs in order to promote nutritional approach and interventions should be implemented according to guildelines with respect of ethical considerations (Pepersack 2003, 2005, 2007, Volkert et al. 2006).

References

Abbasi AA, Rudman D. Observations on the prevalence of protein-calorie undernutrition in VA nursing homes. *J. Am. Geriatr. Soc.* 1993; 41:117-121.

Ahronhein JC, Mulvihill M, Sieger C, Park P, Fries BE. State practice variations in the use of tube feeding for nursing home residents with severe cognitive impairment. *J. Am. Geriatr. Soc.* 2001; 49: 148-152.

Akner G, Cederholm T. Treatment of protein-energy malnutrition in chronic non-malignant disorders. *Am. J. Nutr.* 2001; 74: 6-24.

Amarantos E, Martinez A, Dwyer J. Nutrition and quality of life in older adults. *J. Gerontol.* 2001; 56: (Special Issue 2): 54-64.

Applegate WB, Miller ST, Graney MJ, Elam JT, Burns R, Akins DE. A randomized, controlled trial of a geriatric assessment unit in a community rehabilitation hospital. *N. Engl. J. Med.* 1990; 322: 1572-1578.

Barrocas A, Belcher D, Champagne C, Jastram C. Nutrition assessment: practical approaches. *Clin. Geriatr. Med.* 1995; 11: 675–713.

Beck AM, Ovesen L, Osler M. The "Mini Nutritional Assessment" (MNA) and the "Determine Your Nutritional Health" Checklist (NSI Checklist) as predictors of morbidity and mortality in an elderly Danish population. *Br. J. Nutr.* 1999; 81: 31-36.

Becker PM, McVey LJ, Saltz CC, Feussner JR, Cohen HJ. Hospital-acquired complications in a randomized controlled clinical trial of a geriatric consultation team. *JAMA* 1987; 257: 2313-2317.

Bischoff HA, Stahelin HB, Monsch AU, Iversen MD, Weyh A, von Dechend M, Akos R, Conzelmann M, Dick W, Theiler R. Identifying a cut-off point for normal mobility: a comparison of the timed "up and go" test in community-dwelling and institutionalised elderly women. *Age Ageing* 2003; 32: 315-320.

Blaum CS, Fries BE, Fiatarone MA. Factors associated with low body mass index and weight loss in nursing home residents. *J. Gerontol. Med. Sci.* 1995;50A:M162-M168.

Bortz WM II. A conceptual framework of frailty: a review. *J. Gerontol. Med. Sci.* 2002; 57A:M283-M288.

Borum ML, Lynn J, Zhong ZS, Roth K, Connors AF Jr, Desbiens NA, Phillips RS, Dawson NV. The effect of nutritional supplementation on survival in seriously ill hospitalized adults: an evaluation of the SUPPORT data. *J. Am. Geriatr. Soc* 2000; 48: (5 Suppl S): S33-S38.

Callahan CM, Haag KM, Weinberger M, Tierney WM, Buchanan NN, Stump TE, Nisi R. Outcomes of percutaneous endoscopic gastrostomy among older adults in a community setting. *J. Am. Geriatr. Soc.* 2000; 48: 1048-1054.

Campion EW, Jette A, Berkman B. An interdisciplinary geriatric consultation service: a controlled trial. *J. Am. Geriatr. Soc.* 1983; 31: 792-796.

Chao D, Espeland MA, Farmer D, Register TC, Lenchik L, Applegate WB, Ettinger WH Jr. Effect of voluntary weight loss on bone mineral density in older overweight women. *J. Am. Geriat. Soc.* 2000; 48: 753-759.

Chernoff R. Nutrition and health promotion in older adults. *J. Gerontol.* 2001; 56: (Special Issue 2) 47-53.

Christensson L, Unosson M, Ek AC. Evaluation of nutritional assessment techniques in elderly people newly admitted to municipal care. *Eur. J. Clin. Nutr.* 2002; 56: 810-818.

Chumlea WC, Guo SS, Wholihan K, Cockram D, Kuczmarski RJ, Johnson CL. Stature prediction equations for elderly non-Hispanic white, non-Hispanic black, and Mexican-American persons developed from NHANES III data. *J. Am. Diet. Assoc.* 1998; 98: 137-142.

Chumlea WC, Guo SS. Equations for predicting stature in white and black elderly individuals. *J. Gerontology A Biol. Sci. Med. Sci.* 1992; 47A: M197-M203.

Coats KG, Morgan SL, Bartolucci AA, Weinsier RL. Cohen HJ, Feussner JR. Comprehensive geriatric assessment: mission not yet accomplished. *J Gerontol.* 1989; 44: M175-M177.

Coleman EA, Martau JM, Lin MK, Kramer AM. Pressure ulcer prevalence in long-term nursing home residents since the implementation of OBRA '87. *J. Am. Geriatr. Soc.* 2002; 50: 728-732.

Creditor M. Hazards of hospitalization of the elderly. *Ann. Intern. Med.* 1993; 118: 219-223.

Delmi M, Rapin CH, Bengoa J-M, Delmas PD, Vasey H, Bonjour J-P. Dietary supplementation in elderly patients with fractured neck of the femur. *Lancet* 1990; 335: 1013-1016.

Drewnowski A, Evans WJ. Nutrition, physical activity, and quality of life in older adults: summary. *J. Gerontol.* 2001; 56: (Special Issue 2): 89-94.

Duez M, Solis S, Benoit F, Martin Martinez M, Pegnyemb M, Simonetti C, Pepersack T. Prevention of falls in the elderly and physiotherapy. *Rev. Med. Brux.* 2003; 24: A223-30.

Epstein AM, Hall JA, Besdine R, Cumella E Jr, Feldstein M, McNeil BJ, Rowe JW. The emergence of geriatric assessment units: the "new technology of geriatrics." *Ann. Intern. Med.* 1987;106:299-303.

Flaherty JH, Perry HM 3rd, Lynchard GS, Morley JE. Polypharmacy and hospitalization among older home care patients. *J. Gerontol. A Biol. Sci. Med. Sci.* 2000; 55: M554–9.

Folstein MF, Folstein S, McHuth PR. Mini-Mental State: a practical method for grading the cognitive state of patients for the clinician. *J. Psychiatr. Res.* 1975;12:189-198.

Fretwell MD, Raymond PM, McGarvey ST, Owens N, Traines M, Silliman RA, Mor V. The Senior Care Study: a controlled trial of a consultative/unit-based geriatric assessment program in acute care. *J. Am. Geriatr. Soc.* 1990; 38: 1073-1081.

Fried LP, Tangen CM, Walston J, Newman AB, Hirsch C, Gottdiener J, Seeman T, Tracy R, Kop WJ, Burke G, McBurnie MA, Cardiovascular Health Study Collaborative Research Group. Frailty in older adults: evidence for a phenotype. *J. Gerontol. Med. Sci.* 2001; 56A: M146-M156.

Gazzotti C., Albert A., Pepinster A., Petermans J. Clinical usefulness of the mini nutritional assessment (MNA) scale in geriatric medicine. *J. Nutr. Health Aging* 2000; 4: 176-81.

Gessert CE, Mosier MC, Brown EF, Frey B. Tube feeding in nursing home residents with severe and irreversible cognitive impairment. *J. Am. Geriat. Soc.* 2000; 48: 1593-1600.

Gillick M. Pinning down frailty. *J. Gerontol. Med. Sci.* 2001; 56A: M134-M135.

Guigoz Y, Vellas B, Garry PJ. Assessing the nutritional status of the elderly: the Mini Nutritional Assessment as part of the geriatric evaluation. *Nutr. Rev.* 1996; 54: S59-S65.

Guigoz Y, Lauque S, Vellas B. Identifying the elderly at risk for malnutrition. The Mini Nutritional Assessment. *Clin. Geriatr. Med.* 2002; 18: 737-757.

Guralnik JM, Ferrucci L, Simonsick EM, Salive ME, Wallace RB. Lower-extremity function in persons over the age of 70 years as a predictor of subsequent disability. *N. Engl. J. Med.* 1995; 332: 556-561.

Hirsch CH, Sommers L, Olsen A, Mullen L, Winograd CH. The natural history of functional morbidity in hospitalized older patients. *J. Am. Geriatr. Soc.* 1990; 38: 1296-1303.

Hospital-associated malnutrition: a reevaluation 12 years later. *J. Am. Diet Assoc.* 1993; 93: 27-33.

Jensen GL, Friedmann JM, Coleman CD, Smiciklas-Wright H. Screening for hospitalization and nutritional risks among community-dwelling older persons. *Am. J. Clin. Nutr.* 2001; 74: 201–5.

Katz S, Ford AD, Moskowitz RW, Jackson BA, Jaffe MW. Studies of illness in the aged. The index of ADL: a standardized measure of biological and psychosocial function. *JAMA*. 1963; 185: 914-919.

Katz S, Downs TD, Cash HR, Grotz RC. Progress in the development of the index of ADL. *Gerontology*. 1970;1:20-30.

Kelly M. The omnibus budget reconciliation act of 1987. A policy analysis. *Nurs. Clin. North Am.* 1989; 3: 791-4.

Kyle UG, Morabia A, Slosman DO, Mensi N, Unger P, Pichard C. Contribution of body composition to nutritional assessment at hospital admission in 995 patients: a controlled population study. *Br. J. Nutr.* 2001; 86: 725-31.

Kyle UG, Pirlich M, Lochs H, Schuetz T, Pichard C. Increased length of hospital stay in underweight and overweight patients at hospital admission: a controlled population study. *Clin. Nutr.* 2005; 24: 133-42.

Kyle UG, Unger P, Dupertuis YM, Karsegard VL, Genton L, Pichard C. Body composition in 995 acutely ill or chronically ill patients at hospital admission: a controlled population study. *J. Am. Diet Assoc.* 2002; 102: 944-55.

Landefeld CS, Palmer RM, Kresevic DM, Fortinsky RH, Kowal J. A randomized trial of care in a hospital medical unit especially designed to improve the functional outcomes of acutely ill older patients. *N. Engl. J. Med.* 1995; 332: 1338-1344.

Larsson J, Unosson M, Ek A-C, Nilsson L, Thorslund S, Bjurulf P. Effect of dietary supplement on nutritional status and clinical outcome in 501 geriatric patients - a randomized study. *Clin. Nutri.* 1990; 9: 179-184.

Larsson J. Clinical problem of hospital malnutrition. *Nutrition* 1993; 9: 274-5.

Lipski PS, Torrance A, Kelly PJ, James OFW. A study of nutritional deficits of long stay geriatric patients. *Age Ageing* 1993; 22: 244-255.

MacIntosh C, Morley JE, Chapman IM. The anorexia of aging. *Nutrition* 2000; 16: 983-995.

MacLellan DL, Van Til LD. Screening for nutritional risk among community-dwelling elderly on Prince Edward Island. *Can. J. Public Health* 1998; 89: 342–6.

Margetts BM, Thompson RL, Elia M, Jackson AA. Prevalence of risk of undernutrition is associated with poor health status in older people in the UK. *Eur. J. Clin. Nutr.* 2003; 57: 69-74.

Mayence S, Bayens JP, Dekoninck, Kennes B, Mayence P, Pepersack T. Vers un vieillissement réussi. Observatoire de l'âge - Institut Européen Inter-Universitaire de l'Action Sociale ed. 1996.

McElhaney JE. Nutrition, exercise, and influenza vaccination. *J. Gerontol Med. Sci.* 2002; 57A: M555-M556.

McVey LJ, Becker PM, Saltz CC, Feussner JR, Cohen HJ. Effect of a geriatric consultation team on functional status of elderly hospitalized patients: a randomized, controlled clinical trial. *Ann. Intern. Med.* 1989; 110: 79-84.

McWhirter JP, Pennington CR. Incidence and recognition of malnutrition in hospital. *BMJ* 1994; 308: 945–8.

McWhirter JP, Pennington CR. Incidence and recognition of malnutrition in hospital. *BMJ* 1994; 308: 945-8.

Milne AC, Potter J, Avenell A., Protein and energy supplementation in elderly people at risk from malnutrition. *Cochrane Database Syst Rev*. 2005; April 18: CD003288.

Mitchell SL, Tetroe JM. Survival after percutaneous endoscopic gastrostomy placement in older persons. *J. Gerontol. Med. Sci.* 2000; 55A: M735-M739.

Montuclard L, Garrouste-Orgeas M, Timsit JF, Misset B, De Jonghe B, Carlet J. Outcome, functional autonomy, and quality of life of elderly patients with a long-term intensive care unit stay. *Crit. Care Med.* 2000; 28: 3389–95.

Moreiras O, van Staveren WA, Cruz JA, Nes M, Lund-Larsen K. Intake of energy and nutrients. Euronut SENECA investigators. *Eur. J. Clin. Nutr*. 1991; 45 Suppl 3:105-19.

Morley JE, Silver AJ. Nutritional issues in nursing home care. *Ann. Int. Med.* 1995; 123: 850-859.

Morley JE. Decreased food intake with aging. *J. Gerontol.* 2001; 56: (Special Issue 2) 81-88.

Morley JE, Kraenzle D. Causes of weight loss in a community nursing home. J Am Geriatr Soc 1994; 42: 583-585.

Morley JE, Flaherty JH. It's never too late: health promotion and illness prevention in older persons. *J. Gerontol. Med. Sci.* 2000; 57A: M338-M342.

Morley JE, Perry HM III, Miller DK. Something about frailty. *J. Gerontol. Med. Sci.* 2002; 57A: M698-M704.

Neal RM, Baldwin RC. Screening for anxiety and depression in elderly medical outpatients. *Age Ageing* 1994;23:461-464.

Nelson KJ, Coulston AM, Sucher KP, Tseng RY. Prevalence of malnutrition in the elderly admitted to long-term-care facilities. *J. Am. Diet Assoc.* 1993; 93: 459-461.

Newman AB, Gottdiener JS, McBurnie MA, Hirsch CH, Kop WJ, Tracy R, Walston JD, Fried LP, Cardiovascular Health Study Research Group. Associations of subclinical cardiovascular disease with frailty. *J. Gerontol. Med. Sci.* 2001; 56A: M158-M166.

Newman AB, Yanez D, Harris T, Duxbury A, Enright PL, Fried LP. Weight change in old age and its association with mortality. *J. Am. Geriatr. Soc*. 2001; 59: 1309-1318.

Nikolaus T, Bach M, Siezen S, Volkert D, Oster P, Schlierf G. Assessment of nutritional risk in the elderly. *Ann. Nutr. Metab*. 1995; 39: 340–5.

Payette H, Gray-Donald K, Cyr R, Boultier V. Predictors of dietary intake in a functionally dependent elderly population in the community. *Am. J. Publ. Health* 1995; 85: 677-683.

Pepersack T. Falls in elderly persons: evaluation of risk and prevention. *Rev. Med. Brux* 1997; 18: 227-230.

Pepersack T. Functional rehabilitation in geriatrics. In: *L'Année Gérontologique*, Serdi Edition, Paris 1999; 2: 72-89.

Pepersack T. Prévention du vieillissement. In : Vieillissement : dignité, autonomie, solidarité / Delécluse F, Decharneux P, Pepersack T et al. - Bruxelles: CAL; Bruxelles : Espace de libertés 2000.

Pepersack T. [Recommendations for a nutritional approach in geriatric institutions]. *Revue medicale de Bruxelles* 2001;22(4):A320-9.

Pepersack T. La nutrition des personnes âgées. Kluwer Editions, Brussels, 2002b, pp264.

Pepersack T. [Ethics and artificial nutrition]. *Revue medicale de Bruxelles* 2003;24(6):A491-3.

Pepersack T. Savoir vieillir. Espace de Libertés 2004 ; 321 : 7-8.

Pepersack T. Outcomes of continuous process improvement of nutritional care program among geriatric units. *J. Gerontol. A Biol. Sci. Med. Sci*. 2005; 60: 787-92.

Pepersack T. Minimum Geriatric Screening Tools to Detect Common Geriatric Problems. Accepted in *J. Nutr. Health Ageing* April 2007.

Pepersack T, Bastan M. Prévalence de la dépression et caractéristiques du patient gériatrique déprimé. In: *L'Année Gérontologique*, Serdi Edition, Paris 2001; 15: 103-114.

Pepersack T, Beyer I, and the Study Group on Dependence in the French Community of Belgium. Activities of daily living scales and the needs for care and help among the elderly in Belgium. In: *Facts Research Intervention Gerontology*, 1998a, eds: JP Michel, LZ Rubenstein, BJ Vellas, JL Albarede. Springer Publishing Company, p 455-464.

Pepersack T, Beyer I, and the Study Group on Dependence in the French Community of Belgium. Activities of daily living scales and the needs for care and help among elderly before and after geriatric hospitalization. *Arch. Public Health* 1998b; 56: 291-303.

Pepersack T, Corretge M, Beyer I, Namias B, André S, Benoît F, Mergam A, Simonetti C. Examining the effect of intervention to nutritional problems of hospitalised elderly: a pilot project. *J. Nutr. Health Aging* 2002a; 6: 306-10.

Pepersack T, De Breucker S, Mekongo YP, Rogiers A, Beyer I. Correlates of unrecognized depression among hospitalized geriatric patients. *Journal of psychiatric practice* 2006;12(3):160-7.

Pepersack T, De Breucker S. Could geriatric comprehensive assessment predict the outcome of pneumonia in the very old? *Accepted in Age Ageing* April 2007.

Pichard C, Kyle UG, Morabia A, Perrier A, Vermeulen B, Unger P. Nutritional assessment: lean body mass depletion at hospital admission is associated with an increased length of stay. *Am. J. Clin. Nutr*. 2004; 79: 613-8.

Pinchocofsky-Devin GD, Kaminski NW. Incidence of protein calorie malnutrition in the nursing home population. *J. Am. Coll. Nutr*. 1987; 6: 109-112.

Posner BM, Jette AM, Smith KW, Miller DR. Nutrition and health risks in the elderly: The Nutrition Screening Initiative. *Am. J. Public Health* 1993; 83: 972–8.

Reilly JJ Jr, Hull SF, Albert N, Waller A, Bringardener S. Economic impact of malnutrition: a model system for hospitalized patients. *JPEN J. Parenter Enteral Nutr*. 1988; 12: 371-6.

Reuben DB, Borok GM, Wolde-Tsadik G, Ershoff DH, Fishman LK, Ambrosini VL, Liu Y, Rubenstein LZ, Beck JC. A *randomized trial of comprehensive geriatric assessment in the care of hospitalized patients. N. Engl. J. Med.* 1995; 332: 1345-1350.

Reynish W, Andrieu S, Nourhashemi F, Vellas B. Nutritional factors and Alzheimer's disease. *J. Gerontol. Med. Sci.* 2001; 56A: M675-M680.

Robinson G, Goldstein M, Levine GM. Impact of nutritional status on DRG length of stay. *JPEN J Parenter Enteral Nutr.* 1987; 11: 49-51.

Rubenstein LZ, Josephson KR, Wieland GD, English PA, Sayre JA, Kane RL. Effectiveness of a geriatric evaluation unit: a randomized clinical trial. *N. Engl. J. Med.* 1984; 311: 1664-1670.

Rubenstein LZ, Harker JO, Salva A, Guigoz Y, Vellas B. Screening for undernutrition in geriatric practice: developing the Short-Form Mini-Nutritional Assessment (MNA-SF) 1. *J. Gerontol. Med. Sci.* 2001; 56A: M366-M372.

Sahyoun NR, Jacques PF, Dallal GE, Russell RM. Nutrition Screening Initiative checklist may be a better awareness/educational tool than a screening one. *J. Am. Diet Assoc.* 1997; 97: 760–4.

Salva A, Corman B, Andrieu S, Salas J, Vellas B, and the International Association of Gerontology/International Academy of Nutrition and Aging (IAG/IANA) Task Force. Minimum Data Set for Nutritional Intervention Studies in Elderly People. *J. Gerontology* M S 2004; 59A: 724–729.

Shaver HJ, Loper JA, Lutes RA. Nutritional status of nursing home patients. *J. Parenter Enteral Nutr.* 1980; 4: 367-370.

Silver AJ, Morley JE, Strome LS, Jones D, Vickers L. Nutritional status in an academic nursing home. *J. Am. Geriatr. Soc.* 1988; 36: 487-491.

Solomon DH. Geriatric assessment: methods for clinical decision making. *JAMA* 1988;259:2450-2452.

Stuk AE, Siu AL, Wieland GD, Adams J, Rubenstein LZ. Comprehensive geriatric assessment : a meta-analysis of controlled trials. *Lancet* 1993; 342: 1032-1036.

Sullivan DH, Walls RC, Lipschitz DA. Protein-energy undernutrition and the risk of mortality within 1 y of hospital discharge in a selected population of geriatric rehabilitation patients. *Am. J. Clin. Nutr.* 1991; 53: 599-605.

Thomas DR. Issues and dilemmas in the prevention and treatment of pressure ulcers: a review. *J. Gerontol. Med. Sci.* 2001; 56A: M328-M340.

Thomas DR. The critical link between health-related quality of life and age-related changes in physical activity and nutrition. *J. Gerontol. Med. Sci.* 2001; 56A: M599-M602.

Thomas DR, Verdery RB, Gardner L, Kant AK, Lindsay J. A prospective study of outcome from protein-energy malnutrition in nursing home residents. *J. Parenter Enteral Nutr.* 1991; 15: 400-404.

Thomas DR, Zdrowski CD, Wilson MM, Conright KC, Lewis C, Tariq S, Morley JE. Malnutrition in subacute care. *Am. J. Clin. Nutr.* 2002; 75: 308-313.

Tinetti ME. Performance-oriented assessment of mobility problems in the elderly. *J. Am. Geriatr. Soc.* 1986; 36: 613-616.

Van Marwijk HW, Wallace P, de Bock GH, Hermans J, Kaptein AA, Mulder JD. Evaluation of the feasibility, reliability and diagnostic value of shortened versions of the geriatric depression scale. *Br. J. Gen. Pract.* 1995; 45: 195-199.

Vellas B, Guigoz Y, Garry PJ, Nourhashemi F, Bennahum D, Lauque S, Albarede JL. The Mini Nutritional Assessment (MNA) and its use in grading the nutritional state of elderly patients. *Nutrition* 1999; 15: 116–22.

Vellas B, Guigoz Y, Baumgartner M, Garry PJ, Lauque S, Albarede JL. Relationships between nutritional markers and the mini-nutritional assessment in 155 older persons. *J. Am. Geriatr. Soc.* 2000; 48: 1300-1309.

Volkert A, Berner YN, Berry E, Cederholm T, Coti Bertrand P, Milne A, Palmblad J, Schneider S, Sobotka L, Stanga Z, DGEM: Lenzen-Grossimlinghaus R, Krys U, Pirlich M, Herbst B, Schütz T, Schröer W, Weinrebe W, Ockenga J, Lochs. ESPEN Guidelines on Enteral Nutrition: *Geriatrics. Clinical Nutrition* (2006) 25, 330–360.

Waitzberg DL, Caiaffa WT, Correia MI. Hospital malnutrition: the Brazilian national survey (IBRANUTRI): a study of 4000 patients. *Nutrition* 2001; 17: 573-80.

Wallace JI. Involuntary weight loss in older outpatients: incidence and clinical significance. *J. Am. Geriatr. Soc.* 1995; 43: 329-337.

Wimo A, Winblad B, Stoffler A, Wirth Y, Mobius HJ. Resource utilisation and cost analysis of memantine in patients with moderate to severe Alzheimer's disease. *Pharmacoeconomics* 2003; 21: 327-340.

Winograd CH, Gerety MB, Lai NA. A negative trial of inpatient geriatric consultation: lessons learned and recommendations for future research. *Arch. Intern. Med.* 1993; 153: 2017-2023.

Wouters-Wesseling W, Rozendaal M, Snijder M, Graus Y, Rimmelzwaan G, De Groot L, Bindels J. Effect of a complete nutritional supplement on antibody response to influenza vaccine in elderly people. *J. Gerontol. Med. Sci.* 2002; 57A: M563-M566.

Wright BA. Weight loss and weight gain in a nursing home: a prospective study. *Geriatr. Nurs.* 1993; 14: 156-159.

Wyszynski DF, Perman M, Crivelli A. Prevalence of hospital malnutrition in Argentina: preliminary results of a population-based study. *Nutrition* 2003; 19: 115-9.

Yesavage JA, Brink TL. Development and validation of a geriatric depression scale: a preliminary report. *J. Psychiatr. Res.* 1983; 17: 37-49.

Zuliani G, Romagnoni F, Volpato S, Soattin L, Leoci V, Bollini MC, Buttarello M, Lotto D, Fellin R. Nutritional parameters, body composition, and progression of disability in older disabled residents living in nursing homes. *J. Gerontol. Med. Sci.* 2001; 56A: M212-M216.

In: Nutrition for the Middle Aged and Elderly
Editors: N. E. Bernhardt, A. M. Kasko, pp. 253-269
ISBN: 978-1-60456-146-3

Chapter VIII

I Heard It Through the Grapevine: Beliefs Among College Students and Older Adults Regarding Foods Essential for Building Strength and Muscle

Michael E. Oakes*[*] *and Heather Leeman
University of Scranton, Scranton, PA, USA

Abstract

What kinds of messages are the public receiving concerning food intake and potential to build strength/muscle and how have the public assimilated this information? In the present study 132 college students and 109 older respondents were asked to provide information concerning the nutrients that they believe to be important for building strength/muscle as well as the sources for these messages. A second goal involved determining to what degree food names (e.g., an egg) have reputations for building strength/muscle that are congruent with judgements of the nutrient descriptions of those same foods (e.g., the nutrient profile for an egg). Results revealed that both cohorts believed protein to be most important for building strength/muscle and that this information came from the media more than any other source. Interestingly, heightened familiarity with media messages predicted less stereotypical thinking about foods among the older participants. Cohort differences for food names occurred in seven cases but never for descriptions. Wide disparities between a food's name rating for building strength/muscle and ratings of that same food's nutrient description were common. It appears that we have acquired mistaken beliefs about the strength/muscle building potential (and protein content) of foods but the impact of the popular media on these beliefs is not clear.

[*] Contact Information: Michael E. Oakes, Ph.D. Dept. of Psychology, University of Scranton, Scranton, PA 18510-4596, (570) 941-7895 (office), (570) 941-7899 (fax). email: oakesm2@scranton.edu

In recent years, it has been demonstrated that the average person possesses a wide range of beliefs/expectations concerning common foods. For example, beliefs concerning the satiety/satiation capacity (Green and Blundell, 1996; de Graaf, Stafleu, Staal, and Wijne, 1992), general acceptability (Cardello, 1995; Cardello, 1994), potential to promote weight gain (Oakes and Slotterback, 2005; Oakes, 2005a; Oakes, 2005b; Rozin, Ashmore, and Markwith, 1996), vitamin and mineral content (Oakes, 2005c; Oakes, 2004a; Oakes, 2004b), and general health value of foods have been observed (Oakes, 2003; Oakes and Slotterback, 2001a; Oakes and Slotterback, 2001b). These beliefs have been described as stereotypical (Oakes, 2003; Oakes and Slotterback, 2001a; Oakes and Slotterback, 2001b; Cardello, 1995) and likely influence the types and amounts of foods consumed (Cardello, 1995; Cardello, 1994; Knight and Boland, 1989). Many factors determine and influence our image of specific foods including our past experiences with a particular food (e.g., its taste, texture, color, odor, and packaging; Cardello, 1994) as well as information that we have assimilated regarding the name of the food. This would generally include information on food labels, commercials, television shows, movies, cartoons, and newspaper and magazine articles and advertisements (Cardello, 1995; Goering, 1985). Additionally, a food's reputation for health, vitamin and mineral content, and weight-gain potential may often be based on social/historical events and personalities from the more distant past, e.g., folklore and political trends (Oakes, 2005c; Oakes, 2004a; Oakes, 2004c).

In recent years it has been shown that specific foods names (e.g., apple) often have reputations for (1) health (Oakes, 2003; Oakes and Slotterback, 2001a; Oakes and Slotterback, 2001b), (2) potential to promote weight gain and (3) satiation (Oakes, 2006) that vary in terms of their relationships with ratings of the nutrient contents of those same foods (e.g., the unlabeled nutrient description for an apple). For example, it was recently shown that name and descriptions ratings for potential to promote weight gain were not related while data from those same respondents (rating the same foods) indicated that name and description ratings for satiation were highly correlated (Oakes, 2006). The most likely interpretation of these findings is that a food's reputation for satiation is likely influenced primarily by the food's nutrient content (e.g., calories, fat, protein) while a food's reputation for weight gain is often shaped by non-nutritional factors (e.g., media coverage, food-label information, and folklore).

For the present study, we sought to test this hypothesis by asking respondents to assess food names and descriptions once again on a novel subject that receives media attention. Certain popular media sources (e.g., magazines) often offer advice concerning foods to eat in order to promote muscle growth and/or increase strength (see Appendix A for an example). The goals of the present study were to investigate where college students and older adults get their information on the muscle/strength building capacity of foods and to examine whether the reputation of food names on this subject correspond to ratings of the unlabeled nutrient descriptions of those same foods for a sample of college students and older adults. Further, does a person's familiarity with media sources and messages concerning diet and nutrition predict their ratings of food names or descriptions? A variety of other food scholars have suggested that the number and intensity of diet and nutrition messages, in recent years, have negatively shaped the public's shopping and eating habits (Aarnio and Lindeman, 2004; Dreezens, Martijn, Tenbult, Kok, and de Vries, 2005; Patterson, Satia, Kristal, Neuhouser, and Drewnowski, 2001; Schwartz and Borra, 1997; Rozin, Ashmore, and Markwith, 1996). Finally, we were interested in assessing which nutrients are considered important for building strength/muscle.

It was expected that the respondents would indicate that the media is the primary source of information concerning the muscle/strength building potential of foods. Also, we expected that food-name ratings for muscle/strength building would often differ from ratings of the nutrient descriptions for those same foods: previous work has suggested that this might be most pronounced in the college sample (Oakes, 2003). For example, the general positive image of the apple would cause its name to be rated as having a strong potential to build strength/muscle while the apple's nutrient description would be rated much lower. Finally, it was considered likely that a greater familiarity with diet and nutrition messages and media sources would predict greater use of food stereotypes. For example, respondents who express the greatest familiarity with diet and nutrition media sources (compared to those with less familiarity) will rate the name "apple" as having more potential to build strength/muscle.

Method

Participants

Participants were 132 undergraduate students enrolled in the Fundamentals of Psychology course at the University of Scranton. The mean age (SD) was 18.8 (1.14) years; 49 were male and 83 were female. Participation in the study fulfilled a research requirement for the psychology department (other options were available for the students to fulfill this requirement). Participants were told that they would be asked about their perceptions of foods. The vast majority of the participants were college freshman who were not enrolled in nutritional programs.

The older participants were 109 men (n =39) and women (n = 70) ranging in age from 37 to 78. The mean age (SD) was 50.8 (7.2). Participants were friends and relatives of students involved in course work at the University of Scranton (these students were taking advanced psychology courses and were not the author's students). Students who were engaged in course work were offered extra-credit for having relatives and acquaintances over the age of 35 complete the survey over a holiday break. There was limited extra-credit permitted and other options were available for the students to earn the available extra-credit.

Materials

A written list of 34 food names (with a serving/portion size indicated alongside) and a separate list of the same 34 foods' unnamed nutrient descriptions was presented to each participant. The portion sizes used were considered typical and were provided by Pennington (1998). Each food name and description was followed by a seven-point scale (with 1 = "No Potential," 4 = "Fair potential," and 7 = "Strong Potential"). This method was similar to that used in the past (Oakes, 2003; Oakes and Slotterback, 2001a; Oakes and Slotterback, 2001b), except a seven-point scale was used rather than a five-point scale and the respondents were required to rate each name and description according to "its potential to build strength and/or muscle" rather than "how good it is for you." Participants were also provided with some space to explain why they rated each name and description as they did. All but three of the 34 foods examined were used in previous research (Oakes, 2003; Oakes and Slotterback, 2001a; Oakes and Slotterback, 2001b): the three exceptions were "1 banana" (added because of interest to the authors), "8 oz. whole milk," and "8 oz. of nonfat (skim) milk." The milk beverages were added because one previous study had shown that whole milk was judged to contain more vitamins and minerals than skim milk (Oakes, 2004a). There were several foods represented in each of the four tiers of the old food guide pyramid (USDA, 2002).

Each of the 34 food descriptions contained information about the food's percentage of the recommended daily value (RDV) of protein, % RDV of fiber, number of vitamins and minerals, % RDV of calories, % RDV of fat, % RDV of cholesterol, % RDV of sodium, and % RDV of carbohydrates (presented in this order to the respondents). Vitamins and minerals were counted only if their amounts were equal to or greater than 10% of the daily value for a 2000 calorie diet (Pennington, 1998) and sodium was not included in the number of vitamins and minerals.

Procedure

Internal review board approval for the study was obtained before data collection began. The student participants were surveyed in groups of approximately 30 people per session. Respondents were initially asked to indicate their age and gender. They were then asked to answer the following questions concerning physical activity. (1) Do you routinely do physical activity? (2) Do you engage in strength/muscle building exercise, if yes what exercises and how often? (3) Is it essential to eat certain types of foods in order to build strength and/or muscle, if yes what types of foods? (4) Where do you get information about these foods? Additionally the older adult participants were also asked the following three things (1) "Please list all of the titles of books and magazines that you can recall that discuss diet or nutritional issues" (16 lines were provided). (2) "Please list all of the authors of diet or nutrition books that you can recall" (16 lines were provided). (3) "We often hear information that eating certain foods is helpful and healthy (e.g., eating carrots is good for your eyes) and that eating other foods is dangerous and unhealthy (e.g., eating candy is bad for your teeth). Please list as many of these sorts of messages as you can on the lines provided below" (24 lines were provided). All of the participants were instructed in writing to rate each food name and description in terms of "its potential to build strength and/or muscle." All participants were presented with names and descriptions of the same 34 food items. The respondents evaluated the 34 food names first followed by the descriptions. While evaluating the food descriptions, the respondents were unaware they were rating the same foods that they had previously encountered by name only (Appendix B has the information provided in the food descriptions).

Results

Approximately 82% of the college respondents indicated that they routinely engage in physical activities versus 63% of the older-adult participants (chi-square, $p < .001$). Further, almost 60% of the college respondents (compared to 31% of the older respondents) indicated that they engage in strength/muscle building exercise at least twice a week (chi-square, $p < .001$). Over 93% of the college respondents (and 91% of the older sample) indicated that it is essential to eat certain types of foods in order to build strength and/or muscle (chi-square, $p > .10$). When asked to indicate which types of foods are essential for building strength and/or muscle, most of the college respondents (78%) and older adults (80%) mentioned protein or meat products (chi-square, $p > .10$). About 28% of the college respondents (versus 27% for the older participants) related that carbohydrates or foods that primarily contain carbohydrates (fruits and vegetables) are important for strength and/or muscle growth (chi-square, $p > .10$). Approximately 58% of the college participants (compared to 71% older sample) indicated at least one media source (i.e., internet, television, magazines, newspaper and books) for information on foods to build strength and/or muscle (chi-square, p < .05). About 40% of the college students versus 17% of the older participants indicated authoritative sources (i.e., classes, teachers, doctors, nutritionists, and trainers; chi-square, p < .001). Approximately 30% of the student sample versus 9% of the older respondents indicated friends, peers, and/or family as sources (chi-square, $p < .001$). About 28% of the college students and 13% of the older sample indicated food labels, General Nutrition Center (a chain of stores that sell nutritional products), or some weight loss organization as sources of information (chi-square, $p < .005$).

The mean (SD) number of diet or nutrition books/magazines listed (by the older participants) was 3.5 (2.7). The South Beach Diet was mentioned most often (24% of respondents) followed by Atkins' books (17%), Prevention Magazine (17%), Good Housekeeping (17%), Family Circle (12%), Weight Watchers (10%), Ladies Home Journal (9%), Time (8%), and Shape (8%). The mean (SD) number of authors of diet or nutrition books listed was 1.2 (1.8). Atkins was listed far more than any other author (36% of the respondents) followed by Dr. Phil (9%), Ornish (6%), and Agatston (5%). The older respondents mentioned an average of 4.3 (3.3) specific messages indicating that specific foods or food nutrients (e.g., protein) benefit specific body systems (e.g., heart, bones, muscles) or functioning (e.g., constipation).

The response to the request to list books and magazines that discuss diet or nutritional issues (compared to the requests to list authors or health messages) predicted the food-name ratings best. Eight food names were correlated with the book/magazine responses ($p < .05$): four of the eight were negatively correlated (banana, grapes, carrot, apple), i.e., the higher the rated potential to build muscle the fewer books/magazines listed. Four of the eight (hotdog, Big Mac, fried chicken, and Egg McMuffin) were positively correlated with the book/magazine responses, i.e., a greater number of books/magazines listed predicted higher ratings of potential to build muscle. Somewhat similar results were evident for the health-message responses: negative correlations were evident for banana, grapes, carrot, apple, and rice cake and a positive correlation was evident for fried chicken ($p < .05$). Description ratings were almost never correlated with these responses (e.g., the response to the book/magazines question was correlated only with Egg McMuffin).

Ratings of Potential to Build Strength/Muscle

Between-subjects comparisons. Comparisons were made using t-tests with an alpha level of .01 (to control for Type I errors). Cohort differences were found for seven of the 34 food names examined (see Table 1; $p < .01$): these seven included beer, skim milk, peanut butter, yogurt, ice cream, cottage cheese, and tuna. In all seven cases the older respondents (compared to the college sample) judged food names to have greater potential for building strength/muscle. The asterisks for the tests are adjacent to the older-adult means. No cohort differences were evident for any of the food descriptions.

Table 1. Mean Ratings of Food Names and Descriptions and within- and between-Subject Comparisons

		Name Mean (SD)	Descript Mean (SD)	Paired t-Statistic
Potential for building strength greater for food names than descriptions for both cohorts				
1 hard boiled egg	young	5.35 (1.26)	2.17 (1.12)	23.22*
	old	5.43 (1.26)	2.30 (1.29)	20.60*
1 medium banana	young	4.76 (1.47)	3.05 (1.44)	11.45*
	old	4.90 (1.52)	2.96 (1.76)	10.87*
8 oz. nonfat (skim) milk	young	4.72 (1.44)	4.05 (1.37)	03.85*
	old	5.18 (1.53)**	4.05 (1.42)	05.69*
8 oz. whole milk	young	4.57 (1.53)	3.65 (1.21)	05.12*
	old	4.89 (1.74)	3.68 (1.28)	06.23*
2 Tbsp. peanut butter	young	4.22 (1.63)	2.91 (1.13)	08.06*
	old	5.19 (1.40)**	3.26 (1.44)	11.62*
1 medium apple	young	4.21 (1.42)	2.76 (1.59)	09.18*
	old	4.71 (1.55)	2.65 (1.80)	11.99*
1 cup grapes	young	4.07 (1.48)	2.84 (1.37)	08.12*
	old	4.23 (1.64)	2.86 (1.55)	07.96*
1 medium carrot	young	4.03 (1.45)	2.87 (1.51)	08.25*
	old	4.26 (1.62)	2.47 (1.60)	10.23*
½ cup Romaine lettuce	young	3.82 (1.71)	2.44 (1.74)	07.77*
	old	4.21 (1.81)	2.28 (1.46)	10.47*
1 beef hotdog (no bun)	young	3.81 (1.56)	2.13 (1.09)	10.17*
	old	3.74 (1.72)	2.30 (1.29)	07.41*
1 rice cake	young	3.38 (1.47)	2.15 (1.43)	07.67*
	old	3.36 (1.46)	1.89 (1.26)	08.58*
1 Cup Cheerios	young	4.42 (1.32)	3.71 (1.32)	05.04*
	old	4.15 (1.41)	3.60 (1.43)	03.13*

Table 1. (Continued)

		Name Mean (SD)	Descript Mean (SD)	Paired t-Statistic
Potential for building strength greater for food descriptions than names for both cohorts				
3.5 cups unbut. popcorn	young	2.27 (1.25)	3.53 (1.37)	05.24*
	old	3.03 (1.57)	3.88 (1.63)	04.82*
1 Big Mac	young	2.20 (1.38)	4.23 (1.92)	11.00*
	old	2.47 (1.56)	3.73 (1.86)	05.98*
4 gingersnaps	young	2.17 (1.08)	2.94 (1.31)	05.76*
	old	2.32 (1.20)	2.95 (1.41)	03.85*
1 Snickers bar	young	1.72 (1.06)	2.95 (1.14)	09.36*
	old	1.87 (1.13)	3.25	(1.44)08.03*
1 oz. potato chips	young	1.50 (0.77)	2.67 (1.16)	10.48*
	old	1.54 (0.83)	2.77 (1.24)	08.68*
1 glazed donut	young	1.33 (0.63)	2.82 (1.13)	13.51*
	old	1.19 (0.55)	2.53 (1.04)	12.11*
1 12 oz. beer	young	1.42 (0.98)	2.27 (1.59)	04.91*
	old	1.81 (1.13)**	2.32 (1.65)	02.70*
3.5 oz. fried chicken	young	3.55 (1.42)	4.47 (1.65)	05.01*
	old	3.48 (1.64)	4.02 (1.71)	02.77*
1 raisin bagel	young	3.50 (1.22)	4.07 (1.40)	03.74*
	old	3.45 (1.48)	4.05 (1.40)	03.20*
Potential for building strength greater for names than descriptions for older sample only				
3 oz. tuna canned in water	young	4.92 (1.47)	5.13 (1.39)	01.44
	old	5.66 (1.27)**	5.06 (1.52)	03.76*
8 oz. whole plain yogurt	young	4.38 (1.39)	4.15 (1.20)	01.46
	old	5.15 (1.48)**	4.50 (1.43)	03.95*
I hamburger	young	4.33 (1.45)	4.22 (1.33)	00.68
	old	4.72 (1.61)	3.83 (1.55)	04.89*
Potential for building strength greater for descriptions than names for older sample only				
1 piece of apple pie	young	2.34 (1.09)	2.57 (1.06)	01.96
	old	2.23 (1.16)	2.68 (1.23)	03.19*
Potential for building strength greater for descriptions than names for younger sample only				
I cup 1% fat cottage cheese	young	3.88 (1.55)	5.04 (1.68)	05.91*
	old	5.01 (1.43)**	4.71 (1.67)	01.44
No differences between names and descriptions in potential to build strength				
1 baked potato w/skin	young	4.29 (1.41)	4.09 (1.53)	01.23
	old	4.49 (1.59)	4.16 (1.53)	01.77
1 cup pasta	young	4.24 (1.52)	4.18 (1.47)	00.32
	old	3.95 (1.57)	4.20 (1.68)	01.17
1 pkt. apple/cinn oatmeal	young	4.21 (1.20)	4.05 (1.41)	01.23
	old	4.15 (1.56)	4.03 (1.50)	00.67
1 piece beef jerky	young	3.41 (1.65)	3.00 (1.11)	02.45
	old	3.58 (1.81)	3.06 (1.24)	02.54

Table 1. (Continued)

		Name Mean (SD)	Descript Mean (SD)	Paired t-Statistic
1 Egg McMuffin	young	3.22 (1.26)	3.51 (1.71)	01.65
	old	2.96 (1.47)	3.25 (1.72)	01.38
1 oz. pretzels	young	3.09 (1.27)	2.93 (1.24)	01.26
	old	2.81 (1.39)	2.59 (1.18)	01.50
5 Saltine crackers	young	2.74 (1.20)	2.63 (1.22)	00.80
	old	2.78 (1.36)	2.53 (1.20)	01.49
½ cup vanilla ice cream	young	2.34 (1.14)	2.42 (1.04)	00.62
	old	2.95 (1.46)**	2.52 (1.22)	02.58

Note. Higher scores indicate greater perceived potential to build strength/muscle. The table is divided into six categories. (1) Foods in which both cohorts gave higher ratings to food names than their corresponding unnamed descriptions. (2) Foods in which both cohorts gave higher ratings to food descriptions than their corresponding names. (3) Foods in which higher ratings were given to food names (than descriptions) only by the older sample. (4) Foods in which higher ratings were given to food descriptions (than names) only by the older sample. (5) Foods in which higher ratings were given to food descriptions (than names) only by the younger sample. (6) Foods in which name and description ratings were similar (nonsignificant) for both cohorts.

* $p < .01$ for paired-subjects tests.

** $p < .01$ for between-subjects tests.

Paired-subjects comparisons. Paired sample t-tests using an alpha level of .01 were used to analyze the ratings of potential to build strength/muscle for each of the 34 food items. Of the 34 food items that were examined, in 8 cases no significant differences were observed between the name of each food item and its corresponding description for either cohort (see Table 1). Although name and description ratings were similar in 8 cases, wide discrepancies between ratings of food names and descriptions were common. The overall correlation between name and description ratings was $\underline{r}(33) = .35$, $p < .05$ for the college students and $\underline{r}(33) = .43$, $p < .05$ for the older sample . According to the Kolmogorov-Smirnov Test (a goodness of fit test to determine whether or not a variable is normally distributed), the description ratings are normally distributed while the name ratings are not. However, one would not expect name ratings concerning questions about the health value of foods to be normally distributed: in fact, when asked to rate the general health value and weigh-gain potential of food names a bimodal distribution has been observed indicating stereotypical thinking (Oakes, 2005d, Oakes and Slotterback, 2001a; Oakes and Slotterback, 2001b).

Food names were considered to have more potential for building strength/muscle than their corresponding descriptions in 12 instances for both cohorts (see Table 1). These 12 items included all fruits and vegetables (with the exception of the potato), milk beverages, egg, beef hotdog, Cheerios, and peanut butter.

Food descriptions were judged to have a greater potential for building strength/muscle than their corresponding food names in nine cases (for both cohorts). These 10 included fried and fast foods (i.e., fried chicken and Big Mac), several grain products and snack foods (i.e., bagel, gingersnaps, glazed donut, popcorn, Snickers bar, potato chips) as well as beer.

In three cases only the older sample considered the food name to have a greater potential for building strength/muscle than its corresponding description: these included tuna, yogurt, and hamburger.

Stepwise Regressions

To better understand which factors may have been used by the participants when they evaluated the names and also descriptions of foods, stepwise regression analyses were performed. The regressions used the average rating of participants for names or descriptions of foods as the dependent variable and each food's content of protein, fiber, calories, fat, cholesterol, sodium, carbohydrate as well as the food's status as being derived from animal sources and number of vitamins and minerals as independent variables.

Evaluating names. A food's vitamin and mineral content, as well as whether or not the food was an animal product (i.e., meat or dairy), and calories explained a significant amount of the variance in perceived potential to build strength/muscle for the college students' ratings of food names (adj. $R^2 = .45$; $F(3,33) = 10.13$, $p < .001$). For the older respondents status as an animal product, fat, and fiber explained a significant amount of the variance (adj. $R^2 = .40$; $F(3,33) = 8.43$, $p < .001$) The Beta values (see Table 2) indicated that as calories and fat increased in foods the perceived potential to build strength/muscle decreased. Also, food names with higher vitamin/mineral and fiber content were judged as having a greater potential to build strength/muscle, as were foods that were animal products (e.g., meat and dairy).

Table 2. Statistics for Stepwise Regression

	Adjusted R^2	Beta	t	sig.	Tolerance
Overall Evaluation of Names					
Animal Product	0.45	0.39	2.93	.006	.924
Number of Vit/Min		0.59	3.72	.001	.670
Calories		-0.77	-4.83	.001	.646
Overall Evaluation of Descriptions					
Protein	0.91	1.05	11.77	.001	.354
Fat		-0.35	-5.25	.001	.625
Carbohydrates		0.19	2.79	.009	.637
Cholesterol		-0.31	-4.98	.001	.711
Number of Vit/Min		0.32	4.35	.001	.512
Sodium		-0.21	-2.49	.019	.397

Note. Regressions were performed using the respondents' average strength/muscle building rating for each food name and description as the dependent variable and each food's actual content of protein, fiber, calories, fat, cholesterol, sodium, carbohydrate as well as the food's status as being derived from animal sources and number of vitamins and minerals as independent variables.

Evaluating descriptions. For the college students, protein, fat, carbohydrate, cholesterol, vitamin/mineral, and sodium content explained a significant amount of the variance for the ratings of food descriptions (adj. $\underline{R}^2 = .91$; $\underline{F}(6,33) = 55.17$, $p < .001$). Similar results were found for the older sample (adj. $\underline{R}^2 = .84$; $\underline{F}(7,33) = 25.93$, $p < .001$) The Beta values indicated that as fat, cholesterol, and sodium levels in descriptions of foods increased, ratings of potential for building muscle and strength decreased. As the amount of protein, carbohydrates, and the number of vitamins and minerals in the descriptions of foods increased, participants' ratings of that food's potential to increase muscle and strength also increased.

Open-Ended Questions

In situations where food names were rated as having a greater potential to build strength/muscle than corresponding nutrient descriptions (the first half of Table 3), respondents often commented about the high protein content and general health value of the food names. However, these comments were much less common when respondents evaluated the unnamed nutrient descriptions for those same foods.

Conversely, when nutrient descriptions were rated as better than names (the second half of Table 3), respondents often commented about the high fat content of the food names. However, when evaluating the descriptions of these same foods, respondents often commented about high protein content, the food having balanced amounts of nutrients, as well as the amount of fat being high or low.

Generally, it appears that the older respondents (compared to the younger sample) judged many foods (i.e., their names) to have higher levels of protein, but perhaps less fat.

Table 3. Common responses for several foods with wide discrepancies between food name and descriptions ratings

Names build more strength/muscle than descriptions				
Food	Name resp.	Percent Young Old	Description Resp.	Percent Young Old
1 hard boiled egg	High Protein Good/healthy	78% 93% 11% 0%	High Cholesterol High Protein	68% 67% 16% 17%
1 medium banana	Vitamins/healthy High Potassium Fruit	38% 23% 38% 46% 23% 08%	High Fiber Low Everything Low Protein	33% 33% 29% 08% 19% 33%
2 Tbsp. Peanut butter	High Protein High Fat	64% 98% 20% 17%	High Fat High Protein	86% 75% 18% 50%
1/2 cup Romaine Lettuce	Vitamins/healthy Watery	30% 58% 26% 0%	Low Nut. Value Low Protein	68% 42% 16% 25%
I beef hotdog	High Protein High Fat Processed	69% 85% 16% 23% 16% 08%	High Fat High Sodium High Cholesterol	82% 55% 18% 27% 9% 0%

Table 3. (Continued)

Descriptions build more strength/muscle than names				
Food	Name resp.	Percent Young Old	Description Resp.	Percent Young Old
3.5 cups unbuttered popcorn	High Carb. No Nut. Value Fiber	39% 15% 17% 23% 0% 38%	High Fiber OK/Balanced	42% 67% 32% 08%
1 Big Mac	High Fat High Protein	69% 38% 35% 62%	High Protein Balanced	40% 55% 28% 45%
1 Snickers Bar	High Fat High Sugar Peanut/nut	42% 08% 38% 31% 0% 54%	High Fat High Protein	50% 67% 21% 25%
1 glazed donut	High Fat High Sugar High Carb.	43% 17% 39% 42% 18% 17%	High Fat High Carb. Low Protein	52% 62% 29% 0% 29% 46%
3.5 oz. fried chicken	High fat/grease High Protein Fried	50% 38% 30% 77% 25% 15%	High Protein High Fat High Cholesterol	75% 42% 35% 75% 20% 17%

Note. When food names were rated as having a greater potential to build strength/muscle than corresponding nutrient descriptions, respondents often commented about the high protein content and general health value of the food names. These comments were less common when respondents evaluated the nutrient descriptions. Conversely, when nutrient descriptions were rated as better than names (the second half of the Table), respondents often commented about the high fat content of the food names. However, when evaluating the descriptions of these same foods, respondents often commented about high protein content, the food having balanced amounts of nutrients, as well as the amount of fat being high or low.

Percentages were tallied by determining the number of specific references for a food name or description (e.g., excessive fat in the name Snickers Bar) by the total amount of comments for that food (e.g., number of comments for the name Snickers Bar).

Discussion

It appears that the respondents' primary source for information concerning the strength/muscle building characteristics of foods is the media. When specifically asked to indicate what types of foods build strength/muscle, the vast majority of respondents specifically indicated the importance of high protein foods. However, when asked to evaluate the strength/muscle building characteristics of food names, protein content was not predictive of the ratings at all. It appears that certain food names frequently have reputations for building strength/muscle that are not congruent with judgements of the nutrient descriptions for those same foods. For example, the name "egg" was considered to have a high potential to build strength/muscle (likely due to its perceived protein content) but the nutrient content for the egg was apparently much less impressive in this regard (protein content was much less salient to the respondents than cholesterol content). Also, although surprisingly name and description ratings did not differ for several of the foods examined, wide disparities in name and description ratings were common for most of the foods investigated. The average name and description ratings for the foods examined were only moderately correlated for the students (i.e., r = .35) and the older participants (i.e., r = .43), this relationship was much weaker than name and description ratings for perceived satiation (Oakes, 2006; r = .76) as well as the general health value of foods (Oakes, 2003; Oakes and Slotterback, 2001a; Oakes and Slotterback, 2001b; r's = .68 - .72). However, the average name and description ratings for building strength/muscle were more highly correlated than those for promoting weight gain (Oakes, 2006; r = .27). Perhaps as previously suggested certain food attributes (e.g., perceived satiation capacity) seem to be based more on nutrient content compared to other food attributes (e.g., perceived capacity to promote weight gain and build muscle).

The most surprising finding was that the older respondents who expressed the most familiarity with popular nutritional messages and sources appeared to rely less on the reputation or stereotype of food names. The food names which were considered to have the highest general health value according to Oakes and Slotterback, 2001 (i.e., carrot, apple, and grapes) were actually considered to have less potential to build strength/muscle by the respondents who showed the most familiarity with popular nutrition information (compared to those who showed less familiarity). Also, foods that were considered among the least healthful by Oakes and Slotterback, 2001 (i.e., Big Mac, Egg McMuffin, hotdog, and fried chicken) were judged to have more potential for building strength/muscle by the participants who expressed the most familiarity with popular nutrition information (compared to those who expressed less familiarity). These results would suggest that the assimilation of popular media messages may diminish the use of stereotypical thinking when evaluating foods. However, it may be more the quality rather than the quantity of messages that is influential: these respondents seemed to be most familiar with low-carbohydrate sources.

On the other hand, heightened meticulousness and conscientious may also explain these findings. Perhaps the respondents who expressed the most familiarity about nutritional information were more meticulous and conscientious about completing the survey. This also may explain why they listed more diet and nutrition sources and messages and evaluated the food names somewhat differently than those who expressed less familiarity. Future work should involve exploring food reputations both before and after a nutrition course, dieting regime, or exposure to media messages.

There were several instances where cohort differences were evident for food names. It was clear that the older respondents (compared with the younger sample) considered many dairy products, tuna, peanut butter and beer to have a greater potential to build muscle and strength. This is likely due to cohort differences in the perceived protein content of these foods (information provided in Table 3 would suggest this). With the exception of tuna, cohort differences were not evident for the general-health value of these same foods between samples of young and older women (Oakes, 2003).

Also of interest is the fact that carbohydrates were considered to be a positive characteristic of food descriptions in the current study. This is somewhat surprising given that recent messages coming primarily from popular diet books (e.g., Agatston, 2003; Atkins, 1999) and the food industry have conveyed that high-carbohydrate diets in general should be avoided even for athletes (Sears, 1995). Perhaps the public now considers carbohydrates as somewhat helpful for athletes but negative in terms of their general health value.

Oddly, the food guide pyramid (even when tailored for athletes), as well as other government sources advises Americans to eat less overall and to generally limit food intake of meat, eggs, and dairy products (USDA, 2005; USDA, 2002; Manore and Thompson, 2000). However, it is these very foods that we are advised, in magazines as well as scientific sources (Tipton and Wolfe, 2001; Grandjean,1999), to eat in abundance if the goal is to increase strength/muscle. This likely causes somewhat of a conflict particularly for men who more than ever are receiving messages that muscle mass is attractive and desirable (Clarkson and Rawson, 1999). It would be interesting to assess how older men (i.e., age 30 and over) are balancing these two messages. It has been suggested by some scholars that interest in exercise nutrition is currently at an all time high (Manore and Thompson, 2000). Thus, it seems important to devote more attention to examining the sorts of nutritional information that Americans are assimilating concerning strength and muscle development. Nutritional messages geared toward increasing strength and muscle should be congruent and consistent with those promoting over all health. Also, the current findings indicate that adults believe protein to be important for building strength/muscle, however, the food-name ratings suggest that they have acquired some misleading information regarding the protein content of common foods (e.g., that a single hotdog has high protein content). Perhaps the public would benefit from more specific information concerning the protein content of foods.

Appendix A

The primary nutritional message in magazines geared toward the pursuit of strength and muscular development is to consume more foods derived from animal sources (eggs, poultry, fish, meat, and cheese) as well as protein products, such as, protein shakes, protein powder, and protein bars (e.g., containing oats, nuts, and soy protein; Aceto, 2005; Get Big, 2005; Get Lean, 2005). For example, a recent *Men's Fitness* article unequivocally stated "eat more protein, less of everything else" (Schuler & Williams, 2005, p. 69). An article in *Muscle & Fitness* offered "Consider, for a moment, the egg: so full of protein, so tasty when scrambled, fried, or omeletted, so likely to make you consume fewer calories if eaten for breakfast." And later in that same article "chicken is the most popular protein source for body builders but beef's benefits make it a worthy contender" and "beef and chicken were equally effective protein sources." (Hotline Nutrition, 2005, p. 52). Finally, in addition to the frequent advertisements for protein powders, bars, and shakes *Men's Fitness* recommends a specific protein bar and powder each month (MF Picks, 2005). Conversely, the message is often to reduce carbohydrates (Get Lean, 2005; Schuler & Williams, 2005; Volek, 2005) or at least to "control" or "balance" carbohydrates with protein (Alexander, 2005a) in order to provide energy and maintain muscle glycogen. Magazines that provide nutritional information concerning increasing strength and muscle mass generally indicate that dietary fat does not promote muscle development and should be reduced as much as possible, e.g., recipes they provide often use lean meat and low fat dairy products (Aceto, 2005; Alexander, 2005b).

Appendix B

Food Name	% RDV of protein	% RDV of fiber	# of vitamin & mineral	% RDV of calories	% RDV of fat	% RDV of cholesterol	% RDV of sodium	% RDV of carb.
1 glazed donut	4%	2%	2	12%	21%	2%	12%	10%
1 Egg McMuffin	20%	5%	11	15%	17%	98%	42%	10%
1 12-oz. beer	1%	2%	0	7%	0%	0%	1%	5%
1 cup pasta	7%	8%	4	10%	1%	0%	0%	15%
1 cup Cheerios(dry)	3%	10%	11	6%	3%	0%	16%	8%
1 rice cake	1%	1%	0	2%	0%	0%	1%	3%
8 oz. nonfat (skim) milk	9%	0%	6	4%	1%	2%	7%	4%
1 hamburger	13%	4%	6	12%	13%	16%	27%	10%
3.5 oz. fried chicken	25%	1%	6	14%	27%	38%	16%	3%
1 hard boiled egg	7%	0%	1	4%	8%	92%	3%	0%
1/2 cup Romaine lettuce	1%	2%	3	1%	0%	0%	0%	0%
1 oz. potato chips	2%	4%	4	8%	15%	0%	9%	6%
1 Snickers bar	5%	5%	6	15%	23%	3%	9%	13%
1 raisin bagel	8%	5%	5	10%	2%	0%	13%	14%
1 pkt. apple/cinn oatmeal	4%	8%	10	6%	2%	0%	7%	10%
1 piece beef jerky	7%	1%	1	4%	8%	4%	25%	1%
2 Tbsp peanut butter	8%	7%	5	9%	25%	0%	9%	3%
1 medium apple	0%	12%	1	4%	1%	0%	0%	8%
1 Big Mac	28%	5%	13	28%	50%	45%	53%	16%
1 oz. pretzels	3%	3%	2	5%	2%	0%	27%	8%
3.5 cups unbut. popcorn	4%	14%	1	5%	2%	0%	0%	8%
8 oz. low fat yogurt	10%	0%	7	11%	4%	4%	7%	16%
5 Saltine crackers	2%	2%	0	3%	3%	0%	11%	4%
1 medium carrrot	1%	7%	2	2%	0%	0%	1%	3%
1 cup grapes	1%	5%	3	6%	1%	0%	0%	10%
1/2 cup vanilla ice cream	3%	0%	0	7%	11%	13%	3%	6%

Appendix B (Continued)

Food Name	% RDV of protein	% RDV of fiber	# of vitamin & mineral	% RDV of calories	% RDV of fat	% RDV of cholesterol	% RDV of sodium	% RDV of carb.
1 beef hotdog	7%	0%	1	9%	25%	15%	33%	0%
1 piece apple pie	3%	6%	1	15%	21%	0%	19%	16%
4 gingersnaps	2%	2%	2	6%	4%	0%	10%	8%
1 cup 1% fat cottage cheese	31%	0%	4	8%	4%	5%	52%	2%
3 oz. tuna in water	24%	0%	5	5%	1%	11%	16%	0%
8 oz. whole milk	9%	0%	5	8%	12%	14%	7%	4%
1 baked potato w/skin	5%	15%	11	11%	0%	0%	1%	19%
I banana	1%	9%	3	5%	1%	0%	0%	10%

References

Aarnio, K. and Lindeman, M. (2004). Magical food and health beliefs: a portrait of believers and functions of the beliefs. *Appetite, 43*, 65-74.

Agatston, A. (2003). *The South Beach diet: The delicious, doctor-designed, foolproofplan for fast and healthy weight loss*. Emmaus, PA: Rodale Books.

Atkins, R. C. (1999). *Dr. Atkins' new diet revolution.* New York, NY: Avon books.

Cardello, A. V. (1995). The role of image, stereotypes, and expectations, on the acceptance and consumption of rations. In B. M. Marriott (Ed.), *Not eating enough: Overcoming underconsumption of military operational rations*. Washington, D. C.: National Academic Press.

Cardello, A. V. (1994). Consumer expectations and their role in food acceptance. In H. J. H. MacFie and D. M. H. Thomson (Ed,), *Measurement of food preferences*. New York: Blackie Academic and Professional.

Clarkson, P. M., and Rawson, E. S. (1999). Nutritional supplements to increase muscle mass. *Critical Reviews in Food Science and Nutrition, 39*, 317-328.

de Graaf, C., Stafleu, A., Staal, P., and Wijne, (1992), Beliefs about the satiating effect of bread and spread varying in macronutrient content. *Appetite, 18,* 121-128.

Dreezens, E., Martijn, C., Tenbult, P., Kok, G., and de Vries, N. K. (2005). Food and values: an examination of values underlying attitudes toward genetically modified- and organically grown food products. *Appetite, 44,* 115-122.

Goering, P. A. (1985). Effects of product trial on consumer expectations, demand, and prices. *Journal of Consumer Research, 12*, 74-82.

Grandjean, A. (1999). Nutritional requirements to increase lean mass. *Clinical Sports Medicine, 18*, 623-632.

Green, S. M., and Blundell, J. E. (1996). Subjective and objective indices of the satiating effect of foods. Can people predict how filling a food will be? *European Journal of Clinical Nutrition 50*, 798-806.

Knight, L. J. and Boland, F. J. (1989). Restrained eating: An experimental disentanglement of the disinhibiting variables of perceived calories and food type. *Journal of Abnormal Psychology, 98*, 412-420.

Manore, M., and Thompson, J. (2000). *Sport nutrition for health and performance*. Champaign, IL: Human Kinetics.

Oakes, M. E. (2006). Filling yet fattening: Stereotypical beliefs about the weight gain potential and satiation of foods. *Appetite, 46*, 224-233.

Oakes, M. E. (2005a). Beauty or beast: does stereotypical thinking about foods contribute to overeating? *Food Quality and Preference, 16,* 447-454.

Oakes, M. E. (2005b). Stereotypical thinking about foods and perceived capacity to promote weight gain. *Appetite*, 44, 317-324.

Oakes, M. E. (2005c). Bad company: The addition of sugar, fat, or salt reduces the perceived vitamin and mineral content of foods. *Food Quality and Preference, 16*, 111-119.

Oakes, M. E. (2004a). Good foods gone bad: "Infamous" nutrients diminish perceived vitamin and mineral content of foods. *Appetite, 42*, 273-278.

Oakes, M. E. (2004b). Suspicious minds: perceived vitamin content of ordinary and diet foods with added fat, sugar or salt. *Appetite, 43*, 105-108.

Oakes, M. E. (2004c). *Bad foods: Changing attitudes about what we eat.* Piscataway, NJ: Transaction Publishers.

Oakes, M. E. (2003). Differences in judgments of food healthfulness by young and elderly women. *Food Quality and Preference, 14,* 227-236.

Oakes, M. E., and Slotterback, C. S. (2005). Too good to be true: Dose insensitivity and stereotypical thinking of foods' capacity to promote weight gain. *Food Quality and Preference, 16,* 675-681.

Oakes, M. E., and Slotterback, C. S. (2001a). What's in a name? A comparison of men's and women's judgements about food names and their nutrient contents. *Appetite, 36,* 29-40.

Oakes, M. E., and Slotterback, C. S. (2001b). Judgements of food healthfulness: food name stereotypes in adults over age 25. *Appetite, 37,* 1-8.

Patterson, R. E., Satia, J. A., Kristal, A. R., Neuhouser, M. L., and Drewnowski, A. (2001). Is there a consumer backlash against the diet and health message. *Journal of the American Dietetic Association, 101,* 37-41.

Pennington, J. A. T. (1998). *Bowes and Church's food values of portions commonly used (seventeenth edition).* New York: Lippincott.

Rozin, P., Ashmore, M., and Markwith, M. (1996). Lay American conceptions of nutrition: Dose insensitivity, categorical thinking, contagion, and the monotonic mind. *Health Psychology, 15*, 438-447.

Schwartz, N. E. and Borra, S. T. (1997). What do consumers really think about dietary fat? *Journal of the American Dietetic Association, 97*, S73-S75.

Sears, B. (1995). *The Zone*. New York: HarperCollins.

Tipton, K. D., and Wolfe, R. R. (2001). Exercise, protein metabolism, and muscle growth. *International Journal of Sport Nutrition and Exercise Metabolism, 11*, 109-132.

US Department of Agriculture, Center for Nutrition Policy and Promotion. Home and Garden Bulletin Number 252. The Food Guide Pyramid. http://www.usda.gov/ cnpp/ Pubs/Pyramid/fdgdpyr1.pdf. Accessed: October 16, 2002.

US Department of Agriculture. (2005). *2005 Dietary Guidelines for Americans*. Washington, DC.

Appendix A

Aceto, C. (April 2005). Heavy duty protein. *Muscle and Fitness*, 134-138.

Alexander, D. (April 2005a). Training table: Cook smart, eat better. *Muscle and Fitness*, 72.

Alexander, D. (April 2005b). Training table: Nutrition Rx. *Muscle & Fitness*, 74.

(no author) (April 2005). Get lean. *Men's Fitness*, 32.

(no author) (April 2005). Hotline Nutrition. *Muscle and Fitness*, 52.

(no author) (April 2005). MF Picks. *Men's Fitness*, 38.

(no author). (April 2005). Get big. *Men's Fitness*, 24.

Schuler, L. and Williams, J. (April 2005). Defy your genetics. *Men's Fitness*, 66-71.

Volek, J. (April 2005). Low-carb lies. *Men's Fitness*, 34.

In: Nutrition for the Middle Aged and Elderly
Editors: N. E. Bernhardt, A. M. Kasko, pp. 271-284
ISBN: 978-1-60456-146-3

Chapter IX

Serum Magnesium and Cancer Mortality

Charles J. Everett[1], Dana E. King[1], Brian J. Wells[2], Ivar L. Frithsen[1] and Arch G. Mainous III[1]
[1]Department of Family Medicine, Medical University of South Carolina, Charleston, SC, USA
[2]Department of Quantitative Health Sciences, The Cleveland Clinic Foundation, Cleveland, OH, USA

Dedication

This chapter is dedicated to my parents, who both died of cancer far too young, and to my wife who is a cancer survivor. – CJE.

Abstract

The association of serum magnesium with cancer mortality was investigated prospectively using the Atherosclerosis Risk in Communities (ARIC) Study. Black (N=3,898) and nonblack (N=10,534) participants, aged 45-64 at baseline, were analyzed separately. In a Cox's regression adjusted for gender, age, body mass index, exercise, education, number of cigarettes currently smoked, and smoking history, nonblack participants with serum magnesium $\leq$1.4 meq/l had a hazard ratio of 2.72 (95% CI 1.40-5.29) for all-cancer mortality compared to persons with serum magnesium $\geq$1.9 meq/l. When nonblack participants were classified as $\leq$1.6 meq/l versus $\geq$1.7 meq/l, low serum magnesium had a hazard ratio of 1.53 (95% CI 1.19-1.97) for all-cancer mortality. Significant inverse relationships between nonblack participants' serum magnesium and two types of cancer mortality were found. First, an association with mortality due to malignant neoplasm of respiratory/intrathoracic organs, and second an association with all other types of cancer mortality. For black participants there was no association of serum magnesium and all-cancer mortality. This pattern of a relationship with serum magnesium among nonblack participants, but no association among black participants was similar to previously published research on the development of diabetes and serum magnesium in the ARIC Study.

Introduction

Recent biologic and epidemiologic evidence strongly supports a significant role for magnesium in human health, and in particular, in the relationship between hypertension and inflammation [1-3]. Further, in light of recent evidence that 77% of adults and 84% of adults with hypertension plus inflammation have magnesium intake below the recommended daily allowance (RDA) [4-5], evaluating the possible impact of magnesium intake on human health and cancer is clearly timely.

The association between magnesium and the body's inflammatory response may have implications for the association between magnesium and subsequent cancer. As early as two decades ago, Bloom [6] demonstrated the development of inflammation in the coronary arteries of hamsters fed a magnesium-deficient diet. Affected arteries showed endothelial cell hyperplasia and pleomorphism, chronic inflammation of the media and adventitia, and fibrinoid necrosis. The author concluded that this inflammation response was a significant factor to be considered in the pathophysiology of magnesium-poor diets.

Chronic inflammation has been linked to several solid malignancies, including esophageal, gastric, liver, pancreatic, renal and prostatic cancers [7-9]. Possible mechanisms by which inflammation may contribute to carcinogenesis include elaboration of inflammatory cytokines and growth factors that favor tumor cell growth, induction of cyclo-oxygenase-2 in macrophages and epithelial cells; and promotion of oxidative stress [10].

In support of the inflammatory model linking cancer and magnesium, evidence of inflammation has been found in magnesium-deficient rat models [11]. More recently, Maier [12] found that low serum magnesium concentrations impact the inflammatory response by affecting pro-inflammatory cytokines, such as up-regulation of interleukin-1 (IL-1) and serum vascular adhesion molecule (sVCAM-1). Magnesium deficiency in rats is also associated with an increase in serum levels of tumor necrosis factor-α [13].

In humans, magnesium operates in many enzyme systems, including acting as the rate-limiting enzyme in the cholesterol biosynthesis sequence that is targeted by HMG-CoA reductase inhibitor drugs (statins), which are known to lower systemic inflammation [14]. In this context, magnesium has been shown to inhibit proliferation and migration of vascular smooth muscle cells and macrophages. This effect offers one of several possible mechanisms for the anti-inflammatory effects of magnesium.

Recent studies add human epidemiologic evidence that magnesium may play a role in inflammation. Guerrero-Romero et al. [15] have investigated the association of serum magnesium levels with c-reactive protein (CRP), an inflammatory biomarker, and found the likelihood of having elevated CRP, after adjustment for demographic and other factors, was 2.11 (1.23-3.84) for those in the lowest quintile of serum magnesium compared to the highest. Other researchers have found that magnesium intake and inflammation are inversely related [16, 17]. Inflammation has been theorized to be an important component of carcinogenesis and CRP levels have been associated with cancer risk [18-20].

In a recent study by King et al [4], adults who consumed <50% of the recommended daily allowance (RDA) of magnesium were more likely to have elevated CRP than adults who consumed ≥ RDA (Odds Ratio [OR] = 1.75, 95% CI 1.08-2.87). In a second cross-sectional study, it was found that magnesium supplementation lowers the likelihood of elevated CRP in people with low dietary magnesium intake by 22% [5]. This observation suggests that magnesium supplementation may be a useful strategy for reduction of inflammation. The study also provides important epidemiologic support for the idea that magnesium itself, rather than some component of magnesium-containing food, is responsible for the decreased inflammation.

Magnesium's impact on oxidative stress is another possible mechanism for the association between magnesium and cancer. Several components of oxidative metabolism are dependent upon dietary micronutrients [21]. Accumulating experimental evidence supports the idea that magnesium deficiency promotes an immuno-inflammatory reaction and increased oxidative stress that can damage cells [22-24]. In addition, magnesium-deficient rats demonstrate an increased susceptibility to oxidative stress in organ tissues including the liver [25].

A recent study was undertaken to examine the hypothesis that magnesium deficiency accentuates oxidative stress in experimental rats [26]. Electrically stimulated rat papillary muscle was used for recording the contractile variation. Biochemical variables were assayed in Langendorff-perfused rat hearts. Hydrogen peroxide was used as the source of reactive oxygen species. The negative inotropic response to hydrogen peroxide was significantly higher in Mg deficiency (0.48 mmol Mg/L) than in Mg sufficiency (1.2 mmol Mg/L). Hydrogen peroxide induced an enhancement of oxidative stress in the presence of Mg deficiency.

Evidence in humans suggests that a magnesium-rich diet may enhance antioxidant capacity [27]. In Lopes' study, 24 individuals were studied on their usual diets and after following a magnesium-rich diet and a low-antioxidant diet in random sequence for 4 weeks each. Acute oxidative stress was induced by a 4-hour infusion of intralipid and heparin. Ferric-reducing activity of plasma (FRAP) and plasma F2-isoprostanes were measured as biomarkers of antioxidant capacity and oxidative stress, respectively. F2-isoprostanes increased on the low-antioxidant diet but not in individuals on the magnesium-rich diet. Thus, the magnesium-rich diet made participants more resistant to oxidative stress. In another study, 93 patients with unexplained chronic fatigue were evaluated for magnesium status and oxidant status. Mg deficient patients (47%) had lower total antioxidant capacity in plasma ($p=0.007$) than non-Mg deficient patients.

Magnesium is an abundant element in the human body and is involved in a wide range of metabolic pathways. Magnesium is vital to DNA replication, genomic stability, apoptosis, and cell membrane integrity [28]. Nuclear magnetic resonance spectroscopy has revealed that magnesium is crucial for stabilizing the secondary and tertiary structure of DNA [29], and magnesium protects DNA from oxidative damage [30]. Magnesium's effect on DNA underscores the interest between magnesium and cancer. Magnesium appears to be protective at the early stages of carcinogenesis, while it promotes growth of existing tumors at later stages [13, 31]. Data from animal studies indicate metastases are promoted by low magnesium levels [31]. Hence, studies of magnesium and cancer mortality may have different results than studies of diagnoses of cancer.

The studies reviewed here deal with all-cancer mortality [32, 33], specific cancer mortality [32, 34-44], and specific cancer morbidity [45-48]. Only one study has measured serum magnesium [33] and three have looked at magnesium intake using a food frequency questionnaire [46-48] the other studies deal with magnesium in drinking water or total hardness of drinking water. Magnesium intake from water represents perhaps 10% of total intake, but magnesium in water is thought to be more easily absorbed than magnesium in food [41]. Water hardness is an indicator of calcium and magnesium content of the water.

Colorectal cancer has been studied more than other types of cancer. Larsson et al. [46] looked at magnesium intake and colorectal cancer morbidity in a cohort study with 14.8 years of follow-up. They found the highest quintile of magnesium intake had a relative risk of 0.59 (95% CI 0.40-0.87) compared to the lowest quintile. Folsom et al. [47] found magnesium intake was not related to colorectal cancer morbidity among Iowa women in a cohort study with 17 years of follow-up. However, when looking specifically at colon cancer, they did find a significant inverse relationship between magnesium intake and colon cancer morbidity. Van den Brandt et al. [48] found magnesium intake was not associated with colorectal morbidity in a case-cohort study with 13.3 years of follow-up. They did find a significant inverse relationship between magnesium intake and colon cancer morbidity or proximal colon cancer morbidity among persons with body mass index ≥ 25 kg/m^2. Looking at magnesium in drinking water, Yang and Chiu [37] found no relationship with rectal cancer mortality in a case-control study conducted in Taiwan. Similarly, Yang et al. [34] found no relationship between magnesium in drinking water and colon cancer mortality. The results of two other case-control studies, also conducted in Taiwan, showed significant inverse relationships between total hardness of drinking water and colon cancer mortality [36] or rectal cancer mortality [38].

In addition to magnesium and colorectal cancer, magnesium and breast cancer, prostate cancer, esophageal cancer, liver cancer, ovarian cancer, and gastric or stomach cancer have been studied. Yang et al. [41] found a significant inverse relationship between magnesium in drinking water and breast cancer mortality in a case-control study conducted in Taiwan. Similarly, Yang et al. [40] found a significant inverse relationship between magnesium in drinking water and prostate cancer mortality. Both total hardness and magnesium content of drinking water have been studied with respect to esophageal cancer mortality. Yang et al. [39] found soft water had an odds ratio of 1.42 (95% CI 1.22-1.66) for esophageal cancer mortality compared to hard water. More specific to the question of magnesium, Yang et al. [42] found magnesium in drinking water to be inversely related to esophageal cancer mortality. Using Bayesian modeling, Tukiendorf and Rybak [45] found magnesium in drinking water to be inversely related to liver cancer morbidity in Poland. In Taiwan, Yang et al. [43] found no relationship between magnesium in drinking water and liver cancer mortality. In another case-control study ovarian cancer mortality was found to be inversely related to magnesium in drinking water [44]. In Japan, Sakamoto et al. [32] studied all-cancer mortality and stomach cancer mortality in relation to magnesium in drinking water. They found no significant relationship for all-cancer mortality, but significant inverse relationship, via a covariate analysis, for magnesium in drinking water and stomach cancer mortality.

Another case-control study from Taiwan showed a significant inverse relationship between magnesium in drinking water and gastric cancer mortality [35]. Taken together, these studies show an inverse relationship between magnesium and a wide variety of specific cancer mortalities.

The only study using the best measure of magnesium status, that is serum magnesium, is a cohort study with 18 years of follow-up [33]. The Paris Prospective Study 2 is a cohort of 4,035 men age 30-60 years at baseline. There were a total of 176 deaths due to cancer during follow-up. Leone et al. [33] found the highest quartile of serum magnesium had a relative risk of 0.5 (95% CI 0.3-0.8) for all-cancer mortality compared to the lowest quartile.

The purpose of this study is to assess the role of race as a factor determining the association, or lack of association, between serum magnesium and cancer mortality. None of the studies preceding ours have evaluated the association of serum magnesium and all-cancer mortality in an African American cohort. We compare and contrast the relationship for the African American participants with that of the mostly Caucasian, nonblack participants of the Atherosclerosis Risk in Communities Study. Where we find an association between serum magnesium and all-cancer mortality we further explore the nature of the relationship for two types of cancer mortality.

Methods

The Atherosclerosis Risk in Communities (ARIC) Study is a cohort of 15,792 participants aged 45 to 64, from four US communities. The locations included are Forsyth County, NC; Jackson, MS (African Americans only), the suburbs of Minneapolis, MN; and Washington County, MD. In the public-use data set, participants are classified as either nonblack or black. The nonblack participants are mostly Caucasians, but include 14 American Indians and 34 Asian participants. The baseline examination (Visit 1) was in 1986-89 and follow-up examinations were in 1990-92 (Visit 2), 1993-95 (Visit 3), and 1996-98 (Visit 4). We conducted a longitudinal analysis using information from Visit 1 to classify participants and then following them to December 31, 1998.

We defined 5 smoking history categories using interview information from Visit 1. Participants were first classified as never, former or current smokers. Former and current smokers were then further classified by response to the question: "On the average of the entire time you smoked, how many cigarettes did you usually smoke per day?" Heavy smokers were defined as those who had smoked 15 or more cigarettes per day, and light smokers as those who had smoked less than 15 cigarettes per day. We used a cut-off of 15 cigarettes per day to make our results comparable to Godtfredsen et al. [49] and because 15 cigarettes per day is close to the mean for former and current African American smokers in the ARIC Study.

Serum magnesium level was measured using the metallochromic dye calmagite (1-[1-hydroxy-4-methyl-2-phenylazo]-2-naphthol-4-sulfonic acid), based on the method of Gindler and Heth [50]. Magnesium was measured to the nearest 0.1 meq/l. The coefficient of variation was 3% for specimens blindly sent to the laboratory 1 week apart [51]. Serum magnesium was classified in two ways, first as ≤1.4, 1.5, 1.6, 1.7, 1.8 and ≥1.9 meq/l, the finest increments possible, and second as two categories, $\leq$1.6 and $\geq$1.7 meq/l (split close to the median). We classified magnesium in two ways because it was not possible to use quartiles or quintiles with 0.1 meq/l increments.

We used gender, age, body mass index, exercise and education as control variables due to their associations with cancer and mortality. Body mass index (BMI) was calculated from weight and height measurements as kg/m^2. Exercise was characterized using a sports index derived from answers to a modified version of a questionnaire developed by Baecke et al. [52]. The index was semicontinuous and ranged from 1 (low) to 5 (high). The sports index was a sum of the yearly frequency, weekly duration, and intensity (low, medium, or high) of up to four self-reported sport activities, plus answers to three additional questions about self-rated amount of leisure time activity compared with others of the same age, frequency of sweating, and general frequency of sport play [53]. Exercise physiology research assistants used standard references to assign intensity codes to the types of sports or exercises [54]. Education was classified as three categories: 1) 11 years of schooling or less, 2) High school graduate or vocational school, and 3) College or graduate school or professional school.

To account for current smokers quitting at a later date, and former smokers who resumed smoking at a later date, we included the current number of cigarettes per day a participant smoked as a time-dependent control variable. The current number of cigarettes smoked per day at Visits 1 through 4 was used to create this variable. If a participant was not smoking at a particular visit, the value of this variable was 0 for that time interval.

Participants who died of cancer during the first three years following baseline were excluded from our analyses. These persons may have had undiagnosed cancer at Visit 1, which could introduce misclassification bias due to the association between cancer and hypomagnesaemia.

Our cohort consisted of 14,432 participants age 45-64 at baseline. Events were classified as either all-cancer mortality, mortality due to malignant neoplasm of respiratory and intrathoracic organs (*International Classification of Diseases, Ninth Revision* codes 160-165), or other types of cancer mortality. We excluded from our cohort 873 participants who reported a previous diagnosis of cancer, 90 persons who died of cancer during the first three years following baseline, 206 participants missing magnesium tests, and 191 persons missing smoking, BMI, exercise or education variables. In addition to undergoing clinical examinations, participants were contacted annually to determine their follow-up status. Of the 14,432 persons in our cohort, 1,209 died before December 31, 1998. The remainder had a mean follow-up time of 10.4 years, with the minimum follow-up being 6 years.

We used the statistical package SAS (Statistical Analysis System, Cary, North Carolina) for all analyses. Adjusted Cox's regressions were performed by race. There were 3,898 black participants and 10,534 nonblack participants included in our analyses. Also, there were 131 cases of all-cancer mortality among black participants and 251 cases of all-cancer mortality among nonblack participants.

Results

Demographic data about the participants enrolled in this study are shown in Table 1. A total of 7.8% of the nonblack participants and 21.0% of the black participants had serum magnesium concentrations ≤1.4 meq/l.

Table 1. Demographics of nonblack and black participants

	Nonblack	Black
Serum Magnesium (meq/l) (%)		
≤1.4	7.8	21.0
1.5	14.8	20.8
1.6	26.1	25.3
1.7	27.2	18.3
1.8	16.3	9.9
≥1.9	7.8	4.6
Education (%)		
≤11th Grade	17.1	41.5
High School or Vocational School	45.3	28.2
College or Professional School	37.6	30.2
Smoking (%)		
Never	40.4	47.1
Former Light Smoker	10.4	12.2
Former Heavy Smoker	25.1	11.2
Current Light Smoker	4.6	14.0
Current Heavy Smoker	19.5	15.5
Age (yr) [1]	54.2 (5.7)	53.4 (5.8)
Body Mass Index (kg/m^2)[1]	27.0 (4.9)	29.6 (6.1)
Sports Index[1]	2.5 (0.8)	2.2 (0.7)
[1]Mean (Standard Deviation)		

Results of our Cox's regressions differed substantially between nonblack and black participants. Serum magnesium ≤1.4 meq/l had a hazard ratio of 2.72 (95% CI 1.40-5.29) compared to serum magnesium ≥1.9 meq/l for all-cancer mortality among nonblack participants (Table 2). For black participants, serum magnesium ≤1.4 meq/l had a hazard ratio of 1.36 (95% CI 0.53-3.49) compared to serum magnesium ≥1.9 meq/l for all-cancer mortality (Table 3). The difference between nonblack and black participants was due to a high rate of all-cancer mortality among black participants regardless of magnesium level. For serum magnesium ≥1.9 meq/l there were 2.0 cases per 1,000 person-years among nonblack participants and 4.1 cases per 1,000 person-years among black participants.

When the data for nonblack participants was split nearly in two, 5,133 participants with serum magnesium ≤1.6 meq/l and 5,401 participants with magnesium ≥1.7 meq/l, the hazard ratio for all-cancer mortality was 1.53 (95% CI 1.19-1.97) for serum magnesium ≤1.6 meq/l compared to serum magnesium ≥1.7 meq/l.

Table 2. Adjusted Cox's regressions using serum magnesium to predict all-cancer mortality among nonblack participants[1]

	Hazard Ratio	95% CI	Cases per 1,000 Person-Years[2]
Magnesium[3] (meq/l)			
≤ 1.4	2.72	1.40-5.29	5.9
1.5	1.77	0.93-3.38	3.6
1.6	1.82	0.99-3.34	3.8
1.7	1.28	0.68-2.38	2.7
1.8	1.38	0.72-2.64	2.9
≥ 1.9	1.00	---	2.0
Magnesium[4] (meq/l)			
≤ 1.6	1.53	1.19-1.97	4.1
≥ 1.7	1.00	---	2.7

[1] Adjusted for number of cigarettes smoked per day at most recent visit, smoking history, gender, age, body mass index, exercise and education.
[2] Calculated excluding the first three years of follow-up.
[3] Serum magnesium in six categories.
[4] Serum magnesium in two categories.

Table 3. Adjusted Cox's regressions using serum magnesium to predict all-cancer mortality among black participants[1]

	Hazard Ratio	95% CI	Cases per 1,000 Person-Years[2]
Magnesium[3] (meq/l)			
≤ 1.4	1.36	0.53-3.49	6.5
1.5	1.00	0.38-2.64	4.3
1.6	0.90	0.35-2.35	4.2
1.7	0.96	0.36-2.55	4.3
1.8	1.67	0.62-4.48	7.1
≥ 1.9	1.00	---	4.1
Magnesium[4] (meq/l)			
≤ 1.6	0.92	0.64-1.32	4.9
≥ 1.7	1.00	---	5.1

[1] Adjusted for number of cigarettes smoked per day at most recent visit, smoking history, gender, age, body mass index, exercise and education.
[2] Calculated excluding the first three years of follow-up.
[3] Serum magnesium in six categories.
[4] Serum magnesium in two categories.

Table 4. Adjusted Cox's regressions using serum magnesium to predict mortality due to malignant neoplasm of respiratory and intrathoracic organs among nonblack participants[1]

	Hazard Ratio	95% CI	Cases per 1,000 Person-Years[2]
Magnesium[3] (meq/l)			
≤ 1.4	3.06	0.83-11.34	1.6
1.5	2.54	0.73-8.86	1.3
1.6	3.09	0.95-10.10	1.6
1.7	1.70	0.50-5.75	0.9
1.8	1.34	0.36-4.96	0.7
≥ 1.9	1.00	---	0.5
Magnesium[4] (meq/l)			
≤ 1.6	1.97	1.27-3.06	1.5
≥ 1.7	1.00	---	0.8

[1] Adjusted for number of cigarettes smoked per day at most recent visit, smoking history, gender, age, body mass index, exercise and education.

[2] Calculated excluding the first three years of follow-up.

[3] Serum magnesium in six categories.

[4] Serum magnesium in two categories.

Table 5. Adjusted Cox's regressions using serum magnesium to predict cancer mortality other than respiratory/intrathoracic organ cancer mortality among nonblack participants[1]

	Hazard Ratio	95% CI	Cases per 1,000 Person-Years[2]
Magnesium[3] (meq/l)			
≤ 1.4	2.56	1.18-5.53	4.3
1.5	1.50	0.70-3.21	2.4
1.6	1.38	0.67-2.84	2.2
1.7	1.14	0.55-2.36	1.8
1.8	1.40	0.66-2.97	2.2
≥ 1.9	1.00	---	1.5
Magnesium[4] (meq/l)			
≤ 1.6	1.34	0.98-1.82	2.6
≥ 1.7	1.00	---	1.9

[1] Adjusted for number of cigarettes smoked per day at most recent visit, smoking history, gender, age, body mass index, exercise and education.

[2] Calculated excluding the first three years of follow-up.

[3] Serum magnesium in six categories.

[4] Serum magnesium in two categories.

These results indicate a possible role for magnesium in cancer mortality among the nonblack participants regardless of how the data are categorized. To further investigate magnesium and specific types of cancer mortality we conducted two additional analyses of nonblack participants. In the first analysis (Table 4) we looked at mortality due to malignant neoplasm of respiratory and intrathoracic organs. Using six categories of serum magnesium the results were not significant due to the limited number of cases being analyzed (86 cases). However, when the data were divided into two classes, serum magnesium $\leq$1.6 meq/l had a hazard ratio of 1.97 (95% CI 1.27-3.06) compared to serum magnesium $\geq$1.7 meq/l for mortality due to malignant neoplasm of respiratory and intrathoracic organs. For nonblack cancer mortality other than respiratory/intrathoracic organ cancer mortality, serum magnesium $\leq$1.4 meq/l had a hazard ratio of 2.56 (95% CI 1.18-5.53) compared to serum magnesium $\geq$1.9 meq/l (Table 5). These results indicate magnesium is associated with both respiratory and intrathoracic organ cancer mortality, and other types of cancer mortality among nonblack participants.

Conclusion

Relatively few studies have looked at magnesium and all-cancer mortality. We found inverse relationships between serum magnesium and all-cancer mortality, serum magnesium and mortality due to malignant neoplasm of respiratory and intrathoracic organs, and serum magnesium and cancer mortality other than respiratory/intrathoracic organ cancer mortality, among nonblack participants. There was no relationship between serum magnesium and all-cancer mortality for black participants. This pattern of significant results for the nonblack participants and nonsignificant results for black participants was also observed in a study of serum magnesium and incidence of diabetes conducted using the ARIC Study [55]. In our study, black participants had high rates of all-cancer mortality regardless of serum magnesium levels. The difference between blacks and nonblacks may be due to higher fibrinogen levels among blacks, which has been shown to be associated with cancer mortality, particularly among African Americans [56]. Our results are consistent with those of Leone et al. [33], who evaluated the Paris Prospective Study 2, and confirm a number of studies of magnesium in drinking water and cancer mortality. More studies of magnesium and cancer morbidity are needed as our results, and those of Leone et al. [33], may be due to the promotion of metastases by low levels of magnesium [31].

Acknowledgments

The Atherosclerosis Risk in Communities (ARIC) Study is conducted and supported by the NHLBI in collaboration with the ARIC Study Investigators. This manuscript was prepared using a limited access dataset obtained by the NHLBI and does not necessarily reflect the opinions or views of the ARIC Study or the NHLBI.

References

[1] Boos, CJ; Lip, GY. Is hypertension an inflammatory process? *Current Pharmaceutical Design.* 2006;12(13):1623-1635.

[2] Li, JJ; Chen, JL. Inflammation may be a bridge connecting hypertension and atherosclerosis. *Medical Hypotheses* 2005;64(5):925-9.

[3] Guerrero-Romero, F; Rodriguez-Moran, M. Hypomagnesemia, oxidative stress, inflammation, and metabolic syndrome. *Diabetes-Metabolism Research and Reviews* 2006;22(6):471-476.

[4] King, DE; Mainous, AG III; Geesey, M; Woolson, RF. Dietary magnesium and C-reactive protein levels. *Journal of the American College of Nutrition* 2005;24(3):166-171.

[5] King, DE; Mainous, AG III; Geesey, M; Egan, BM; Rehman, S. Magnesium supplement intake and C-reactive protein levels in adults. *Nutrition Research* 2006;26(5):193-196.

[6] Bloom, S. Coronary arterial lesions in Mg-deficient hamsters. *Magnesium* 1985;4(2-3):82-95.

[7] Tan, TT; Coussens, LM. Humoral immunity, inflammation and cancer. *Current Opinion in Immunology* 2007;19(2): 209-216.

[8] Nelson, WG. Prostate cancer prevention. *Current Opinion in Urology* 2007;17(3):157-167.

[9] Budhu, A; Wang, XW. The role of cytokines in hepatocellular carcinoma. *Journal of Leukocyte Biology* 2006;80(6):1197-1213.

[10] Lucia, MS; Torkko, KC. Inflammation as a target for prostate cancer chemoprevention: Pathological and laboratory rationale. *Journal of Urology* 2004;171(2 Pt 2):S30-S34.

[11] Walsh, RJ; Weglicki, WB; Correa-de-Araujo, R. Distribution of specific substance P binding sites in the heart and adjacent great vessels of the Wistar white rat. *Cell and Tissue Research* 1996;284(3):495-500.

[12] Maier, JA; Malpuech-Brugere, C; Zimowska, W; Rayssiguier, Y; Mazur, A. Low magnesium promotes endothelial cell dysfunction: implications for atherosclerosis, inflammation and thrombosis. *Biochimica et Biophysica Acta* 2004:13-21.

[13] Anastassopoulou, J; Theophanides, T. Magnesium-DNA interactions and the possible relation of magnesium to carcinogenesis. Irradiation and free radicals. *Critical Reviews in Oncology Hematology* 2002;42(1):79-91.

[14] Rosanoff, A; Seelig, MS. Comparison of mechanism and functional effects of magnesium and statin pharmaceuticals. *Journal of the American College of Nutrition* 2004 ;23(5) :501S-505S.

[15] Guerrero-Romero, F; Rodriguez-Moran, M. Relationship between serum magnesium levels and C-reactive protein concentration, in non-diabetic, non-hypertensive obese subjects. *International Journal of Obesity* 2002;26(4):469-74.

[16] Song, Y ; Ridker, PM ; Manson, JE ; Cook, NR ; Buring, JE ; Liu, S. Magnesium intake, c-reactive protein, and the prevalence of metabolic syndrome in middle-aged and older US women. *Diabetes Care* 2005;28(6):1438-44.

[17] Barbagallo, M; Dominguez, LJ. Magnesium metabolism in type 2 diabetes mellitus, metabolic syndrome and insulin resistance. *Archives of Biochemistry and Biophysics* 2007;458(1):40-47.

[18] Erlinger, TP; Platz, EA; Rifai, N; Helzlsouer, KJ. C-reactive protein and the risk of incident colorectal cancer. *JAMA* 2004;291(5):585-590.

[19] McSorley, MA; Alberg, AJ; Allen, DS; Allen, NE; Brinton, LA; Dorgan, JF; Pollak, M; Tao, Y; Helzlsouer, KJ. C-reactive protein concentrations and subsequent ovarian cancer risk. *Obstetrics and Gynecology* 2007;109(4):933-941.

[20] Siemes, C; Visser, LE; Coebergh, JW; Splinter, TA; Witteman, JC; Uitterlinden, AG; Hofman, A; Pols, HA; Stricker, BH. C-reactive protein levels, variation in the C-reactive protein gene, and cancer risk: The Rotterdam Study. *Journal of Clinical Oncology* 2006;24(33):5216-5222.

[21] Evans, P; Halliwell, B. Micronutrients: oxidant/antioxidant status. *British Journal of Nutrition* 2001;85(Suppl 2):S67-74.

[22] Shivakumar, K. Pro-fibrogenic effects of magnesium deficiency in the cardiovascular system. *Magnesium Research* 2002;158(3-4):307-15.

[23] Pandhi, P; Saha, L; Malhotra, S. Effect of oral magnesium supplementation on experimental pre-eclampsia induced by prolonged blockade of nitric oxide syntheses in pregnant rats. *Indian Journal of Experimental Biology* 2002;40(3):349-851.

[24] Dickens, BF; Weglicki, WB; Li, YS; Mak, IT. Magnesium deficiency in vitro enhances free radical-induced intracellular oxidation and cytotoxicity in endothelial cells. *FEBS Letters* 1992;311(3):187-191.

[25] Busserolles, J; Gueux, E; Rock, E; Mazur, A; Rayssiguier, Y. High fructose feeding of magnesium deficient rats is associated with increased plasma triglyceride concentration and increased oxidative stress. *Magnesium Research* 2003;16(1):7-12.

[26] Manju, L; Nair, RR. Magnesium deficiency augments myocardial response to reactive oxygen species. *Canadian Journal of Physiology and Pharmacology* 2006;84(6):617-624.

[27] Lopes, HF; Martin, KL; Morrow, JD; Goodfirend, TL; Egan, BM. DASH diet lowers blood pressure and lipid-induced oxidative stress in obesity. *Hypertension* 2003; 41: 422-430.

[28] Hartwig, A. Review: Role of Magnesium in genomic stability. *Mutation Research* 2001;475:113-21.

[29] Pelletier, H; Sawaya, MR; Kumar, A; Wilson, SH; Kraut, J. Structures of ternary complexes of rat DNA polymerase beta, a DNA template-primer, and ddCTP. *Science* 1994;264(5167):1891-1903.

[30] Sclavi, B; Sullivan, M; Chance, MR; Brenowitz, M; Woodson, SA. RNA folding at millisecond intervals by synchrotron hydroxyl radical footprinting. *Science* 1998;279(5358):1940-1943.

[31] Wolf, FI; Maier, JAM; Nasulewicz, A; Feillet-Coudray, C; Simonacci, M; Mazur, A; Cittadini, A. Magnesium and neoplasia: From carcinogenesis to tumor growth and progression or treatment. *Archives of Biochemistry and Biophysics* 2007;458:24-32.

[32] Sakamoto, N; Shimizu, M; Wakabayashi, I; Sakamoto, K. Relationship between mortality rate of stomach cancer and cerebrovascular disease and concentrations of

magnesium and calcium in well water in Hyogo prefecture. *Magnesium Research* 1997;10:215-223.

[33] Leone, N; Courbon, D; Ducimetiere, P; Zureik, M. Zinc, copper, and magnesium and risks for all-cause, cancer, and cardiovascular mortality. *Epidemiology* 2006;17:308-314.

[34] Yang, CY; Chiu, HF; Chiu, JF; Tsai, SS; Cheng, MF. Calcium and magnesium in drinking water and risk of death from colon cancer. *Japanese Journal of Cancer Research* 1997;88:928-933.

[35] Yang, CY; Cheng, MF; Tsai, SS; Hsieh, YL. Calcium, magnesium, and nitrate in drinking water and gastric cancer mortality. *Japanese Journal of Cancer Research* 1998;89:124-130.

[36] Yang, CY; Hung, CF. Colon cancer mortality and total hardness levels in Taiwan's drinking water. *Archives of Environmental Contamination and Toxicology* 1998;35:148-151.

[37] Yang, CY; Chiu, HF. Calcium and magnesium in drinking water and risk of death from rectal cancer. *International Journal of Cancer* 1998;77:528-532.

[38] Yang, CY; Tsai, SS; Lai, TC; Hung, CF; Chiu, HF. Rectal cancer mortality and total hardness levels in Taiwan's drinking water. *Environmental Research* 1999;80:311-316.

[39] Yang, CY; Chiu, HF; Cheng, MF; Tsai, SS; Hung, CF; Lin, MC. Esophageal cancer mortality and total hardness levels in Taiwan's drinking water. *Environmental Research* 1999;81:302-308.

[40] Yang, CY; Chiu, HF; Tsai, SS; Cheng, MF; Lin, MC; Sung, FC. Calcium and magnesium in drinking water and risk of death from prostate cancer. *Journal of Toxicology and Environmental Health Part A* 2000;60:17-26.

[41] Yang, CY; Chiu, HF; Cheng, MF; Hsu, TY; Cheng, MF; Wu, TN. Calcium and magnesium in drinking water and the risk of death from breast cancer. *Journal of Toxicology and Environmental Health Part A* 2000;60:231-241.

[42] Yang, CY; Chiu, HF; Tsai, SS; Wu, TN; Chang, CC. Magnesium and calcium in drinking water and the risk of death from esophageal cancer. *Magnesium Research* 2002;15:215-222.

[43] Yang, CY; Chiu, HF; Tsai, SS; Chang, CC; Chuang, HY. Magnesium in drinking water and the risk of death from liver cancer. *Magnesium Research* 2002;15:223-228.

[44] Chiu, HF; Chang, CC; Yang, CY. Magnesium and calcium in drinking water and risk of death from ovarian cancer. *Magnesium Research* 2004;17:28-34.

[45] Tukiendorf, A; Rybak, Z. New data on ecological analysis of possible relationship between magnesium in drinking water and liver cancer. *Magnesium Research* 2004;17:46-52.

[46] Larsson, SC; Bergkvist, L; Wolk, A. Magnesium intake in relation to risk of colorectal cancer in women. *JAMA* 2005;293:86-89.

[47] Folsom, AR; Hong, CP. Magnesium intake and reduced risk of colon cancer in a prospective study of women. *American Journal of Epidemiology* 2006;163:232-235.

[48] van den Brandt, PA; Smits, KM; Goldbohm, RA; Weijenberg, MP. Magnesium intake and colorectal cancer risk in the Netherlands Cohort Study. *British Journal of Cancer* 2007;96:510-513.

[49] Godtfredsen, NS; Prescott, E; Osler, M. Effect of smoking reduction on lung cancer risk. *JAMA.* 2005;294:1505-1510.

[50] Gindler, EM; Heth, DA. Colorimetric determination with bound "Calmagite" of magnesium in human blood serum [abstract]. *Clinical Chemistry* 1971;17:662.

[51] Ma, J; Folsom, AR; Melnick, SL; Eckfeldt, JH; Sharrett, AR; Nabulsi, AA; Hutchinson, RG; Metcalf, PA. Associations of serum and dietary magnesium with cardiovascular-disease, hypertension, diabetes, insulin and carotid arterial-wall thickness – The ARIC Study. *Journal of Clinical Epidemiology* 1995;48:927-940.

[52] Baecke, JAH; Burema, J; Fretters, JER. A short questionnaire for the measurement of habitual physical activity in epidemiologic studies. *American Journal of Clinical Nutrition.* 1982;36:936-942.

[53] Schmitz, KH; Arnett, DK; Bank, A; Liao, DP; Evans, GW; Evenson, KR; Stevens, J; Sorlie, P; Folsom, AR. Arterial distensibility and physical activity in the ARIC study. *Medicine and Science in Sports and Exercise.* 2001;33:2065-2071.

[54] Folsom, AR; Arnett, DK; Hutchinson, RG; Liao, FZ; Clegg, LX; Cooper, LS. Physical activity and incidence of coronary heart disease in middle aged women and men. *Medicine and Science in Sports and Exercise.* 1997;29:901-909.

[55] Kao, WHL; Folsom, AR; Nieto, FJ; Mo, JP; Watson, RL; Brancati, FL. Serum and dietary magnesium and the risk for type 2 diabetes mellitus – The Atherosclerosis Risk in Communities Study. *Archives of Internal Medicine* 1999;159:2151-2159.

[56] Everett, CJ; Wells, BJ; Frithsen, IL; Koopman, RJ. Smoking, fibrinogen and cancer mortality. *Journal of the National Medical Association* 2007;99:328-333.

In: Nutrition for the Middle Aged and Elderly
Editors: N. E. Bernhardt, A. M. Kasko, pp. 285-298
ISBN: 978-1-60456-146-3

Chapter X

Nutrition in Older Adults: An Overview

Rossana Salerno-Kennedy*
School of Medicine
University College Cork,
Cork, Ireland

Abstract

The aging process alters body composition so that nutritional status changes as one gets older. The nutritional problems of older adults are not only related to physiological decline but also to socio-economic changes and to a multitude of disease processes and the therapeutic regimens prescribed to cure or treat those illnesses. The gap between actual nutrient consumption among older adults and the recommended intakes for diets associated with health promotion and the prevention of chronic disease is large. Undernutrition, which leads to the "anorexia of aging", and obesity are critical factors of disease and death in the middle-aged and elderly.

This article gives a brief overview of the factors which can contribute to malnutrition and suggests strategies for improvement.

Keywords: *malnutrition, undernutrition, obesity, elderly, middle-aged.*

Introduction

In reviewing the importance of nutrition in older adults, both malnutrition and the role of nutrition in the management of health conditions must be considered. Malnutrition is defined

* Contact details: Dr. Rossana Salerno-Kennedy, School of Medicine, Brookfield Health Sciences Complex, University College Cork, Cork, Ireland, Email:r.kennedy@ucc.ie

more specifically by nutrition professionals as *poor nutrition* which encompasses not only inadequate intake but also excess intake of nutrients [1]. Obesity is a common nutritional disorder in the middle-aged and elderly and is often linked with other clinical conditions such as dyslipidemia, hypertension, and diabetes [2]. The prevalence of obesity in older American adults [3], as well as in Mediterranean countries [4], will likely continue to increase.Therefore, preventing obesity by good dietary habits is a key to achieving longevity. However, a lean body is not always good for health. In the hospital setting, underweight, but not overweight or obesity, predicts mortality [5, 6], and the relative risk of death associated with overweight has been reported to decline with age in population-based studies [3, 7, 8, 9, 10]. Data from the "Gruppo Italiano di Farmacovigilanza nell'Anziano" (GIFA) [9] has shown that the prevalence of obesity-related diseases was significantly associated with increasing BMI values and high BMI values are not associated with, but rather likely protect from, mortality and dependency [5-7]. Infact, total mortality was lower in overweight (3.1%) and obese (2.8%) patients than in underweight (12.3%) subjects [9]. Moreover, a length of hospital stay greater than 14 days was recorded in 38.9% of underweight and 35.3% of obese patients [9]. Thus, obesity, if not extreme, should not be considered a major health problem in elderly patients requiring hospital care. The available evidence suggests that visceral obesity and overweight dating from middle age but not overweight developed in the older age could affect survival [11, 12]. Research is needed to verify whether a comparable conclusion applies to the general population.

It seems that, the prevention of weight loss in elderly is a more important issue for maintaining health and longevity instead [1]. Older people are more likely than younger ones to have a variety of chronic conditions and functional impairments that may adversely affect their nutritional status; they are therefore more likely than younger adults to have a higher risk of nutrient deficiencies [13] Undernutrition, which leads to the 'anorexia of ageing' and gradual weight loss, is associated with increased demands on health services, lengthier hospital stays and immune dysfunction and it is recognized as an important predictor of morbidity and mortality [14]. Undernutrition has been found in a variety of settings: community, care home and hospital residents. In particular, the prevalence of malnutrition is 5–10% of independently living older individuals, 30–60% of institutionalized patients, ≤ 35–65% of hospitalized patients [15, 16, 17] and ≤ 85% of nursing home patients. [18] This picture has lead to the development of guidelines and policy initiatives on treating and preventing malnutrition. [10, 20, 21].

This chapter examines dietary requirements for older adults as well as factors which can contribute to poor nutrition and strategies for improvement.

Dietary Requirements for Older Adults

The macronutrient, vitamin and trace element requirements for a healthy adult diet are summarized in Tables 1, 2 and 3 below, respectively. They follow the recommendations of the Institute of Medicine, Dietary Reference Intakes: Applications in Dietary Assessment, 2000 and Dietary Reference Intakes for Energy, Carbohydrates, Fiber, Fat, Protein and Amino Acids 2002 [22, 23, 24].

Table 1. Dietary Reference Intakes (DRIs) for Older Adults

Macronutrients

	Energy (Kcal)	Protein (g)	Carbo-hydrates (g)	Total Fat (%Kcal)	n-6 PUFA (g)	n-3 PUFA (g)	Total Fiber (g)	Drinking water, Beverages, Water in food (L)
RDA or AI [1]								
Age 51-70 Male	2204	**56**	**130**		14*	1.6*	30*	3.7*
Female	1978	**46**	**130**		11*	1.1*	21*	2.7*
Age 70+ Male	2054	**56**	**130**		14*	1.6*	30*	2.6*
Female	1873	**46**	**130**		11*	1.1*	21*	2.1*
		10-35%	45-65%	20-35%	5-10%	0.6-1.2%		

[1] Recommended Dietary Allowances (RDAs) are in **bold type** and Adequate Intakes (AIs) are in ordinary type followed by an asterisk (*).

Table 2. Dietary Reference Intakes (DRIs) for Older Adults

Vitamins

	Vit A (μg)	Vit C (mg)	Vit D (μg)	Vit E (mg)	Vit K (μg)	Vit B6 (mg)	Vit B12 (μg)	Folate (μg)
RDA or AI [1]								
Age 51-70 Male	**900**	**90**	10*	**15**	120*	**1.7**	**2.4**	**400**
Female	**700**	**75**	10*	**15**	90*	**1.5**	**2.4**	**400**
Age 70+ Male	**900**	**90**	15*	**15**	120*	**1.7**	**2.4**	**400**
Female	**700**	**75**	15*	**15**	90*	**1.5**	**2.4**	**400**

	Riboflavin (mg)	Niacin (mg)	Pantothenic Acid (mg)	Biotin (μg)	Cholin (mg)	Thiamin (mg)
RDA or AI [1]						
Age51-70 Male	**1.3**	**16**	5*	30*	550*	**1.2**
Female	**1.1**	**14**	5*	30*	425*	**1.1**
Age 70+ Male	**1.3**	**16**	5*	30*	550*	**1.2**
Female	**1.1**	**14**	5*	30*	425*	**1.1**

1 Recommended Dietary Allowances (RDAs) are in bold type and Adequate Intakes (AIs) are in ordinary type followed by an asterisk (*).

Table 3. Dietary Reference Intakes (DRIs) for Older Adults

Trace Elements

Nutrient	Age group#	RDA/AI* g/d	UL[a]
Boron (mg/d)	a b	ND ND	20 20
Calcium (mg/d)	a b	1,200* 1,200*	2,500 2,500
Chromium (μg/d)	a b	20 20	ND ND
Copper (μg/d)	a b	900 900	10,000 10,000
Fluoride (mg/d)	a b	3* 3*	10 10
Iodine (μg/d)	a b	150 150	1,100 1,100
Iron (mg/d)	a b	8 8	45 45
Magnesium (mg/d)	a b	320 320	350 350
Manganese (mg/d)	a b	1.8* 1.8*	11 11
Molybdenum (μg/d)	a b	45 45	2,000 2,000
Nickel (mg/d)	a b	ND ND	1.0 1.0
Phoshorous (mg/d)	a b	700 700	4,000 4,000
Selenium (μg/d)	a b	55 55	400 400
Vanadium (mg/d)	a b	ND ND	1.8 1.8
Zinc (mg/d)	a b	8 8	40 40

Age group: a: 50-70; b: >70.

The table is adapted from the DRI reports (2001) (see www.nap.edu). It represents Recommended Dietary Allowances (RDAs) in bold type, Adequate Intakes (AIs) in ordinary type followed by an asterisk (*), and Tolerable Upper Intake (ULs).. RDAs and AIs may both be used as goals for individual intake. UL = the maximum level of daily nutrient intake that is likely to pose no risk of adverse effects. Unless otherwise specified, the UL represents total intake from food, water, and supplements

ND = Not determinable due to lack of data of adverse effects in this age group and concern with regard to lack of ability to handle excess amounts. Source of intake should be from food only to prevent high levels of intake.

Factors Affecting the Nutritional Status in Older Adults

Aging is accompanied by a variety of economic, psychological and social changes that can compromise an individual's nutritional status [25]. Aging also produces physiological changes that affect the need for several essential nutrients [25]. Moreover, older people have a higher prevalence of chronic disease, take multiple medications and tend to be sedentary. While obesity is one of the most important causes of lifestyle-related disease and often occurs linked with other clinical conditions such as dyslipidemia, hypertension, and diabetes, undernutrition is the major concern in the elderly [2]. People eat less and make different food choices as they get older [26]. Lower food intake among the elderly has been associated with lower intakes of calcium, iron, zinc, B vitamins and vitamin E. Low energy intakes or low nutrient density of the diet may increase the risk of diet-related illnesses and so pose a health problem [26]. Several factors may influence this observed decline in energy intake. Older adults tend to consume less energy-dense sweets and fast foods, and consume more energy-dilute grains, vegetables and fruits [26]. Daily volume of foods and beverages also declines as a function of age [26]. The causes of undernutrition in older people are likely to be multifactorial as summarized below [27]:

- Ageing:
  - Changes in body composition: sarcopenia
  - Changes to the gastrointestinal tract
  - Oral changes and food intake
  - Atrophic gastritis
  - Changes in sensory function
  - Changes in fluid and electrolyte regulation
- Chronic illness
- Medication and hospitalization
- Drug-diet interactions
- Social and economic determinants

Changes in Body Composition

The major age-related physiological change in older people is a decline in skeletal muscle mass, known as sarcopenia [27, 28]. The nutritional consequences of a reduced lean body mass are reduced metabolic rate together with a proportional decline in total energy requirements [29]. A reduction in energy expenditure is also associated with sedentary behaviour and a loss of mobility related to systemic (e.g., cardiovascular, pulmonary) or bone and joint disease [27]. Reduced energy intakes can lead to inadequate consumption of protein, vitamins, and minerals. Data from the NHANES III data have shown potentially important decreases with age in median protein and zinc intakes as well as intakes of calcium, vitamin E, and other nutrients [30]. In addition, the nutrient density of the diet (i.e., consumption of a given nutrient expressed per 1000 kcal) also falls with age [30]. Low nutrient density and inadequate intakes of protein, vitamins, and minerals are thus important areas of concern. Other notable changes in body composition with aging are decreases in intracellular fluid and an increase in the amount of and change in the distribution of fat stores [31]. These changes predispose older people to dehydration, falls and injury, and central weight gain. Nutrition plays a role in the progression and attenuation of these changes [27, 28, 29].

Gastrointestinal Changes

Poor nutritional status is also related to decreased efficiency of the gastrointestinal tract [32]. Nutrients may not be digested or absorbed well due to a number of causes including atrophic gastritis, a decrease in hormone and enzyme production, senescent changes in the cells of the bowel surface, and interactions among drugs and nutrients [33, 34].

Chewing and swallowing may also be impaired for a variety of reasons [34]. Poor oral health, edentulousness, dentures that may not fit properly, or lesions in the oral cavity will interfere with the consumption of a well-balanced diet [35]. Mortality is increased as a result, as evidenced by a study of 829 women aged 70-79 years in Baltimore [36]. Women who used dentures and reported difficulty chewing or swallowing had lower five-year survival (H.R. 1.43, 95% C.I. 1.05-1.97).

Up to 40% of older people complain of having a dry mouth. While this might be due to medical conditions, medication, inadequate fluid intake and/or dehydration, 80% of the medications most commonly used by older people reduce salivary secretion [30, 37, 38]. The observed deficits in taste and smell may also lead to a reduced sensory enjoyment of foods and therefore to the adoption of a restricted diet.

Compounding these changes is the effect of both chronic and acute illness [39]. As they are usually on medication, interactions between drugs and diet are more likely to cause additional problems for the elderly. Drugs can affect nutrition by altering appetite, absorption, metabolism, action on target tissues, or excretion of macronutrients and micronutrients, thereby causing a deficiency [40]. Malnutrition may also affect drug metabolism and hence the required dosage and possible toxicity [40].

Social and Economic Changes

Dietary intakes in elderly may also decrease due to challenges associated with their environment, social and financial status, and their level of functional ability. Social determinants include facilities for food storage and preparation, opportunities for and access to shopping, and the ability to prepare food and eat in the company of others. [19]. Many older adults have been widowed, have had their children move to other geographical areas, are living on a fixed income, and/or experience disability. Cooking for one may not be a motivating activity after years of shopping and preparing food and meals for a spouse and family. Surveys of independently living older people indicate that those living alone, or eating alone, eat less and are at higher risk of poor nutritional status [41]. Limited income has its own financial challenges leading to prioritization of expenditure which may not include food as a main concern. Thus, overall dietary quality decreases. The elderly are more likely to consume foods which fall into the category of "favourite and comfort", and are frequently those that are high in fat and carbohydrate. The challenge is to obtain an adequate nutrient intake, and in particular sufficient amounts of micronutrients, within the complex nature of the human aging process [35].

Strategies to Improve Malnutrition in Older Adults

Strategies to improve malnutrition in older adults range from health promotion, including health diet guidelines and changing dietary components, to reducing social isolation.

Health Promotion

Good nutrition is ageless and the message to older people must be that the quality of their nutrition is central to the quality of their life. Therefore, more information should be given on how to improve the nutritional intake of elderly people particularly to those affected by limited income, disability, and institutionalization. Longitudinal studies have shown that health promotion activities extend the number of years of health in older people, although the relationship weakens in older age [42]. Changes in diet and exercise patterns are most effective when they are instituted early in life, particularly in the prevention of nutrition-related conditions, but positive effects can occur at any age.

Dietary Recommendations

The current adult guidelines for a healthy diet make no distinctions between adults aged 25-50 and those aged 51 and over [43]. The USDA Food Guide Pyramid has been suggested as one of the key tools for communicating dietary advice to consumers [43]. It gives a science-based advice on food and physical activity choices for health. The Dietary Guidelines describe a healthy diet as one that emphasizes fruits, vegetables, whole grains, and fat-free or low-fat milk and milk products; includes lean meats, poultry, fish, beans, eggs, and nuts; and it is low in saturated fats, *trans*- fats, cholesterol, salt (sodium), and added sugars.

Researchers at Tufts University have instead produced a 70+ pyramid to reflect specifically the nutrient needs of elderly adults [43]. The base of this revised pyramid is narrowed, signifying the reduced energy intake common among seniors. Most people eat fewer calories as they get older. With a typical energy (calorie) intake of 1200 to 1600 calories per day, elderly consumers have to make every calorie count in order to get enough of the essential nutrients [25]. The 70+ pyramid, therefore, outlines the "nutrient dense" choices in each food category, emphasizing whole grain or enriched breads and cereals (e.g., folate); a variety of different colored fruits and vegetables; low-fat dairy foods; and lean meats, fish, poultry, and legumes. It also highlights the importance of fiber, water and supplements [43]. Adequate dietary fiber works to control constipation, and a fiber-rich diet may help reduce the risk of heart disease and some types of cancer [43]. As adequate hydration is another chronic problem for many seniors, this alternative pyramid advises seniors to drink at least eight glasses of fluids a day.

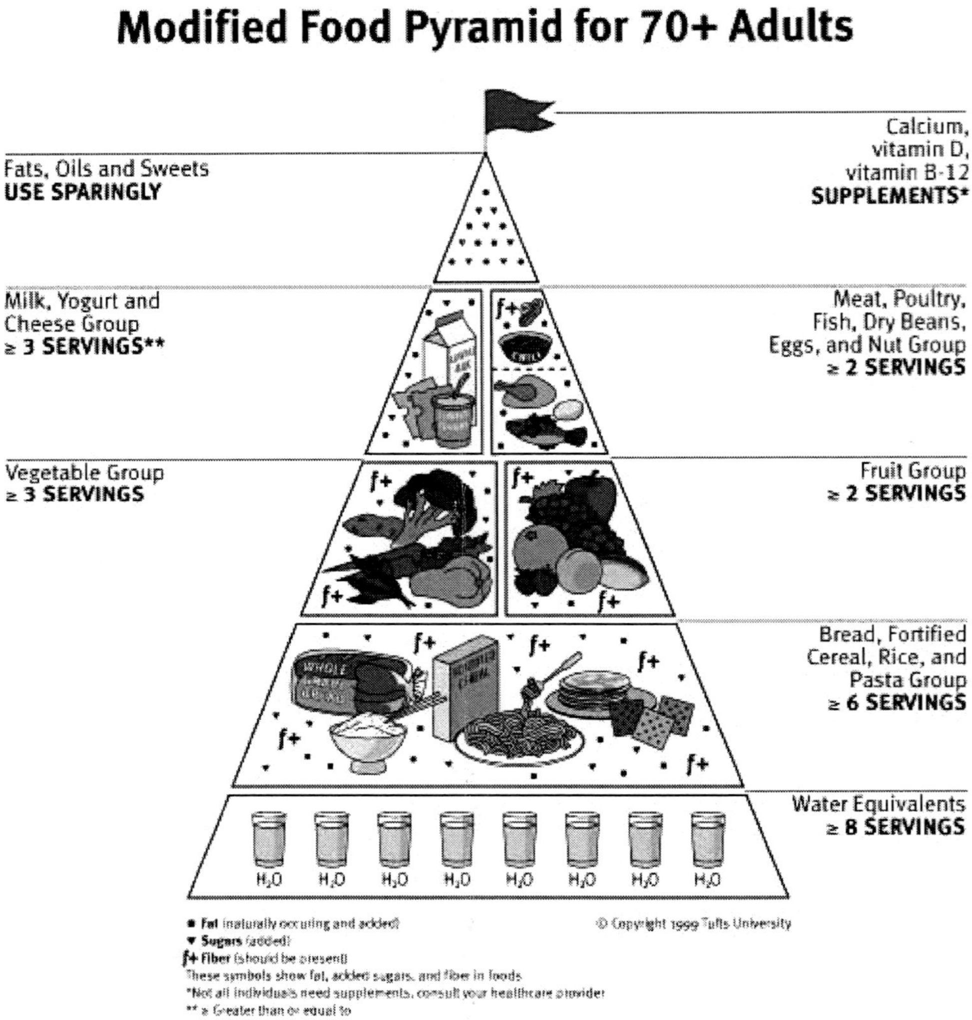

The Tufts researchers point out that these dietary recommendations, as well as the USDA Food Guide Pyramid recommendations, are aimed at healthy, mobile seniors with the resources needed to prepare adequate meals. The 70+ pyramid is not designed to consider the special dietary needs of those with significant health problems, nor does it address the socioeconomic factors—such as decreased income and mobility—that can make it harder for many seniors to meet nutrient needs.

The Mediterranean Diet

Studies consistently support the view that the Mediterranean diet is also compatible with healthier ageing and increased longevity. It may also lower the risk of Alzheimer's disease [44]. The Mediterranean diet is characterized by a high intake of vegetables, legumes, fruits and cereals (in the past largely unrefined); a moderate to high intake of fish; a low intake of saturated lipids but a high intake of unsaturated lipids, particularly olive oil; a low to moderate intake of dairy products, mostly cheese and yogurt; a low intake of meat; and a modest intake of alcohol, mostly as wine. Mediterranean and modified Mediterranean diets are associated with reductions in mortality [45, 46]. The benefit of the diet does not seem to be limited to Mediterranean countries and can be exported to others [46].

Dietary Supplements

Another important issue in older adults is represented by the possible need for dietary supplements. Both calcium and vitamin D absorption decrease with age; this has adverse effects on bone health, and increases the risk of fractures. The SENECA study [47] has shown that in Europe a low calcium intake and a suboptimal vitamin D status are very common in the elderly. In about one third of subjects, the dietary calcium intake was between 300 and 600 mg/day in women and 350-700 mg/day in men. The optimal way to achieve adequate calcium intake is through the diet. However, when dietary sources are scars or not well tolerated, calcium supplementation may be used. Evidence supports routine supplementation for these people at risk of osteoporosis, by providing a daily intake of 700-800 mg of calcium and 400-800 IU of vitamin D [47]. This is an effective, safe and cheap means of preventing osteoporotic fractures.

The ability to absorb the amount of vitamin B12 needed for normal nerve function also decreases with age, making this another key nutrient in the diet. A deficiency of vitamin B_6, B_{12} or folate [48] can result in hyperhomocysteinemia, which is very prevalent condition in elderly subjects, and increases with age [49]. There is evidence from recent observational studies that high levels of homocysteine (Hct), which is a risk factor for atherosclerotic cardiovascular disease, stroke, peripheral arterial occlusive disease, venous thrombosis, osteoporosis and more recently associated with cardiovascular fitness in women [50, 51], are also associated with cognitive impairment in old age, including Alzheimer's Diseas (AD) and Vascular Dementia (VD) [52, 53, 54]. Blood levels of Hct can be reduced by increasing the intake of folic acid (or folate) and vitamins B_6 and B_{12}. The effective daily dose of folic acid for achieving normal homocysteine levels has been determined for young adults (400 μg/day) [55, 56]. While homocysteine levels appear to plateau at folate intakes greater than approximately 350-400 μg/day in the elderly [23], recent data suggest that, if vitamin B_{12} intake is adequate, an intake of about 900 μg/day of folate would be required to ensure that 95% of the elderly population would be without increased cardiovascular risk attributable to folate deficiency [56]. This corresponds to a daily supplement of 600 μg/day of folic acid in addition to usual dietary intakes [56].

The data available [33, 57, 58] suggest that multivitamin and mineral supplements are beneficial particularly where there is evidence of a deficiency state and in certain specific risk groups, e.g. institutionalized elderly. Therefore, in the absence of readily available and cost effective tests for specific deficiencies, this is an issue that older adult consumers should discuss with their health care providers; practitioners should consider routine multivitamin supplementation in the elderly.

Reducing Social Isolation

Studies undertaken in hospitals and residential and nursing homes have shown that the eating environment and fellowship at meal times affect appetite. Older acute care patients in hospital who eat in a supervised dining room improve their food intake but not their weight in comparison to those eating from a tray at the bedside [59]. Buffet-style dining in long term care improves older residents' satisfaction with meals but yielded no significant difference in weight or biochemical markers of nutritional status [60]. A cluster quasi-randomized trial of family-style dinners versus tray service in nursing home residents with an average age of 77 years found that the quality of life, physical functioning, energy intake, and body weight were all improved in the former group [60].

Conclusion

Aging is associated to a marked increase risk of malnutrition. The extremes of malnutrition are obesity and undernutrition. Obesity is a common nutritional disorder in older adults and often occurs linked with other clinical conditions such as dyslipidemia, hypertension, and diabetes. The available evidence suggests that visceral obesity and overweight dating from middle age but not overweight developed in the older age, could affect survival. Under nutrition, which leads to the 'anorexia of ageing' and gradual weight loss, is instead a more important issue for maintaining health and longevity. It is associated with increased demands on health services, lengthier hospital stays and immune dysfunction and it is recognized as an important predictor of morbidity and mortality.

Aging produces physiologic changes that affect the need for several essential nutrients; these changes include slower gastric emptying, altered hormonal responses, decreased basal metabolic rate, and altered taste and smell which may also contribute to lowered energy intake. Other factors such as marital status, income, education, socioeconomic status, diet-related attitudes and beliefs, and convenience likely play a role as well.

Good nutrition is therefore essential to the health, self-sufficiency, and quality of life of older adults. Maintaining good nutrition, following recommendation for a healthy adult diet, should be an essential part of medical care and should be promoted by health professionals. Many age-related nutritional problems may be remedied to some extent by providing nutrient-dense meals through home delivery or meal congregate programs. Management of medical and dental problems and the provision of vitamin and mineral supplements may also be effective. Research needs to be expanded to identify the most effective and acceptable interventions and to determine the impact of diet on nutrition, health, and overall quality of life.

References

[1] The Role of nutrition in Maintainig Health in the Nation's Elderly: Evaluating Coverage of Nutrition Services for the Medicare Beneficiaries, Food and Nutrition Board. ISBN:978-0-309-06846-8 (2000) (free http://www.nap.edu/catalog/9741.html)

[2] Shimokata, H. Dietary habit and longevity. *Nippon Ronen Igakkai Zasshi*, 2007; Mar 44(2): 209-11.

[3] Arterburn, DE; Crane PK; Sullivan SD. The Coming Epidemic of Obesity in Elderly Americans. *Journal of the American Geriatrics Society*. 2004; Nov 52 (11) 1907-1912.

[4] Gutierrez JL; Lopez E; Banegas R *et al*. Prevalence of Overweight and Obesity in Elderly People in Spain. *Obesity Research* 2004; 12:710-715.

[5] Antonelli Incalzi R; Landi F; Cipriani L *et al*. Nutritional assessment: A primary component of multidimensional geriatric assessment in the acute care setting. *J Am Geriatr. Soc.* 1996; 44: 166–174.

[6] Landi F; Onder G; Gambassi G *et al*. Body mass index and mortality among hospitalized patients. *Arch. Intern. Med.* 2000;160: 2641–2644.

[7] Stevens J; Cai J; Pamuk ER *et al*. The effect of age on the association between body-mass index and mortality. *N. Engl. J. Med.* 1998;338: 1–7.

[8] Bender R; Jockel KH; Trautner C *et al*. Effect of age on excess mortality in obesity. *JAMA* 1999;281: 1498–1504.

[9] Carosella L; Pahor M; Pedone C *et al*. Pharmacosurveillance in hospitalized patients in Italy. Study design of the 'Gruppo Italiano di Farmacovigilanza nell'Anziano' (GIFA). *Pharmacol. Res.* 1999; 40: 287–295.

[10] Rossner S. Obesity in the elderly—a future matter of concern? *Obes. Rev.* 2001;2: 183–188.

[11] Folsom AR; Kushi LH; Anderson KE *et al*. Associations of general and abdominal obesity with multiple health outcomes in older women. The Iowa Women's Health Study. *Arch. Intern. Med.* 2000;160: 2117–2128.

[12] Harris TB; Launer LJ; Madans J *et al*. Cohort study of effect of being overweight and change in weight on risk of coronary heart disease in old age. *BMJ* 1997;314: 1791–1794.

[13] Jensen GL; McGee M; Binkley J. Nutrition in the elderly. *Gastroenterology Clinics of North America* 2001; 30: 313–334.

[14] Chernoff R. Micronutrient requirements in older women. *American Journal of Clinical Nutrition.* 2005 May; Vol. 81, No. 5, 1240S-1245S.

[15] Chen CC; Schilling LS; Lyder CH. A concept analysis of malnutrition in the elderly. *Journal of Advanced Nursing* 2001; 36: 131–142.

[16] Gilford A; Khun RK. Development of nutritional risk screening in the community. *British Journal of Community Health Nursing* 1996; 1: 335–336.

[17] Vellas B; Lauque S; Andrieu S *et al.* Nutrition assessment in the elderly. *Current Opinion in Clinical Nutrition and Metabolic Care* 2001; 4: 5–8.

[18] Mion LC; McDowell JA; Heaney LK. Nutritional assessment of the elderly in the ambulatory care setting. *Nurse Practitioner Forum* 1994; 5: 46–51.

[19] National Institute of Clinical Excellence. Nutrition support in adults: oral nutrition support, enteral tube feeding and parenteral nutrition. 2006. www.nice.org.uk/pdf/CG032NICEguideline.pdf (accessed 1 May 2006).

[20] NHS Quality Improvement Scotland. Food, fluid and nutritional care. Clinical Standards. Glasgow: NHS Quality Improvement Scotland. 2003. http://www.nhshealthquality.org/(accessed 1 May 2006).

[21] Council of Europe. Food and nutritional care in hospitals: how to prevent undernutrition. *Report and recommendations of the Committee of Experts on Nutrition, Food Safety and Consumer Protection.* Strasbourg: Council of Europe Publishing; 2002.

[22] Institute of Medicine. *Dietary reference intakes for energy, carbohydrates, fiber, fat, fatty acids, cholesterol, protein, and amino acids.* Washington DC: National Academy Press, 2002;1–450.

[23] Institute of Medicine. Dietary Reference Intakes for Thiamin, Riboflavin, Niacin, Vitamin B_6, Folate, Vitamin B_{12}, Pantothenic Acid, Biotin, and Choline. Washington DC: National Academy Press, 2001;1–564.

[24] Institute of Medicine. Dietary reference intakes for vitamin A, vitamin K, arsenic, boron, chromium, copper, iodine, manganese, molybdenum, nickel, silicon, vanadium, and zinc. Washington DC: National Academy Press, 2001.

[25] Blumberg J. Nutritional needs of seniors. *J. Am. Coll Nutr.* 1997; 16(6):517-23.

[26] Drewnowski A; Shultz JM. Impact of aging on eating behaviors, food choices, nutrition, and health status. *J. Nutr. Health Aging.* 2001; 5 (2):75-9.

[27] Evans WJ. Exercise, nutrition and aging. *Clinics in Geriatric Medicine* 1995; 11: 725–734.

[28] Haller J. The vitamin status and its adequacy in the elderly: An international overview. *International Journal for Vitamin and Nutrition Research* 1999; 69: 160–168.

[29] Jensen GL; McGee M; Binkley J. Nutrition in the elderly. *Gastroenterology Clinics of North America* 2001; 30: 313–334.

[30] Wakimoto P; Block G. Dietary intake, dietary patterns and changes with age: epidemiological perspective. *J. Gerontol. Biol. Sci. Med. Sci.* 2001; 56A: (Special Issue II) 65-80.

[31] Brownie S. Why are elderly individuals at risk of nutritional deficiency? *International Journal of Nursing Practice* 2006; 12: 110–118.

[32] Blechman MB; Gelb AM. Aging and gastrointestinal physiology. *Gastroenterology* 1999; 15: 429–438.

[33] Pilotto A. Aging and the gastrointestinal tract. *Italian Journal of Gastroenterology and Hepatology* 1999; 31: 137–153.

[34] Kim Y-I; Saltzman JR. The aging gut. In: Chernoff R, ed. *Geriatric nutrition: the health professional's handbook.* 3rd ed. Boston: Jones and Bartlett (in press).

[35] Martin WE; Saunders MJ. Oral health in the elderly. In: Chernoff R, ed. *Geriatric nutrition: the health professional's handbook.* 3rd ed. Boston: Jones and Bartlett (in press).

[36] Semba RD; Blaum CS; Bartali B *et al.* Denture use, malnutrition, frailty, and mortality among older women living in the community. *J. Nutr. Health Aging.* 2006 Mar-Apr; 10(2):161-7.

[37] Finkelstein JA; Schiffman SS. Workshop on taste and smell in the elderly: An overview. *Physiology and Behavior* 1999; 66: 173–176.

[38] Rolls BJ; Phillips PA. Aging and disturbances of thirst and fluid balance. *Nutrition Reviews* 1990; 48: 137–143.

[39] Suter PM. Vitamin metabolism and requirements in the elderly: Selected aspects. In: Chernoff R, ed. *Geriatric nutrition: the health professional's handbook.* 3rd ed. Boston: Jones and Bartlett (in press).

[40] Neuvonen PJ; Kivistö KT. The clinical significance of food-drug interactions: a review. *Medical journal of Australia* 1989; 150:36-40.

[41] Wright L; Hickson M; Frost G. Eating together is important: using a dining room in an acute elderly medical ward increases energy intake. *J. Hum. Nutr. Dietet* 2006; 19: 23-6.

[42] Chernoff R. Nutrition and health promotion in older adults. *Journals of Gerontology Biological Sciences and Medical Sciences.* 2001; 56A (Suppl. 2):47-53.

[43] Drewnowski A; Warren-Mears VA. Does aging change nutrition requirements? *J. Nutr. Health Aging.* 2001; 5(2): 70-4.

[44] Salerno-Kennedy R, Cashman KD. The role of nutrition in dementia: an overview. *J. Br. Menopause Soc.* 2006 Jun; 12(2):44-8.

[45] Knoops KT; de Groot LC; Kromhout D *et al.* Mediterranean diet, lifestyle factors, and 10-year mortality in elderly European men and women: the HALE project. *JAMA* 2004; 292:1433-9.

[46] Trichopoulou A ; Orfanos P ; Norat T *et al.* Modified Mediterranean diet and survival: EPIC-elderly prospective cohort study. *BMJ* 2005; 330: 991.

[47] Gennari C. Calcium and Vitamin D nutrition and bone disease of the elderly. *Public Health Nutr.* 2001; 4 (2B):547-59.

[48] Fuchs D; Jaeger M; Widner B et al. Is hyperhomocysteinemia due to the oxidative depletion of folate rather than to insufficient dietary intake? *Clin. Chem. Lab. Med.* 2001; 39: 691-694.

[49] Deschamps V; Barberger-Gateau P; Peuchant E et al. Nutritional factors in cerebral aging and dementia: epidemiological arguments for a Role of oxidative stress. *Neuroepidemiol.* 2001; 20: 7-15.

[50] Herrmann W. The importance of hyperhomocysteinemia as a risk factor for diseases: an overview. *Clin. Chem. Lab. Med.* 2001; 39: 666-674.

[51] Kuo HK; Yen CJ; Bean JF. Levels of homocysteine are inversely associated with cardiovascular fitness in women, but not in men: data from the National Health and Nutrition Examination Survey 1999-2002. *Journal of Internal Medicine* 2005; 258: 328-335.

[52] Joosten E. Homocysteine, vascular dementia and Alzheimer's disease. *Clin. Chem. Lab. Med.* 2001; 39: 717-720.

[53] Prins ND, den Heijer T, Hofman A *et al*. Homocysteine and cognitive function in the elderly. *Neurology*. 2002; 59: 1375-1380.

[54] Seshadri S, Beiser A, Selhub J et al. Plasma homocysteine as a risk factor for Dementia and Alzheimer's disease's. *N. Engl. J. Med*. 2002; 346: 476-483.

[55] Quinlivan EP, McPartlin J, Mcnulty H et al. Importance of both folic acid and vitamin B12 in reduction of risk of vascular disease. *Lancet* 2002; 359: 227-228.

[56] Rydlewicz A, Simpson JA, Taylor RJ *et al*. The effect of folic acid supplementation on plasma homocysteine in an elderly population. *Q. J. M.* 2002; 95: 27-35.

[57] Blechman MB; Gelb AM. Aging and gastrointestinal physiology. *Gastroenterology* 1999; 15: 429–438.

[58] Kim Y-I; Saltzman JR. The aging gut. In: Chernoff R, ed. *Geriatric nutrition: the health professional's handbook*. 3rd ed. Boston: Jones and Bartlett (in press).

[59] Remsburg RE ; Lukin A ; Baran P *et al*. Impact of a buffet-style dining program on weight and biochemical indicators of nutritional status in nursing home residents. *J. Am. Dietet. Assoc.* 2001; 101: 1460-3.

[60] Nijs KAND; de Graaf C; Kok FJ *et al*. Effect of family-style mealtimes on quality of life, physical performance, and body weight of nursing home residents: cluster randomised controlled trial. *BMJ* 2006:332: 1180-3.

In: Nutrition for the Middle Aged and Elderly ISBN: 978-1-60456-146-3
Editors: N. E. Bernhardt, A. M. Kasko, pp. 299-317

Chapter XI

Fruit and Vegetable Consumption among Mid-Age and Older Women in Australia

Zumin Shi **and** ***Julie Byles***
Research Centre for Gender, Health and Ageing
The University of Newcastle, Newcastle, Australia

Abstract

Fruits and vegetables are essential components of a healthy diet. However, only limited information is available about the fruit and vegetable intake of older women. This study describes the socio-demographic and health correlates of intake of fruit and vegetables among two large cohorts of Australian women – one group aged 50-55 years and one aged 79-84 years. Almost all women ate some amount of fruit and vegetables each day. In each cohort, around 8-9% of the women ate five or more serves of vegetables each day, and 30% ate four or more serves each day. In the Mid-age cohort, around 60% of the women ate two or more servings of fruit each day, and the corresponding proportion for the Older cohort was 70%. Around 7-8% of each cohort could be considered to eat the national recommended intake of two serves of fruit and five serves of vegetables. Eating higher levels of fruit and vegetables was associated with country of birth, education, marital status, and with functional abilities and oral health. Longitudinal analyses describe trends in BMI, health-related quality of life and survival according to women's fruit and vegetable intakes.

Observational studies have shown that high intake of fruit and vegetables is associated with a lower risk of cancers [1], cardiovascular disease [2], stroke [3], and diabetes [4].

* Research Fellow, Newcastle Institute of Public Health – Hunter Medical Research Institute, Faculty of Health, The University of Newcastle, phone 49138643, 49138321 or 49138142. fax 49138323. email: julie.byles@newcastle.edu.au

Positive association has also been found between intake of fruit and vegetables and mental and physical function. It is suggested that these effects are mediated through the antioxidant effects of micronutrients in fruits and vegetables such as vitamin C, vitamin E, and carotenoids [5]. Dietary fiber from fruits and vegetables may also add health benefits [4]. However, antioxidant supplement trials on the prevention of cancer and cardiovascular disease show inconsistent or discouraging results, including the Alpha-Tocopherol Beta-Carotene (ATBC) study and the CARET study [6, 7]. It is still debatable whether vitamin supplementation should be used for the prevention of chronic disease [8]. At present, data do not justify the use of antioxidant vitamin supplements for diabetes and CVD risk reduction [9-11]. The beneficial effects of fruits and vegetables can not be explained only by known chemicals, and available studies suggest that the whole diet or food is more important rather than single nutrients. For disease prevention and health promotion we ought to focus on these foods as a whole.

It is recommended by the World Health Organisation that adults should eat 400-500 grams fruits and vegetables everyday [4]. Intervention programs focusing on increasing intakes of fruit and vegetables have been implemented in many countries. For instance Australia has been running a "go for 2 and 5 campaign" to encourage consumption of at least two serves of fruit and five serves of vegetables each day (http://www.gofor2and5.com.au). However, many individuals do not consume enough fruit and vegetables to meet recommended dietary requirements. In Australia, it has been estimated that only around 11% of adults consume the recommended two serves of fruit and five serves of vegetables a day [12] and women living alone are less likely to meet recommendations for vegetable intake [13].

Socioeconomic characteristics are high among the many factors that are associated with fruit and vegetable intake [14]. However, the association between socio-economic factors and intake of fruit and vegetable varies in developed and developing countries. In developed countries, high intake of fruit and vegetable is seen in high socio-economic groups; while the opposite association is found in developing countries. Findings in the USA, Australia and some European countries have shown that individuals with low education, working in blue-collar occupations or with low incomes have less healthy diets that are lower in fruits and vegetables than those with higher education, in professional occupations and with high incomes [15, 16]. In Europe, the difference in the intake of fruit is 24.3g/person/day between men in the highest level of education and those in the lowest level of education; this difference was 33.6g/person/day for women [16]. One study of Australian women shows that individual and social factors only partly mediated socioeconomic variations in fruit and vegetable consumption [17]. Lifestyle factors are also associated with fruit and vegetable intake. Healthy lifestyles like physical activity and non-smoking usually cluster with high intake of fruit and vegetable [18].

A number of studies have examined whether area-level socio-economic characteristics influence diet. Research in the USA, the UK and Finland has shown that people residing in prosperous areas have healthier dietary behaviours and nutrient intakes than those in disadvantaged areas, independent of their individual-level socioeconomic position. However, studies in the Netherlands and Australia did not show any variation between areas differing in their socio-economic characteristics [19]. The density of fruit and vegetable stores in the local neighborhoods was not associated with fruit intakes in Australia women [17].

Age is another socioeconomic factor that is likely to have an impact on fruit and vegetable consumption. Older people are known to be at risk of malnutrition for a variety of reasons, including reduced appetite, eating alone, disability in food preparation, and reduced access to food [20-22]. Older women may be especially vulnerable to poor intakes since they are likely to be widowed and living alone and because they have high rates of disability on activities of daily living.

From the evidence to hand, it is widely accepted that fruits and vegetables are essential components of a healthy diet, and that understanding the determinants of fruit and vegetable consumption is important to promote healthy eating and good health in the population. However, at present, only limited information is available about the fruit and vegetable intake among older people in the community. This study describes the socio-demographic and health correlates of intake of fruit and vegetables among two large cohorts of Australian women – one group aged 50-55 years and one aged 79-84 years.

Method

Women in this study were from the Australian Longitudinal Study on Women's Health (ALSWH). Two cohorts of women were involved: "Mid-age" women aged 45-50 years, and "Older" women aged 70-75 years, at the start of the study in 1996 (Survey 1 - S1). These two cohorts of women were randomly sampled from the Health Insurance Commission (HIC) database, and have each completed four surveys between 1996 and 2005. More details of the study have been published elsewhere [23] and are available from www.alswh.org.au. Characteristics of the women have been compared with each national census since 1996. These comparisons show that, at baseline the women in the study were roughly representative of women of their age in the Australian population with some over-representation of women with tertiary education and under-representation of immigrant women of non-English speaking background [24].

The overall aim of the study is to determine "factors that affect the health of women". The main measures of health are survival and health-related quality of life (QoL). Deaths were ascertained annually from the National Death Index with matching on name, address and date of birth information [25]. All phone calls and correspondence notifying of death or withdrawal from the study were also logged by the study office and compared with the National Death Index notifications to ensure completeness of follow-up for mortality. For survivors, QoL is measured at each survey using the Medical Outcomes Study SF-36 Health Survey (SF-36) [26], a widely used and well validated generic profile measure examines eight dimensions of quality of life including physical, mental and social well-being [27].

Questions about fruit and vegetables were asked at Survey 1 (S1), when women were asked whether they "eat fruit and vegetables most days", and at S4 when women were asked: "How many serves of fruit do you eat each day?" and "How many serves of vegetables do you eat each day?" Response options were; "none", "1 serve", "2-3 serves", "4 serves", "5 serves or more". For this analysis, we defined "higher" intake as two or more serves of fruit, four or more serves of vegetables and six or more serves of fruit or vegetables each day based on the distribution of total intakes. This definition is conservative since the national recommended intake is two serves of fruit and five serves of vegetables (www.nhmrc.gov.au), but is to allow adequate group sizes for analysis.

Other survey items inquire about health circumstances and conditions such as need for help with daily tasks, and use of support services such as meal delivery services. Comorbid diseases were measured at S2-S4 as self-reported doctor-diagnoses including arthritis, diabetes, heart disease, hypertension, stroke, thrombosis, low iron level, osteoporosis, cancer, depression, anxiety, and Alzheimer's/dementia. Other self-reported health conditions (breathing difficulty, chest pain, tiredness, stiff or painful joints, back pain, foot problems, dysuria, nocturia, urinary urgency, incontinence, constipation, poor memory, clumsiness, dizziness) were also reported at each survey as occurring "often", "sometimes", "rarely" or "never" in the past year. A specific item was added at S4 to enable women to rate the condition of their "teeth, mouth or gums", and the five response options were dichotomised as "good" (excellent, very good, good) and" poor" (fair or poor) [28]. Alcohol intake was measured according to quantity (number of standard drinks – 10 grams of alcohol) and frequency (number of days per week). Alcohol intake was classified as Non-Drinkers (no alcohol), Rare drinkers (less than weekly), Low Risk (up to 14 drinks per week), Risky drinkers (15-28 drinks per week), and High Risk (> 28 drinks per week).

Statistical Analyses

Data analysis was performed using SAS 9.1 (SAS Institute Inc, Cary, NC), and STATA 9.2 (Stata Corp, College Station, TX) statistical packages. Initial analyses assessed the effect of fruit and vegetable intake at S1 on survival and withdrawal and loss to follow-up using Cox Proportional Hazards techniques. Frequency tables were used to describe response frequencies for fruit and vegetable intakes at S4. Relative risk (RR) ratios and 95 % confidence intervals (CI) were used to compare the prevalence of other health problems and comorbidities according to fruit and vegetable intake. The association between fruit and vegetable intake and other health conditions and circumstances was assessed using Chi-square tests. The cell contribution to Chi-square was used to examine the effects within different categories where differences were statistically significant with more that 1 degree of freedom. All variables of interest where $P<0.2$ were entered into sets of multivariable polychotomous reqression models. Separate models were used to identify factors associated with intake of fruit, intake of vegetables, and "higher" fruit and vegetable intake (six or more serves of fruit and vegetables per day). In each set, a manual backwards selection process was used to identify variables that could be removed from the model without significantly affecting the significance of the model or goodness of fit. Statistical significance for interpreting these models was set at $P=0.01$.

Longitudinal modeling techniques using SAS Proc Mixed were employed to assess within-individual changes in health related quality of life (based on SF-36) according to fruit and vegetable intake. Change in the log likelihood and Akaike Information criteria [29] were used to compare models.

Results

In 1996, 13716 Mid-age women completed S1 in 1996, and 10903 of these women (72%) completed S4 in 2004. Between Surveys 1 and 4, 204 women died[1], a further 946 women withdrew and 1663 were missing at follow up from the study due to other reasons. Compared to women who stayed in the study, Mid-age women who did not complete the survey were more likely to be separated, divorced or widowed. Of the 12432 Older women who completed S1, 7088 (58%) completed their S4 in 2005; 1838 women died,[2] a further 2101 women withdrew and 1405 were missing at follow up due to other reasons. Women who did not remain in the study at S4 tended to be in poorer health on previous surveys.

At S1, 97.2% of the Older women said they eat fruit and vegetables most days. Survival analyses indicate that Older women who did not eat fruit and vegetables most days were significantly more likely to die between S1 and S4. After adjustment for potential confounding factors (number of comorbidities, education, area, of residence, smoking and BMI),[3] the relative risk of death for women reporting "no" to this item was 1.38(95% CI: 1.03-1.85). Proportional hazards models of withdrawal or other loss to follow-up from the study indicate that this outcome was not associated with fruit and vegetable intake (p=0.204).

Fruit and Vegetable intakes for women who survived and completed Survey 4 are shown in Table 1. Almost all women ate some amount of fruit and vegetables each day. In each cohort, around 8-9% of the women ate five or more serves of vegetables each day, and around 30% could be considered to eat four or more serves each day. In the Mid-age cohort, around 60% of the women ate two or more serves of fruit each day, and the corresponding proportion for the Older cohort was around 70%. Approximately 7.9% of the mid-age women and 7.4 % of the older women could be considered to consume adequate amounts of fruit and vegetables combined if the national standard of two serves and fruit and five serves of vegetables was applied. Applying our less stringent definition of six or more serves of fruit and vegetables approximately 29.3% of the mid-age women and 31.5% of the older women could classified as having "higher" fruit and vegetable intake.

Social and personal factors associated with fruit and vegetable intake in the older women in the multivariable models are shown in Table 2. Area of residence classification was not significantly associated with fruit and vegetable consumption but was retained in the model to adjust for sampling strategy. Older women were more likely to consume two or more serves of fruit if they had higher education levels, and if they had eaten out in the past month. Women were less likely to consume four or more serves of vegetables if they were born overseas, were separated, divorced or widowed. Difficulty preparing meals was associated with lower intake of both fruit and vegetables. The probability that a woman would consume six or more serves of fruit and vegetables a day was positively associated with higher education, eating out in the past month, and "good" condition of teeth, and negatively associated with being born overseas, widowed, and having difficulty preparing meals. There was no association between fruit and vegetable intake and income, needing help with daily

[1] Death recorded prior to 30th June 2004

[2] Death recorded prior to 30th June 2005

[3] High rates of missing data on BMI resulted in reduced sample size for these analyses and so analyses were repeated with and without BMI. There was no impact on the relative risk estimate.

tasks, receiving food services, and difficulty getting to shops. These factors were removed during backward regression with no significant impact on model fit. Odds ratios for the final model were not significantly affected by removing these variables (data not shown).

Table 1. Reported fruit and vegetable intake for Mid-age and Older cohorts of women (Survey 4)

	Mid-age women 53-58 years N= 10,903	Older women 79-84 years N= 7088
Serves of Vegetables % None	 0.7	 0.8
One	14.9	21.0
Two-Three	53.9	50.4
Four	21.5	19.5
Five or more	8.9 Miss=0.5	8.4 Miss = 0.7
Serves of Fruit % None	 5.0	 1.4
One	35.2	27.4
Two-Three	50.1	58.4
Four	7.5	9.7
Five or more	2.2 Miss=0.3%	3.1 Miss=0.6

More and stronger associations were apparent in the mid-age group (see Table 3). A more rural area of residence was associated with higher intakes of vegetables, and higher education levels were associated with higher intakes of fruit and vegetables separately and combined. Country of birth was also associated with intake with those born in Europe being more likely to consume adequate levels of fruit and less likely to consume adequate levels of vegetables. Women born in Asia were less likely to consume adequate levels of vegetables and less likely to consume adequate levels of fruit and vegetables combined. Separated women were less likely to consume fruit, vegetables and fruit and vegetables combined, and widowed women were less likely to consume vegetables and fruit and vegetables combined. Difficulty managing on income was associated with all measures of fruit and vegetable intake. Needing help with daily tasks was not associated with fruit and vegetable intake among women in this age group.

Table 4 shows the association between fruit and vegetable intakes and BMI, physical activity, drinking, and smoking in each cohort. Among both cohorts higher fruit and vegetable consumption was associated with more physical activity, and lower rates of current smoking and risky and high risk drinking. While there were statistical associations between fruit and vegetable intakes and weight, the differences were mostly due to only a few cells in the table.

Table 2. Sociodemographic and personal variables associated with adequate fruit and vegetable intake among Australian women aged 79-84

Factors in area adjusted multivariable model	Fruit(>=2servings/day)		Vegetable (>=4servings/day)		Fruit and vegetable(>=6servings/day)	
	OR (95%CI)	P	OR (95%CI)	P	OR (95%CI)	P
	N = 6505		N = 6501		N = 6484	
Education						
No formal qualification	1		1		1	
School or intermediate	1.14(1.00-1.30)	0.053	1.11(0.97-1.27)	0.144	1.13(0.98-1.29)	0.087
High school	1.37(1.13-1.65)	0.001	1.16(0.96-1.40)	0.136	1.28(1.06-1.54)	0.009
Trade	0.89(0.66-1.20)	0.442	0.83(0.59-1.17)	0.281	0.89(0.64-1.23)	0.477
Certificate/diploma	1.82(1.45-2.29)	<0.001	1.35(1.10-1.67)	0.004	1.55(1.26-1.90)	<0.0001
University or above	1.87(1.38-2.54)	<0.001	1.11(0.84-1.46)	0.477	1.56(1.19-2.03)	0.001
Missing	1.06(0.80-1.41)	0.681	1.01(0.75-1.36)	0.951	1.19(0.89-1.60)	0.233
Country of birth						
Australian born	1		1		1	
Other ESB (English Speaking Background)	0.92(0.78-1.09)	0.363	0.68(0.57-0.81)	<0.001	0.85(0.72-1.00)	0.054
Europe	1.41(1.10-1.81)	0.007	0.25(0.18-0.36)	<0.001	0.46(0.35-0.61)	<0.001
Asia	2.09(0.99-4.38)	0.052	0.26(0.10-0.66)	0.005	0.29(0.12-0.70)	0.006
Other	1.53(0.68-3.40)	0.301	1.30(0.64-2.66)	0.464	1.77(0.89-3.52)	0.102
Missing	0.89(0.70-1.14)	0.347	0.75(0.57-0.97)	0.032	0.81(0.63-1.05)	0.119
Marital status						
Married/Defacto	1		1		1	
Separated/Divorced	0.89(0.68-1.17)	0.394	0.73(0.55-0.97)	0.033	0.82(0.62-1.08)	0.166
Widowed	0.90(0.80-1.01)	0.064	0.78(0.70-0.88)	<0.001	0.77(0.69-0.86)	<0.001
Never married	0.98(0.69-1.39)	0.913	0.80(0.58-1.12)	0.195	0.79(0.57-1.10)	0.165

Table 2. (Continued)

	Fruit(>=2servings/day)		Vegetable (>=4servings/day)		Fruit and vegetable(>=6servings/day)	
Difficulty Managing on income						
No	1		1		1	
Yes	0.96(0.84-1.09)	0.513	0.84(0.73-0.97)	0.016	0.88(0.76-1.01)	0.065
Difficult in preparing meal						
No difficult	1		1		1	
Some difficult	0.70(0.59-0.84)	<0.001	0.57(0.46-0.70)	<0.001	0.55(0.45-0.68)	<0.001
Unable to do	0.45(0.34-0.60)	<0.001	0.56(0.39-0.80)	0.002	0.38(0.25-0.57)	<0.001
Eating out last month						
No	1		1		1	
Yes	1.35(1.20-1.51)	<0.001	1.15(1.02-1.30)	0.026	1.26(1.12-1.43)	<0.001
Teeth condition						
Bad	1		1		1	
Good	1.18(1.05-1.33)	0.006	1.23(1.09-1.40)	0.001	1.27(1.12-1.43)	<0.001

Model adjusted for area of residence to correct for sampling strategy.

Table 3. Sociodemographic and personal variables associated with adequate fruit and vegetable intake among Australian women aged 53-58 years

	Fruit(>=2servings/day)		Vegetable (>=4servings/day)		Fruit and vegetable(>=6servings/day)	
Factors in mutlivariable model	OR (95%CI)	P	OR (95%CI)	P	OR (95%CI)	P
	N = 10404		N = 10390		N = 10374	
Area of residence						
Capital/Other metro	1		1		1	
Large Rural	0.92(0.81-1.05)	0.205	1.12(0.98-1.29)	0.096	1.04(0.90-1.19)	0.626
Small rural	0.91(0.81-1.03)	0.154	1.25(1.10-1.42)	0.001	1.14(1.00-1.30)	0.045
Remote/Other remote/rural	0.90(0.82-0.99)	0.031	1.23(1.11-1.36)	<0.001	1.08(0.98-1.20)	0.135
Education						
No formal qualification	1		1		1	
School or intermediate	1.16(1.03-1.31)	0.015	1.29(1.13-1.47)	<0.001	1.33(1.16-1.52)	<0.001
High school	1.23(1.07-1.41)	0.003	1.18(1.01-1.37)	0.036	1.22(1.04-1.43)	0.014
Trade	1.31(1.04-1.65)	0.021	1.28(1.00-1.65)	0.047	1.31(1.02-1.70)	0.037
Certificate/diploma	1.80(1.57-2.07)	<0.001	1.57(1.35-1.82)	<0.001	1.76(1.51-2.06)	<0.001
University or above	1.83(1.58-2.12)	<0.001	1.44(1.24-1.69)	<0.001	1.75(1.49-2.05)	<0.001
Country of birth						
Australian born	1		1		1	
Other (English Speaking)	0.94(0.83-1.05)	0.279	0.82(0.72-0.93)	0.001	0.85(0.75-0.97)	0.014
Europe	1.46(1.22-1.75)	<0.001	0.50(0.40-0.61)	<0.001	0.81(0.67-0.98)	0.03
Asia	0.89(0.67-1.18)	0.408	0.27(0.18-0.40)	<0.001	0.38(0.26-0.56)	<0.001
Other	1.28(0.79-2.07)	0.317	0.36(0.19-0.67)	0.001	0.70(0.41-1.20)	0.196

Table 3. (Continued)

	Fruit(>=2servings/day)		Vegetable (>=4servings/day)		Fruit and vegetable(>=6servings/day)	
Marital status						
Married/Defacto	1		1		1	
Separated/Divorced	0.67(0.55-0.82)	<0.001	0.59(0.47-0.74)	<0.001	0.67(0.53-0.85)	0.001
Widowed	0.91(0.79-1.04)	0.165	0.58(0.50-0.68)	<0.001	0.65(0.55-0.76)	<0.001
Never married	1.15(0.93-1.42)	0.205	0.62(0.49-0.79)	<0.001	0.75(0.59-0.96)	0.02
Difficulty Managing on income						
No	1		1		1	
Yes	0.81(0.75-0.88)	<0.001	0.87(0.79-0.95)	0.002	0.81(0.74-0.89)	<0.001
Need help in daily tasks						
Yes	1		1		1	
No	0.99(0.78-1.25)	0.931	1.07(0.82-1.38)	0.628	1.19(0.90-1.57)	0.217

Table 4. Association between intake of fruit and vegetables and BMI and health behaviours in Australian women at survey 4

		Fruit (servings/day) %				Vegetable (servings/day) %				FV (servings/day) %			
		<=1	2-3	>=4	p	<=1	2-3	>=4	p	<=2	2-5	>=6	p
Old cohort													
BMI	n												
<20	659	**36.0**	**52.3**	11.7		21.2	48.5	30.4		**13.0**	56.4	30.5	
20-25	2,703	28.8	58.9	12.4		19.6	49.9	30.6		9.5	58.8	31.7	
25-30	2,070	26.6	59.4	14.0	<0.001	20.2	51.3	28.5	0.220	8.4	60.6	31.0	0.016
>30	872	28.5	60.5	10.9		23.1	49.4	27.6		11.0	59.6	29.5	
Physical activity													
Sedentary	2864	**35.9**	54.5	**9.6**		**23.7**	51.9	**24.4**		**13.3**	**61.9**	**24.8**	
Low	1677	25.9	60.3	13.8	<0.001	19.2	49.0	31.8	<0.001	7.8	58.4	33.8	<0.001
Moderate	887	24.5	59.6	15.9		16.8	49.0	34.2		**6.2**	56.8	37.0	
High	1052	**21.3**	62.8	15.9		17.2	49.7	33.1		7.7	55.5	36.8	
Smoking													
Non-smoker	4354	28.2	58.6	13.2		19.4	49.9	30.8		9.5	57.9	32.6	
Ex-smoker	1936	29.4	58.5	12.1	<0.001	22.0	50.9	27.1	<0.001	10.3	60.9	28.8	<0.001
Current smoker	379	45.4	48.0	6.6		31.0	48.5	20.4		**17.6**	63.6	**18.9**	
Alcohol drinking													
Low risk	2,471	28.2	59.1	12.8		**18.3**	51.3	30.4		**8.6**	59.4	32.0	
Non-drinkers	2,177	30.7	57.4	11.9		**23.2**	47.8	29.0		**11.7**	58.8	29.5	
Rarely drinks	1,978	28.4	58.5	13.1	0.004	21.2	51.1	27.7	0.007	10.4	58.8	30.8	0.007
Risky	222	**38.3**	50.9	10.8		21.6	50.9	27.5		10.4	63.5	26.1	
High risk	25	**56.0**	36.0	8.0		24.0	56.0	20.0		**24.0**	56.0	20.0	

Table 4. (Continued)

		<=1	2-3	>=4	p	<=1	2-3	>=4	p	<=2	2-5	>=6	p
Mid cohort													
BMI													
<20	436	39.0	48.9	**12.2**		**20.4**	50.3	29.3		**13.6**	56.8	29.7	
20-25	3571	39.5	49.8	10.7	<0.001	15.3	52.7	32.1	0.005	9.9	60.0	30.1	0.001
25-30	3298	39.8	50.9	9.2		14.0	51.8	34.2		8.4	60.7	30.9	
>30	2515	**43.5**	47.9	8.6		16.1	52.8	31.1		10.2	62.3	27.5	
Physical activity													
Sedentary	1669	**55.6**	**39.4**	**5.0**		**23.1**	51.8	**25.1**		**16.0**	64.6	**19.4**	
Low	2981	46.1	46.3	7.6	<0.001	15.0	55.1	29.9	<0.001	10.0	64.8	**25.2**	<0.001
Moderate	2312	34.8	54.8	10.4		13.1	52.6	34.3		**7.5**	59.7	32.8	
High	3189	**33.0**	**54.6**	**12.5**		13.3	49.6	**37.1**		**7.9**	**56.1**	**36.1**	
Smoking													
Non-smoker	6424	**37.9**	51.8	10.3		**13.9**	52.0	**34.1**		**8.2**	60.2	**31.6**	
Ex-smoker	2934	39.8	50.3	9.9	<0.001	13.8	53.7	32.6	<0.001	8.4	61.4	30.2	<0.001
Current smoker	1449	**58.5**	**36.6**	**5.0**		**25.5**	50.2	**24.3**		**19.6**	62.4	**18.0**	
Alcohol drinking													
Low risk	5834	41.0	50.6	8.5		**13.1**	54.0	32.9		**8.4**	62.2	29.4	
Non-drinkers	1651	39.7	47.6	**12.8**		**20.1**	47.7	32.3		**12.6**	56.0	31.5	
Rarely drinks	2564	39.7	49.9	10.4	<0.001	**18.6**	51.1	30.3	<0.001	**11.2**	60.6	28.2	<0.001
Risky	614	**49.5**	44.3	6.2		**10.3**	53.6	36.1		7.7	63.4	28.9	
High risk	97	**69.1**	**25.8**	5.2		14.3	42.9	42.9		14.4	56.7	28.9	

Figures in bold indicate significant cell contribution to Chi square.

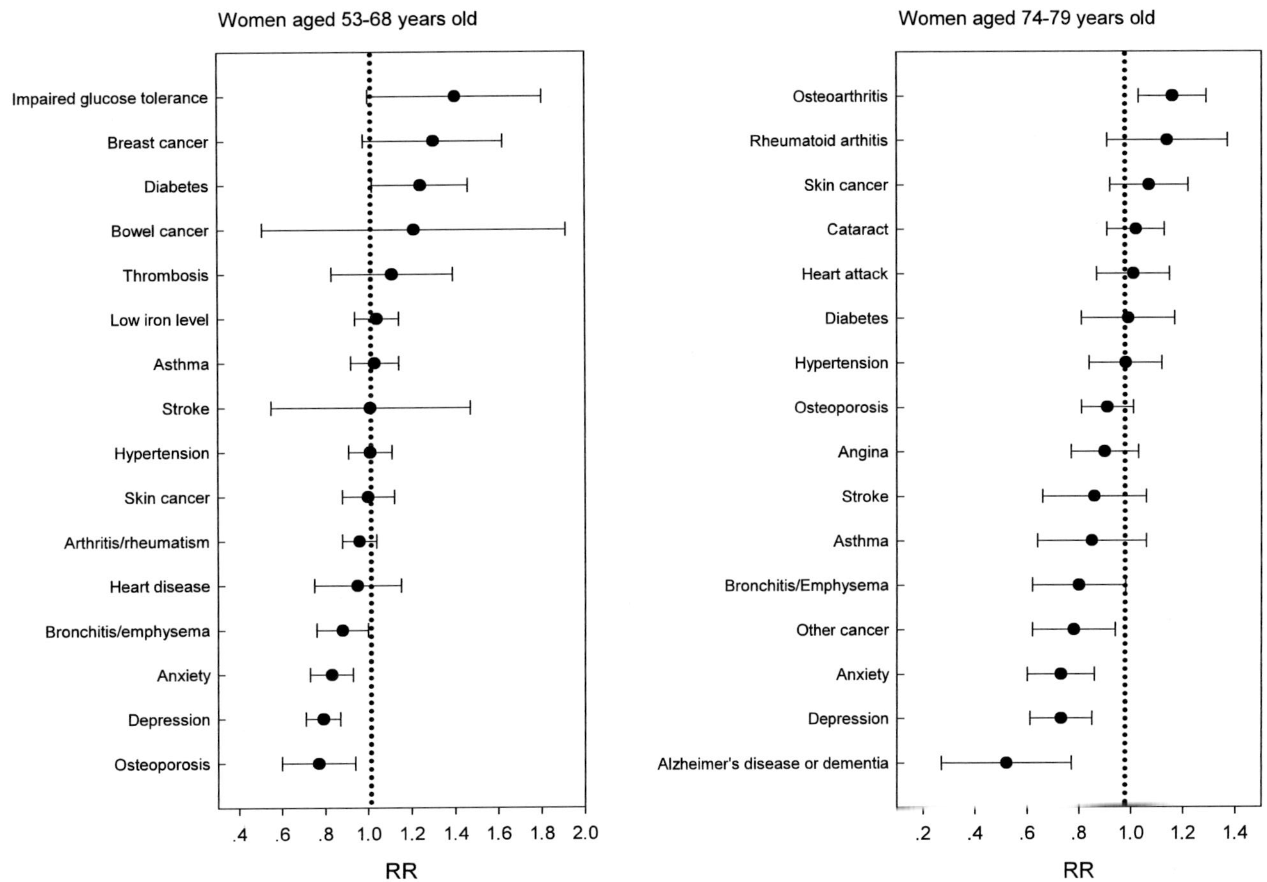

Figure 1a. Univariate Relative Risks for self reporting diagnosed conditions for women reporting six or more serves of fruit and vegetables compared with women reporting less than six serves/day.

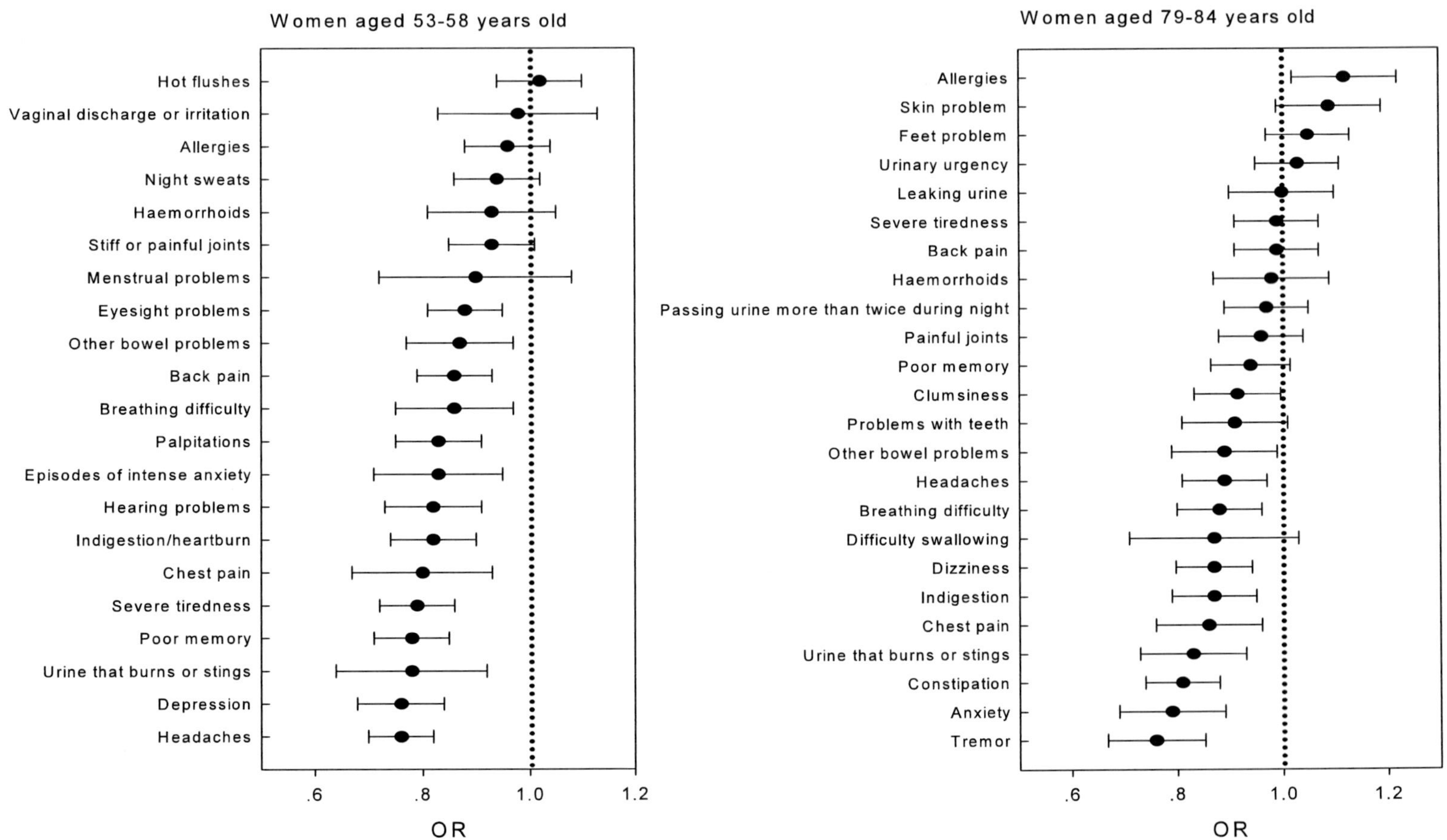

Figure 1b. Univariate Odds Ratios for self reporting diagnosed conditions for women reporting six or more serves of fruit and vegetables compared with women reporting less than six serves/day.

Among the older women, those who were underweight were more likely to consume low amounts of fruit; whereas underweight women in the mid-age group were more likely to consume more fruit and fewer vegetables, and obese women were more likely to consume low levels of fruit.

Figure 1a presents relative risk of comorbid conditions diagnosed during the observation period (S1-S4) for women according to their fruit and vegetable intake, and Figure 1b presents relative risks for reporting other health conditions and symptoms at S4. A number of conditions were less likely to be reported by women who also report higher intakes of fruit and vegetables. However these associations were not strong and upper confidence limits were close to 1.0. Women reporting adequate fruit and vegetable intake were also less likely to report many of the symptoms/complains shown in figure 1b.

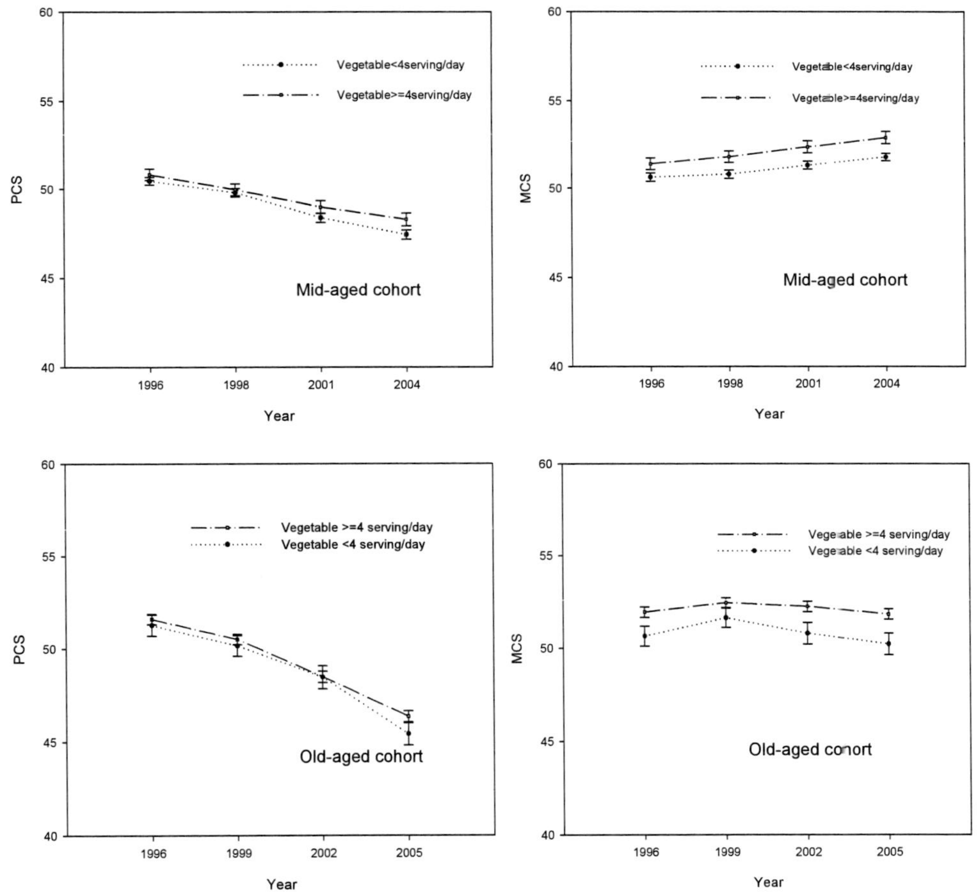

Figure 2. Adjusted (marginal) means and 95% CI for PCS and MCS for women having four or more serves of vegetables and women having less than four serves of vegetables/day. Means are adjusted for age, area, education, marital status, smoking and alcohol drinking status.

Longitudinal analyses described trends in health-related quality of life according to women's vegetable intakes, and the marginal means resulting from these analyses are graphed in Figure 2. In the mid-aged cohort, women who report eating four or more serves of vegetables per day had higher Physical Component Summary scores (PCS) at S4, and higher

Mental Health Component Summary scores (MCS) at all Surveys. In the Older cohort these differences were not so clear but the trends were similar. MCS scores were higher at all surveys except S2, and there was a non-significant trend for women consuming four or more vegetables to have higher PCS scores at S4.

Discussion

Fruit and vegetables are deemed to be important components in a healthy diet. The data from this large longitudinal study of two age cohorts of women demonstrate the prevalence of adequate intake among two cohorts of women, and show the strong association between these dietary factors and other health and social circumstances. The longitudinal analyses show the different nine-year trends in health-related quality of life scores for women who do and do not have higher intakes of vegetables the dietary components.

A limitation of this study is that the data can only represent those women who survived and stayed in the study. Older women with poor fruit and vegetable intake at baseline were more likely to die, but were not more likely to withdraw. The association between fruit and vegetable intake and survival is limited by the fact that the women were asked very scant details of their dietary intake at the time of the baseline survey, and the item did not allow much differentiation between different levels of intake.

At S4, the ascertainment of fruit and vegetable intake allowed greater differentiation between women according to different levels of fruit intake and different levels of vegetable intake. The lack of repeated measures of this item over the course of the study prevents an analysis of change in fruit and vegetable consumption and the temporal association between diet and health factors.

It is also a problem that this measure relies on self-report, but this is the method used by most studies of fruit and vegetable intake.

Despite these limitations, the study does provide a large amount of information on women's reported fruit and vegetable intakes and the circumstances surrounding women with inadequate intake and how these women differ from other women of their age group. These contextual factors are important in considering ways to promote higher intakes among mid-age and older women.

Despite national recommendations for two serves of fruit and five serves of vegetables each day (www.nhmrc.gov.au), very few women report intake levels that would meet these standards. There appears to be less of a problem in relation to consumption of fruit than of vegetables. Less than 10% of women in either cohort consumed adequate amounts of vegetables to meet the recommendation. In these data we also do not know what types of vegetables the women consumed and it is possible that one or more of these serves of vegetables could be potatoes which have less micro-nutrient and fibre benefit than many other vegetables. The recommended daily intake does acknowledge that potatoes may make up one serve of vegetables, but if women are consuming more than one serve of potatoes a day then their reported intakes of more beneficial vegetables may be inflated. Australians are known to have high potato consumption and fried potato "chips" are particularly popular among certain cohorts, including mid-age women.

Our categorization of high combined fruit and vegetable intake did not differentiate between proportions of fruits and vegetables in the diet. A large proportion of women would have met this criterion on the basis of high consumption of fruit and low consumption of vegetables, with many women consuming four or more serves of fruit a day. This is not necessarily a desirable behaviour as fruits are higher in sugar and have higher glyceamic index and so may contribute to problems of glucose metabolism (among women with diabetes) and obesity.

The data also indicate that there are clear socioeconomic and personal factors that affect women's consumption of fruit and vegetables. These factors are important to consider if health promotion messages are to be equitable. As it stands, women who are able bodied and who have better levels of education and income may have more ability to consume a healthy diet. The barriers that prevent other women from also protecting their health in this way need to be more carefully understood. It is noteworthy that women who have lower fruit and vegetable consumption are also likely to have other health risk behaviours such as smoking and low levels of physical activity.

While associations between fruit and vegetable intake and the prevalence of chronic conditions were not great, there are more and stronger associations with current symptoms. These immediate benefits may be a stronger selling point for promoting healthy eating than the more distal benefits of disease prevention. Constipation, other bowel problems and urinary problems are particular examples of conditions that are common among mid-age and older women and that may benefit from higher intakes of fruit and vegetables.

Conclusion

The data present a case for further promotion of fruit and vegetable intakes among mid-age and older women who show low intakes of these nutritional components. However in promoting these dietary behaviours some consideration needs to be given to the capacity of women of different socio-economic background to respond to this advice, and to the potential for an unwanted increase in the increase in less beneficial vegetables (such as potatoes) and/or an excess consumption of fruit as an alternative to the vegetable component.

References

[1] Riboli, E. and T. Norat, Epidemiologic evidence of the protective effect of fruit and vegetables on cancer risk. *Am. J. Clin. Nutr.,* 2003. 78(3 Suppl): p. 559S-569S.

[2] Hu, F.B., Plant-based foods and prevention of cardiovascular disease: an overview. Am *J. Clin. Nutr.,* 2003. 78(3 Suppl): p. 544S-551S.

[3] Dauchet, L., P. Amouyel, and J. Dallongeville, Fruit and vegetable consumption and risk of stroke: A meta-analysis of cohort studies. *Neurology*, 2005. 65(8): p. 1193-1197.

[4] WHO/FAO, Diet, nutrition and the prevention of chronic diseases: report of a Joint WHO/FAO Expert Consultation. WHO technical report series 916. 2003, Geneva: World Health Organization. X, 149 s.

[5] Montonen, J., et al., Dietary Antioxidant Intake and Risk of Type 2 Diabetes. *Diabetes Care*, 2004. 27(2): p. 362-366.
[6] Clarke, R. and J. Armitage, Antioxidant vitamins and risk of cardiovascular disease. Review of large-scale randomised trials. *Cardiovasc. Drugs Ther.*, 2002. 16(5): p. 411-5.
[7] Greenwald, P., et al., Clinical trials of vitamin and mineral supplements for cancer prevention. *Am. J. Clin. Nutr.,* 2007. 85(1): p. 314S-317S.
[8] Hemila, H. and E.R. Miller, 3rd, Evidence-based medicine and vitamin E supplementation. *Am. J. Clin. Nutr.,* 2007. 86(1): p. 261-2; author reply 262-4.
[9] Kris-Etherton, P.M., et al., Antioxidant Vitamin Supplements and Cardiovascular Disease. *Circulation*, 2004. 110(5): p. 637-641.
[10] American Diabetes, A., Nutrition Recommendations and Interventions for Diabetes-2006: A position statement of the American Diabetes Association. *Diabetes Care,* 2006. 29(9): p. 2140-2157.
[11] Hasanain, B. and A.D. Mooradian, Antioxidant vitamins and their influence in diabetes mellitus. *Curr. Diab. Rep.*, 2002. 2(5): p. 448-56.
[12] Magarey, A. McKean, S. and Daniels, L. Evaluation of fruit and vegetable intakes of Australian adults: the National Nutrition Survey 1995. *Aust. NZ J. Public Health* 2006 30(1):32-7.
[13] Ball, K., et al., How well do Australian women comply with dietary guidelines? *Public Health Nutr.*, 2004. 7(3): p. 443-52.
[14] Kamphuis, C.B., et al., Environmental determinants of fruit and vegetable consumption among adults: a systematic review. *Br. J. Nutr.*, 2006. 96(4): p. 620-35.
[15] Giskes, K., et al., Socio-economic differences in fruit and vegetable consumption among Australian adolescents and adults. *Public Health Nutr.*, 2002. 5(5): p. 663-9.
[16] Irala-Estevez, J.D., et al., A systematic review of socio-economic differences in food habits in Europe: consumption of fruit and vegetables. *Eur. J. Clin. Nutr.,* 2000. 54(9): p. 706-14.
[17] Ball, K., D. Crawford, and G. Mishra, Socio-economic inequalities in women's fruit and vegetable intakes: a multilevel study of individual, social and environmental mediators. *Public Health Nutr.,* 2006. 9(5): p. 623-30.
[18] Johansson, L., et al., Healthy dietary habits in relation to social determinants and lifestyle factors. *Br. J. Nutr.,* 1999. 81(3): p. 211-20.
[19] Giskes, K., et al., A multilevel study of socio-economic inequalities in food choice behaviour and dietary intake among the Dutch population: the GLOBE study. *Public Health Nutr.*, 2006. 9(1): p. 75-83.
[20] Patterson, A.J., et al., Relationships between nutrition screening checklists and the health and well-being of older Australian women. *Public Health Nutr.,* 2002. 5(1): p. 65-71.
[21] Lipski, P., *The consequences of undernutrition in the elderly.* Nutrition Society Australia, 1995. 19: p. 146-51.
[22] McCormack, P., Undernutrition in the elderly population living at home in the community: a review of the literature. *J. Adv. Nurs.*, 1997. 26(5): p. 856-63.

[23] Brown, W.J., et al., Women's Health Australia: recruitment for a national longitudinal cohort study. *Women Health*, 1998. 28(1): p. 23-40.

[24] Lee, C., et al., Cohort Profile: the Australian Longitudinal Study on Women's Health. *Int. J. Epidemiol.,* 2005. 34(5): p. 987-91.

[25] Powers, J., et al., Effectiveness of the National Death Index for establishing the vital status of older women in the Australian Longitudinal Study on Women's Health. *Aust. NZ J. Public Health*, 2000. 24(5): p. 526-8.

[26] Ware, J.E., Jr. and C.D. Sherbourne, The MOS 36-item short-form health survey (SF-36). I. Conceptual framework and item selection. *Med. Care*, 1992. 30(6): p. 473-83.

[27] Haywood, K.L., A.M. Garratt, and R. Fitzpatrick, Quality of life in older people: a structured review of generic self-assessed health instruments. *Qual. Life Res.*, 2005. 14(7): p. 1651-68.

[28] Benyamini, Y., H. Leventhal, and E.A. Leventhal, Self-rated oral health as an independent predictor of self-rated general health, self-esteem and life satisfaction. *Soc. Sci. Med.*, 2004. 59(5): p. 1109-16.

[29] Akaike, H., A new look at the statistical model identification.IEEE Trans. *Automat. Contr.* AC-19:716-23. Institute of Statistical Mathematics, Minato-ku, Tokyo, Japan, 1974.

In: Nutrition for the Middle Aged and Elderly
Editors: N. E. Bernhardt, A. M. Kasko, pp. 319-331
ISBN: 978-1-60456-146-3

Chapter XII

Nutrition in the Critically Ill Older Person

Suzie Ferrie
Intensive Care Service, Royal Prince Alfred Hospital,
Sydney, Australia

Abstract

Critical illness poses special challenges for the middle-aged or elderly patient. Increasing age correlates with an increased length of stay in intensive care, and older patients are more likely to experience complications that increase morbidity and mortality. There are several key contributing factors. A smaller lean body mass may mean that many older people lack the physical reserve to withstand a prolonged period of critical illness, where more than 1% of body protein may be lost each day even when adequate energy and protein are being provided. Age-related changes in lean body tissue metabolism may mean that the catabolism of critical illness is much greater in older patients, and losses are more difficult to regain, even with optimal nutrition support and intensive rehabilitation. Pre-existing deficiencies, and an increased baseline level of inflammation, may contribute to early depletion of the body's protective antioxidant system and increase demands for particular vitamins, minerals and trace elements. Lastly, changes in absorption and digestion in older people may reduce micronutrient bioavailability, so that deficiencies become more likely, especially with the uniquely altered requirements of critical illness.

Introduction

Older people tend to have a longer stay in the intensive care unit (ICU), [1] and have increased mortality both in ICU [2, 3] and afterwards. Why? Older people are at higher risk for many different reasons. Firstly, reductions in organ function may mean that they are more vulnerable to organ impairment during stress [4] (see Table 1). For example, age-related reductions in heart function [5] and renal function [6] increase the risk of mortality and morbidity.

Table 1. Effect of aging on physiological processes

Function	Percentage decline from age 20-30 years to age 60-80 years
Anthropometry/body composition	
height	5%
body weight	10%
total body water	15%
lean body mass	35%
Gastrointestinal/metabolic function	
basal metabolic rate	15%
serum albumin	15%
tissue oxygen delivery	20-30%
hepatic blood flow	40-50%
Renal function	
renal mass	20%
creatinine clearance	35%
glomerular filtration rate	40-50%
Respiratory function	
total lung capacity	10%
arterial oxygen tension (PaO2)	15%
FEV1	20%
tissue oxygen delivery	20-30%
cardiac index, vital capacity	30-50%
maximum oxygen uptake	35-70%
number of alveoli	30-40%

Sources: Shock NW. Aging and physiological systems. *J Chron Dis* 1983; 36:137-142 and Professor A.B. Baker, Nuffield Professor of Anaesthetics, University of Sydney (reproduced with permission).

Compared with younger adults, the elderly have a higher incidence of ICU-acquired infections [7] and double the risk of fatal acute lung injury [8] They have poorer outcomes from sepsis compared to younger patients [9], and poorer recovery from injuries to the head [10] and chest [11]. It has been argued that these phenomena have little to do with age *per se*, instead reflecting merely the increased statistical likelihood of comorbidities in the aged, such as pre-existing organ dysfunctions, neurological impairments or functional disabilities. It certainly appears to be the case that age alone does not strongly predict outcome once it is controlled for illness severity, comorbidities and functional status [12, 13, 14]. As injury severity increases, age becomes less of a predictive factor [15]. This can be seen in the weighting that age is given in the illness-severity scoring system APACHE III where it represents only 3% of the variance [16]. Nevertheless, it is certainly the case that the older intensive care patient *does* have many extra problems and these *do* affect outcomes. In wealthy countries, the older patient may come to ICU having reached the limits of a long period of high-level medical management, with little margin for further improvement, with multiple comorbidities and polypharmacy. It is not possible to 'control for comorbidities and functional status' in an individual patient, who is still likely to do less well after an ICU admission, [17, 18, 19] and age remains an important determinant of long-term survival after ICU discharge [20, 21]. This should not be viewed as a reason to deny older people the possible benefits of intensive care, as other factors still remain of vital importance in predicting outcome [22]. Additionally, the elderly survivors of critical illness are more likely to report satisfaction with their outcome than younger patients. They report higher quality of life [23, 24, 4] compared with younger survivors, possibly because of a greater acceptance of a reduced functional status [25]. It is nevertheless important to acknowledge that they may present with pre-existing disadvantages and increased awareness of these will help to improve the care they receive.

Protein

Both height and weight decrease with aging, [26] so that there may be minimal change in body mass index (BMI) despite significant changes in body composition, with a steady loss of lean tissue [27, 28]. An older person will have a lower lean body mass than a younger person at the same BMI, and this may be reflected in decreased strength, function and mobility even within the lower limits of the 'healthy' range for BMI [29]. This has serious implications even in community-dwelling active older people, [30, 31] but gains far more significance in illness, [32] and is of crucial importance in critical illness [33] which can be a profoundly catabolic state. A prolonged period of critical illness can have a devastating impact on the patient's lean tissue stores, with possible losses of 1% of muscle protein for each day of illness. Hill et al [34] found a loss of 14% of total body nitrogen and 19% of fat-free mass (of which nearly half was limb muscle) over 21 days in septic patients despite nutritional support. Losing about 40% of total body weight appears to be inevitably fatal when lean tissue is not conserved, and losses of 10-15% have significant effects on functioning, [35] affecting respiratory muscles as well as other organs, skeletal muscle strength, and also mental status. This means that even a week's admission to the intensive care unit poses a high risk of morbidity or even mortality if optimal nutritional support is not provided.The lean body mass is therefore a key determinant of survival in the context of critical illness.

The recommendations for protein intake in critical illness are generally about 1.2 – 1.5 g / kg body weight, based on studies indicating that nitrogen balance fails to improve above that level [36, 37]. However, protein requirements appear to be about 20-25% higher in the healthy elderly compared to younger adults, [38,39,40] and this may mean that the increased requirements of a critically ill patient need to be boosted even further in the critically ill older person and that closer attention needs to be paid to preventing delays and interruptions to nutrition support. Early initiation of nutritional support is essential in minimising nutritional deficits that can accumulate due to such delays and interruptions, which is important as these appear to have a deleterious effect on outcomes [41].

After a hospital admission, nutrition and muscle mass continue to exert a significant influence on longer-term outcomes [42, 43, 44, 45]. If there has been significant depletion of lean tissue stores as a result of critical illness, it may take months to regain even part of this. The classic Minnesota experiment of Keys *et al* showed that even young fit university-aged men took more than a year to return to their previous body composition, although they had regained significant weight (mostly fluid and fat) much earlier [46]. Older people have greater difficulty in maintaining lean body mass even in health, and intensive rehabilitation is needed to regain function after hospitalisation. This includes a structured increase in physical activity, [47] and optimal nutrition support [48, 49]. As older people have a reduced response to normal stimuli for protein synthesis (such as increased glucose, insulin, whole-protein supplements) it may be important to focus on the particular protein source, and on essential amino acids. Extra protein should be of high biological value. In comparison to whey protein, casein is retained longer in the splanchnic bed. In younger people this means that it is better utilised, as the stored amino acids are able to complement one another, resulting in a complete amino acid profile across more than one meal. In the elderly, whey protein may instead be more beneficial, as the faster absorption and release into the bloodstream means reduced losses, and improved inhibition of body protein breakdown [50]. Consuming protein *before* exercise, and concentrating the bulk of the day's protein intake into one main high-quality meal, may also improve protein utilization [51].

Micronutrients

Critical illness increases the requirements for many vitamins, minerals and trace elements, while at the same time, the inflammatory response may cause disturbances in the body's normal processes for releasing micronutrients from their stores and transporting them to where they are needed. The increase in requirements is multifactorial. Firstly, there is an increased demand for micronutrients as metabolic cofactors, during the hypermetabolism of critical illness.

Secondly, micronutrients are required in increased amounts as part of the body's protective anti-oxidant system, [52] because exposure to free radicals, which can cause oxidative damage to cells, is increased by hypermetabolism, by injury and inflammation, by ischaemia-reperfusion, and also by treatments such as artificial ventilation and continuous dialysis (renal replacement therapy). This includes minerals and trace elements such as selenium, zinc, copper and manganese, and vitamins C and E. [46, 53]. These may become rapidly depleted in severe stress. Because they work together as a coordinated system, a deficiency in just one component may affect the working of the whole system [46].

Thirdly, falls in serum levels may reflect the body's need to relocate micronutrients as part of the acute phase response, [54] for example to the liver for synthesis of acute phase proteins (in the case of zinc) [55] or redistributing from the serum to any site of oxidative stress (in the case of selenium) [47]. Serum levels of many vitamins decrease, reflecting a shift into the cell where they are cofactors in metabolic pathways [48].

Fourth, micronutrient losses may often be increased in critical illness, due to complications such as diarrhoea, vomiting or gastric aspirate losses, losses from wounds [56] or fistulae, or due to treatments such as continuous dialysis. For example, continuous dialysis (renal replacement therapy) may significantly deplete thiamine, selenium and copper, more than doubling requirements [57] Fifth, intake of micronutrients may be compromised if enteral feeding is poorly tolerated, or if incomplete parenteral nutrition is provided (by omitting some micronutrients).

Selective supplementation of some micronutrients, particularly selenium, may lead to better outcomes in critical illness, [58, 59, 60] but at present it is unclear exactly what should be supplemented, and by how much [61, 62]. Care is required, as large doses of any antioxidant, or even more moderate doses given in isolation (independent of other components of the body's antioxidant system) can act as oxidants in their own right [46, 63, 64].

Immunonutrition is a relatively recent development in nutrition support which remains somewhat controversial [65, 66]. Although clear benefits are seen when immunonutrients are given preoperatively, there seems to be a difference in effect once the body enters the acute phase response. Individual responses to immunonutrition during inflammation may be genetically determined, which may explain the rather mixed clinical trial results when used in an intensive care setting, particularly when there is sepsis.

There appear to be significant changes in the immune function and inflammatory response with aging [67]. In particular, cell-mediated immunity exhibits age-related changes such as reduced mature T lymphocyte numbers and impaired responses to stimuli, as well as slower and less specific humoral antibody responses [68]. Such changes are similar to those which occur in protein malnutrition and in deficiencies of individual micronutrients such as zinc, selenium and vitamin B6, which are also more likely in the elderly. Another contributor to some of these lymphocyte effects may be the loss of proinflammatory cytokine regulation, [69] possibly due to the decrease in sex hormones with aging [70] An increased baseline cortisol level also appears to be predictive of mortality and length of hospital stay, [71, 72, 73] and older people tend to have higher cortisol levels as production increases with age [74]. In the case of inflammation, being overweight is a disadvantage for the elderly, as adipose tissue generates its own low-level inflammatory state [75, 76]. Ongoing inflammation appears to increase mortality risk [77]. This means that older people are simultaneously at increased risk of immune impairment (with the result that they are more vulnerable to infections) *and* chronic inflammation (which may deplete body protein and micronutrients, reduce bone mass and contribute to a deterioration in cognitive function). This may mean that older people respond unpredictably to immunonutrition, but may benefit from micronutrient supplementation more profoundly than younger people [78, 79].

Complicating matters is the fact that the patient may have pre-existing micronutrient deficiencies which exacerbate the situation, and older people are more likely to be in this group. The aged are at increased risk of poor nutritional intakes, and already have higher requirements for many micronutrients such as thiamine, [80] riboflavin, [81] folate, [82, 83, 84] and vitamin B6. [53] Reduced absorption of vitamin B12 in older people may be due to common gastric pathologies, or merely a decrease in secretion of gastric acid and intrinsic factor [85]. Calcium absorption also decreases with age [86]. Vitamin D status may be compromised as older people are more likely to be housebound, and less likely to expose significant areas of bare skin to the sun. In addition, their skin synthesis of vitamin D is less efficient for the same amount of exposure [87] The older patient may therefore require additional supplementation of a variety of micronutrients just to reach repletion levels, while also being confronted with increased requirements due to critical illness itself.

These increases in micronutrient needs pose a challenge for nutrition prescription in critical care, since it is difficult to establish the extent of supplementation required (since serum levels do not accurately indicate the body's overall micronutrient status), and the risk of overfeeding is simultaneously increased because energy requirements are reduced with age. This reduction in energy requirements is not just due to a decrease in habitual activity, which becomes irrelevant when the critically ill patient is paralysed and/or sedated, but is also a function of reduced basal metabolic rate (due to smaller muscle mass). Nutrient-dense nutrition is therefore required, to meet the patient's needs without exceeding energy requirements, and close attention to supplementation is also indicated. Early feeding is also important. Prevention of some oxidant damage may be possible if adequate amounts of the relevant micronutrients are provided early [88].

Nutritional Assessment in Critical Illness

It is essential to identify nutritional problems early, as nutrition makes such a vital difference to outcome [89]. There are several simple tools that have been developed for nutritional screening and assessment of the hospital patient, some specifically targeted towards older people [90]. Screening tools are often designed to be used by staff who are not trained in nutrition, and while these can help to identify patients requiring more detailed evaluation, they do not replace a more formal process of nutritional assessment. One reason is that many such tools fail to distinguish between nutritional *status* and nutritional *risk* [91]. . To clarify this distinction: nutritional status refers to the body's stores of essential substrates for energy, metabolism, normal organ function, and for processes such as healing and immune function, while nutritional risk refers to the patient's likelihood of significantly depleting these body stores and becoming malnourished, resulting in compromised organ function and impaired healing and immunity, as a result of increased nutrient demand or losses due to inflammation, infection or injury. The appropriate response is different for each. Nutritional status, when suboptimal, can usually be corrected by nutritional means, since the primary cause is a nutritional one. Nutritional risk, on the other hand, cannot be modified by nutrition alone, since the primary cause of the increased demand is *not* nutritional. The underlying causes (inflammation, infection, or injury) must be addressed and the priority for nutrition care is to provide adequate maintenance and support, avoiding over- and under-feeding, during this time. It is usually not appropriate to aim for changes in body weight at such a time, and often it may be difficult even to achieve repletion of nutritional deficiencies.

Serum levels of hepatic proteins such as albumin and prealbumin have traditionally been regarded as an essential component of nutritional assessment, and certainly albumin has been widely used as an indicator of nutritional status, particularly in studies of the elderly. During critical illness, however, serum proteins cannot be used in the same way, and a failure to distinguish between nutritional status and nutritional risk may cause confusion and misinterpretation [92]. Because they are affected by the acute phase response, in critical illness they become indicators of illness severity (that is, nutritional *risk*) rather than of nutritional status, and do not respond significantly to nutrition input *per se*. [93, 94, 95, 96]. That is, increasing protein or energy delivery above the patient's actual requirement does not cause an increase in protein utilisation or lead to any extra improvement in hepatic protein levels, [97] and levels will remain low even with adequate nutrition, if there is an ongoing acute phase response to inflammation, infection or injury. This does not mean that the serum protein levels are useless, however: as indicators of nutritional risk, they can help in identifying situations where early, preventive, nutrition intervention is most needed, and where frequent monitoring may be required.

To assess nutritional *status* in critical illness, there is no substitute for a clinical examination that takes into account current signs and symptoms relevant to nutritional status, as well as examining the patient's actual body tissue stores rather than using surrogate markers (such as laboratory tests) to make a guess. A simple physical assessment looks at lean tissue and adipose stores, particularly identifying depletion of body protein or reduction in muscle tone, and noting skin, hair and nail condition and the presence of oedema [98] Body tissue stores may be important in estimating the patients' nutritional requirements [99] as well as in categorising the patient's nutritional status.

Conclusion

Although critical illness is a gruelling experience for the middle-aged or elderly patient, there are strategies that may improve outcome. Careful attention to nutritional screening and assessment enables early identification of those with a depleted lean body mass who require more aggressive nutritional support. Prompt diagnosis of pre-existing micronutrient deficiencies may make it possible to achieve repletion, or at least provide the required level of supplementation that critical illness demands. And post-discharge care, with a targeted increase in protein intake and regular physical activity, may allow the ICU survivor to regain satisfying quality of life and independent function, regardless of age.

References

[1] Carson SS. The epidemiology of critical illness in the elderly. *Critical Care Clinics* 2003; 19(4):605-617.

[2] Kaarlola A, Tallgren M, Pettila V. Long-term survival, quality of life and quality-adjusted life-years among critically ill elderly patients. *Critical Care Medicine* 2006; 34(8):2120-2126.

[3] Fakhry SM, Kercher KW, Rutledge R. Survival, quality of life, and charges in critically ill surgical patients requiring prolonged ICU stays. *J. Trauma* 1996; 41(6):999-1007.

[4] Wood KA, Ely EW. What does it mean to be critically ill and elderly? *Curr. Opin. Crit. Care* 2003; 9(4):316-320.

[5] Suttner SW, Piper SN, Boldt J. The heart in the elderly critically ill patient. *Curr. Opin. Crit. Care* 2002; 8(5):389-394.

[6] Linderman RD. Changes in renal function with aging: implications for treatment. *Drugs Aging* 1992; 2:423-431.

[7] Rellos K, Falagas ME, Vardakas KZ, Sermaides G, Michalopoulos A. Outcome of critically ill oldest-old patients (aged 90 and older) admitted to the intensive care unit. *J. Am. Geriatrics Soc.* 2006; 54(1):110-114.

[8] Ely EW, Wheeler AP, Thompson BT et al. Recovery rate and prognosis in older persons who develop acute lung injury and the acute respiratory distress syndrome. *Ann. Intern. Med.* 2002; 136:25-36.

[9] Martin GS, Mannino DM, Moss M. The effect of age on the development and outcome of adult sepsis. *Crit. Care Med.* 2006; 34(1):15-21.

[10] Vollmer DG, Torner JC, Jane JA, *et al.* Age and outcome following traumatic coma: why do older patients fare worse? *J. Neurosurg.* 1991; 75: S37-S49.

[11] Shorr RM, Rodriguez A, Indeck MC, Crittenden MD, Hartunian S, Cowley RA. Blunt chest trauma in the elderly. *J. Trauma* 1989; 29:563-573.

[12] Kleinpell RM, Ferrans CE. Factors influencing intensive care unit survival for critically ill elderly patients. *Heart Lung* 1998;27(5):337-343.

[13] Rodriguez-Reganon I, Colomer I, Frutos-Vivar F, Manzarbeitia J, Rodriguez-Manas L, Esteban A. Outcome of older critically ill patients: a matched cohort study. *Gerontology* 2006; 52(3):169-173.

[14] Soares M, Carvalho MS, Salluh JI, *et al.* Effect of age on survival of critically ill patients with cancer. *Critical Care Medicine* 2006; 34(3):912-913.

[15] Nicolas F, Le Gall JR, Alperovitch A, *et al.* Influence of the patient's age on survival, length of therapy and length of stay in intensive care unit. *Intensive Care Med.* 1987; 13:9-13.

[16] Knaus WA, Wagner DP, Draper EA, *et al.* The APACHE III prognostic system: risk prediction of hospital mortality for critically ill hospitalized adults. *Chest* 1991; 100:1619-1636.

[17] Hennessy D, Juzwishin K, Yergens D, Noseworthy T, Doig C. Outcomes of elderly survivors of intensive care: a review of the literature. *Chest* 2005; 127(5):1764-1774.

[18] Hamel MB, Davis RB, Teno JM, *et al.* Older age, aggressiveness of care, and survival for seriously ill, hospitalized adults. *Ann. Int. Med.* 1999;131(10):721-728.

[19] Topeli A, Cakir B. Hospital survival of older patients admitted to a medical intensive care unit. *Aging – Clinical and Experimental Research* 2007; 19(1):69-74.

[20] Marik PE. Management of the critically ill geriatric patient. *Critical Care Medicine* 2006; 34(9 Suppl): S176 – S182.

[21] Chelluri L, Im KA, Belle SH, *et al.* Long-term mortality and quality of life after prolonged mechanical ventilation. *Crit. Care Med.* 2004; 32: 61–69.

[22] Thomas DR, Ritchie CS. Preoperative assessment of older adults. *J Am Geriatr Soc* 1995; 43:811-821.

[23] Udekwu P, Gurkin B, Oller D, Lapio L, Bourbina J. Quality of life and functional level in elderly patients surviving surgical intensive care. *J. Am. Coll Surgeons* 2001;193(3):245-249.

[24] Marik PE. Should age limit admission to the intensive care unit? *American Journal of Hospice and Palliative Care* 2007; 24(1): 63-66.

[25] Chenaud C, Ricou B, Merlani P. [What about quality of life in elderly intensive care survivors?] [French]. *Revue Medicale Suisse* 2006; 2(91):2845-2849.

[26] Dey DK, Rothenberg E, Sundh V, Bosaeus I, Steen B. Height and body weight in the elderly. I. A 25-year longitudinal study of a population aged 70–95 years. *Eur. J. Clin. Nutr* 1999; 53: 905–914.

[27] Tzankoff SP, Norris AH. Longitudinal changes in basal metabolic rate in man. *J. Appl. Physiol.* 1978;33:536–539.

[28] Hughes VA, Frontera WR, Roubenoff R, Evans WJ, Fiatarone-Singh MA. Longitudinal changes in body composition in older men and women: role of body weight change and physical activity. *Am. J. Clin. Nutr.* 2002;76:473–481.

[29] Janssen I, Heymsfield SB, Ross R. Low relative skeletal muscle mass (sarcopenia) in older persons is associated with functional impairment and physical disability. *J. Am. Geriatr Soc.* 2002; 50(5): 889–896.

[30] Landi F, Zuccala G, Gambassi G, *et al.* Body mass index and mortality among older people living in the community. *J. Am. Geriat. Soc.* 1999;47:1072–1076.

[31] Calle EE, Thum MJ, Petrelli JM, Rodriguez C, Heath CW. Bodymass index and mortality in a prospective cohort of US adults. *New Engl. J. Med.* 1999;341:1097–1105.

[32] Thomas DR, Kamal H, Azharrudin M, *et al.* The relationship of functional status, severity of illness, and nutritional markers to in-hospital mortality and length of stay. *J. Nutr. Health Aging* 2005;9:169–175.

[33] Galanos AN, Pieper CF, Kussin PS, *et al.* SUPPORT investigators (The Study to Understand Prognoses and Preferences for Outcome and Risks of Treatments). Relationship of body mass index to subsequent mortality among seriously ill hospitalized patients. *Crit. Care Med.* 1997;25:1962–1968.

[34] Hill AA, Plank LD, Finn PJ, *et al.* Massive nitrogen loss in critical surgical illness: effect on cardiac mass and function. *Ann. Surg.* 1997; 226:191-197.

[35] Allison SP. The uses and limitations of nutritional support. *Clin. Nutr.* 1992; 11:319-330.

[36] Ishibashi N, Plank LD, Sando K, Hill GL. Optimal protein requirements during the first 2 weeks after the onset of critical illness. *Crit. Care Med.* 1998; 26:1529-1535.

[37] Shaw JHF, Wildbore M, Wolfe RR. Whole body protein kinetics in severely septic patients. *Ann. Surg.* 1987; 205:288-294.
[38] Campbell WW, Evans WJ. Protein requirements of elderly people. *Eur. J. Clin. Nutr.* 1996;50:S180–S185.
[39] Hansen RD, Raja C, Allen BJ. Total body protein in chronic diseases and in ageing. *Ann. N Y Acad. Sci.* 2000;904:345–52.
[40] Campbell WW, Trappe TA, Wolfe RR, Evans WJ. The recommended dietary allowance for protein may not be adequate for older people to maintain skeletal muscle. *J. Gerontol A Biol. Med. Sci. 2001*;56:M373–M380.
[41] Villet S, Chiolero RL, Bollmann MD, *et al.* Negative impact of hypocaloric feeding and energy balance on clinical outcome in ICU patients. *Clin. Nutr.* 2005; 24:502-509.
[42] Dardaine V, Dequin P, Ripault H, Constans T. Outcome of older patients requiring ventilatory support in intensive care: impact of nutritional status. *J. Am. Geratrics Soc.* 2001; 49(5):564-570.
[43] Walter LC, Brand RJ, Counsell SR, *et al.* Development and validation of a prognostic index for 1-year mortality in older adults after hospitalization. *JAMA* 2001; 285:2987-2994.
[44] Visvanathan R, Penhall R, Chapman I. Nutritional screening of older people in a sub-acute care facility in Australia and its relation to discharge outcomes. *Age Ageing* 2004; 33:260-265.
[45] Espaulella J, Arnau A, Cubí D, Amblàs J, Yánez A. Time-dependent prognostic factors of 6-month mortality in frail elderly patients admitted to post-acute care. *Age Ageing* 2007; 36:407-413.
[46] Keys A, Brozek J, Henschel A, *et al. Biology of human starvation.* (2 vols.) Minneapolis: University of Minnesota Press, 1950.
[47] Evans WJ. Protein nutrition, exercise and aging. *J. Am. Coll Nutr.* 2004; 23: 601S–9S.
[48] Campbell SE, Seymour DG, Primrose WR. A systematic literature review of factors affecting outcome in older medical patients admitted to hospital. *Age Ageing* 2004; 33:110-115.
[49] Lee SJ, Lindquist K, Segal MR, Covinsky KE. Development and validation of a prognostic index for 4-year mortality in older adults. *JAMA* 2006; 295:801-808.
[50] Dangin M, Guillet C, Garcia-Rodenas C, *et al.* The rate of protein digestion affects protein gain differently during aging in humans. *J. Physiol.* 2003; 549(2): 635-644.
[51] Walrand S, Boirie Y. Optimizing protein intake in aging. *Curr. Opin. Clin. Nutr. Metab. Care* 2005; 8(1):89-94.
[52] Evans P, Halliwell B. Micronutrients: oxidant / antioxidant status. *Br. J. Nutr.* 2001; 85(Suppl 2): S67 – S74.
[53] Berger MM. Can oxidative damage be treated nutritionally? *Clin. Nutr.* 2005; 24(2):172-183.
[54] Louw JA, Werbeck A, Louw ME, Kotze TJ, Cooper R, Labadarios D. Blood vitamin concentrations during the acute-phase response. *Crit. Care Med.* 1992;20:934–41.
[55] Shenkin A. The key role of micronutrients. *Clin. Nutr.* 2006; 25(1):1-13.
[56] Berger MM, Cavadini C, Chiolero R, Dirren H. Copper, selenium, and zinc status and balances after major trauma. *J. Trauma* 1996;40:103–9.

[57] Berger MM, Shenkin A, Revelly JP, *et al.* Copper, selenium, zinc, and thiamine balances during continuous venovenous hemodiafiltration in critically ill patients. *Am. J. Clin. Nutr.* 2004; 80(2):410-416.
[58] Angstwurm MW, Schottdorf J, Schopohl J, Gaertner R. Selenium replacement in patients with severe systemic inflammatory response syndrome improves clinical outcome. *Crit. Care Med.* 1999;27:1807–1813.
[59] Crimi E, Liguori A, Condorelli M, Bontempo P, *et al.* The beneficial effects of antioxidant supplementation in enteral feeding in critically ill patients: a prospective, randomized, double-blind, placebo-controlled trial. *Anesth. Analg.* 2004;99:857–863.
[60] Galley HF, Howdle PD, Walker BE, Webster NR. The effects of intravenous antioxidants in patients with septic shock. *Free Radic. Biol. Med.* 1997;23:768–774.
[61] Mishra V. Oxidative stress and role of antioxidant supplementation in critical illness. *Clin. Laboratory* 2007; 53(3-4):199-209.
[62] Berger MM, Shenkin A. Update on clinical micronutrient supplementation studies in the critically ill. *Curr. Opin. Clin. Nutr. Metab. Care* 2006; 9:711–716.
[63] Chandra RK, McBean LD. Zinc and immunity. *Nutrition* 1994;10:79–80.
[64] Angstwurm MW, Schottdorf J, Schopohl J, *et* al. Bench-to-bedside review: iron metabolism in critically ill patients. *Crit. Care* 2004;8:356–362.
[65] Heyland DK, Novak F, Drover JW, Jain M, Su X, Suchner U. Should immunonutrition become routine in critically ill patients? *JAMA* 2001; 286:944-953.
[66] Zaloga GP. Immune-enhancing enteral diets: where's the beef? *Crit. Care Med.* 1998; 25:66-72.
[67] De Martinis M, Franceschi C, Monti D, Ginaldi L. Inflammation markers predicting frailty and mortality in the elderly. *Experimental and Molecular Pathology* 2006; 80(3):219-227.
[68] Lesourd BM. Nutrition and immunity in the elderly: modification of immune responses with nutritional treatments. *Am. J. Clin. Nutr.* 1997; 66(2 Suppl):478S – 484S.
[69] Hager K, Machein U, Krieger S, *et al.* Interleukin-6 and selected plasma proteins in healthy persons of different ages. *Neurobiol Aging* 1994; 6:771-772.
[70] Ershler W, Keller E. Age-associated increased interleukin-6 gene expression, late-life diseases, and frailty. *Ann. Rev. Med.* 2000; 51:245-270.
[71] Elminger MW, Dengler T, Weinstock C, *et al.* Endocrine alteration in the aging male. *Clin. Chem. Lab. Med.* 2003; 41:934-941.
[72] Beale E, Zhu J, Belzberg H. Changes in serum cortisol with age in critically ill patients. *Gerontology* 2002; 48:84-92.
[73] Rotman-Pikielny P, Roash V, Chen O, Limor R, Stern N, Gur HG. Serum cortisol levels in patients admitted to the Department of Medicine: prognostic correlations and effects of age, infection and comorbidity. *Am. J. Med. Sci.* 2006; 332(2):61-67.
[74] Purnell JQ, Brandon DD, Isabelle LM, *et al.* Association of 24-hour cortisol production rates, cortisol-binding-globulin, and plasma free cortisol levels with body composition, leptin levels, and aging in adult men and women. *J. Clin. Endocrinol. Metab.* 2004; 89;281-287.

[75] Black PH. The inflammatory response is an integral part of the stress response: implications for atherosclerosis, insulin resistance, type II diabetes and metabolic syndrome X. *Brain Behav. Immun.* 2003; 17:350-364.

[76] Visser M, Bouter LM, McQuillan GM, Wener MH, Harris TB. Elevated C-reactive protein levels in overweight and obese adults. *JAMA* 1999; 282(22):2131-2135.

[77] Bruunsgaard H, Pederson M, Pederson BK. Aging and proinflammatory cytokines. *Curr. Opin. Hematol.* 2001; 8:131-136.

[78] Walston J, Xue Q, Semba RD, *et al.* Serum antioxidants, inflammation, and total mortality in older women. *Am. J. Epidemiol.* 2006; 163(1):18-26.

[79] Moroni F, Di Paolo ML, Rigo A, *et al.* Interrelationship among neutrophil efficiency, inflammation, antioxidant activity and zinc pool in very old age. *Biogerontology* 2005; 6(4):271-281.

[80] Hoorn RK, Flikweert JP, Westerink D. Vitamin B1, B2 and B6 deficiencies in geriatric patients, measured by coenzyme stimulation activities. *Clin. Chim. Acta* 1975;61: 151–162.

[81] Madigan SM, Tracey F, McNulty H, *et al.* Riboflavin and vitamin B-6 intakes and status, and biochemical response to riboflavin supplementation, in freeliving elderly people. *Am. J. Clin. Nutr.* 1998; 68:389–395.

[82] Bates CJ, Fleming M, Paul AA, Black AE, Mandal AR. Folate status and its relation to vitamin C in healthy elderly men and women. *Age Ageing* 1980;9:241–248.

[83] Garry PJ, Goodwin JS, Hunt WC. Folate and vitamin B12 status in a healthy elderly population. *J. Am. Geriatr. Soc* .1984;32:719–726.

[84] Jagerstad M. Folate intake and blood folate in elderly subjects, a study using the double sampling portion technique. *Nutr. Metab.* 1977;21:29–31.

[85] Scarlett JD, Read H, O'Dea K. Protein-bound cobalamin absorption declines in the elderly. *Am. J. Hematol.* 1992; 39:79–83.

[86] Need AG, Morris HA, Horowitz M, Scopasa F, Nordin BEC. Intestinal calcium absorption in men with spinal osteoporosis. *Clin. Endocrinol.* 1998;48:163–168.

[87] Need AG, Morris HA, Horowitz M, Nordin B. Effects of skin thickness, age, body fat, and sunlight on serum 25-hydroxyvitamin D. *Am. J. Clin. Nutr.* 1993;58:882–885.

[88] Schiller HJ, Reilly PM, Bulkley GB. Antioxidant therapy. *Crit Care Med* 1993;21:S92–102.

[89] Reid MB, Allard-Gould P. Malnutrition and the critically ill elderly patient. *Crit. Care Nurs. Clinics of North America* 2004; 16(4): 531-536.

[90] Guigoz Y, Vellas B, Garry PJ. Mini Nutritional Assessment: a practical assessment tool for grading the nutritional status of elderly patients. *Facts Res. Gerontology* 1994; Suppl 2: 15-59.

[91] ASPEN Board of Directors. Guidelines for the use of parenteral and enteral nutrition in adult and pediatric patients. Section III: Nutrition Assessment. *JPEN.* 26(suppl 1):9 SA – 12 SA.

[92] Fuhrman MP, Charney P, Mueller CM. Hepatic proteins and nutrition assessment. *JADA.* 2004; 104(8):1258-1264.

[93] Phang PT, Aeberhardt LE. Effect of nutritional support on routine nutrition assessment parameters and body composition in intensive care unit patients. *Canadian J. Surg.* 1996; 39(3):212-219.

[94] Casati A, Muttini S, Leggieri C, *et al.* Rapid turnover proteins in critically ill ICU patients. Negative acute phase proteins or nutritional indicators? *Minerva Anestesiol.* 1998; 64:345-350.

[95] Bauer P, Charpentier C, Bouchet C, Nace L, Raffy F, Gaconnet N. Parenteral with enteral nutrition in the critically ill. *Int. Care Med.* 2000; 26:893-900.

[96] Clark MA, Hentzen BTH, Plank LD, Hill GL. Sequential changes in insulin-like growth factor 1, plasma proteins, and total body protein in severe sepsis and multiple injury. *JPEN* 1996; 20(5):363-370.

[97] Phang PT, Aeberhardt LE. Effect of nutritional support on routine nutrition assessment parameters and body composition in intensive care unit patients. *Canadian J. Surg* 1996; 39(3):212-219.

[98] Detsky A, Smalley PS, Chang J. Is this patient malnourished? *JAMA* 1994; 271(1):54-58.

[99] Ferrie S, Ward M. Back to basics: estimating energy requirements for hospitalised adults. *Nutrition and Dietetics* 2007; 64(3):192-199.

In: Nutrition for the Middle Aged and Elderly ISBN: 978-1-60456-146-3
Editors: N. E. Bernhardt, A. M. Kasko, pp. 333-352

Chapter XIII

Magnesium in Aging: Facts or Myths?

Davidovic Mladen, Djurica Snezana, Dragoslav P. Milosevic, Nebojsa Despotovic and Predrag Erceg
KBC Zvezdara, Clinic Department for Geriatrics, Serbia

Introduction

About Magnesium

The name originates from "magnesia"- a district in Thessaly, Greece. There are 711 minerals with Mg in the Mineralogy Database. The atomic mass of magnesium is 24.305, and the atomic number is 12. Until recent days, there are three stabile magnesium`s isotopes. Magnesium was discovered in early 1755, recognized by Joseph Black at Edinburgh, Scotland, and isolated by Sir Humphry Davy in 1808. This is the silvery white, lustrous, relatively soft metal, obtained by electrolysis of fused $MgCl_2$, which burns in air and reacts with hot water. It is used as a bulk metal and in lightweight alloys with magnesium for engines, also as a sacrificial electrode to protect other metals [1].

A growing number of publications stress magnesium as a life important electrolyte.

Magnesium is second most important intracellular cation, the "natural" calcium channel blocker and is involved in different metabolic processes [2]:

- ion channel translocation
- stimulus-contraction coupling and stimulus-secretion coupling
- peptide hormone receptor signal transduction
- cellular glucose metabolism

Numerous clinical studies and case reports document a growing interest for magnesium as a therapeutic agent in coronary disease, arrhythmias, arterial hypertension, and asthma.

The range of magnesium in the elderly can be in disorder for two reasons: a deficit of magnesium or changes of metabolism of magnesium (the loss of magnesium) [3].

The results of the study [4] showed, there are more frequent deficiencies of magnesium in organisms then it is generally assumed.

Some experimental results have demonstrated the constancy of magnesium status throughout the adult lifetime .[5] There were no significant differences in total magnesium concentration of various tissues (plasma, erythrocytes, brain, testicles, heart, skeletal muscle, gastrointestinal tract, kidney, femoral bone) in Wistar male rats of different ages. The oldest group of rats tended to decreased intestinal magnesium absorption. Also, hypomagnesaemia is associated with the increased production of free oxygen radicals. Low levels of magnesium increase platelets agreeability and adhesives [6].

Magnesium Deficiency

Possible Genetic Basis of Magnesium Deficit

Despite the critical role of magnesium handling, the exact mechanisms mediating transepithelial transport remained obscure. According the study [7], focused on TRPM6, an ion channel of the "transient receptor potential (TRP) gene family, which, when mutated, causes a combined defect of intestinal magnesium absorption and renal magnesium conservation as observed in primary hypomagnesaemia with secondary hypocalcaemia.

Mainly primary defects of epithelial magnesium transport, disorders associated with defects in Ca(2+)/ Mg(2+) sensing, as well as diseases characterized by renal salt wasting and hypokalemic alkalosis.

Magnesium is an essential cation playing a crucial role in many physiological functions. It is critical in energy-requiring metabolic processes, in protein synthesis, membrane integrity, nervous tissue conduction, neuromuscular excitability, muscle contraction, hormone secretion, and in intermediary metabolism. Approximately half of the total Mg in the body of a normal adult human is present intracellularly in soft tissues, and the other half is found in bone, either as exchangeable, surface-bound, divalent cations, which may serve as a reservoir for maintaining normal extra cellular Mg level, or as an integral component of the hydroxyapatite lattice in bone matrix, which may be released during bone resorption.

Serum magnesium concentration is maintained within a narrow range by the small intestine and kidney which both increase their fractional magnesium absorption under conditions of magnesium deprivation. If magnesium depletion continues, the bone store helps to maintain serum magnesium concentration by exchanging part of its content with extracellular fluid. The abundance of magnesium within cells is consistent with its relevant role in regulating tissue and cell functions. Large fluxes of magnesium can cross the cell plasma membrane in either direction following a variety of hormonal and non-hormonal stimuli, resulting in major changes in total and, to a lesser extent, in free magnesium content within tissues.

Imbalances of magnesium are common and are associated with a great number of pathological situations responsible for human morbidity and mortality.

A large part of the population may have an inadequate magnesium intake, and in particular elderly subjects and may be prone to chronic latent magnesium deficiency.

Magnesium deficit is frequently observed in alcoholics and diabetic patients, in whom a combination of factors contributes to its pathogenesis. Dietary magnesium (Mg) deficiency is more prevalent than generally suspected. According to a recent fact, older adults are at increased risk of magnesium (Mg) deficiency. A potential magnesium deficiency is a matter of concern for many individuals of all ages, but for the elderly, it could be particularly serious. through primary and secondary magnesium deficiency and depletion, ageing constitutes one major risk factor for magnesium deficit [1].

Iatrogenic Secondary Magnesium Deficit

Long term treatment with loop diuretics rather than thiazides may induce magnesium depletion due to an excess urinary loss Although the loop diuretics are the main offenders in treatment of congestive heart failure, patients receiving long-term treatment with such agents as the thiazides, are at risk, especially the elderly. Diuretics and digitalis can intensify an underlying Mg deficiency in elderly people [8, 9]. A patient with renal Mg wasting developed hypokalemic hypochloremic alkalosis while being treated with a diuretic for edema of unknown derivation, despite administration of KCl. Alkalotic patients had greater vulnerability to digitalis toxicity, even though they had therapeutic digitalis blood levels lower than the nonalkalotic patients. Only when MgCl2 was added was normal electrolyte status restored [10].

Magnesium Deficiency Influence the Aging Process

Based on the some recent studies, magnesium deficiency can influence the aging process in many different ways:

- Genetic stability plays an important role in individual longevity. Magnesium deficiency can cause inadequate DNA repair and lead to genetic instability, accelerated aging, and many diseases [11].
- Magnesium deficiency influences different cell functions and ends with senescence [12].
- Magnesium supplements can prolong the life span of rats [13].

In order to clarify if the need for magnesium increased with aging, two age-different rats groups were orally supplemented with two magnesium acetate solutions and mineral water rich with magnesium during several weeks [6]. The magnesium supplementation did not affect magnesium content in any rat tissue, as well as proteins and high-density lipoproteins concentrations in serum.

On the other hand, the beneficial effect of magnesium supplementation on serum cholesterol concentration is noticed, expressed more in younger animals, and on triglycerides, observed only in younger ones again, suggesting that older animals needed increased amounts of magnesium compared to younger rats to attain the similar consequence.

Although the results are in accordance with some literature data, having in mind to establish more exactly the effect of rats aging on magnesium contents and distribution in tissues as well as on possible pharmacological magnesium potency, it is necessary to experiment with older rats that are more age different, to use other supplements of higher magnesium concentrations during longer periods and finally to determine any other biochemical constituents.

If we accept as a fact that a deficit of magnesium is essential in the disorder of the lipid status and development of atherosclerosis, it would play a significant role in early aging.

Magnesium deficit accelerates ageing through its various effects on the neuromuscular, cardiovascular and endocrine apparatus, kidney and bone, immunity, antistress and anti-oxidant systems [14]. Poor nutritional status, impaired gastrointestinal (GI) status and polypharmacy are other factors that put the elderly at greater risk for magnesium deficiency [15, 16, 17].

A magnesium deficit in the elderly can occur due to inadequate nutrient intakes, multiple drug use, or altered gastrointestinal function. Magnesium has been targeted as a risk factor for elderly people and has been implicated in the aging process.

Therapy with thiazide or loop diuretics for hypertension or congestive heart failure - and the consequent diuresis - may further stress their mineral balance. Hypokalemia can be a problem in the elderly population. It has been reported finding hypomagnesaemia in 38% to 42% of hypokalemic patients. Because the correction of a potassium deficit may be difficult to achieve unless the magnesium deficit is also corrected, patients with hypokalemia should also be evaluated for magnesium deficiency. The elderly are also vulnerable to hypomagnesaemia-induced malabsorption syndromes and nephrolithiasis [18].

Absorption of Magnesium in the Elderly

Magnesium is the second most abundant intracellular cation in vertebrates. Magnesium ion is a critical cofactor in more than 300 enzymatic reactions involving energy metabolism, and protein and nucleic acid synthesis. Mg is essential for various normal tissue and organ functions . The primary source of Mg in humans is from the diets. Magnesium absorption appears to be greatest within the duodenum and ileum and occurs by both passive and active processes Excessive Mg is rapidly excreted into the urine Factors that contribute to this are lower dietary intakes of magnesium, decreased intestinal absorption of magnesium in older people and a greater excretion of it by the kidneys. Whether long-standing Mg deficiency affects the health of the aged, and increases their susceptibility to adverse cardiac reactions to disease and drugs that cause Mg-wasting deserves investigation. Transient ischemic cerebral attacks, to which the elderly are particularly prone, might be intensified by Mg deficiency. Subjects who have Mg added to their diets have been reported to be less likely to have transient ischemic events [14, 19, 20]. Through primary and secondary magnesium deficiency and depletion, ageing constitutes one major risk factor for magnesium deficit. The efficiency with which magnesium is absorbed declines in elderly subjects. Elderly patients are susceptible to illness predisposing to two types of magnesium deficit: either pathological magnesium deficit induced by disease or iatrogenic magnesium deficit due to the side effects of medical treatments (secondary magnesium deficit of ageing). The diseases to which the elderly are vulnerable, and some of the drugs used in therapy, also contribute to magnesium loss. The efficiency of magnesium absorption can vary greatly depending on magnesium intake. One study showed that 25% of magnesium was absorbed when magnesium intake was high compared with 75% when intake was low [21]. There are homeostatic capacity of the body to adapt to a wide range of magnesium intakes. High intakes of dietary fiber (40–50 g/day) lower magnesium absorption. The effects of dietary components such as phytate on magnesium absorption are probably critically important only when magnesium intake is low. Consumption of phytate- and cellulose-rich products increases magnesium intake which often compensates the decrease in absorption. There is no consistent evidence that modest increases in the intake of calcium, iron, or manganese affect magnesium balance. In contrast, high intakes of zinc (142 mg/day) decrease magnesium absorption. Active reabsorption of magnesium takes place in the loop of Henle in the proximal convoluted tubule and is influenced by both the urinary concentration of sodium and probably by acid–base balance. So, the kidney has a very significant role in magnesium homeostasis.

Increased urinary pH and decreased titratable acidity reduce urinary magnesium output by 35% despite marked increases in magnesium input from vegetable protein diets. Calcium intake in excess of 2600mg/day, particularly contributes to negative magnesium balance or enhance its urinary output.

Magnesium and Atherosclerosis

With aging, alterations in the structure and functioning of the cardiovascular system usually occur [22]. These changes result in increased peripheral resistance and arterial stiffness with significant impact on blood pressure, leading to acceleration of atherosclerosis. Inadequate magnesium (Mg) intake may exacerbate age-related diseases commonly encountered in industrialized countries, such as cardiovascular disease, diabetes, and hypertension [23].

Nutritional status deteriorates in elderly in whom the blood levels of some vitamins and trace minerals prove low. This is the result of reduced dietary intakes, poor intestinal absorption or increased consumption of the antioxidants due to accelerated lipid peroxidation. Also, nutrition is associated with socioeconomic conditions, health status and functional capacity [24-26].

Magnesium as a Natural Calcium Antagonist

Fifty years ago it was registered that in the accelerated body metabolism like in thireotoxicosis the expenditure of Mg was also accelerated by increasing the rate of oxidative fosforilation in mitochondria [27]. Several years after, the Mg medications showed inverse effect on atherosclerosis provoked in rats on the diet rich by cholesterol [28]. Also, Mg has been showed that could successfully antagonize the effect of calcium on realizing catecholamines after sympathetic stimulation [29]. After another 40 years Mg has been described as a calcium antagonist agent capable of displacing calcium of intracellular sites and blocking the voltage-dependent L- and T-type Ca-channels and receptor-mediated Ca-permeable non-selective cation currents in vascular smooth muscle cells [30]. It was suggested that magnesium may have a favorable role avoiding vasoconstrictor responses mediated by calcium [31].

Magnesium Influences Serum Lipid Levels

The relationship between Mg status and lipids in healthy individuals may be different from that in patients with chronic conditions, such as obesity, diabetes and hypertension. Magnesium is necessary for the activity of lecithin cholesterol acyltransferase (LCAT) and lipoprotein lipase (LPL), which lowers triglyceride levels and raises HDL-cholesterol levels. Moreover, Mg-ATP is also the controlling factor for the rate-limiting enzyme in the cholesterol biosynthesis, which associated with cholesterol levels [32].

The low plasma levels of magnesium accelerate atherogenesis by promoting inflammation and increasing LDL concentration and oxidative modification [33, 34]. Also, the hypercholesterolemic state may cause the loss of Mg from soft tissues to the serum, masking an underlying Mg deficiency [35].

Magnesium Deficiency and Atherosclerosis

It was found that serum Mg concentration was decreased in atherosclerosis obliterans and aortic aneurysm. Also, the ratio Mg/Cu was found lower in both serum and arterial wall of these patients as a result of aging and vascular disease [36, 37]. The concentrations of Ca, Mg, Zn and Cu were higher in plaque than in the surrounding tissue. Copper chlorophyllin and its Mg analog could function as potent antagonists of atherogenic LDL modification. [38] Although the hypomagnesaemia is often associated with the imbalance of sodium, potassium and calcium ions, Ca-antagonizing effects are the main among all other electrolytes.

The magnesium deficiency was important for developing carotid atherosclerosis in healthy middle-age adults [39]. The low Mg serum levels in patients with periphery arterial disease were associated with an increased risk of neurological events [40]. Thereafter, it was suggested that low Mg is mainly a risk factor for stroke based macrovascular disease.

Do Magnesium Rich Diet Influence Atherosclerosis?

Magnesium serum levels express only 1% of the total Mg pool. Magnesium supplementation in the diet did not lead to significant increase on its serum level However, in rats receiving a normal or low Mg diet, the injured arteries showed decreased endothelium-dependent relaxing responses to acetylcholine when compared to their respective controls

[32]. An increased amount of dietary Mg was found to suppress the development of atherosclerotic lesions in the aorta of cholesterol-fed rabbits without affecting plasma total cholesterol and HDL-cholesterol concentrations [40].

The inverse association between dietary intake and the risk of stroke has been demonstrated. This association was stronger in hypertensive then normotensive men hypertensive men [41]. Magnesium intake from drinking water was suggested to exert a significant protective effect on the risk of cerebrovascular disease and death from stroke [42]. The possible mechanism of neuroprotective effects of magnesium are: noncompetitive blockade of the NMDA receptors, enhanced regional cerebral blood flow to ischemic areas, inhibition of the Ca entry into the cells through leak, voltage-operated and receptor-operated channels, and favorable recovery of cellular energy metabolism after restoration of perfusion [43].

Magnesium substitution improved endothelial function and exercise tolerance in patients with stable coronary artery disease as well as after acute myocardial infarction [44, 45].

Suggested Mechanism of Magnesium Influence on Vessels

In injured vessels, Mg has a favorable role avoiding vasoconstriction responses mediated by calcium. Also, Mg can reduce free radicals in occlusion-reperfusion model. It also decreases intracellular calcium due to: the blockade of Ca-channels, disruption of agonist-receptor interaction and by its mobilization to cellular organelles. It seems also that Mg is essential for the G-protein activation which is an early step in the cascade for nitric-oxide formation. Magnesium decreases the homocysteine-induced matrix metalloproteinase-2 secretion [46, 47].

Magnesium and Diabetes Mellitus

Diabetes mellitus (DM) is disease characterized by the metabolic disorders related to high levels of serum glucose [48], and it is strongly associated with Mg depletion in intra and extra-cellular compartments [49]. DM is common disease in the elderly, with 20 percent of population affected by the age of 75 [50]. Magnesium (Mg) is an important cofactor for numerous enzymes involved in glucose metabolism and it is hypothesized that Mg plays an important role in glucose homeostasis, insulin action and in the development of type 2diabetes [51-54]. Londono and Rosenbloom first described relationship between Mg and diabetes in 1971 [55]. They found that glucagon injection in diabetic children significantly reduces plasma magnesium level. From that time, a significant body of research about relation between Mg and diabetes has been published.

Role of Magnesium in the Glucose Metabolism

Magnesium is an essential cofactor in over 300 enzymatic reactions and it is involved in processes that engage the utilization and transfer of adenosine triphosphate (ATP). Therefore, intracellular Mg, as part of the activated Mg-ATP complex, is a significant cofactor for several enzymes in carbohydrate metabolism [56]. It is required for all of the rate-limiting enzymes of glycolysis, and regulates the activity of enzymes involved in phosphorylation reactions [56]. Magnesium concentration is important in the phosphorylation of the tyrosine-kinase of the insulin receptor. Mg deficiency results in disorder of tyrosine-kinase activity on the insulin receptor, leading to the development of post-receptorial insulin resistance and decreased cellular glucose utilization [54].

Old age is frequently associated with insulin resistance and glucose intolerance [56, 57]. Continuous age-dependent fall of intracellular Mg levels has been found in healthy elderly subjects [58]. Intracellular free magnesium levels quantitatively predict the fasting and post - glucose levels of hyperinsulinemia, as well as peripheral insulin sensitivity [56]. Evidence exist that intra-cellular Mg depletion contributes to the insulin resistance in peripheral tissues and may lead to the glucose intolerance in healthy aged persons [54, 56].

Magnesium Deficiency in Type 2 Diabetes Mellitus

Type 2 diabetes is characterized by the cellular and extra-cellular magnesium depletion. Numerous epidemiological studies have shown high prevalence of hypomagnesaemia and lower intracellular Mg concentrations in diabetic patients [54]. Magnesium deficiency in diabetics is frequently observed in patients with poor metabolic control or in those with chronic complications [59, 60].

Hypomagnesaemia in diabetic patients is caused by the low dietary intake and/or increased urinary losses [61-63]. Low dietary Mg intake is associated with a significant impairment of insulin-mediated glucose uptake [64], and it aggravates metabolic control in diabetics. On the other hand, hyperglycemia and hyperinsulinemia in type 2 diabetics is associated with increased urinary Mg excretion and leads to the Mg depletion. Treatment with loop and thiazide diuretics, drugs frequently used in the elderly, promotes Mg wasting and eventually worsens Mg depletion [56].

Magnesium deficiency has been recently proposed as a factor involved in the pathogenesis of vascular diabetes complications. Several studies have shown that magnesium supplementation could prevent development and progression of vascular complications [65-68].

Deficient Mg status in old population is not just a secondary consequence of diabetes. Actually, it may cause insulin resistance and altered glucose tolerance, and even type 2diabetes [49].

Magnesium Supplementation in Diabetic Patient

The role of magnesium supplementation in diabetics is still unclear [69]. While some studies have shown the positive effects of Mg supplements on metabolic profile in DM patients [70-72], other reports failed to confirm the benefit of such treatment [73-75].

Data reported in one large prospective study (ARIC) suggest that there is no association between dietary magnesium intake and increased risk for developing type 2 diabetes [76]. However, the same study reported inverse correlation between low serum Mg and the incidence of DM in white population. In addition, ffindings from recent meta-analysis study indicates that increased intake of magnesium may reduce the incidence of type 2 diabetes [77]. According to the recommendations from American Diabetes Association, magnesium supplementation in diabetic patients is warranted only in the case of the proven hypomagnesaemia [78]. In diabetics with normal Mg laboratory values, magnesium-rich foods such as whole grains, beans, nuts, and green leafy vegetables is recommended.

The Methods for Magnesium Detection

Assessment of Mg status in patients is extremely difficult, since less than 1% of total body Mg is stored in the blood, and only 0.3% in the serum [79]. It is impossible to determine the exact Mg status of persons, because it is a sum of intra- and extra cellular concentrations of ionized magnesium and magnesium bound to proteins and inorganic ligands. Routine measurement of total serum magnesium concentration gives a little information about Mg status of subjects, because only ionized fraction possesses the biological activity [51]. Further more, it is not useful in clinical practice, because important Mg depletion is required before total serum levels decrease [56]. Thus, it is imperative to determine not only the total magnesium concentration, but also to measure the free ionized intra and extra -cellular magnesium concentrations. Alternative methods could be Mg loading tests, which measures magnesium retention percentage, and correlates well with Mg bone stores [79].

Development of new techniques, such as P-NMR spectroscopy and Mg-specific ion-selective electrodes, that measure intra and extra-cellular Mg , respectively, are major advance in the field, and have a higher sensitivity in detecting Mg deficits [56]. While P-NMR technique is a research based test due to the expenses in setting up and maintaining the NMR equipment, the development of an Mg-selective electrode apparatus may be particularly useful in routine clinical practice.

Analysis of intracellular Mg is usually performed in erythrocytes, but recent data suggests that lymphocytes and platelets may be more appropriate cells than erythrocytes for such purpose [80]. Another method for assessing the Mg status is tissue sampling such as muscle biopsy, or non-invasive measurement of Mg in sublingual epithelial cells. It is interesting that ionized intracellular Mg concentration in epithelial cells correlates well with Mg in cardiac atria, but not with serum magnesium [81]. However, tthese techniques are too time consuming, too invasive and/or too expensive for routine measurement [79].

It seems reasonable to recommend measurement of ionized serum Mg in assessing magnesium status in elderly, when possible. Testing should be done by the analyzers with ion-selective electrodes, according to the guidelines from International Federation of Clinical Chemistry and Laboratory Medicine [82].

Magnesium Therapy

Magnesium is inexpensive, natural, easy to handle and reasonably safe element. Although, there is generally accepted guidelines for magnesium therapy, considering doses and duration of treatment.

Acute Myocardial Infarction

It is estimated that two-thirds that two thirds of acute myocardial infarction (AMI) patients do not receive reperfusion therapy (patients ineligible for thrombolysis and the elderly) [83]. Their in-hospital mortality rate, particularly in elderly, is in the high range of 14-20% [84]. In those patients, the additional pharmacological therapy is of the most importance in reducing the mortality rate.

Seven possible ways were suggested for influence on infarct size by magnesium (Mg) supplementation: reduction of the toxic calcium overload in the mitochondria of myocytes, reduction of the risk of arrhythmias, the promotion of coronary vasodilatation, the reduction of the catecholamine secretion in the myocardium, the prevention of intramyocardial lipolysis, the influence on the healing and re-endothelization of vascular injuries, the protection of viable cells against oxygen-derived free radicals and the inhibition of platelet thrombosis in patients with coronary artery disease [85].

Magnesium administration should be applied as early as possible, in the first few hours of the AMI [86, 87]. Usually the first dose is given as a slow intravenous bolus (during 15 minutes) 2 gram of magnesium sulphate, followed by 17 gram of continuous infusion over 24-hours [88]. The long-term outcome (for at least 4.8 years) is better, along with preserved LVEF, if the administration of magnesium sulphate is extended to the first 48 hours of AMI [85].

Magnesium and Ventricular Arrhythmia

According to ACC/AHA/ESC 2006 guidelines for management of patients with ventricular arrhythmias and the prevention of sudden cardiac death [89], the magnesium therapy is needed in: torsades de pointes (if QT interval is prolonged), endocrine disorders, diabetes and end-stage renal failure where the ventricular arrhythmias are the result of electrolyte disbalance, in patients with long QT who received drugs that lead to hypomagnesaemia (diuretics), in patients with structurally normal hearts with ventricular tachycardia due to digoxin toxicity, in AIM, in patients arterial hypertension and congestive cardiac failure (precipitated with diuretic use), acute starvation, and acute alcohol toxicity/withdrawal. Intravenous magnesium sulphate in ventricular arrhythmias are efficacious even when the serum level of magnesium is normal (torsades de pointes).

Magnesium as a Neuroprotective Agent

Magnesium is safe and feasible for even prehospital treatment by paramedics in the field in focal stroke patients [90]. Magnesium reverses cerebral vasospasm and reduces infarct volume after experimental subarachnoid hemorrhage (SAH) in rats [91]. In humans, started within 4 days after SAH (continuous intravenous dose of 64 mmol/l magnesium sulphate per day) and continued another 14 days, the incidence of a new hypodense lesions on computed tomography was less often in patients receiving magnesium [92]. The risk reduction of magnesium is added to the risk reduction already achieved with the routinely administrated N-type calcium channel antagonist nimodipine.

However, the results of IMAGES trial showed that magnesium given within 12 hours of acute stroke did not reduce the risk of poor outcome [93]. In this study, magnesium has been administrated only for 24 hours. Since the ischemic cascade continues for > 24 hours, this leaves the possibility that secondary brain damage was not counteracted with short magnesium usage.

Magnesium Supplementation for Inadequately Dietary Intake

Elderly [94], especially diabetics [95] and those with malabsorbtive disorders [96] are at the risk of hypomagnesaemia due to inadequate magnesium intake. The magnesium estimated average requirement (EAR) and recommended dietary allowance (RDA) for men aged ≥ 31 years are 330 mg and 400 mg respectively, and for women aged ≥ 31 years is 265mg and 320 mg respectively. Thereafter, in USA the magnesium intake from dietary sources remains suboptimal and supplement use can be important source of magnesium intake [97]. Green vegetables such as spinach are good sources of magnesium because the center of the chlorophyll molecule (which gives green vegetables their color) contains magnesium. Some legumes (beans, peas), nuts, seeds and Bread made from whole grain are also rich with magnesium. "Hard" water contains more magnesium then "soft" water. The daily value (DA) for magnesium is 400 mg. The food sources with the percent DV (%DV) 10-19% provides a good Mg source (halibut, almonds, cashews, soybeans, spinach, nuts, cereal, oatmeal, potato, peanuts) [98].

When blood levels of magnesium are very low, intravenous magnesium replacement is usually recommended. Magnesium tablets can also be used, although some forms can cause diarrhea. The most commonly used preparation of magnesium as a supplement to dietary intake is multivitamin preparations, containing 100 mg of magnesium.

Clinical Forms of Chronic Magnesium Deficit

Clinical forms of chronic magnesium deficit are polymorphous and without specificity, but the clinical and paraclinical consequences on the nervous system should be studied first. Subjective symptomatology includes non-specific central, peripheral and autonomic manifestations. Central symptoms seem: anxiety, hyperemotionality, fatigue, headaches, insomnia, light-headedness, dizziness, nervous fits, sensation of 'a lump in the throat', 'nuchalgia' and 'blocked breathing'. Peripheral signs are common: acroparathesiae, cramps, myalgias. Functional disorders include chest pain, *sine materia* dyspnoea, precordialgia, palpitations, extrasystoles, dysrhythmias and Raynaud's syndrome. The dysautonomic disturbances involve both the sympathetic and parasympathetic nervous systems causing orthostatic hypotension or borderline hypertension. In elderly patients hyperemotivity, tremor, asthenia, sleep disorders and amnesic and cognitive disturbances are particularly important.

Chronic magnesium deficit may be associated with benign senescent forgetfulness, but not with malignant senescent forgetfulness usually associated with cognitive functional alterations. On physical examination one should systematically look for a genuine Chvostek sign as well as a non-ejection systolic click or a mid-to-end systolic or parasystolic murmur. An electromyogram is useful to look for repetitive tetanic stigmata and an echocardiogram to define mitral valve prolapse. In cardiovascular and renal forms of magnesium deficit, various magnesium-dependent changes may be sought, for example the blood lipid profile, basal glycaemia and insulin sensitivity, albumin, fibrinogen, and in the urine creatinine and microalbuminuria. These classical data should be supplemented by investigations of oxidative stress such as malonedialdehyde and thiobarbituric acid reactive substances and of various magnesium-dependent elements of the antioxidant systems, *i.e.* taurine, reduced glutathione, glutathione-peroxidase, Se, vitamin A, vitamin E and by studies on adrenergic receptivity. There is discussion about the role of magnesium deficit in the pathophysiology of senile osteoporosis, in immunodepression of aged persons and in oncology.

Influences on Parathornone, Vitamine D3 and Bone Mineral Density

Mg deprivation is regularly associated with hyperparathyroidism, low production of 1,25-dihydroxyvitamin D3 [1,25-(OH)2D3], and resistance to PTH and vitamin D. The combined effects of Mg deficiency on PTH and 1,25-(OH)2D3 synthesis and secretion could lead to hypocalcaemia without the compensatory increase in PTH secretion These could impair bone growth and mineralization and reduce bone quality, strength, and bone mineral density. Mg deficiency has been suggested to be a potential risk factor for osteoporosis. Women with postmenopausal osteoporosis are frequently associated with low dietary Mg intake and reduced serum and bone Mg levels. Daily oral magnesium supplementation suppresses bone turnover [17] and prevent the osteoporosis.

Influences on the Others Hormone

The symptoms of magnesium deficiency are identical with many of the symptoms of thyroid disease, especially hyperthyroidism. The symptoms of magnesium deficiency are identical with many of the symptoms of thyroid disease, especially hyperthyroidism. The condition is called hypokalemic periodic paralysis and is highly associated with hyperthyroidism. It's possible that the origin of the disease is not from low potassium (hypokalemia) but from low magnesium, which we know is a factor in hyperthyroidism. Magnesium is depleted in the hyperthyroid state and treatment by Methimazole increases the magnesium content of both erythrocytes (red blood cells) and serum. This emphasizes the need for magnesium supplementation in hyperthyroidism. In Graves' disease, the magnitude of magnesium metabolism alteration is closely related to the extent of the increase in thyroid hormones in plasma. Supplementation the magnesium can control rapid and irregular heartbeat experienced in hyperthyroidism, due to the effect of magnesium on the sodium-potassium pump in the heart [18]. The principal function of magnesium that is critical in thyroid disease is that it enables muscles to relax. With inadequate magnesium, the muscles cramp. When this happens to the heart muscles the heart does not go through a complete relaxation phase, and the next calcium-driven contraction begins before the relaxation is complete. This results in rapid heart beat and irregular heart rate known as arrhythmia chronic fatigue symptoms and fibromyalgia have magnesium deficiencies.

Stress increases the secretion of adrenalin and corticosteroid hormones. These stress hormones mobilize Mg from the cells and increase its renal excretion. It is paradoxical that Mg inadequacy increases secretion of stress hormones.

The consequences of hyperadrenoglucocorticism may concern immunosuppression, muscle atrophy, centralization of the fat mass, osteoporosis, hyperglycemia, hyperlipidaemia, arteriosclerosis, and disturbances of mood and mental performance, through accelerated hippocampal ageing particularly. It seems very important to point out that magnesium deficit aggravate each other problem in ageing.

Fibromyalgia, muscle pain are associated with magnesium deficiency. Very importantly it also indicates that magnesium deficiency may be a consequence of thiamine (vitamin B-1) deficiency and that selenium status is slightly correlated with magnesium levels. This shows that there is some interdependence of selenium and magnesium and that thiamine may be critical for magnesium metabolism and possibly selenium metabolism.

It is not known to what extent suboptimal intakes may affect the aging process; however, magnesium-deficient conditions have been associated with neuromuscular and cardiovascular disorders, endocrine disturbances, insulin resistance and Alzheimer's disease.

The original symptoms which may have been due to magnesium deficiency include weakness and night cramps. Muscle cramps are often due to calcium deficiency, but magnesium controls the secretion of parathyroid hormone and often calcium supplements will not correct nocturnal cramps without concurrent magnesium supplementation.

Literature

[1] Emsley, J., 1991; *THE ELEMENTS*: Sec. Ed., Clarendon Press, Oxford, 251 p.

[2] Dominguez L. J, Barbagallo M., Lauretani F., Bandinelli S., Bos A., Corsi A. M., Simonsick E. M, and Ferrucci L.- Magnesium and muscle performance in older persons: the InCHIANTI study1–3 . *Am. J. Clin. Nutr*. 2006;84:419 –26.

[3] Davidovic, M., Trailov, D., Milosevic, D., Radosavljevic, B., Milanovic, P., Djurica, S., Loncar-Stevanovic, H., and Stevic, R. (2004) Magnesium, aging, and the elderly patient. *TheScientificWorldJOURNAL* 4, 544–550.

[4] Wilhelm Z, Hegyi P, Kleinova J, Kalabova R, Pechova A, and Urbanova R-Diagnosis of magnesium deficiency in the body, personal experience- *Vnitr Lek*, 2004;50(4): 291-9.

[5] de Valk, H.W., Kok, P.T., Struyvenberg, A., van Rijn, H.J., Haalboom, J.R., Kreukniet, J., and Lammers, J.W. (1993) Extracellular and intracellular magnesium concentrations in asthmatic patients. *Eur. Respir. J.* 6(8), 1122–1125.

[6] B.Radosavljevic, Z.Vujovic, H.Loncar-Stevanovic,A.Rasic- Magnezium and maturation process in rats- *Arch. Gerontol. Geriatr. Suppl.* 8 (2002) 291_/294.

[7] Schlingmann KP, Konrad M. and Seyberth HW-Genetics of hereditary disorders of magnesium homeostasis.- *Pediatr. Nephrol.,* 2004; 19(1): 13-25.

[8] Seelig MS: Magnesium requirements in human nutrition. *Magnesium Bull.* 1981;3 (Suppl 1A):26-47.

[9] Fehlinger R, Fauk D, Seidel K. Hypomagnesemia and transient ischemic cerebral attacks. *Magnesium Bull.* 1984;6:100-104.

[10] Brater DC, Morrelli HF. Systemic alkalosis and digitalis related arrhythmias. Acta Med Scand 1981;647:79-85. Wacker WEC. "*Magnesium and Man*", Harvard University Press, Cambridge, MA 1980.

[11] Hartwig, A. (2001) Role of magnesium in genomic stability. *Mutat. Res.* 475(1–2), 113–121.

[12] Li,Y. and Liu, X. (2002) Effects of magnesium deficiency on senescence of Dimocarpus longana leaves. *Ying Yong Sheng Tai Xue Bao* 13(3), 311–314.

[13] Chlebovska, K., Chlebovsky, O., Ahlers, I., Ahlersova, E., and Bacenkova, D. (2002) Effect of K, MG aspartate on some biological parameters of aging rats. *Arch. Ital. Biol.* 140(2), 91–100.

[14] Rayssiguier, Y., Durlach, J., Gueux, E, Rock, E. and Mazur, A. (1993): Magnesium and ageing: 1. Experimental data: importance of oxidative damage. *Magnes. Res.* 6, 373-382.

[15] Klein M (1994), Magnesium therapy in cardiovascular disease. *Cardiovasc. Rev. Rep.* 15(10):9-56.

[16] Kawano Y, Matsuoka H, Takishita S, Omae T (1998), Effects of magnesium supplementation in hypertensive patients: assessment by office, home, and ambulatory blood pressures. *Hypertension* 32(2):260-265.

[17] L. Gullestad, M. Nes, R. Ronneberg, K. Midtvedt, D. Falch and J. Kjekshus: Magnesium status in healthy free-living elderly Norwegians. *Journal of the American College of Nutrition*, Vol 13, Issue 1 45-50, Copyright © 1994 by American College of Nutrition.

[18] White J, Massey L, Gales SK et al. (1992), Blood and urinary magnesium kinetics after oral magnesium supplements. *Clin. Ther.* 14(5):678-687.

[19] Abdulla, M., Behbehani, A. and Dashti. H. (1989): Marginal deficiency of magnesium and suggested treatment. In: *Magnesium in health and disease*, eds. Y. ltokawa and J. Durlach, pp. 111-117. London, Paris: John Libbey.

[20] Costello, R.B. and Moser-Veillon, P.B. (1992): A review of magnesium intake in the elderly. A cause for concern? *Magnes. Res.* 5, 61-68.

[21] Kesteloot H, Joosens JV. The relationship between dietary intake and urinary excretion of sodium, potassium, calcium and magnesium. *Journal of Human Hypertension*, 1990, 4:527–533.

[22] Marin J, Rodriguez-Martinez MA. Age-related changes in vascular responses. *Exp. Gerontl.* 1999;34:503-512.

[23] Bloomgarden ZT. Magnesium deficiency, atherosclerosis and health Care. *Diabetes Care* 1995;18:1623-7.

[24] Morgan DB, Newton HB, Schorach CJ, Jewitt MA, Hancock MR. Abnormal indices of nutrition in the elderly: a study of differential clinical groups. *Age Aging* 1986;1:165-77.

[25] Heseker H, Schneider R. requirement and supply of vitamin C, E and beta-carotene for elderly men and women. *Eur. J. Clin. Nutr.* 1994;48:118-27.

[26] Bianchetti A, Rozzini R, Carabellese C, Yanetti O, Trabucci M. Nutritional intake, socioeconomic conditions and health status in large elderly poplation. *J. Am. Geriatr. Soc.* 1990;38:521-6.

[27] Vitale JJ, White PL, Nakamura M, Hegsted DM, Zamcheck N, Hellerstein EE. Interrelationships between experimental hypercholesterolemia, magnesium requirement and experimental atherosclerosis. *J. Exper. Med.* 1957;106:757-777.

[28] Jankelson OM, Vitale JJ, Hegsted DM. Serum magnesium, cholesterol and lipoproteins in patients with atherosclerosis and alcoholism. *Am. J. Clin. Nutrit.* 1959;7:23-29.

[29] Burn JH, Gibbons WR. Part played by calcium in sympathetic stimulation. *Br. Med. J.* 1964;(5396):1482-1483.

[30] Nakajima T, Iwasawa K, Hazama H, et al. Extracellular Mg 2+ inhibits receptor-mediated Ca 2+-permeabile non-selective cation currents in aortic smooth muscle cells. *Eur. J. Pharmacol.* 1997;320:81-6.

[31] Fonseca FA, Paiva TB, Silva EG, Ihara SS, Kasinsky N, Martinez TL, Filho EE. Dietary magnesium improves endothelial dependent relaxation of balloon injured arteries in rats. *Atherosclerosis* 1998;139:237-242.

[32] Inoue I. Lipid metabolism and magnesium. *Clin. Calcium*. 2005;15(11):65-76.

[33] Maier JA. Low magnesium and atherosclerosis: an evidence-based link. *Mol. Aspects Med.* 2003;24:137-146.

[34] Malpuech-Brugere C, Nowacki W, Daveau, Gueux E, Linard C, Rock E, Lebreton J, Mazur A, Rayssiguier Y. Inflammatory response following acute magnesium deficiency in the rat. *Biochem. Biophys. Acta* 2000;1501:91-98.

[35] Altura BT, Brust M, Bloom S, Barbour RI, Stempak JG, Altura BM. Magnesium dietary intake modulates blood lipid levels and atherogenesis. *Proc. Natl. Acad. Sci. USA* 1990;87:1840-1844.

[36] Iskra M, Baralkiewicz D, Majewski W, Piorunska-Stoizmann M. Serum magnesium, copper and zinc concentration changes in lower limb ischemia and postoperative treatment. *Magnes. Res.* 2005;18(4):261-7.

[37] Iskra M, Majewski W, Piorunska-Stoizmann M. Modifications of magnesium and cooper concentrations in serum and arterial wall of patients with vascular diseases

related to aging, atherosclerosis and aortic aneurysm. *Magnes. Res*. 2002;15(3-4):279-85.

[38] Kapiotis S, Hermann M, Exner M, Laggner H, Gmeiner BM. Copper- and magnesium protophyrin complexes inhibit oxidative modification of LDL induced by hemin, transition metal ions and tyrosyl radicals. *Free Radic. Res*. 2005;39(11):1193-202.

[39] Ma J, Folsom AR, Melnick SL, Eckfeldt JH, Sharrett AR, Nabulsi AA, Hutchinson RG, Metcalf PA. Association of serum and dietary magnesium with cardiovascular disease, hypertension, diabetes, insulin, carotid arterial wall thickness: the ARIC study. *J. Clin. Epidemiol.* 199;48:927-940.

[40] Amighi J, Sabeti S, Schlager O, Mlekusch W, Exner M, Lalouschek W, Ahmadi R, Minar E, Schillinger M. Low serum magnesium predicts neurological events in patients with advanced atherosclerosis. *Stroke* 2004;35:22-27.

[41] Orimo H, Ouchi Y. The role of calcium and magnesium in the development of atherosclerosis. Experimental and clinical evidence. *Ann. NY Acd. Sci.* 1990;598:444-457.

[42] Ascherio A, Rimm B, Hernan MA, Giovannucci EL, Kawachi I, Stampfer MJ, Willet WC. Intake of potassium, magnesium, calcium and fiber and risk of stroke among US men. *Circulation* 1998;98:1198-1204.

[43] Yang CY. Calcium and magnesium in drinking water and risk of death from cerebrovascular disease. *Stroke* 1998;29:411-414.

[44] Saris NE, Mervaala E, Karppanen H, Khawaja JA, Lewenstam A. Magnesium. An update on physiological, clinical and analytical aspects. *Clin. Chim. Acta* 2000;294:1-26.

[45] Shechter M , Merz CNB, Stuehlinger GH, Slany J, Pachinger O, Rabinowitz B. Effects of oral magnesium therapy on exercise tolerance, exercise-induced chest pain, and quality of life in patients with coronary artery disease. *Am. J. Cardiol*. 2003;91:517-521.

[46] Pokan R, Hofmann P, von Duvillard SP, Smekal G, Wonisch M, Lettner K, Schmid P, Shechter M, Silver B, Bachl N. Oral magnesium therapy, exercise heart rate, exercise tolerance, and myocardial function in coronary artery disease patients. *Br. J. Sports Med.* 2006;40(9):773-778.

[47] Guo H, Lee JD, Uzui H, Yue H, Wang J, Tovoda K, Geshi T, Ueda T. Effects of folic acid and magnesium on the production of homocysteine-induced extracellular matrix metalloproteinase-2 in cultured rat vascular smooth muscle cells. *Circ. J.* 2006;70(1):141-6.

[48] American Diabetes Association. Diagnosis and classification of diabetes mellitus. *Diabetes Care.* 2004;27(Suppl. 1):S5–S10.

[49] Paolisso G, Barbagallo M. Hypertension, diabetes mellitus, and insulin resistance. The role of intracellular magnesium. *Am. J. Hypertens* 1997;10(3):346–55.

[50] Meneilly GS, Tessier D. Diabetes in elderly adults. *J. Gerontol. A Biol. Sci. Med. Sci.* 2001;56(1):M5-13.

[51] Saris NE, Mervaala E, Karppanen H, Khawaja JA, Lewenstam A. Magnesium. An update on physiological, clinical and analytical aspects. *Clin. Chim. Acta* 2000; 294: 1–26.

[52] Paolisso G, Scheen A, D'Onofrio F, Lefebvre P. Magnesium and glucose homeostasis. *Diabetologia* 1990; 33: 511–4.

[53] Barbagallo M, Dominguez LJ, Galioto A et al. Role of magnesium in insulin action, diabetes and cardio-metabolic syndrome X. *Mol. Aspects. Med.* 2003; 24: 39–52.

[54] Barbagallo M, Dominguez LJ. Magnesium metabolism in type 2 diabetes mellitus, metabolic syndrome and insulin resistance. *Arch. Biochem. Biophys*. 2007;458(1):40-7.

[55] Londono JH, Rosenbloom AL. Serum calcium and magnesium levels after glucagon in children with diabetes. *Diabetes* 1971;20:365.

[56] Barbagallo M, Dominguez LJ, Brucato V, et al. Magnesium metabolism in insulin resistance, metabolic syndrome, and type 2 diabetes mellitus. In: Nishizawa Y, Morii H, Durlach J, editors. *New Perspectives in Magnesium Research. Nutrition and Health.* London: Springer-Verlag Limited; 2007. p 213-23.

[57] Stevic R, Zivkovic TB, Erceg P, Milosevic D, Despotovic N, Davidovic M. Oral glucose tolerance test in the assessment of glucose-tolerance in the elderly people. *Age Ageing* 2007;36(4):459-62.

[58] Barbagallo M, Gupta RK, Dominguez LJ, Resnick LM. Cellular ionic alterations with age: relation to hypertension and diabetes. *J. Am. Geriatr. Soc.* 2000;48:1111–6.

[59] Tosiello L. Hypomagnesemia and Diabetes Mellitus. *Arch Intern. Med.* 1996;156:1143–8.

[60] Sales CH, Pedrosa Lde F. Magnesium and diabetes mellitus: their relation. *Clin. Nutr.* 2006;25(4):554-62.

[61] McNair P, Christensen MS, Christiansen C, Madsbad S, Transbol I. Renal hypomagnesaemia in human diabetes mellitus: its relation to glucose homeostasis. *Eur. J. Clin. Invest* 1982;12:81–5.

[62] Djurhuus MS, Klitgaard NA, Pedersen KK, et al. Magnesium reduces insulinstimulated glucose uptake and serum lipid concentrations in type 1 diabetes. *Metabolism* 2001;50:1409–17.

[63] Djurhuus MS. New data on the mechanisms of hypermagnesuria in type I diabetes mellitus. *Magnes. Res.* 2001;14:217–23.

[64] Matsunobu S, Terashima Y, Senshu T, Sano H, Itoh H. Insulin secretion and glucose uptake in hypomagnesemic sheep fed a low magnesium, high potassium diet. *J. Nutr. Biochem*. 1990;1:167–71.

[65] De Leeuw I, Engelen E, De Block C, Van Gaal L. Long term magnesium supplementation influences favourably the natural evolution of neuropathy in Mg-depleted type 1 diabetic patients (T1dm), *Magnes. Res.* 2004;17(2):109–14.

[66] Rodriguez-Moran M, Guerrero-Romero F. Low serum magnesium levels and foot ulcers in subjects with type 2 diabetes. *Arch. Med. Res*. 2001 Jul-Aug;32(4):300-3.

[67] Mahaba HM, Ben Thabet EA, el-Ghazali S, el-Ebiari H, Abd el-Aziz HF. Magnesium deficiency and other risk factors for diabetic retinopathy. *J. Egypt Public Health Assoc.* 2000;75(3-4):323-33.

[68] Whang R, Sims G. Magnesium and potassium supplementation in the prevention of diabetic vascular disease. *Med. Hypotheses*. 2000;55(3):263-5.

[69] Guerrero-Romero F, Rodriguez-Moran M. Complementary therapies for diabetes: the case for chromium, magnesium, and antioxidants. *Arch. Med. Res.* 2005;36:250–7.

[70] Rodriguez-Moran M, Guerrero-Romero F. Oral magnesium supplementation improves insulin sensitivity and metabolic control in type 2 diabetic subjects: a randomized double-blind controlled trial. *Diabetes Care* 2003;26:1147–1152.

[71] Yokota K, Kato M, Lister F, et al. Clinical effi cacy of magnesium supplementation in patients with type 2 diabetes. *J. Am. Coll Nutr.* 2004;23:506S–509S.

[72] Paolisso G, Scheen A, Cozzolino D, et al. Changes in glucose turnover parameters and improvement of glucose oxidation after 4-week magnesium administration in elderly noninsulin-dependent (type II) diabetic patients. *J. Clin. Endocrinol. Metab.* 1994;78:1510–1514.

[73] de Valk HW, Verkaaik R, van Rijn HJ, Geerdink RA, Struyvenberg A. Oral magnesium supplementation in insulin-requiring Type 2 diabetic patients. *Diabetes Med.* 1998;15:503–507.

[74] Lima Mde L, Cruz T, Pousada JC, Rodrigues LE, Barbosa K, Cangucu V. The effect of magnesium supplementation in increasing doses on the control of type 2 diabetes. *Diabetes Care* 1998;21:682–686.

[75] Gullestad L, Jacobsen T, Dolva LO. Effect of magnesium treatment on glycemic control and metabolic parameters in NIDDM patients. *Diabetes Care* 1994;17:460–461.

[76] Kao WH, Folsom AR, Nieto FJ, Mo JP, Watson RL, Brancati FL. Serum and dietary magnesium and the risk for type 2 diabetes mellitus: the Atherosclerosis Risk in Communities Study. *Arch. Intern. Med.* 1999;159(18):2119-20.

[77] Larsson SC, Wolk A. Magnesium intake and risk of type 2 diabetes: a meta-analysis. *J. Intern. Med.* 2007;262(2):208–214.

[78] American Diabetes Association. Evidence-based nutrition principles and recommendations for the treatment and prevention of diabetes and related complications. *Diabetes Care* 2002;25(1):202-12.

[79] Rob PM, Dick K, Bley N, Seyfert T, Brinckmann C, Höllriegel V, et al. Can one really measure magnesium deficiency using the short-term magnesium loading test? *J. Intern. Med.*1999;246(4):373-8.

[80] Feillet-Coudray C, Coudray C, Gueux E, Mazur A, Rayssiguier Y. A New In Vitro Blood Load Test Using a Magnesium Stable Isotope for Assessment of Magnesium Status. *J. Nutr.* 2003;133:1220-3.

[81] Haigney MC, Silver B, Tanglao E, Silverman HS, Hill JD, Shapiro E, et al. Noninvasive measurement of tissue magnesium and correlation with cardiac levels. *Circulation.* 1995;92(8):2190-7.

[82] Rayana MC, Burnett RW, Covington AK, D'Orazio P, Fogh-Andersen N, Jacobs E, et al. Guidelines for sampling, measuring and reporting ionized magnesium in undiluted serum, plasma or blood: International Federation of Clinical Chemistry and Laboratory Medicine (IFCC): IFCC Scientific Division, Committee on Point of Care Testing. *Clin. Chem. Lab. Med.* 2005;43(5):564-9.

[83] Eagle KA, Goodman SG, Avezum A, Budaj A, Sullivan CM, Lopez-Sendan J. Practice variation and missed opportunities for reperfusion in ST segment elevation myocardial infarction: Findings from the Global Registry of Acute Coronary Events (GRACE). *Lancet* 2002;359:373-377.

[84] Behar S, Gilat D, Reicher-Reiss H, Kaplinsky E, Zion M, Mandelzweig L, Goldbourt U. Myocardial infarction in patients older than 75 years of age: the short- and long-term prognosis in 653 consecutive patients. *Cardiol. Elderly* 1993;1:103-111.

[85] Shechter M, Hod H, Rabinowitz B, Boyko V, Chouraqui P. Long-term outcome of intravenous magnesium therapy in thrombolysis-ineligible acute myocardial infarction patients. *Cardiology* 2003;99:205-210.

[86] ISIS-4: A randomised factorial trial assessing early oral captopril, oral mononitrate, and intravenous magnesium sulphate in 58050 patients with suspected acute myocardial infarction. *Lancet* 1995;345:669-685.

[87] Woods KL, Fletcher S. Long-term outcome after intravenous magnesium sulphate in suspected acute myocardial infarction: the second Leicester Intravenous Magnesium Intervention Trial (LIMIT-2). *Lancet* 1994;343:816-19.

[88] MAGIC Trial Investigators. Early administration of intravenous magnesium to high-risk patients with acute myocardial infarction in the Magnesium in Coronaries (MAGIC) trial: a randomised controlled trial. *Lancet* 2002;360:1189-96.

[89] American College of cardiology/American Heart Association Task Force and the European Society of Cardiology Committee for Practice Guidelines. ACC/AHA/ESC 2006 guidelines for the management of patients with ventricular arrhythmias and the prevention of sudden cardiac death. http://www.escardio.org/knoledge/guidelines /Rules/

[90] Saver JL, Kidwell C, Eckstein M, Starkman S, for the FAST-MAG Pilot Trial Investigators. Prehospital neuroprotective therapy for acute stroke. *Stroke* 2004;35:e106-110.

[91] Ram Z, Sadeh M, Shacked I, Sahar A, Hadani M. Magnesium sulphate reverses experimental delayed cerebral vasospasm after subarachnoid hemorrhage. *Stroke* 1991;22:922-927.

[92] Van den Bergh WM, for the MASH Study Group. Magnesium sulphate in aneurysmal subarachnoid hemorrhage. *Stroke* 2005;36:1011-1114.

[93] Muir KW, Lees KR, Ford I, Davis S. Magnesium for acute stroke (intravenous magnesium efficacy in stroke trial): randomised controlled trial. *Lancet* 2004;363:439-445.

[94] Vaquero MP. Magnesium and trace elements in the elderly: intake, status and recommendations. *J. Nutr. Health Aging* 2002;6:147-153.

[95] Whang R, Sims G. Magnesium and potassium supplementation in the prevention of diabetic vascular disease. *Med. Hypotheses* 2000;55:263-265.

[96] Hamerman D. Molecular-based therapeutic approaches in treatment of anorexia of aging and cancer cahexia. *J. Geront.* 2002;57A(8):M511-516.

[97] Ford ES, Mokdad AM. Dietary magnesium intake in a national sample of U.S. adults. *J. Nutr.* 2003;133:2879-2882.

[98] Orimo H, Ouchi Y. The role of calcium and magnesium in the development of atherosclerosis. Experimental and clinical evidence. *Ann. NY Acad. Sci.* 1990;598:1444-457.

[99] Dimai H.-P, S. Porta, G. Wirnsberger , M. Lindschinger, I. Pamperl,H. Dobnig, M. Wilders-Truschnig, K.-H. W. Lau: Daily Oral Magnesium Supplementation Suppresses

Bone Turnover in Young Adult Males. *J. Clin. Endocrinol. Metab.* 1998: 83: 2742–2748.

[100] Disashi T; Iwaoka T; Inoue J; Naomi S; Fujimoto Y; Umeda T; Tomita K Magnesium metabolism in hyperthyroidism. *Endocr. J.,* 1996: 43(4):397-402.

In: Nutrition for the Middle Aged and Elderly ISBN: 978-1-60456-146-3
Editors: N. E. Bernhardt, A. M. Kasko, pp. 353-369

Chapter XIV

Nutrition for the Middle-Aged and Elderly: Improving Quality of Life over Adulthood

Maria Bernarda Cordeiro*[*1] and Marly Augusto Cardoso[2]
[1]Department of Medicine Internal,
Nutrition Division, University Federal of Triângulo Mineiro (UFTM),
Uberaba, MG, Brazil. Rua Frei Paulino,
30. 38025-180. Uberaba, MG
[2]Department of Nutrition,
School of Public Health, University of São Paulo (USP),
São Paulo, SP, Brazil. Av Dr. Arnaldo,
715. 01246-904. São Paulo, SP

Abstract

The reviewed literature indicates that even in industrialized countries the nutrition of mature and aged persons is often inadequate, which may lead to premature or pathological senescence. Nutritional research on aging laboratory animals shows that dietary restriction may be the most effective procedure to achieve a long and disease-free life span, probably due to a better protection against mitochondria-linked to oxygen stress. Nowadays, the evidences suggest that diets enriched in micronutrients, including antioxidants vitamins, polyphenols, and essential fatty acids, maintain cellular antioxidant status and stress response enzymes, which otherwise decrease with age. However, at present, there are insufficient data from randomized controlled trials to justify establishment of population wide recommendations for use of antioxidant vitamins supplementation in chronic disease prevention and prolong maximal life span. Instead, the current dietary guidelines recommend a balanced diet with an emphasis on antioxidant-rich fruits and vegetables and whole grains. The beneficial impact of antioxidants on various age-related degenerative diseases may forecast an improvement

* Phone/fax: +55-34-33185840. E-mail: mbcfmtm@mednet.com.br

in life span and enhance quality of life over adulthood in both the developed and developing world.

Introduction

A good health status during the continuing aging process depends on the improvement of several factors: hygiene, nutritional status, sanitary conditions, and prevention of some chronic diseases. In this age group, the elderly person often has several pathologies that require the use of multiple-drug therapy. In addition, due to several reasons that lead to inadequate diets, elderly people are more vulnerable to malnutrition and micronutrient deficiencies (Akamine et al., 2007).

In this regard, many studies suggest that diet, along with genetic and environmental factors, is a major factor affecting longevity. However, inadequate food intake is rampant among the elderly and may strongly influence health status in both young and older persons in developed and in developing countries, contributing to premature or pathological senescence (De Groot et al., 2002). While many socio-economic characteristics are closely related to this phenomenon, pathological factors also significantly contribute to malnutrition in the aged. Smoking, malabsorption syndromes, iatrogenic disease, e.g. dysphagia, nausea, constipation or diarrhea associated with the increased use of medication result in inadequate intake of both macronutrients and micronutrients. Anorexia is also common among elders and, even though it is normally associated with aging, it is often a consequence of depression. Malnourished in aging, associated with impairment in food intake and drug metabolism, leads to many complications. Malnutrition may exacerbate the appearing of the chronic disease associated with aging, heightening the risk for morbidity and mortality (Visvananthan, 2003). Thus, a nutritionally adequate diet, with a good balance for dietary antioxidants, has been considered a critical component of a lifestyle aimed at promoting healthful and active aging (Amarantons et al., 2001).

Oxidative Stress and Ageing

The process of ageing may be defined as a progressive decline in the physiological functions of an organism after the reproductive phase of life. The free radical theory of ageing, was first introduced in 1956 by Denham Harman who proposed the concept of free radicals playing a role in the ageing process (Harman, 1956). His work has gradually triggered intense research into the field of the role of free radicals in biology systems. Harman defines aging as the progressive "accumulation of diverse deleterious changes in cells and tissues with advancing age that increase the risk of disease and death" (Harman, 2001). This definition illustrates two widely recognized and equally important aspects of the aging process: 1) aging is characterized as a progressive decline in biological functions with time, and 2) aging results in a decreased resistance to multiple forms of stress, as well as an increased susceptibility to numerous diseases (Kregel and Zhang, 2007).

Even with a well-described definition and a familiar set of characteristics, aging remains one of the most poorly understood of all biological phenomena, due in large part to its inherently complex and integrative nature, as well as the difficulty in dissociating the effects of normal aging from those manifested as a consequence of age-associated disease conditions (Kregel and Zhang, 2007).

The "free radical approach" is one of the prevalent theories in current literature based on the fact that the random deleterious effects of free radicals produced during aerobic metabolism cause damage to DNA, lipids, and proteins and accumulate over time. Harman proposed in the 1950s that the damage to cellular macromolecules via free radical production in aerobic organisms is a major determinant of life span (Harman, 1956). It was subsequently discovered that reactive oxygen species (ROS) contribute to the accumulation of oxidative damage to cellular constituents. Thus, an "oxidative stress theory" of aging, which holds the increase in ROS accompany aging, will lead to functional alterations, pathological conditions, and even death. Oxidative stress in a physiological setting can be defined as an excessive bioavailability of ROS, which is the net result of an imbalance between production and destruction of ROS (Droge, 2002; Lin and Holbrook, 2003).

It has long been recognized that high levels of ROS can inflict direct damage to macromolecules, such as lipids, nucleic acids, and protein. Due to the bisallylic structures of polyunsaturated fatty acids, lipids are one of the most sensitive oxidation targets for ROS. Once lipid peroxidation is initiated, a propagation of chain reactions will take place until termination products are produced. Therefore, end products of lipid peroxidation, such as malondialdehyde (MDA), 4-hydroxy-2-nonoxidation (4-HNE), and F2-isoprostanes are accumulated in biological systems. These oxidative modifications lead to functional changes in various types of proteins, which can have substantial physiological impact (Blumberg, 2004). In addition to elevations in vivo ROS levels and redox balance in aged organism, one of the most common types of evidence presented by investigators is the strong correlation between aging and the increase in damage oxidative to tissues throughout the body in species ranging from C. elegans to humans (Navarro and Boveris, 2004). However, despite a large body of evidence supporting the notion that ROS produced in cells can manifest damage, a causal link between ROS and aging has not been established clearly, yet.

Antioxidants Vitamin and Chronic Disease Prevention

Vitamin E

Potential biological mechanisms by which vitamin E supplementation may inhibit atherosclerosis have been identified and overall human observational data are compatible with the possibility that vitamin E intake, either from food or supplements may reduce the risk of cardiovascular disease (Gaziano, 2004; Marchioli et al., 2001; Bleys et al., 2006; Törnwall et al., 2004).

Antioxidant vitamins represent one of the many nonenzymatic antioxidant defense mechanisms. Vitamin E (of which α-tocopherol is the major component) is among the most abundant and most widely studied natural antioxidants. However, there are hundreds or thousands of other dietary compounds that may function as antioxidants. In vitro data have demonstrated the possible role of these antioxidants in preventing or slowing various steps in atherogenesis by inhibiting the oxidation of LDL or other free radical reactions (Williams et al., 1992). The major dietary sources of vitamin E are vegetable oils, nuts, whole grains and green leafy vegetables (Visioli and Hagen, 2007).

Many cross-sectional, case-control and cohort studies have found an association between antioxidant consumption and reduced risk of developing heart disease, with the strongest data in favor of vitamin E. Conversely, several large-scale, epidemiological and clinical randomized trials of antioxidant supplements have now been completed, but their results are not entirely consistent (Gaziano, 2004; Visioli and Hagen, 2007).

Whereas some studies show an association between high dietary vitamin E intakes, and lower rates of cardiovascular disease (CVD), other controlled trials examining vitamin E intakes in populations with different risk levels for CVD did not confirm such observations (Gaziano, 2004; Marchioli et al., 2001). The causes for these discrepancies are not clear, and might be due to subject compliance, study design, dosage regime, timing of therapy, and the form of vitamin E used, i.e. natural versus synthetic (Visioli and Hagen, 2007). Completed randomized clinical trials have demonstrated results conflicting. For example, the Primary Prevention Project (PPP) (De Gaetano, 2001), an open-label 2 x 2 factorial trial of 300 mg of synthetic vitamin E and/or 100 mg of low dose aspirin daily in 4,495 Italian men and women with at least one major risk factor for heart disease, observed no effect of vitamin E on reducing the incidence of cardiovascular events. Regarding the secondary prevention effects, the Cambridge Heart Antioxidant Study (CHAOS), a double-blind, placebo-controlled randomized trial using 2,002 patients with coronary artery disease, found a reduced incidence of nonfatal myocardial infarction (MI) by 77% (955 CI, -53 to -9%) among patients allocated to experimental arm with 400 or 800 IU/day during a median period of 510 days – de 400 e 800 IU/day) (Stephens et al., 1996). The combined end point of any major cardiovascular event was also significantly reduced in vitamin E recipients (-53%; 95% CI, -17 to -66%).

In another investigation, The Study of Middle-Aged French-Canadian Men, the use of vitamin and mineral supplements in relation to risk factors for ischemic heart disease were assessed in a cohort of 2,313 men (Meyer; Bairati and Dagenais, 1996). A total of 23% participants reported regular use of supplements; of them, 5.1% were using vitamin E supplements. After a follow-up of 5 years, men taking supplements had a statistically significant lower risk of ischemic heart disease and MI when compared to non-users. The results suggested that vitamin E was more strongly and consistently associated with a lower incidence of ischemic heart disease events.

Finally, the Heart Outcomes Prevention Evaluation (HOPE) Study Trial randomized 9,541 participants with high risk men and women according to their previous vascular or diabetes event associated with one risk factor (vitamin E (400 IU/day) had no effect on death from CVD or ischemic heart disease (IHD), nonfatal MI or stroke events (Yusuf, 2000). In addition, among the large-scale trials, the Alpha-Tocopherol Beta Carotene Cancer Prevention Study (ATBC trial), with almost 30,000 participants taking 50 IU/day of vitamin E, showed a modest association with a lower risk onset of angina and no clear reduction at all in CVD death (The ATBC, 1994).

Vitamin C

A wealth of experimental and clinical trial data have showed a decline in tissue vitamin C with age in a gender-dependent response, i.e. men are more affected than women (Van der Loo et al, 2003; Lykkesfeldt and Ames, 1999; Rikans, Lopez, Hornbrook, 1996). A meta-analysis of 36 studies reported a strong correlation between age and plasma ascorbic acid (AA) concentrations following oral administration. Thus, older persons would probably require double oral intakes when compared with younger subjects to maintain plasma vitamin C concentrations over adulthood (Brubacher et al., 2000). One explanation for the lower tissue vitamin C concentrations, reported in the elderly, might be related to the reduced uptake of ascorbic acid by an active transport mechanism (Michels et al., 2003). Nevertheless, the lifestyle, socio-economic status, poor diet, and physical disabilities may also play an important role in the maintenance of vitamin C status, which can decline to near scurvy (<5.6μmol/L). Studies suggest that, elderly subjects with clinical pathologies, including diabetes mellitus (Birlouez-Aragon et al., 2001), and Alzheimer's disease (Riviere et al., 1998) tend to have lower plasma AA. These effects can be further magnified by smoking, which also affects plasma AA concentration (Birlouez-Aragon et al., 2001).

Regarding the effect of the vitamin C supplementation and prevention of CVD, a number of epidemiological studies have suggested an inverse association between dietary intake of fresh fruit and vegetables, which are rich in antioxidant substances, and CVD mortality. The largest cohort studies failed to find any association between vitamin C intake and CVD mortality (Kushi et al., 1996; Rimm et al. 1993; Stampfer et al., 1993). In addition, a small randomized clinical trial (578 geriatric patients) found that dietary vitamin C supplementation with 200 mg/day did not reduce mortality rates at 6 months of follow-up (Wilson et al., 1973).

On the other hand, the National Health and Nutrition Examination Survey (Enstrom et al., 1992), a large prospective study conducted in the United States among 11,348 adults followed for 10 years found a 34% lower standardized mortality ratio (95% CI, -18.1 to -47.1%) among subjects consuming at least 50 mg of vitamin C per day from diet or supplements compared with those with lower intakes. In another study, higher AA intakes (> 45 mg/day) were associated with lower mortality rate, regardless of social class or other dietary variables (Gale et al., 1995). Ascorbic acid has also been considered essential to wound healing due to its role in collagen synthesis. Older individuals with diets deficient in this nutrient may have impaired wound healing (Hirschmann and Raugi, 1999).

Carotenoids

Observational studies on consumption and serum levels of β-carotene have showed inverse associations with cancer and CVD (Van Poppel, 1996). In 1989, Steinberg et al. verified the potentially important role of oxidation of low-density lipoprotein-cholesterol (LDL) in atherogenesis. This laboratory work led epidemiologists to examine the association between intake of antioxidants in the diet of free-living humans and subsequent CVD.

Observational studies reported a significantly lower risk of cardiovascular death in those who ate diets rich in β-carotene. In meta-analysis pooled relative risk reduction was 31% (95% CI: 41-20%, $p < 0.0001$) for individuals with high β-carotene intakes or serum β-carotene concentrations when compared with those with lower intakes or serum concentrations (Egger et al, 1998). Therefore, several trials with β-carotene, which had been set up to examine the effect of antioxidants on cancer incidence, then reported their results in the mid 1990s. However, the randomized trials did not confirm the beneficial association seen in observational studies. Instead, they reported a moderate adverse increase in risk of cardiovascular death of 12% (95% CI : 4-21%, $p < 0.005$).

In contrast, observational studies on the five other major carotenoids showed that lycopene and its main dietary sources (tomato products) were inversely associated with prostate cancer (Giovannucci, 1998). Plasma concentrations of β-cryptoxantin were also reduced in cases with upper aerodigestive tract cancer when compared with matched controls (Nomura et al., 1997). The outcomes of these studies suggest that individual carotenoids, or the products from which they are derived, in isolation or combination, are potentially protective against disease process involving free radical damage (Martinez-Cayuela, 1995).

Antioxidants and Immune System

A deficient nutritional status may be superimposed on the age-related intrinsic dysregulation in order to cause immune decline. Therefore, an adequate supply of micronutrients, including antioxidants, seems to be essential for an optimal immune response and concomitant health preservation in later life (Miquel, 2001).

Evidences suggest an age-related impairment in the antioxidant defense mechanisms in immune cells, supporting the attempts on the key role that dietary antioxidants play in immune function preservation (Ito et al., 1998). The dietary antioxidants increase several immunological parameters, including neutrophil mobility, delayed-type hypersensitivity response, and stimulated lymphocyte proliferation. There is compelling evidence that intervention with dietary antioxidants such as vitamin E (Meydani, 1999) and C (De la Fuente, 1998) enhances immune function in the elderly and may reduce infection, thus improving the quality of life. The greater production of ROS and the age related oxidative stress occur at a time in life when malnutrition often occurs. There is a decrease in antioxidant defense. Therefore, it seems evident that antioxidant supplementation might have an effect favorable, neutralizing oxygen stress and normalizing the antioxidant/oxidant balance (De la Fuente, 2000).

Caloric Restriction and Increase Life Span

Caloric restriction (CR), an intervention involving a prolonged reduction in caloric intake while maintaining adequate nutrition, is known to increase life span and retard age-associated physiological deterioration in species ranging from yeast to mammals (Masoro, 2000; Sohal and Weindruch, 1996; Yu, 1994). Traditionally, experimental mammalian models of caloric restriction involve a reduction in caloric intake by ~40% of the ad libitum diet throughout the lifespan of the animal, which results in a 30-40% increase in maximum lifespan (Drew et al., 2003; Dirks and Leeuwenburgh, 2006).

Rodents, various strains of rats and mice, are the most commonly used animal model, in which much of the current literature is based upon (Dirks and Leeuwenburgh, 2006). Ongoing studies involving caloric restriction (CR) in non-human primates are accumulating data and thus far support the life-extensive physiological effects as show in rodents (Kemnitz et al., 1994). However, there are currently no well-controlled long-term studies showing the effects of CR in humans. Although scarce, data concerning the short-term effects in humans have shown health benefits (Fontana et al., 2004; Weyer at al., 2000).

It is difficult to determine whether calorie restriction has beneficial effects on longevity in humans because there are no validated biomarkers that can serve as surrogate markers of aging and because it is impractical to conduct randomized, diet-controlled, long-term survival studies in human (Johnson, 2006). Nonetheless, data from epidemiologic studies suggest that caloric restriction can have beneficial effects on the factors involved in the pathogenesis of primary and secondary aging and life expectancy in humans. Many the effects of prolonged CR have been characterized but the mechanism by which CR increases life span is still under debate. Food shortages during World War II in some European countries were associated with a sharp decrease in coronary heart disease mortality, which increased again after the war ended (Fontana and Klein, 2007). In addition, the Okinawa island population is renowned greatest percent of centenarians anywhere in the world. Inhabitants of Okinawa, who ate ~30% fewer calories than average Japanese residents, had ~35% lower rates of CVD and cancer mortality than the average Japanese population (Kagawa, 1978). However, these associations do not prove causality between decreased calorie intake and increased survival (Fontana and Klein, 2007).

Data from a series of studies conducted in members of the Caloric Restriction Society, which is a group that practices self-imposed calorie restriction to extend their life span, has recently been reported. The calorie restriction group consisted of lean (mean BMI, 19.6 ± 1.6) adult men and women (mean age, 51± 12 years; range, 35-82 years) who had been eating about 1800 kcal/d for an average of 6.5 years, which ~30%fewer calories than age and sex-matched individuals consuming a typical Western diet. The calorie-restricted group ate a diet of nutrient-rich foods, such as vegetables, fruits, nuts, daily products, eggs whites, wheat and soy proteins and meat, which supplied more than 100% of the recommended daily intake for all essential nutrients; processed foods, which are rich in refined carbohydrates and partially hydrogenated oils, were avoid (Fontana et al., 2004). Compared with control individuals consuming a Western diet, the members of the Calorie Restriction Society showed many of the same alterations in metabolic and organ functions previously reported in caloric-restricted rodents, including: (1) Low percentage of body fat, (2) low systolic and diastolic blood pressures, (3) markedly improved lipid profile, (4) increased insulin sensitivity, (5) low plasma concentrations of inflammatory markers, (6) low levels of circulating growth factors, and (7) low serum concentrations of T_3 (Fontana et al., 2004; Meyer et al., 2006).

Caloric Restriction and Cardiovascular Disease

Recent data suggest that elevated levels the oxidation of low-density lipoprotein (LDL) cholesterol, excessive reactive oxygen species generation, hypertension and diabetes are all potential causes for development of endothelial dysfunction, a precipitating event in progression of atherosclerosis. These factors are believed to initiate an inflammatory response in injured endothelial tissue. Although studies on short-term energy restriction are inconclusive, long-term calorie restriction is associated with sustained reductions in factors related to endothelial dysfunction in human, such as decreased blood pressure (Fontana et al., 2004; Meyer et al., 2006; Velthuis-te Wierik, et al., 1994), reduced levels of total plasma cholesterol and triglycerides (Walford et al., 2002), and reduced markers of inflammation such as C-reactive protein and interleukin-6 (Bastard et al., 2000). A long-term calorie restriction study in human supports the feasibility of using calorie restriction as a protective effect against atherosclerosis by showing a 40% reduction in carotid artery intima-media thickness in calorie restriction participants relative to a control group (Fontana et al., 2004).

Caloric Restriction and Oxidative Stress

In humans, the level of oxidative DNA damage, as measured by urinary biomarkers, can be modulated by caloric restriction (CR) and dietary composition. Consequently, longevity may depend not only on the basal metabolic rate but also on dietary caloric intake (Valko et al., 2007).

It is widely accepted that the metabolic rate of an organism is a major factor in the rate of the aging, and is inversely related to its lifespan (Sohal and Allen, 1985). In addition, since 2-5% of consumed oxygen is associated with the production of reactive oxygen is associated with the production of ROS, namely superoxide (O_2^-), hydrogen peroxide (H_2O_2) and the hydroxylion (OH), the production of these highly reactive molecules from normal aerobic metabolism is also in direct proportion to an organism's metabolic rate (Smith et al., 2004).

Studies have shown that modulation of the oxidative stress of an organism through prolonged calorie restriction is able to retard the aging process in various species, including mammals (Jung et al., 2004). Recently, Bevilacqua et al. (2004) has verified that the beneficial effects observed with even short and medium-term calorie restriction include decreased mitochondrial proton leaks, with consequential decreases in VO_2, ROS production and cellular damage.

Demographic Evolution and Nutrition Transition

A projection for 2050, using the 1950s as a reference, estimates an increase of 20% in the older population of the world. This estimate considers both an increase in elderly people compared with the total population, and an increase in the proportion of people aged 80 and over, in the elderly group (United Nations, 2006). Data from 10 countries (USA, Japan,

Germany, United Kingdom, France, Italy, China, India, Indonesia and Brazil) accounted for about 55% of the world population in the year 2000 and provide an overview on demography projection changes for 2025 (Shah, 2004).

In developing countries, over the past century most nutrition research and policies focused on poverty and under-nutrition. Nowadays, there is a growing evidence of a major shift towards overweight, obesity and micronutrients deficiencies amongst the elderly. The SABE Study has provided data on BMI in the elderly from Santiago, Chile and other five cities in Latin America and the Caribbean (Abdala et al., 2005). In Santiago, the highest prevalence of obesity was found in the group aged 60-64 years for both men (35.6%) and women (44.1%), decreasing to 18.3% and 25.7%, respectively, in group aged 75 years and older. On the older hand, a very low prevalence of underweight was observed, increased with age. In Brazil, a large-scale representative data, based on three cross-sectional studies conducted in the 1970s, 80s, and 90s found a rapid increase in adult overweight and obesity, showing that the rates doubled or tripled in adult men and women (Doak et al., 2005). Excluding the majority poor geographic areas, such as rural Northeast, malnutrition prevalence in adult women dropped to acceptable rates (about 5%) since 1989. In contrast, anemia continued to display a high prevalence and there is indication of an epidemic trend (Batista Filho and Rissin, 2003). Strategies to control anemia based exclusively on iron supplementation are likely to fail in this population. Although small studies of specific nutrients have been reported, the deficiency of micronutrients other than iron, such as vitamin B12, folic acid and vitamins A, C and E, seems to be an important determinant of nutritional status to the Brazilian elderly.

The Table 1 shows the proportion of elderly people and type of current health problem, according to their age and gender in Brazil in 1998. In the youngest group (aged between 60 and 80 years), the three worst problems detected were spine or back disease, hypertension and arthritis. No significant differences were observed between genders. For the oldest people, in general, the percentage of diseases described increased when compared with the youngest (especially arthritis or rheumatism, depression and diabetes). However, the incidence of cancer, cirrhosis and tuberculosis were unchanged.

Concerning the nutritional status of hospitalized elderly, Vannucchi et al. (1994) measured the serum concentrations of carotenoids, zinc and vitamins A, E, C and B2 in elderly patients in different wards of the hospital. The study was conducted among 130 men and 72 women with a mean age of 67.8 years (range: 60 to 88 years). The percentage of individuals with nutritional deficiencies were 59.5% for zinc, 56.5% for vitamin C, 34.5% for vitamin B2, 25.9% for vitamin E, 13.2% for vitamin A, and 6.8% for carotenoids. Elderly patients with leucoses, megaesophagus, chronic obstructive pulmonary disease, and congestive heart failure represent a group with a high prevalence of deficiency both of zinc and of the vitamins under study. These results show the importance of detecting deficiencies of these micronutrients and provide a basis for a more rational approach to the treatment of elderly patients.

In another study, Cunha et al. (2001) analyzed serum concentrations of vitamins A, E, C, B2 and carotenoids in protein-energy malnourished (PEM) and non-PEM hospitalized elderly patients (age $\geq$ 65 years). Low serum concentrations of vitamin A and vitamin E were similarly observed in PEM and non-PEM groups, respectively. The prevalence of low serum concentrations of water in soluble vitamins was higher in malnourished elderly than in the non-PEM group ($p<0.01$; Table 2), a phenomenon possibly linked to decreased food intake, especially fruits and vegetables. In addition, Cordeiro et al. (2005) investigated the relation between oxidative stress and the occurrence of the acute-phase response with serum ascorbic acid and α-tocopherol levels in elderly patients with pressure sores. Concentrations of ascorbic acid and α-tocopherol were significantly decreased in patients who had pressure sores or infections ($p< 0.05$), whereas malondialdehyde (MDA) concentrations were significantly increased ($p< 0.05$) when compared with control patients (Table 3).

Table 1. Proportion of elderly people and the type of health problem according to their age and sex, Brazil 1998

	60-80 years		Over 80 years	
	Men (%)	Women (%)	Men (%)	Women (%)
Spine or back disease	42.1	40.8	48.3	46.2
Hypertension	36.7	36	49.9	48.8
Arthritis or rheumatism	29	38.2	42.7	49.2
Heart disease	16.2	20.1	20.1	26.5
Depression	8	8.7	15.4	14.1
Diabetes	8.1	7.2	12	12.7
Bronchitis or asthma	7.3	12	7.5	9.1
Chronic renal disease	7	6.7	6.6	7.3
Tendinitis or tenosynovitis	3.6	2.9	5.6	5.3
Cancer	1.4	1.9	0.8	1.4
Cirrhosis	0.5	0.6	0.2	0.4
Tuberculosis	0.2	0.3	0.1	0.1

Adapted from Camarano, 2002.

Table 2. Median, range values and prevalence of low vitamin serum concentrations of elderly patients with or without protein-energy malnutrition (PEM)

Parameter	PEM elderly ($n = 21$)		Non-PEM elderly ($n = 106$)	
	Values	% low values	Values	% low values
Vitamin A (μg/dL)	39.6(16.5-78.4)	28.6	41.9(9.3-132.2)	29.6
Vitamin E (μg/dl)	0.97(0.45-2.15)	18.7	1.0(0.26-11.0)	25
Carotenoids (μg/dL)	121(35.3-298.3)	14.3(*)	106(27.2-416.2)	3
Vitamin C (mg/dL)	0.21(0.06-1.17)	80.9(*)	0.26(0.04-0.95)	56.7
EGRAC	1.42(1.0-2.57)	58.8	1.285(1.0-3.34)	56.2

EGRAC: erythrocyte glutathione reductase activation coefficient. *χ^2 test; $p < 0.01$.

Table 3. Indicators of nutritional status and oxidative stress in patients in the PS, IC, and C groups*

Parameter	Patient groups		
	PS (n = 11)	IC (n = 12)	C (n = 12)
Hemoglobin (g/dL)	8.0 ± 2.0[†]	12.5 ± 1.8	13.4 ± 1.2
Serum iron (μg/dL)	27.0 ± 18.9[‡]	55.0 ± 44.7	79.2 ± 30.5
Total iron-binding capacity (mg/dL)	120.7 ± 36.8[†]	195.6 ± 55.6	281.7 ± 44.9
Transferrin (mg/dL)	87.0 ± 35.9[†]	138.7 ± 45.9	169.6 ± 78.6
Ferritin (ng/mL)	497.8 ± 289.4	306.4 ± 268.6	226.9 ± 198.7
Ascorbic acid (μmol/L)	39.7 (19.9- 80.6)[§]	28.1 (17.6-45.5)	60.2 (41.7- 97.1)
α-Tocopherol (μmol/L)	17.3 ± 4.1[§]	15.7 ± 4.8	26.2 ± 4.0
Malondialdehyde (nmol/L)	0.9 ± 0.2[§]	0.9 ± 0.1	0.4 ± 0.2

C, patients who did not develop pressure sores or any type of infection (control); IC, patients who had infectious pneumonia; PS, patients who had pressure sores.

* Values are presented as mean ± standard deviation or median (range).

[†] $p < 0.05$, PS versus IC and C.

[‡] $p < 0.05$, PS versus C.

[§] $p < 0.05$, PS and IC versus C.

Five of 11 patients (55.56%) with pressure sores and 10 of 12 patients (83.33%) with pneumonia presented serum ascorbic acid concentrations below the reference value (34 to 91 μmol/L). Concentrations of ascorbic acid and α-tocopherol versus malondialdehyde were significantly correlated in the three patient groups ($r = -0.44$, $p < 0.05$; $r = -0.55$, $p < 0.01$, respectively). Thus, patients with pressure sores and acute infections, present a systemic inflammatory response accompanied by an increase in lipid peroxidation, that is associated with decreased serum ascorbic acid and α-tocopherol levels, suggesting that these patients may be at risk for important nutritional deficiencies even achieving the current recommendations for dietary antioxidant vitamins.

Nutritional Strategies for Health Aging

Adequate dietary intake is essential to preserve health and improve life quality in adulthood (Miquel, 2001), being considered the major aspect affecting longevity as well as vascular disease outcome (Visioli, 2007). On the other hand, inadequate nutritional intake is rampant among the elderly, affecting nearly 44% of otherwise health, community-dwellers in developed countries. The malnutrition, in both qualitative and quantitative terms and especially as related to micronutrient intake, may exacerbate the appearing of chronic disease associated with aging. Conversely, there is an accumulation of evidences that diets enriched in micronutrients, including antioxidant vitamins, polyphenols, and essential fatty acids, maintain cellular antioxidants status and stress response enzymes, which otherwise decreases with age (De Groot et al., 2002; Visvanathan, 2003).

However, at present, there are insufficient data efficacy from completed randomized controlled trials to justify the statement of antioxidant vitamins supplementation in chronic disease prevention for the wide population (Bleys et al., 2006; Gaziano, 2004; NIH, 2006;

The HOPE-the HOPE TOO, 2005; Visioli and Hagen, 2007) and prolong maximal life span (Bonnefoy et al., 2002). Instead, the American Heart Association (AHA) dietary guidelines recommended a balanced diet with an emphasis on antioxidant-rich fruits and vegetables and whole grains (Gaziano, 2004). The beneficial impact of antioxidants on various age-related degenerative diseases may forecast an improvement in life span and enhance quality of life (Bonnefoy et al., 2002).

Even if future clinical trials demonstrate that antioxidant vitamins supplementation, reduces the risk of chronic diseases, the use of these supplements should be considered an adjunct, not an alternative, to other established protective measures, such as smoking abstention, avoidance of obesity, adequate physical activity, and control of high blood pressure and dyslipidemia.

Consuming a wide variety of food is considered the best way to ensure balance of nutrients and consumption of appropriate amounts of healthful food components. When dietary selection is limited, nutrient supplementation with low-dose multivitamin-mineral supplements can be useful for meeting Recommended Dietary Intakes (Position ADA, 2000). Altered ability to taste and smell, poor oral health, dysphagia and failure-to-thrive syndrome can contribute to decrease nutrients intake, involuntary weight loss and malnutrition (Position ADA, 1996; Schiffman, 1999). Many older adults, especially the oldest-old and those in institutions, do not consume enough food at meals to meet their energy and nutrient requirements. An energy- and nutrient-dense supplements provided between meals can benefit these older adults (Turic et al., 1998).

Therapeutic nutrient supplementation would be indicated to treat or prevent nutrient deficiency when nutrient requirements are increased; nutrient consumption, absorption or utilization is decreased or nutrition excretion is increased (Position ADA, 2000).

Conclusion

Nutritional research on aging laboratory animals shows that dietary restriction may be the most effective procedure to achieve a long and disease-free life span, probably due to a better protection against mitochondria linked to oxygen stress. Likewise, human studies indicate that age-dependent changes of the cardiovascular and immune systems are linked to oxygen stress, and an adequate intake of dietary antioxidants may protect those systems against chronic degenerative syndromes in which reactive oxygen species (ROS) play a key role. Recent studies suggest that intervention with dietary antioxidants, such as vitamin C and E, are involved in defending the above systems against ROS attack, enhancing immune responses, and reducing infection in the elderly. Consumption of an adequate intake of antioxidants in diet is essential to preserve health and improve life quality in adulthood. Proactive education of the older adults, and early recognition and treatment of nutritional deficiencies are key strategies to achieve ideal nutritional status and healthy aging.

References

Akamine D, Filho MK, Peres CM. Drug – nutrient interactions in elderly people. *Current Opinion in Clinical Nutrition and Metabolic Care* 2007,10:304-310.

Albala C, Lebrao ML, Leon Diaz Em, Ham-Chande R, Hennis AJ, Palloni A, et al. The health, well-being, and aging ('SABE') survey: methodology applied and profile of the study population. *Revista Panamericana de Salud Pública* 2005;17: 307-322.

Amarantos E, Martinez A, Dwyer J. Nutrition and quality of life in older adults. *J. Gerontol. A Biol. Sci. Med. Sci.* 2001;56:54-64.

Bastard JP, Jardel C, Bruckert E, et al. Elevated levels of interleukin 6 are reduced in serum and subcutaneous adipose tissue of obese women after weight loss. *J. Clin. Endocrinol. Metab*. 2000;85:3338-33342.

Batista Filho M, Rissin A. A. Nutritional transition in Brazil: geographic and temporal trends. *Cad Saude Publica.* 2003; 19 (Suppl 1): S181-191 (in Portuguese).

Birlouez-Aragon I, Delcourt C, Tessier F, et al. Associations of age, smoking habits and diabetes with plasma vitamin C of elderly of the POLA study. *Int. J. Vitam. Nutr. Res.* 2001;71:53-59.

Bleys J, Miller III ER, Pastor-Barriuso R, Appel LJ, Guallar E. Vitamin-mineral supplementation and the progression of atherosclerosis: a meta-analysis of randomized controlled trials. *Am. J. Clin. Nutr*. 2006;84:880-887.

Blumberg J. Use of biomarkers of oxidative stress in research studies. *J. Nutr*. 2004; 134:3188S-3189S.

Bonnefoy M, Drai J, Kostka T. Antioxidants to slow aging, facts and perspectives. *Presse Med*. 2002;31:1174-1184.

Brubacher D, Moser U, Jordan P. Vitamin C concentrations in plasma as a function of intake: a metaanalysis. *Int. J. Vitam Nutr. Res*. 2000;70:226-237.

Camarano AA. Envelhecimento da população brasileira: uma contribuição demográfica. Instituto de Pesquisa Econômica Aplicada (IPEA). Texto para discussão n° 858. Ministério do Planejamento, Orçamento e Gestão. http://www.ipea.gov.br. [Accessed 13 August 2007].

Cordeiro MB, Antonelli EJ, da Cunha DF, Júnior AA, Júnior VR, Vannucchi H. Oxidative stress and acute-phase response in patients with pressure sores. *Nutrition* 2005;21:901-907.

Cunha DF, Cunha SF, Unamuno MR, Vannucchi H. Serum levels assessment of vitamin A, E, C, B2 and carotenoids in malnourished and non-malnourished hospitalized elderly patients. *Clin. Nutr*. 2001;20:167-170.

De Gaetano G. Low-dose aspirin and vitamin E in people at cardiovascular risk: a randomized trial in general practice. Collaborative Group of the Primary Prevention Project. *Lancet* 2001;357:89-95.

De Groot CP, van Staveren WA. Undernutrition in the European SENECA studies, *Clin. Geriatr. Med.* 2002;18:699-708.

De la Fuente M. Ferrández MD, Burgos MS, Soler A, Prieto A, Miquel J. Immune function in aged women is improved by ingestion of vitamins C and E. *Can. J. Physiol. Pharmacol.* 1998;76:373-380.

De la Fuente M. Role of antioxidants in the nutrition of the elderly. *Rev. Esp. Geriatr. Gerontol.* 2000;35:63-71.

Dirks AJ, Leeuwenburgh C. Caloric restriction in humans: potential pitfalls and health concerns. *Mechanisms of Ageing and Development* 2006;127:1-7.

Doak CM, Adair LS, Bentley M, Monteiro C, Popkin BM. The dual burden household and the nutrition transition paradox. *Int. J. Obes*. 2005; 29: 129-136.

Drew B, Phaneuf S, Dirks A, Selman C, Gredilla R, Lezza A, Barja G, Leeuwenburgh C. Effects of aging and caloric restriction on mitochondrial energy production in gastrocnemius muscle and heart. *Am. J. Physiol: Regul Integr. Comp. Physiol.* 2003;284:R474-R480.

Droge W. Free radicals in the physiological control of cell function. *Physiol. Rev.* 2002;82:47-95.

Egger M, Scneider M. Davey Smith G. Spurious precision? Meta-analysis of observational studies. *BMJ* 1998;316:140-144.

Enstrom JE, Kanim LE, Klein MA. Vitamin C intake and mortality among a sample of the United States population. *Epidemiology* 1992;3:194-202.

Fontana L, Klein S. Aging, adiposity, and calorie restriction. *JAMA* 2007; 297:986-994.

Fontana L, Meyer TE, Klein S, Holloszy JO. Long-term calorie restriction is highly effective in reducing the risk for atherosclerosis in humans. *Proc. Natl. Acad. Sci. USA*. 2004;101:6659-6663.

Gale CR, Martyn CN, Winter PD, et al. Vitamin C and risk of death from stroke and coronary heart disease in cohort of elderly people. *BMJ*. 1995;310:1563-1566.

Gaziano JM. *Vitamin E and Cardiovascular Disease*. New York Academy of Sciences 2004;1031:280-291.

Giovannucci E, Clinton SK, Tomatoes, Iycopene, and prostate cancer. *Proc. Soc. Exp. Biol. Med.* 1998;218:129-139.

Harman D. Aging – A theory based on free-radical and radiation-chemistry. *J. Gerontl.* 1956;11:298-300.

Harman D. Aging: overview. *Ann. NY Acad. Sci.* 2001;928:1-21.

Hirschmann JV, Raugi GJ. Adult scurvy. *J. Am. Acad. Dermatol.* 1999;895-906.

Ito Y, Kajkenova O, Feuers RJ, Udupa KB, Desai VG, Epstein J et al. Impaired glutathione peroxidase activity accouts for the age-related accumulation of hydrogen peroxides in activated human neutrophils. *J. Gerontol.* 1998;53:M169-175.

Johnson TE. Recent results: biomarkers of aging. *Exp. Gerontol*. 2006;41:1243-1246.

Jung KJ, Ishigami A, Maruyama N, Takahashi R, Goto S, Yu BP, Chung HY. Modulation of gene expression of SMP-30 by LPS and calorie restriction during aging process. *Exp. Gerontol.* 2004;39:1169-1177.

Kagawa Y. Impact of Westernization on the nutrition of Japanese: changes in physique, cancer, longevity and centenarians. *Prev. Med.* 1978;7:205-217.

Kemnitz JW, Roecker EB, Weindruch R, Elson DF, Baum ST, Bergman RN. Dietary restriction increases insulin sensitivity and lowers blood glucose in rhesus monkeys. *Am. J. Physiol*. 1994; 266:E504-E547.

Kimball MJ, Williams-Burgess C. "Failure to Thrive" in older adults. *Arch. Psych. Nurs.* 1995;9:99-105.

Kregel KC, Zhang HJ. An integrated view of oxidative stress in aging: basic mechanisms. Functional effects, and pathological considerations. *Am. J. Physiol. Regul. Integr. Comp. Physiol.* 2007;292:18-36.

Kushi LH, Folsom AR, Prineas RJ, Mink PJ, Wu Y, Bostick RM. Dietary antioxidant vitamins and death from coronary heart disease in postmenopausal women. *N. Engl. J. Med.* 1996; 334:1156-1162.

Lin J, Holbrook NJ. Common mechanisms for declines in oxidative stress tolerance and proliferation with aging. *Exp. Gerontol.* 2003;35:292-299.

Lykkesfeldt J, Ames BN. Ascorbic acid recycling in rat hepatocytes as measurement of antioxidant capacity: decline with age. *Mech. Ageing Dev.* 1999;299:83-88.

Marchioli R, Schweiger C, Levantesi G, Tavazzi L, Valagussa F. Antioxidant vitamins and prevention of cardiovascular disease: epidemiological and clinical trial data. *Lipids* 2001;36:S53-S63.

Martinez-Cayuela M. Oxygen free radicals and human disease. *Biochimie* 1995;77:147-161.

Masoro EJ. Caloric restriction and aging: an update. *Exp. Gerontol.* 2000;35:299-305.

Meydani M. Dietary antioxidants modulation of aging and inmmune-endothelial cell interaction. *Mech. Ageing Dev.* 1999;11:123-132.

Meyer FI, Bairati and GR Dagenais. Lower ischemic heart disease incidence and mortality among vitamin supplement users. *Can. J. Cardiol.* 1996;12:930-934.

Meyer TE, Kovács SJ, Ehsani AA, Klein S, Holloszy JO, Fontana L. Long-term caloric restriction ameliorates the decline in diastolic function in humans. *J. Am. Coll. Cardiol.* 2006;47:398-402.

Michels AJ, Joisher N, Hagen TM. Age-related decline of sodium-dependent ascorbic acid transport in isolated rat hepatocytes. *Arch. Biochem. Biophys*. 2003;410:112-120.

Ministry of Health and National Institute of Statistics. *National Health Survey* (ENS) 2003. Santiago: Ministry of Health, 2004.

Miquel J. Nutrition and ageing. *Public Health Nutrition* 2001;4:1385-1388.

National Institutes of Health State-of-the-Science Conference Statement: multivitamin/mineral supplements and chronic disease prevention. *Annals of Internal Medicine* 2006;145:364-371.

Navarro A, Boveris A. Rat brain and liver mitochondria develop oxidative stress and lose enzymatic activities on aging. *Am. J. Physiol. Regul. Integr. Comp. Physiol.* 2004;287:R1244-R1249.

Nomura AMY, Ziegler RG, Stemmermann GN, Chyou PH, Craft NE. Serum micronutrients and upper aerodigestive tract cancer. *Cancer Epidemiol. Biomarkers Prev.* 1997;6:407-412.

Position of the American Dietetic Association: nutrition, aging, and the continuum of care. *J. Am. Diet Assoc.* 2000;100:580-595.

Position of the American Dietetic Association: oral health and nutrition. *J. Am. Diet Assoc.* 1996;96:184-189.

Rikans LE, Lopez TR, Hornbrook KR. Age and gender differences in hepatic ascorbic acid concentrations and NADPH-dehydroascorbic acid reductase activity. *Mech. Ageing Dev.* 1996;91:165-169.

Rimm EB, Stampfer MJ, Ascherio A, Giovannucci E, Colditz GA, Willett WC. Vitamin E Consumption and the risk of coronary heart disease in men. *N. Engl. J. Med.* 1993; 328:1450-1456.

Riviere I, Birlouez-Aragon, Nourhashemi F, et al. Low plasma vitamin C in Alzheimer patients despite an adequate diet. *Int. J. Geriatr. Psychiatry.* 1998;13:749-754.

Schiffman SS. Taste and smell losses in normal aging and disease. *JAMA*.1997;278:1357-1362.

Shah RR. Drug development and use in the elderly: search for the right dose and dosing regimen (Parts I and II). *Br. J. Clin. Pharmacol.* 2004;58:452-469.

Smith JV, Heilbronn LK, Ravussin E. Energy restriction and aging. *Current Opinion in Clinical Nutrition and Metabolic Care* 2004;7:615-622.

Sohal RS, Allen RG. Relationship between metabolic rate, free radicals, differentiation and aging: a unified theory. *Basic Life Sci*. 1985;35:75-104.

Sohal RS, Weindruch R. Oxidative stress caloric restriction, aging. *Science* 1996;273:59-63.

Stampfer MJ, Hennekens CH, Manson JE, Colditz GA, Rosner B, Willett WC. Vitamin E Consumption and the risk of coronary disease in women. *N. Engl. J. Med.* 1993;328:1444-1449.

Stephens NG, et al. Randomised controlled trial of vitamin E in patients with coronary disease: Cambridge Heart Antioxidant Study (CHAOS). *Lancet* 1996;347:781-786.

The HOPE and HOPE-TOO Trial Investigators. Effects of long-term vitamin E supplementation on cardiovascular events and cancer. A randomized controlled trial. *JAMA* 2005;293: 1338-1347.

The Alpha-Tocopherol Beta Carotene Cancer Prevention Study Group. The effect of vitamin E and beta-carotene on the incidence of lung cancer and other cancers in male smokers: the Alpha-Tocopherol, Beta-Carotene Cancer Prevention Study Group. *N. Engl. J. Med.* 1994;330:1029-1035.

Törnwall ME, Virtamo J, Korhonen PA, Virtanen MJ, Taylor PR, Albanes D, et al. Effect of □-tocopherol and □-carotene supplementation on coronary heart disease during the 6-year post-trial follow-up in the ATBC study. *The European Society of Cardiology* 2004;25:1171-1178.

Turic A, Gordann KL, Craig LD, Ataya DG, Voss AC. Nutrition supplementation enables erderly residents of long term care facilities to meet or exceed RDAs without displacing energy or nutrition intakes from meals. *J. Am. Diet Assoc*. 1998;98:1457-1459.

United Nations. World population prospects: the 2004 revision population database. United Nations Department of Economic and Social Affairs/Population Division/Living Arrangements of Older Persons Around the World. [online publication] 2004. http://esa.un.org/unpp/p2kOdata.asp. [Accessed july 2007].

Valko M, Leibfritz D, Moncol J, Cronin MTD, Mazur M, Telser J. Free radicals and antioxidants in normal physiological functions and human disease. *The international Journal of Biochemistry and Cell Biology* 2007;39:44-84.

Van der Loo B, Bachschmid M, Spitzer V, Brey L,, Ullrich V, Lüscher TF. Decreased plasma and tissue levels of vitamin C in a rat model of aging: implications for antioxidative defense: *Methods Enzymol.* 2003;303:483-487.

Van Poppel G. Epidemiological evidence for □-carotene in prevention of cancer and cardiovascular disease. *Eur. J. Clin. Nutr.* 1996;50:S57-S61.

Vannucchi H, da Cunha DF, Bernardes MM, Unamuno MR. Serum levels of vitamin A, E, C and B2, carotenoid and zinc in hospitalized elderly patients. *Rev. Saúde Pública* 1994;28:121-126.

Velthuis-te Wierik EJ, van den Berg H, Schaafsma G, et al. Energy restriction, a useful intervention to retard human ageing? Results of a feasibility study. *Eur. J. Clin. Nutr.* 1994;48:138-148.

Vio F, Abdala C, Kain J. Nutrition transition in Chile revisited: mid-term evaluation of obesity goals for the period 2000-2010. *Public Health Nutrition* 2007, 1-8. [Epub ahead of print].

Visioli F, Hagen TM. Nutritional strategies for healthy cardiovascular aging: Focus on micronutrients. *Pharmacological Research* 2007;55:199-206.

Visvanathan R., Under-nutrition in older people: a serious and growing global problem! *J. Postgrad. Med.* 2003;49:352-360.

Walford RL, Mock D, Verdery R, MacCallum T. Calorie restriction in biosphere 2: alterations in physiologic, hematologic, hormonal, and biochemical parameters in humans restricted for a 2-year period. *J. Gerontol. A Biol. Sci. Med. Sci.* 2002;57:B211-B224.

Weyer C, Walford RL, Harper IT, Milner M, MacCallum T, Tataranni PA, Ravussin E. Energy metabolism after 2 years of energy restriction: the biosphere 2 experiment. *Am. J. Clin. Nutr.* 2000;72:946-953.

Williams RJ, et al. Dietary vitamin E and the attenuation of early lesion development in modified Watanabe rabbits. *Atherosclerosis* 1992;94:153-159.

Wilson TS, Datta SB, Murrel JS, Andrews CT. Relation of vitamin C levels to mortality in a geriatric hospital: a study of the effect of vitamin C administration. *Age Aging* 1973;2:163-171.

Yu BP. How diet influences the aging process of the rat. *Proc. Soc. Exp. Biol. Med.* 1994;205:97-105.

Yusuf S, et al. Vitamin E supplementation and cardiovascular events in high-risk patients: the Heart Outcomes Prevention Evaluation Study Investigators. *N. Engl J. Med.* 2000; 342:154-160.

In: Nutrition for the Middle Aged and Elderly
Editors: N. E. Bernhardt, A. M. Kasko, pp. 371-387
ISBN: 978-1-60456-146-3

Chapter XV

Bioindicators of Malnutrition and Inflammation in the Elderly

Dana Hrnciarikova[1], Zdenek Zadak[2], Bozena Juraskova[1], Radomir Hyspler[1] and Petr Klemera[3]

[1]Clinic of Gerontology and Metabolism,
Faculty Hospital in Hradec Kralove,
Czech Republic
[2]Center for Science and Research of the Faculty Hospital and
Faculty of Medicine, Charles University,
Hradec Kralove, Czech Republic,
[3]Faculty of Pharmacy, Charles University,
Hradec Kralove, Czech Republic

Abstract

At present there are varying views on the interpretation of biochemical markers of malnutrition and there is ongoing research on the mutual influence of nutritional indicators during a concurrent inflammatory reaction. Establishing the levels of serum proteins so far remains the basic examination in the diagnosis of malnutrition since its formation in the liver is closely related to the nutritional state of the organism. During malnutrition the proteosynthetic function of the liver is diminished and a resultant decline in serum proteins can be observed. The levels of serum proteins can also be reduced during an inflammatory reaction (negative acute phase proteins) with a concurrent rise in inflammatory markers, such as C-reactive protein (positive acute phase protein). This is a so-called prioritization of inflammation and malnutrition of the organism. Along with the strong influence of the inflammatory process on plasma proteins, the age of the individual also plays a significant role. Studies have shown a statistically significant relationship between age, plasma proteins and positive reactants of inflammation. A valuable bio-indicator of malnutrition and inflammation are certain parameters of lipid metabolism. During inflammatory processes and in the old age a rise in the urinary levels of neopterin has been observed.

Revising the interpretation of malnutrition and inflammation bioindicators reveals the necessity of not using only absolute values of plasma proteins, lipoproteins and other components, but rather the indices that integrate bioindicators of malnutrition, inflammation, sex and age.

In our chapter we aim to convey a comprehensive review of malnutrition bioindicators (serum proteins, lipids, basic immunological parameters etc.) and indicators of inflammatory reaction (sedimentation, C-reactive protein, urine neopterin etc.). Furthermore we will analyze the influence of advancing age and finally compare the behavior of nutritional markers in the presence of inflammation. Concurrently we will be analyzing recently used nutritional indices and expressing novel possibilities of their interpretation.

Introduction

Disorders in nutrition take place in the elderly more frequently than in younger people; nearly every human being over 80 suffers from a certain degree of malnutrition. It is caused by the specific factors of the advanced age, when there are changes in the body composition with a physiological decrease in the muscular mass and an increase in the percentage of fat in the organism resulting form the so-called involutional sarcopenia. This process, in combination with the pathological conditions typical of the old age such as, e.g., polymorbidity, polypragmasia, loss of dentition, bad economic, social and psychic conditions, results very rapidly in the development of malnutrition.

Malnutrition in the elderly is an important problem resulting in a further rapid decrease in the remaining muscular mass including the respiratory muscles with a consequent hypoventilation deterioration of mobility, hypoproteinemia with impairment of the transport of substances bound to plasma proteins, decelerated wound healing, and immunosupression with an increased risk of infection complications [18].

These changes result in significant deterioration of the quality of life and self-sufficiency of seniors, prolong hospitalization due to an increased number of complications, increase the cost of treatment, and intensify the risk of institutionalization and mortality of geriatric patients.

Malnutrition is a complex problem affecting many organ systems, and thus when evaluating the state of nutrition there is not just one universal marker, which itself would unambiguously demonstrate malnutrition and would not be affected by other factors [20]. In order to be able to determine the disorders in nutrition, it is therefore necessary to use a combination of various methods (nutrition anamnesis, anthropometric laboratory and functional examinations). Biochemical markers rank among the principal examinations in malnutrition diagnostics both independently and as part of nutrition indices and other scoring systems [6]. In the diagnostics of malnutrition in the elderly it should be taken into consideration that the geriatric patient differs from a younger adult, and therefore the employed examinations may have certain limits, which should be recognized (e.g., a different setting of pathological values etc.).

A review of the most commonly used bioindicators of malnutrition and inflammation is presented in Table 1.

Table 1. Bioindicators of malnutrition and indices of inflammation

Bioindicators of malnutrition	Indices of inflammation
albumin	C-reactive protein
prealbumin (transthyretin)	fibrinogen
transferin	orosomucoid
cholinesterase	α_1-antitrypsin
protein-binding retinol	neopterin in urine
total protein	sedimentation of erythrocytes
lipids – cholesterol, HDL, LDL and leptin	lipoprotein (a)
some hematological an immunological examinations – absolute number of lymphocytes, immunoskin tests etc.	

Bioindicators of Malnutrition

Bioindicators of malnutrition include not only recently often discussed serum proteins (albumin, prealbumin, transferin) and the enzyme cholinesterase, but also lipids and some other hematological and immunological examinations, which are part of nutritional schemes.

At present, serum proteins are the most widely used bioindicators indicating a possibility of malnutrition [4]. The formation of serum proteins takes place in the liver and is connected with the state of nutrition of the organism; in malnutrition, proteosynthetic function of the liver is decreased and a decrease in serum proteins takes place. In the old age there also occurs a mild physiological decrease in plasma proteins still within the framework of the normal range of values [17]. From the half-life of the individual plasma proteins it is possible to subsequently infer the length of malnutrition [6].

Albumin

Determination of the level of serum albumin was formerly considered to be the gold standard in the evaluation of the nutritional state. At present, however, its role as a nutritional marker is doubted. Nevertheless, it is still a suitable marker for screening and long-term monitoring of malnutrition (if inflammation can be excluded); due to its longer half-life it is not suitable for monitoring acute changes in nutritional state. Its informative value is increased in combination with prealbumin, transferin or cholinesterase. A decrease in serum albumin level correlates with the total prognosis of patients, and it is an independent indicator of seriousness of a clinical state. The values of plasma albumin are also part of the majority of nutritional indices [11].

Albumin possesses a relatively long half-life of 20 – 21 days. The normal range of albumin is 35 - 45g/l, the values giving evidence of significant malnutrition in seniors lie below 28g/l [24]. Albumin decreased below 35g/l does not have to be associated with malnutrition. In seniors with a normal test of ordinary activities of ADL [19-20] and medium decreased ADL [2-18], correction between the levels of serum albumin and other nutritional markers was demonstrated, whereas in patients with a significant decrease in ADL (0 - 1), a decrease in albumin below 35g/l was not demonstrated as a suitable indicator of malnutrition and led to its overestimation [13]. This, however, does not hold true for the shift of evaluation of albumin below 28g/l. Albumin concentration may be influenced by the state of hydration, shifts between the intravascular and extracellular spaces, and liver or renal diseases. It is also a negative acute phase protein and it is necessary to relate its values to the values of CRP.

Prealbumin (transthyretin)

The role of prealbumin is particularly the transfer of thyroxin and collaboration in the transport of retinol-binding protein (RBP), with which it forms a complex in the ratio 1:1. It contains also a high concentration of tryptophane, which significantly participates in proteosynthesis. Of all serum proteins, prealbumin possesses the shortest biological half-life of 1 – 2 days; therefore it is most suitable for the evaluation of acute protein malnutrition and immediate success of possible nutritional therapy in the initial stages of realimentation. Prealbumin is capable to capture part of patients already at risk of malnutrition because at least 44% of patients with decreased prealbumin still has normal values of albumin [23]. At present it is an advantageous marker as well as for monitoring the nutritional state, when the trend of its development is more important than the absolute values [3]. The normal values of prealbumin are 0.2 - 0.4g/l, within a range of 0.10 - 0.20g/l it is a mild degree of malnutrition, and serious malnutrition is signaled by the values below 0.10g/l. But it also belongs to the negative acute phase proteins (its synthesis is suppressed by anti-inflammatory cytokines) and it is necessary to evaluate it in relation with CRP (25). Lower values may occur also in the affections of liver functions (hepatitides, liver cirrhosis) and zinc deficit [2, 9].

Transferin

Transferin is the principal transport protein for iron in plasma. It is a beta-globulin synthesized mainly in the liver, in a small amount also in the reticuloendothelial system, testes and ovaries. The half-life of transferin is 5 – 7 days, and it is an early marker of protein malnutrition, but it is less reliable, having lower specificity and sensitivity [16]. On the other hand, an increase in the transferin level sensitively indicates the onset of a positive nitrogen balance. The physiological range of transferin is 2 - 3.6g/l, the serum concentration giving evidence of malnutrition is below 1.5g/l, but it may be significantly influenced by the amount of iron in the organism, an acute inflammatory disease (negative acute phase protein), malignity in progress, a surgery or chronic hepatopathy. When evaluating transferin, it is suitable to know the state of iron metabolism, C-reactive protein and proteosynthetic liver function [19]. In patients with malnutrition and concurrent sideropenic anemia it is unsuitable as a single marker.

Cholinesterase

Cholinesterase is an enzyme produced by hepatocytes and secreted to blood plasma. It influences the neuromuscular junction of skeletal bones. The normal range is 88 - 215 µkat/l. The half-life of cholinesterase is 5 – 7 days, its level correlates well with the albumin level. Due to its relatively short half-life and low price, cholinesterase can be employed to monitor the nutritional state [16]. A decrease in cholinesterase can be demonstrated in malnutrition (the risk level is that below 88 µkat/l), but also in hypercatabolic states in severe infections and its level is dependent on the function of the liver and on some medicaments (physostigmine, cyclophosphamide, lithium etc.). A decrease in cholesterol level is usually significant in the affection of the hepatic parenchyma most frequently in chronic diseases of the liver thanks to inhibition of the synthesis and number of producing cells [18]. In more severe affection of the liver, it is not possible to take into account the values of cholinesterase in nutritional evaluation, because a low level rather than the state of nutrition reflects a deficit of liver proteosynthesis.

Retinol-Binding Protein (RBP)

Retinol-binding protein is a polypeptide chain synthesized in the liver and its principal role is the transfer of vitamin A from the liver to the peripheral tissues. In plasma it circulates as a complex with prealbumin. The prealbumin-RBP complex is an early marker of the risk of malnutrition, because RBP possesses a very short half-life (12 hours) and its body reserves are extraordinarily low [16]. In the case of using RBP as a marker of the state of nutrition it is more reliable to monitor rather the changes in its levels than the absolute values. RBP levels are significantly influenced in the disorders of hepatic and renal functions [27]. An increase in RBP values is demonstrated in renal diseases due to its decreased catabolism. On the other hand, a decrease in RBP takes place in chronic liver diseases, a vitamin A deficit, hyperthyroidism and also in stress.

Total Protein

At present, total protein is practically not used as a marker of malnutrition. Its disadvantage is its long biological half-life, and therefore it is rather a late marker of protein malnutrition and provides only an orientational idea. Low levels of total protein may give evidence of a long-term protein deficit, but they do not demonstrate acute changes in the nutritional state [16]. The physiological values of total protein are 65 - 80g/l, a decrease below 55g/l is considered serious. The value of total protein is usually significantly influenced particularly by hepatic or renal disorders, degree of dehydration, and a concurrent inflammatory process [18].

Lipids

Significant bioindicators of malnutrition and inflammation are some parameters of lipid metabolism. An increase in plasma, but particularly erythrocytic omega-6 fatty acids, can be considered a marker of inflammation, whereas a decrease in total cholesterol, LDL and HDL indicate an energetic deficit and specific manifestations of malnutrition [10].

Infection and inflammation induce an acute inflammatory reaction, which is reflected in the metabolism of lipids and lipoproteins in a very varied manner. There occur the following changes: a) in the synthesis and consumption of cholesterol, b) in the metabolism of triacylglycerols and the kinetics of free fatty acids, c) in the metabolism, synthesis and receptor uptake of lipoproteins.

a) In an inflammatory reaction, in spite of its increased synthesis, the consumption of cholesterol in the organism is increased to such a degree that in the peripheral circulating lipoproteins its significant depletion is found to the values deep below 2mmol/l. An increased consumption of cholesterol is caused by its intensive incorporation into the cell membranes of the elements of the white blood series, which are increased during acute inflammation in a multiple way. In addition, consumption of cholesterol in the damaged tissues during inflammation and during their subsequent reparation is increased. An increased requirement for cholesterol for the synthesis of corticoids is of importance in stress till the complete exhaustion of adrenal steroids, e.g. in a generalized inflammatory reaction and sepsis.
b) An increase in VLDL during an inflammatory reaction results from stimulated lipolysis in the liver tissue, increased synthesis of free fatty acids in the liver in a generalized inflammatory reaction and suppression of their oxidation mainly in the muscle. During intensification of the inflammatory reaction the removal of VLDL (and thus TAG) from circulation is further decreased by the action of toxic mechanisms.
c) Metabolism of lipoproteins is significantly altered by the influence of the changes in their structures by a reaction with lipopolysaccharides and endotoxin, which is bound to lipoproteins and changes their interaction with membrane receptors.

Changes in the metabolism of cholesterol and lipoproteins as bioindicators of malnutrition are much less defined. Though it is generally accepted that in serious malnutrition cholesterolemia is decreased (manifestations of an energetic deficit, worse availability of acetyl-coenzyme-A), it does not generally hold true. In severely cachectic individuals with mental anorexia, cholesterolemia is often increased up to grossly pathological values. It can be explained by stimulation of the synthesis of cholesterol in deprivation of the absorption of cholesterol from the gastrointestinal tract. Interpretation of plasma concentrations of triacylglycerols in malnutrition is even less unambiguous. This parameter reflects rather the topical state of the intake of nutrients than long-term consequences of malnutrition.

Total Cholesterol

The level of total cholesterol is a relatively sensitive marker of energy malnutrition and correlates better with the body-mass index than the level of albumin. At the same time, however, the levels of total cholesterol and albumin do not have to correlate with each other. The normal range is 2.2 - 5.2mmol/l, the levels below 2.0mmol/l indicate, after the exclusion of the influencing factors, long-term energetic insufficiency [16]. For evaluation of cholesterol it is necessary to know at the same time the values of thyreoideal enzymes, liver functions and the concurrently administered medication (hypolipidemics).

Leptin

Leptin is a protein hormone produced by the fat tissue, which by suppressing neuropeptide Y decreases appetite. It is a feedback between the amount of fat tissue and appetite. Concentration of leptin in serum is increased with the increasing amount of fat tissue in the organism, and it is approximately three times higher in women than in men. On the other hand, a decreased level of leptin accompanies starvation, when a decrease in leptin precedes a decrease in the concentration of plasma proteins (prealbumin and albumin). When malnutrition deteriorates, there is no further decrease in the leptin level [27]. In realimentation, the values of leptin are increased again and their increase indicates the efficacy of nutrition.

Of other biochemical examinations, malnutrition may be also indicated by lower values of thyroid gland hormones, and decreased creatinine may draw attention to a low volume of the muscular mass.

Hematological and Immunological Examinations

The hematological and immunological examinations include particularly the determination of the absolute number of lymphocytes; malnutrition may be indicated by anemia (due to deficiency of iron, folic acid or vitamin B12). In the elderly, there is often an anergic reaction to immunological intradermal skin tests [18, 27]. To evaluate the state of immunity in connection with the state of nutrition, it is possible to employ special immunological examinations such as the determination of the level of immunoglobulins and the examination of the subpopulations of CD4, CD8 lymphocytes (at present rather as part of research tasks, in common clinical practice these examinations are not routinely used).

Absolute Number of Lymphocytes

Malnutrition results in a decrease in the function of the immunity system first at the level of cellular and subsequently also humoral immunity [19, 27]. The absolute number of lymphocytes is evaluated, whose normal value should not decrease below 1 500/μl; below this limit the risk of malnutrition is increased and a decrease below 900/μl means a significant affection of immunity with a high risk of severe malnutrition [14]. It is necessary to first exclude other etiology of decreased lymphocytes (hematooncological diseases, TBC, viroses etc.).

Markers of Inflammation

The best known and most frequently employed markers of inflammation are acute phase proteins (C-reactive protein, fibrinogen, orosomucoid, α_1-antitrypsin), sedimentation of erythrocytes and neopterin in urine (27).

Acute phase proteins are produced in an increased degree in the cells of the hepatic parenchyma mostly de novo up to the inducement of synthesis by an inflammatory noxious substance, therefore it is not only mere washing from the store in the liver tissue [6]. In the course of inflammation, acute phase proteins have specific functions preventing damage to the tissues as regulators of inflammatory process, mediators of various biological reactions, immunomodulant agents, „scavengers“ or inhibitors binding proteolytic ferments released from phagocytes.

C-Reactive Protein (CRP)

CRP is the dominant acute phase protein. It ranks among pentraxins – a group of proteins occurring in all vertebrates and ensuring defense of the organism. CRP activates the complement system by both the classic and alternative way, and by binding to various ligands (proteins from disintegrated cells, polysaccharide envelope of pneumococci C, etc.) it protects the organism from the action of necrotic products from disintegrated cells [16]. Another capacity of CRP is regulation of acute inflammatory processes by influencing thrombocytes by the effect on the metabolism of prostaglandins and also hindrance of stimulation of T-lymphocytes and release of lymphokines. It also acts on phagocytosis by influencing granulocytic and monocytic macrophages. An important task of CRP is also opsonization and rapid removal of fragments of nucleic acids and histones, which prevents the development of autoantibodies against these elements.

CRP is produced by the liver and after stimulation there is an increase after 6 - 8 hours and the maximal values are achieved in 24 - 48 hours. The normal range is below 5 mg/l. Elevation of CRP values is accompanied by acute inflammatory diseases, in the case of malignant diseases and the majority of rheumatic diseases the increase is smaller. It is important to continuously monitor the serum level in the course of therapy, which correlates with the activity of the disease [5, 21]. After successful treatment with antibiotics there is a rapid decrease in CRP, in the case of unsuccessful treatment the increased level persists or it may even rise. Viral infection, in contrast to a bacterial one, is not usually accompanied by an increase in CRP.

Fibrinogen

Fibrinogen belongs to the group of coagulating factors (factor I). It is produced in the liver, which are, together with lymph, also its reservoir. Its main function is conversion to fibrin, which seals up the cracks in the damaged intima of the vessels and prevents further bleeding. It further forms the fibrin matrix making possible the movement of fibroblasts and other cells, stimulates their production in wound healing and tissue damage [16]. The physiological values are 2.8 - 4.8g/l. Increased values of fibrinogen are found after surgeries, in acute inflammations, malignant and rheumatological diseases etc.

Orosomucoid

It is an α_1-protein produced in the liver and occurring in plasma, liquor, gastric juice, and urine. In acute inflammation, there is its increase in 12 - 24 hours with the maximum up to 4 days and reverse normalization within 3 weeks. It suppresses basic conversion of lymphocytes induced by mitogens. The normal values are 0.48 - 1.26 g/l. The values of orosomucoid are increased not only in acute inflammation, but a persistent increase is an indicator of chronicity of the inflammatory process [22]. Besides inflammation, higher values are found in malignant and rheumatological diseases.

α_1-Antitrypsin

α_1-Antitrypsin is a plasmatic protein produced in the liver, whose principal function is to inactivate the proteinases released from lysosomes to extracellular fluid during the disintegration of cells and the elastase released from the granules of neutrophilic leukocytes [16]. The physiological range is 0.78 - 2.00g/l. Nonspecific acute inflammations with disintegration of leukocytes, tissue necrosis and phagocytosis result in an increase in the synthesis of α_1-antitrypsin in the liver and an increase in its plasma concentrations from 12 - 24 hours with the maximum on days 4 to 5. Elevation of α_1-antitrypsin level also accompanies hepatitides and tumor diseases [27].

Neopterin in Urine

Neopterin is produced by human macrophages after stimulation with interferon gamma secreted by activated T-lymphocytes, and therefore it is possible to make use of the change in its serum concentrations to monitor immunity activation [16]. Increased levels of neopterin have been demonstrated in diseases connected with cellular immunity response particularly in patients with autoimmune diseases, infectious diseases (particularly of viral and parasitic origin, furthermore in infections with intracellularly surviving bacteria – e.g. tuberculosis), some types of tumor proliferation (e.g. carcinoma of the pancreas and colorectal carcinoma), and rejections of transplants, and a certain increase takes place physiologically in the old age [6]. High values of neopterin are also an unfavorable mortality prognostic factor. Concentration of neopterin in urine is expressed as the ratio neopterin/creatinine (μmol/mol creatinine). The normal range of neopterin differs in the literature, the values above 200 μmol/mol creatinine can be considered pathological.

Sedimentation of Erythrocytes

Examination of the rate of sedimentation of erythrocytes is a simple and cheap laboratory test with high sensitivity, but low specificity. Under normal circumstances, erythrocytes carry on their surfaces negative charges causing their mutual repulsion and slow sedimentation. In the case of a pathological state in progress, aggregates of erythrocytes are formed, which settle more rapidly. Increased rate of sedimentation is caused by an increase in the concentration of fibrinogen, orosomucoid and C-reactive protein. The values of sedimentation mutually differ in men and women, in both sexes they are physiologically increased with increasing age [16]. The average rate of sedimentation at the age of twenty in men is 4.3 mm/h and in women 7.1 mm/h, whereas in seniors over 80 years of age the values are doubled (men 9.5 mm/h, women 14.5 mm/h). Increased sedimentation is found not only in inflammatory diseases, but also in systemic rheumatic diseases, malignant diseases or nephropathies. Approximately in 4% of cases there is high sedimentation without any obvious cause.

Lipoprotein (a)

The physiological function of lipoprotein (a) is not quite clear. Thanks to the similarity of its structure (a specific antigen of apoprotein (a)) with plasminogen it possesses the capacity to bind to fibrin and makes possible the supply of cholesterol molecules into the thrombus which is being organized and plays its role in wound healing [10]. In the organism lipoprotein (a) exerts a dual risk effect: it acts antifibrinolytically (due to the presence of apoprotein (a)) and as an atherogenic risk factor (via apolipoprotein B100). The physiological values of lipoprotein (a) are 0.10 - 0.20g/l, an increased risk of undesirable effects begins at the levels above 0.30g/l. Lipoprotein (a) can be considered the reactant of the acute phase, its values are temporarily increased after major surgeries, in acute myocardial infarction or during stress [16].

Inflammatory Disease, Stress Starvation and Mutual Relationships between Bioindicators of Malnutrition and Markers of Inflammation

An inflammatory disease is a catabolizing state resulting, in particular in groups of population at risk, including seniors, in a rapid development of malnutrition of the kwashiorkor-like type (the so-called stress starvation). An even worse situation takes place in the case of inflammation in patients undernourished already at admittance due to the transition of the marantic (protein-energy) type of malnutrition to the kwashiorkor one. This group of patients faces much more increased risk of the development of complications and higher mortality. In seniors it is necessary to take this situation into account, as roughly 50% of them suffer from a certain degree of protein-energy malnutrition [19].

The classic symptoms of stress starvation are decreased serum proteins and the development of edema. The cause is the affection of capillary permeability by the action of numerous hormonal factors, cytokines and the predominance of thromboxanes with vasoconstrictive and permeability effects. It results in the transition of serum proteins (mostly albumin, but also all others) and sodium from the intravascular to the interstitial space, which is followed also by transition of water. A decrease in the content of the blood bed results in stimulation of secretion of aldosterone and antidiuretic hormone, resulting in further retention of water and sodium with intensification of the edematous state [27].

During inflammation there develops the hypermetabolic state with an increase in stress hormones (catecholamines, cortisol and glucagon). The result is significant intolerance of glucose with a decrease in its utilization, but gluconeogenesis in the liver persists and stress hormones, in addition, induce insulin resistance, which results in hyperglycemia and simultaneously in a decrease in the oxidation of fatty acids even during stimulated lipolysis. These metabolic processes decrease or even block the obtaining of energy from glucose and fatty acids. An important alternative source of energy becomes amino acids, in particular those with branched chains (valine, leucine, isoleucine) and also glutamine. That is why there occurs catabolism of body proteins from the visceral (plasma proteins, parenchymatous organs, tissues in the gastrointestinal tract) as well as the somatic (muscles) regions [15]. In the case of plasma proteins, catabolism results in a rapid decrease in serum albumin and in a lesser extent also in other transport proteins (transferin, prealbumin).

Beside the mechanism in which proteins are consumed as a source of energy, in the case of inflammatory reaction there is a rapid transfer of proteins to the regions of essential importance for the survival of the individual. After proteolysis, a portion of amino acids is transformed into acute phase proteins and a portion is transferred into the damaged regions, where it ensures reparation of the damaged tissues. It is prioritization of inflammation (synthesis of acute phase proteins) to the detriment of nutrition (decreased synthesis and degradation of visceral proteins). For this reason the level of serum proteins is significantly decreased also in satisfactory nutrition and sufficient supply of proteins, because the organism prefers proteosynthesis of the reactants of the acute phase and their levels rise. Cytokines released from macrophages, lymphocytes and other cells significantly contribute to the increase in the synthesis of acute phase proteins. They are mainly the tumor necrosis factor (TNF), interleukins 1 and 6 (IL-1, IL-6). But in long-term duration of this state with continuing mobilization of protein reserves there occurs weakening of the defensive reaction and a decrease in reparation of the damaged tissues [5]. If malnutrition preceded the development of the disease, exhaustion of the reserves is more rapid (Figure 1).

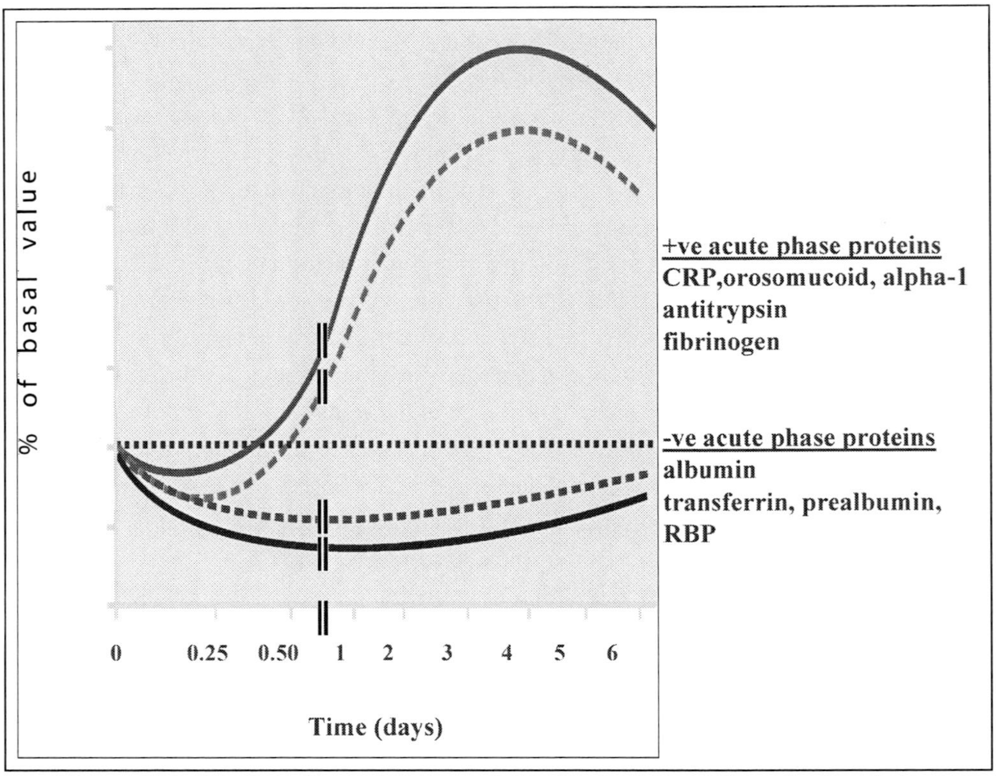

Source: Mayers MA, Fleck A, Saampson B *et al.*: Early plasma protein and mineral changes after surgery: a two stage process. J Clin Pathol 1984.

Figure 1. Reaction of positive and negative acute phase proteins.

The inflammation in progress influences also the lipidogram. Reesterification of triacylglycerols (TAG) is increased. In inflammation there is increased consumption of cholesterol in the formation of a large number of the cells of the white blood series, steroid stress hormones and the construction of new repairing tissues. Significant changes in inflammatory diseases or malnutrition are also shown by some apoproteins, because they act to a certain degree as the acute phase reactants [10]. With the change in the synthesis and degradation of apoproteins also the concentration of C-reactive protein is changed, and in addition it can interfere with lipoproteins rich in triacylglycerols and containing apoprotein B. Disorder in the function of apoprotein C-II originates in serious protein catabolism and it deteriorates the removal of lipoproteins rich in triacylglycerols from plasma. Apoprotein E is produced in many body tissues also by, besides others, activated macrophages in reparatory response in tissue damage.

Nutritional Indices

Revision of the interpretation of protein and other bioindicators of malnutrition and the markers of inflammation leads to the necessity of not using only the absolute values of plasma levels of proteins, lipoproteins and other components, but the formulae (indices), which integrate the bioindicators of malnutrition, inflammation, sex and age into one index (Table 2).

Table 2. A survey of nutritional indices

Prognostic nutritional index (PNI, Mullen and Buzby) PNI=158–1.66xalbumin–0.78xskinfold above the triceps–20xtransferrin–5.8xskin reaction PNI below 40% - low risk PNI of 40 – 49% medium risk PNI over 49% - high risk
Prognostic inflammatory and nutritional index (PINI, Ingenbleek and Carpentier) PINI = $\frac{\text{orosomucoid x C-reactive protein}}{\text{albumin x prealbumin}}$ PINI below 1 – without signs of acute disease PINI of 1 – 10 – low risk PINI of 11 – 20 – medium risk PINI of 21 – 30 – high risk PINI over 30 – life endangering risk
Nutritional risk index (NRI, Buzby) NRI = 1.519 x albumin + 41.7 x topical weight /ideal weight NRI over 100% - normal state of nutrition NRI of 97.5 – 100% – mild malnutrition NRI of 83.5 – 97.5% – medium malnutrition NRI below 83.5% – severe malnutrition
Geriatric nutritional risk index (GNRI) GNRI = 1.489 x albumin + 41.7 x topical weight /ideal weight GNRI over 98% - normal state of nutrition GNRI of 92 – 98% - mild malnutrition GNRI of 82 – 92% - medium malnutrition GNRI below 82% - severe malnutrition
Explanations and units: albumin in g/l, skinfold above the triceps in mm, transferrin in mm, orosomucoid in mg/l, C-reactive protein in mg/l, prealbumin in mg/l, weight in kg skin reaction after application of skin tests (0 – without reaction, 1 – induration to 5 mm, 2 – induration over 5 mm)

Prognostic Nutritional Index According to Mullen and Buzby (PNI)

This index after calculation directly shows the percentage of the risk of complications of a surgery. The critical value is 40%, patients with a higher value of PNI had a substantially increased number of complications versus the group of patients with the PNI value below 40%. The PNI range of 40 - 49% means a medium risk and over 50% a high risk. In patients with medium and high risks, a marked improvement of the condition took place after nutritional intervention [11].

Prognostic Inflammatory and Nutritional Index According to Ingenbleek and Carpentier (PINI)

As the concentration of the majority of serum proteins is not dependent only on the state of nutrition, PINI evaluates simultaneously also inflammatory activity and is suitable for the evaluation of the activity of the disease. The determination of PINI consists in simultaneous examination of the concentration of acute phase proteins (orosomucoid and C-reactive protein) and the concentration of visceral proteins (albumin and prealbumin) in serum [12].

The values of PINI below 1 do not show the signs of acute inflammation or activity of disease, without the risk of vital danger; these are found in the patients with good nutritional states without the signs of protein catabolism in progress and with good prognosis. The values of PINI of 1 - 10 mean a low risk of vital risk in patients with possible inflammatory disease taking place subacutely, with a mild degree of malnutrition and good prognosis in sufficient nutritional intervention. The values of PINI of 11 - 20 indicate a medium degree of vital risk in patients with acute inflammation in progress and a medium degree of malnutrition without functional manifestations. When acute inflammation abates and adequate nutritional support is provided, the version is possible. The range of PINI of 21 - 30 means patients at high risk with acute inflammation in progress and advanced degree of malnutrition with functional manifestations. These patients necessarily require intensive nutritional intervention, as there is high risk of operational and post-operational complications, high percentage of deteriorated healing with subsequent secondary manifestations. The values of PINI over 30 represent immediate danger to life in patients at high risk with severe acute inflammatory disease in progress and serious protein catabolism [11, 19].

Nutritional Risk Index According to Buzby (NRI)

NRI was elaborated directly for the needs of surgical clinics for differentiation of the seriousness of malnutrition and indication of nutritional support in operated patients, because in patients in the condition of severe malnutrition artificial nutrition markedly reduces the risk of surgery in comparison with the group without nutritional intervention [26]. NRI evaluates the nutritional state by a percent value; the normal state of nutrition is over 100%, within the range of 97.5 - 100% it is mild, within 83.5 - 97.5% it is medium malnutrition, and below 83.5% it is severe malnutrition [1, 20].

Geriatric Nutritional Risk Index (GNRI)

This nutritional risk index elaborated particularly for geriatric patients can very well predict the seriousness of muscular dysfunction and identify patients suitable for nutritional support and physical activity. GNRI over 98% means normal nutrition, the values of 92-98% mild, 82-92% medium, ad below 82% serious malnutrition [1, 2].

Blackburn's Scheme

This scheme can be employed for complex evaluation of nutritional status. It includes the examination of weight and height (weight-height index), the skinfold above the triceps, the perimeter of the arm muscles, the values of serum albumin and prealbumin, creatinine-height index, the absolute number of lymphocytes, and the skin tests [11]. Measurements are subsequently compared with normal values and the total index is calculated. The values of 90 - 110% give evidence of normal nutrition, 60 - 90% of malnutrition, and the values below 60% indicate severe malnutrition.

Creatinine-Height Index

Creatinine is a degradation product of creatine and creatine phosphate, which is produced in a constant amount in the skeletal muscular tissue. It is approximately 1.7% of total muscular creatine. The waste of creatinine into urine may thus be used to calculate total muscular mass. Excretion of 1g of creatinine a day corresponds to 17 - 20kg of muscles. Normal values of creatinine in urine in men are 20 - 26mg/kg of ideal body weight for men; in women the creatinine values are lower, being 16 - 22mg/kg of ideal body weight for women.

Measurement of daily excretion of creatinine into urine has also its limits. Excretion of creatinine may be influenced by renal insufficiency, long-term immobilization, emotional and physical stress. The intake of meat as food also significantly participates. Acute states such as sepsis or trauma very markedly increase excretion of creatinine into urine – by 20 - 100%. Wrong results may occur in imprecise collection of urine. Physiological decrease in excretion of creatinine into urine takes place with increasing age, as there occur a gradual decrease in muscular mass, decreased content of creatine in the muscles, and probably also smaller intake of meat in the old age.

Dependence of excretion of creatinine into urine on age is expressed by the following relations:

creatinine in men (mg/kg/den) = 28.2 – 0.172 x age

creatinine in women (mg/kg/den) = 21.9 – 0.115 x age

Creatinine-height index is expressed as the percentage of preserved muscular mass in comparison with the norm. The values considered normal are the values of healthy individuals with the corresponding muscular mass and the same height as the measured patient, which can be found in tables.

$$\text{Creatinine-height index} = \frac{\text{measured excretion of creatinine within 24 hours (mg)}}{\text{tabulated excretion of creatinine within 24 hours (mg)}} \times 100$$

The values of 90 - 100% correspond to the normal muscular mass, 80 - 90% to a mild, 60 - 80% to a medium severe, and below 60% to a severe decrease in muscular mass already with significant functional affection [27].

References

[1] Cereda, E., Limonta, D., Pusani, C., Vanotti, A. Assessing elderly at risk of malnutrition: The new Geriatric Nutritional Risk Index versus Nutritional Risk Index. N*utrition* 2006; 22: 680-682.

[2] Cereda, E., Vanotti, A. The new Geriatric Nutritional Risk Index is a good predictor of muscle dysfunction in institutionalized older patients. *Clin. Nutr*. 2007; 26: 78-83.

[3] Devoto, G., Gallo, F., Marchello, C., Racchi, O., Garbarini, R., Bonassi, S. et al. Prealbumin serum levels as a useful tool in the assessment of malnutrition in hospitalized patients. *Clin. Chem.* 2006; 52: 2281-5.

[4] Fuhrman, M.P., Charney, P., Mueller C.M. Hepatic proteins and nutrition assessment. *J. Am. Diet Assoc*. 2004; 104: 1258-64.

[5] Harris, T.B., Ferrucci, L., Tracy, R.P., Corti, M.C., Wacholder, S., Ettinger, W.H. et al. Associations of elevated Interleukin-6 and C-Reactive protein levels with mortality in the elderly. *Am. J. Med.* 1999; 106: 506-512.

[6] Hrnciarikova, D., Juraskova, B., Zadak, Z., Hronek, M. *Present state of evaluating malnutrition in the elderly – analysing indicators*. Biomed. Pap. Med. Fac. Univ. Palacky Olomouc Czech Repub 2006; 150 (2): 217-221.

[7] Hronek M., Zadak Z., Solichova D., Jandik P., Melichar B.: Choice nutrition factors in colorectal carcinogenesis. *Physiological Research*, 49(4), 2000, P18.

[8] Ingenbleek, Y., Young, V.R. Significance of prealbumin in protein metabolism. *Clin. Chem. Lab. Med.* 2002; 40: 1281-91.

[9] Johnson, A.M., Merlini, G., Sheldon, J., Ichihara, K. Clinical indications for plasma protein assays: transthyretin (prealbumin) in inflammation and malnutrition. *Clin. Chem. Lab. Med.* 2007; 45 (3): 419-426.

[10] Khovidhunkit, W., Kim, M.S., Memon, R.A., Shigenaga, J.K., Moser, A.H., Feingold, K.R., Grunfeld, C. Effects of infection and inflammation on lipid and lipoprotein metabolism: mechanisms and consequences to the host. *J. Lip. Res*. 2004; 45: 1169-96.

[11] Kohout, P. *Dokumentace a hodnocení nutričního stavu pacientů*. Praha: Maxdorf; 2004.

[12] Kohout, P. et al. *Výživa u pacientů s idiopatickými střevními záněty*. Praha: Maxdorf Jessenius; 2004.

[13] Kuzuya, M., Izawa, S., Enoki, H., Okada, K., Iguchi, A. Is serum albumin a good marker for malnutrition in the physically impaired elderly? *Clin. Nutr.* 2007; 26: 84-90.

[14] Kuzuya, M., Kanda, S., Koike, T., Suzuki, Y., Iguchi, A. Lack of correlation between total lymphocyte count and nutritional status in the elderly. *Clin. Nutr.* 2005; 24: 427-432.

[15] Macallan, D. Malnutrition and infection. *Medicine* 2005; 33: 14-16.

[16] Masopust, J. *Klinická biochemie požadování a hodnocení biochemických vyšetření I.* a II. část. Praha: Karolinum; 1998.

[17] Mayers, M.A., Fleck, A., Saampson, B. et al.: Early plasma protein and mineral changes after surgery: a two stage process. *J. Clin. Pathol.* 1984; 37: 862-866.

[18] Navrátilová, M., Češková, E., Sobotka, L. *Klinická výživa v psychiatrii*. Praha: Maxdorf Jessenius; 2000.

[19] Omran, M.L., Morley, J.E. Assessment of protein energy malnutrition in older persons, Part II: laboratory evaluation. *Nutrition* 2000; 16: 131-40.

[20] Pirlich, M., Lochs, H. Nutrition in the elderly. *Best Pract. Res. Clin. Gastroenter.* 2001; 15: 869-884.

[21] Ravaglia, G., Forti, P., Maioli, F., Brunetti, N., Martelli, M., Talerico, T. et al. Peripheral blood markers of inflammation and functional impairment in elderly community-dwellers. *Exp. Geront* 2004; 39: 1415-1422.

[22] Raynaud-Simon, A., Lafont, S., Berr, C., Dartigues, J.F., Le Bouc, Y. Orosomucoid: a mortality risk factor in elderly people living in the community? *Clin. Nutr.* 2002; 21: 45-50.

[23] Robinson, M.K., Trujillo, E.B., Mogensen, K.M., Rounds, J., McManus, K., Jacobs, D.O. Improving nutritional screening of hospitalized patients: the role of prealbumin. *JPEN J. Parenter. Enteral. Nutr.* 2003; 27: 389-95.

[24] Seiler, W.O. Clinical pictures of malnutrition in ill elderly subjects. *Nutrition* 2001; 17: 496-8.

[25] Shenkin A. Serum Prealbumin: Is It a Marker of Nutritional Status or of Risk of Malnutrition? *Clin. Chem.* 2006; 52(12): 2177-79.

[26] Sungurtekin, H., Sungurtekin, U., Hanci, V., Erdem, E. Comparison of Two Nutrition Assessment Techniques in Hospitalized Patients. *Nutrition* 2004; 20: 428-432.

[27] Zadák, Z. *Výživa v intenzivní péči.* Praha: Grada Publishing; 2002.

In: Nutrition for the Middle Aged and Elderly
Editors: N. E. Bernhardt, A. M. Kasko, pp. 389-445
ISBN: 978-1-60456-146-3

Chapter XVI

Pulmonary Emphysema: Not Just a Matter of Alveolar Destruction

Simonetta Baldi
S. Maugeri Foundation I.R.C.C.S, Scientific Institute of Montescano, Rehabilitative Pulmonology Unit and Respiratory Pathophysiology, Montescano (Pavia), ITALY

Abstract

Pulmonary Emphysema is part of the spectrum of Chronic Obstructive Pulmonary Disease (COPD). Classical concepts of its pathogenesis have relied on a paradigm set by inflammation and protease/anti-protease imbalance. Inflammation has been equated with cigarette smoke-induced molecular damage on lung cells. Alternatively, alterations elicited by chronic cigarette smoke on lung cells might relate to critical molecular signals involved in lung development, maturation and aging.

Drawing a parallel between pathophysiological responses to aging and those involved in COPD, particularly the emphysematous type, leads to a new conceptual framework for the pathogenesis of emphysema, in which cigarette smoke constitutes an environmental hazard that causes alveolar destruction by the interaction of apoptosis, oxidative stress, and protease/anti-protease imbalance. Hence, evidence is growing that this disease condition relates to a systemic inflammatory damage targeting the lung as well as skeletal and respiratory muscles.

Emphysema is a condition defined in anatomical terms. Thus, its diagnosis *in vivo* constitutes a challenge, in that it deals with the probability that physiological tests and radiological signs correctly identify the presence of pathological emphysema.

Assessment of severity and extent of emphysema has been one of the goals of the research during this century. Correlation studies that link structural imaging and physiological measurement, particularly loss of lung elastic recoil and CO diffusing capacity have offered over the last twenty years the unique opportunity to phenotype emphysema.

For almost one-century weight loss has been recognized as a clinical feature characterizing the emphysematous type of COPD. Studies dealing with the pathogenesis of nutritional differences between COPD phenotypes have tended to deflect some attention away from the impact of nutritional status itself on quality of life, disability and handicap of COPD. The impact of a wide range of diseases (co-morbidities) on different aspects of nutritional status, e.g. appetite, diet quality, body composition, ability to metabolize nutrients, has been underestimated even more. All together COPD, nutritional status and co-morbidities impact physical, mental and social health.

The evidence that nutritional status marks the emphysematous process independent of severity of airflow obstruction suggests complex metabolic alterations related to disturbed energy balance, systemic inflammation, hypoxia and metabolic adaptation targeting lung as well as skeletal and respiratory muscles. Loss of muscle mass and/or impaired skeletal muscle performance is an important determinant of exercise capacity in COPD. Morphologic and metabolic abnormalities in skeletal muscles are multi-factorially determined; each factor represents a key point for better definition of rehabilitative intervention.

A comprehensive clinical assessment looking at patient centered outcomes, exercise capacity and metabolic assessment should be tailored. It should evaluate the effects of nutrition-rehabilitation programs to obtain new insights into systemic impact of a respiratory disease of middle aged and elderly, which imposes a heavy economic burden on individual and society world-wide.

Introduction

Pulmonary Emphysema, Chronic Bronchitis, and in most of cases association of the two conditions are part of the spectrum of Chronic Obstructive Pulmonary Disease (COPD). This is defined as a progressive limitation of expiratory flow that is not fully reversible [1].

Pulmonary emphysema is a condition defined as the abnormal permanent enlargement of air spaces distal to terminal bronchioles as the result of mechanisms leading to destruction of their walls and reduction of capillary exchange area [2]. Phenotyping emphysema constitutes a challenge, in that its diagnosis in vivo deals with the probability that physiologic tests and radiological signs correctly identify the presence of pathological emphysema. Furthermore, due to different mechanisms contributing to airflow limitation, the relationship between emphysema and the severity of airflow obstruction in patients with COPD has not always been consistently demonstrated [3-5]. Despite the explosion of knowledge based upon multidisciplinary research, mechanisms leading to this unique pattern of alveolar destruction are not adequately understood, and another significant challenge remains in that no novel or even currently effective treatment is available.

Emphysema, chronic bronchitis and COPD have overlapping features. The interaction of host and environmental factors produces clinical pictures that reflect these features to a greater and lesser extent from patient to patient.

For almost one-century weight loss has been recognized as a clinical characteristic of the emphysematous type of COPD [6]. Several studies dealing with the pathogenesis of nutritional differences between COPD phenotypes have tended to deflect some attention away from the impact of nutritional status itself on quality of life, disability and handicap of COPD. The evidence that nutritional status marks emphysematous process independent of severity of airflow obstruction suggests complex metabolic alterations related to disturbed energy balance, systemic inflammation, hypoxia and metabolic adaptation targeting lung as well as skeletal and respiratory muscles [7]. Furthermore, different aspects of nutritional status," what we eat", i.e. our appetite and quality of diet, "what we are", i.e. our body and tissue composition, and "what we can do", i.e. our ability to metabolize nutrients, is affected by a wide range of diseases. Nevertheless, the impact of co-morbid diseases on nutritional status is largely underestimated.

This review is focused to the current challenges related to pulmonary emphysema assessment and management.

We start analyzing the reasons for considering a new conceptual framework of its pathogenesis. We then review the reliability of imaging techniques in the quantitation of emphysema extent and severity, and how the structural damage fits into pathophysiology of airflow obstruction. Finally, we look at studies that have tried to analyze the nutritional differences between COPD phenotypes. We emphasize the importance of measuring how much nutritional status itself impacts on quality of life, disability and handicap of COPD, as well as of weighting the impact of co-morbid diseases on different aspects of nutritional status.

Altogether the above findings forward the conclusion that a comprehensive clinical assessment looking at patient centered outcomes, exercise capacity, and metabolic assessment should be tailored. It would help evaluating the effects of nutrition-rehabilitation programs and to obtain new insights into systemic impact of a respiratory disease of middle aged and elderly, which imposes a heavy economic burden on individual and society world-wide.

References

[1] Pawels RA, Buist AS, Calverly PM, Jenkins CR, Hard SS. Global strategy for the diagnosis, management and prevention of chronic obstructive pulmonary disease. NHLI/WHO Global Initiative for chronic obstructive pulmonary disease (GOLD) Workshop summary. *Am J Respir Crit Care Med.* 2001; 163: 1256-1276.

[2] Snider GL, Kleinerman JL, Thurlbeck WM, Bengali ZH. The definition of emphysema. Report of National Heart, Lung and Blood Institute, Division of Lung Disease Workshop. *Am Rev Respir Dis* 1988; 132: 182-183.

[3] Macklem PT. Airway obstruction and collateral ventilation. *Physiol Rev* 1971; 51: 368-436.

[4] Hogg JC, Macklem PT, Thurlbeck WM. Site and nature of airway obstruction in chronic obstructive lung disease. *N Engl J Med* 1968; 278:1355-1360.

[5] Verbeken EK, Cauberghs M, Van De Woestijne KP. Membranous bronchioles and connective tissue network of normal and emphysematous lung. *J Appl Physiol* 1996; 81: 2468-2480.

[6] Fowler J, Godllee R. Emphysema of the lungs. In *Diseases of the lungs*. London: Longmans, Green and Co. 1898; 171.

[7] Baldi S, Pinna GD, Crotti P, Montemartini S, Dacosto E, Fanfulla F, Fracchia C and Bruschi C. Nutritional status and airflow obstruction: two independent contributors to

CO diffusing capacity impairment in COPD. *Monaldi Arch Chest Dis* 2005; 63: 1, 13-16.

1. An Evolutionary Perspective of Alveolar Destruction

Classical concepts of the pathogenesis of emphysema have relied on a paradigm set by inflammation and protease/anti-protease imbalance [1]. The inflammation has been equated with cigarette smoke-induced molecular alteration on lung cells. Three-dimensional reconstruction of cell to cell contacts in the virtual syncitial network among alveolar type I and II, endothelial and fibroblastic cells has provided evidence for potential cellular pathways damaging alveolar septal cells as the result of cigarette smoke exposure [2, 3]. Nevertheless, the equation: inflammation = cigarette smoke induced lung disease is a daunting prospect as one examines the pathology of lung injury caused by pathogens compared with the prototypic loss of structural septa and progressive decrease in capillary exchange area of emphysematous lung. Thus, the molecular alteration elicited by chronic cigarette smoke on lung cells may rather relate to critical molecular signals involved in lung development, maturation and aging with inflammation representing the response to un-repaired organ injury, rather than the first line of response to environmental stresses [4].

Emphysema bears a remarkable resemblance to the aged lung, where alveolar enlargement is associated with increased airflow resistance [5]. Compared to non aged adult profile, pressure-volume curve, i.e. lung compliance, shifts to the left as a result of fragmentation of elastin fibers in alveoli [6]. Morphologically aged lung has expanded air ducts and shallow alveolar tissue. Although these changes are more uniform than those seen in cigarette smoke-induced emphysema, they are associated with an increase in mean linear intercept (i.e., the measurement of inter-alveolar septal distance), and a decrease in the surface-volume ratio, indicating a decrease in air capillary exchange area. In contrast to emphysema, these changes are not considered to be destructive, and are not generally believed to be associated to inflammation [4].

Figure 1 shows the results of exponential analysis of static elastic recoil pressure-volume curves in 24 patients with COPD. (reproduced with permission from reference 5). reference 5). Emphysema bears a remarkable resemblance to the aged lung, where alveolar enlargement is associated with increased airflow resistance [6]. Compared to non aged adult profile, pressure-volume curve, i.e. lung compliance, shifts to the left as a result of fragmentation of elastin fibers in alveoli [7]. Morphologically aged lung has expanded air ducts and shallow alveolar tissue. Although these changes are more uniform than those seen in cigarette smoke-induced emphysema, they are associated with an increase in mean linear intercept (i.e., the measurement of inter-alveolar septal distance), and a decrease in the surface-volume ratio, indicating a decrease in air capillary exchange area. In contrast to emphysema, these changes are not considered to be destructive, and are not generally believed to be associated to inflammation [4].

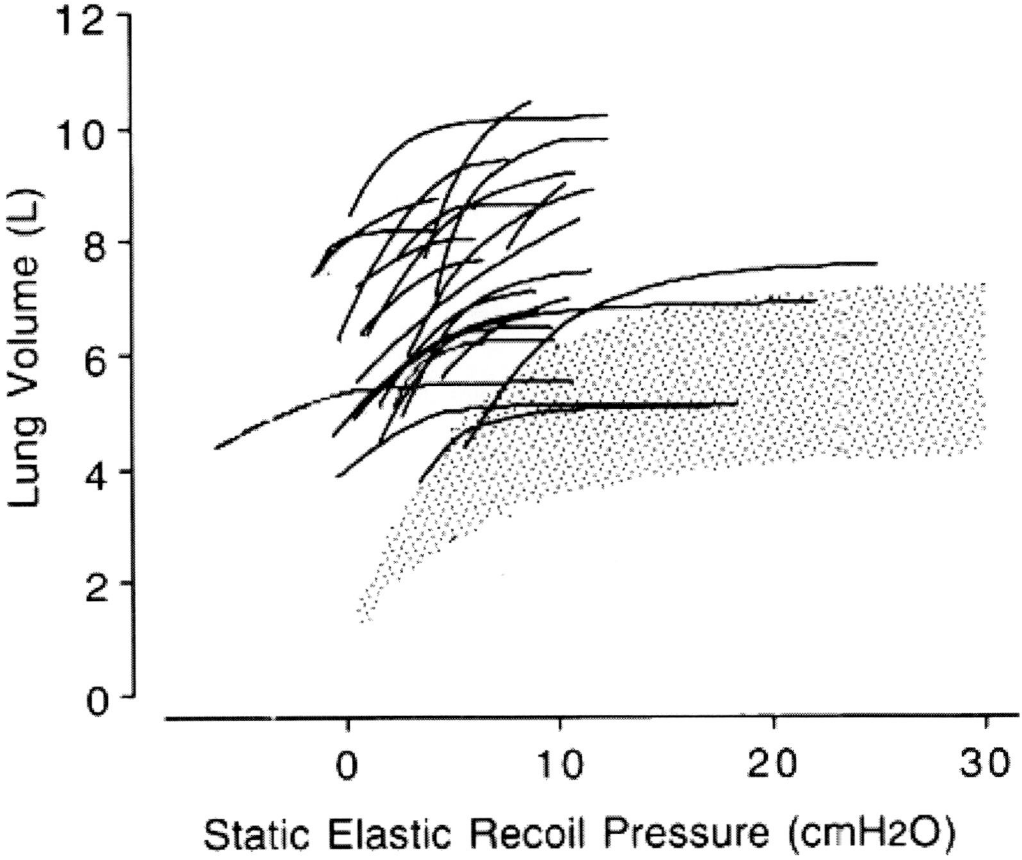

Figure 1. Static lung elastic recoil pressure-volume curves in 24 patients with COPD. Individual pressure-volume curves are obtained by exponential fitting of experimental data point measured in the interval from TLC to 70% of TLC. Shaded area is the confidence interval at 95% of pressure-volume data predicted according to Colebatch et al. [18]

Drawing a parallel between pathophysiological responses to aging and those involved in COPD, particularly emphysema, leads to a new conceptual framework, in which cigarette smoke constitutes an environmental hazard that causes alveolar destruction by the interaction of apoptosis, oxidative stress, and protease/anti protease imbalance [7]. To the extent that aging results from the stochastic interaction between injury and repair to maintain organ integrity, emphysema may recapitulate one of the events underlying accelerated lung aging process [8].

There is compelling evidence that VEGF is a lung maintenance factor throughout lung development [9-11], as well as during the all life span [12-14], and that VEGF gene expression is decreased in human emphysema [15]. Blockade of VEGF receptor, markers of oxidative stress and apoptosis (active caspase-3), co-localized in the central part of alveolar lobule, causes emphysema in rodent, while administration of superoxide dismutase mimetic abrogates alveolar cell apoptosis and emphysema [16]. These data support the evidence that failure of lung maintenance and repair due to significant and sustained lung injury imposed by cigarette smoke, exposure to air particulate, or to pollutants leads to emphysema through the hub process of oxidative stress linked with inflammation, protease/anti-protease imbalance and apoptosis.

The understanding of how the stochastic interaction between environmental hazards and the effort of a particular organ to fend off these hazards results in the accumulation of cellular damage is intriguing. It leads to important insights on novel processes related to senescence and stress response, and possibly addressed to therapeutic targeting of COPD.

References

[1] Shapiro SD. The pathogenesis of emphysema: the elastase:anti-elastase hypothesis 30 years later. *Proc Assoc Am Physicians* 1995; 107: 346-352.

[2] Kuebler WM, Parthasarathi K, Wang PM, Bhattacharia J. A novel signaling mechanism between gas and blood compartments of the lung. *J Clin Invest* 2000; 105:905-913.

[3] Ichimura M, Parthasarathi K,Quadric S, Isekutz AC, Bhattacharia J. Mechano-oxidative coupling by mithocondria induces oxidative proinflammatory responses in venular capillary. *J Clin Invest* 2003; 111: 691-699.

[4] Tuder RM, Yoshida T, Arap W, Pasqualini R, and Petrache I. Cellular and molecular mechanisms of alveolar destruction in emphysema. An evolutionary perspective. *Proc Am Thorac Soc* 2006; 3: 503-511.

[5] Janssens JP, Pache JC, Nicod LP. Physiological changes in respiratory function associated with ageing. *Eur Respir J* 1999; 13: 197-205.

[6] Setnikar I. Origine e significato delle proprietà meccaniche del polmone. *Arch Fisiol* 1955; 55: 349-374.

[7] Kirkwood WBL. Understanding the odd science of aging. *Cell* 2005; 120: 437-447.

[8] Tuder RM, Petrache I, Elias JA, Voelkel NF, Henson PM. Apoptosis and emphysema the missing link. *Am J Respir Mol Cell Biol.* 2003; 28: 551-554.

[9] Gerber HP, Hillian KJ, Ryan AM, Kowalski J, Keller JA, Rangell L, Wright BD, Radtke F, aguet M Ferrara N. VEGF is required for growth an survival in neonatal mice. *Development* 1999; 126: 1149-1159.

[10] Gebb SA, Shannon JM. Tissue interactions mediated early events in pulmonary vasculogenesis. *Dev Dyn* 2000; 217: 159-169.

[11] Compernolle V, Brusselmans K, Acker T, Hoet P, Tjwa M Beck H, Plaisance S Dor Y, Keshet E, Lupu F, et al. Loss of HIF-2alfa and inhibition of VEGF impair fetal lung maturation, whereas treatment with VEGF prevent fatal respiratory distress in premature mice. *Nat Med* 2002; 97:1559-1566.

[12] Mc Grath-Morrow SA, Cho C, ChoC, Zhen L, Hicklin DJ, Tuder RM. Vascular endothelia growth factor receptor 2 blockade disrupts post-natal lung development. *Am J Respir Cell Mol Biol* 2005; 32: 420-427.

[13] Tang K, Rossiter HB, Wagner PD, Breen EC. Lung-targeted VEGF inactivation leads to an emphysema phenotype in mice. *J Appl Physiol* 2004; 97: 1559-1566.

[14] Kasahara Y, Tuder RM, Taraseviciene-Stewart L, Le Cras TD, Abman SH, Hirth P, Waltenberger J, Voelkel NF. Inhibition of vascular endothelial growth factor receptors causes lung cell apoptosis and emphysema. *J Clin Invest* 2000; 106: 1311-1319.

[15] Ferrara N, Gerber HP, LeCouter J. The biology of VEGF and its receptors. *Nat Med* 2003; 9: 669-676.
[16] Kanazawa H, Asai K, Hirata K, Yohikawa J. Possible effects of vascular endothelial growth factor the pathogenesis of chronic obstructive pulmonary disease. *Am J Med* 2003; 114: 354-358.

2. Phenotyping Emphysema

Phenotyping emphysema, a condition defined in anatomical terms, constitutes a challenge, in that its diagnosis *in vivo* is always indirect and deals with the probability that physiologic tests and radiological signs correctly identify the presence of pathological emphysema. Furthermore, due to different mechanisms contributing to airflow limitation, the relationship between emphysema and the severity of airflow obstruction in patients with COPD has not always been consistently demonstrated [1-3]. Emphysema, chronic bronchitis and COPD have overlapping features. The interaction of host and environmental factors produces clinical pictures, which reflect these features to a greater and lesser extent from patient to patient.

Assessment of severity and extent of pulmonary emphysema by means of both physiologic measurement and imaging techniques has been one of the goals of the research during this century. It originates from the unique opportunity to link structure imaging with physiological function, particularly loss of lung elastic recoil and CO transfer capacity. In patients with airflow obstruction ($FEV_1/FVC<70\%$), those physiologic measurements have been regarded as the functional hallmarks of emphysema [4].

Chest radiography is currently part of clinical evaluation to detect the presence and severity of underlying emphysema. Figure 1 and Figure 2 show representative chest radiographs of emphysema in elderly. Do roentgen signs enable diagnosis of pulmonary emphysema?

The choice of radiological signs of emphysema and the accuracy of the radiological diagnosis of emphysema has been matter of some dispute. Laws and Hard [5] stated that the reduction in number and caliber of peripheral and pulmonary vessels was the most reliable radiological sign to predict emphysema post-mortem. They thought that overinflation of the lung was not a reliable sign of severe emphysema, which could be present in the absence of overinflation. They also felt that severe emphysema could be recognized radiologically, but mild emphysema was undetectable. Sensitivity of the chest radiograph in making the diagnosis of emphysema has been reported, varying from 24.3% to 81.8% [6-11].

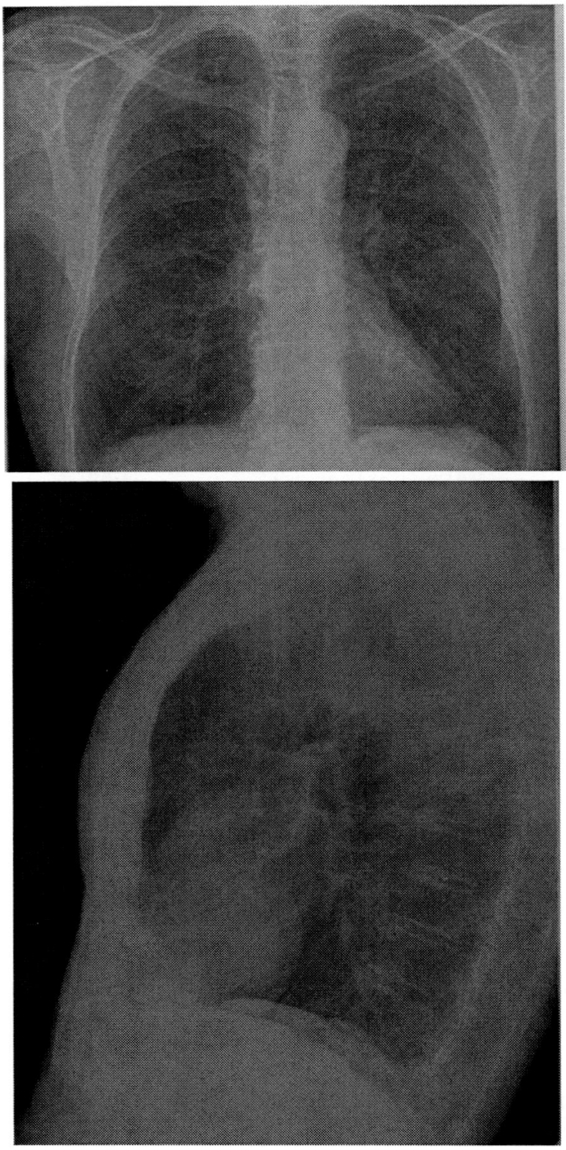

a

b

Figure 1. Standard Chest X-ray: A) PA projection; B) LL projection in a 73 year-old man, ex heavy smoker with occasional sputum, and no chronic cough; Body Mass Index: 19.4 Kg/m^2 — (Courtesy of Dr. Paolo Poggi).

1. What's chest radiograph like, according to the anthropometric and clinical piece of information? Chest X-ray, clinical and anthropometric data suggest pulmonary emphysema in elderly. To notice that "senile emphysema" is sometime a misleading term. It usually refers to pulmonary changes accompanying thoracic cage alteration with age, without no significant pulmonary function impairment. In this case spirometry and CO diffusing capacity resulted severely impaired.

2. Which roentgen signs would raise suspicion of pulmonary emphysema?
In PA projection hyperlucency of right upper lobe, prominency of the lower half of right hilum, and abrupt attenuation in calibre of branches in central pulmonary zone, would be signs suggestive of pulmonary emphysema, prevailing in the right upper lobe. In LL projection, increase of the AP thoracic diameter, due to kyphosis and sternal bowing. Both findings have been shown to be function of weight loss. The smaller abdomen makes the chest appear relatively large. The dimensions of the retrosternal space and heart also vary with body build.

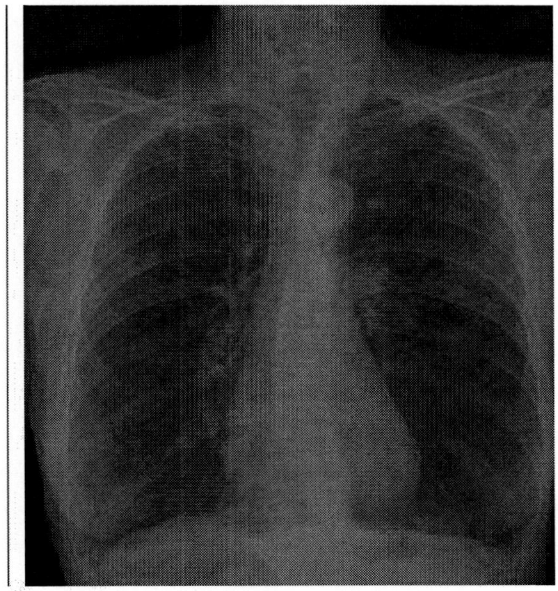

Figure 2. Standard Chest X-ray: A) PA projection in a 72 year-old woman, ex heavy smoker with occasional sputum, and chronic cough; BMI 17.3 (Courtesy of Dr. Paolo Poggi) — What's chest radiograph like, according to the anthropometric and clinical piece of information?
1. Chest X-ray, clinical and anthropometric is diagnostic for advanced pulmonary emphysema.
2. Which roentgen signs would raise suspicion of pulmonary emphysema?
Diminished vascularity in central and peripheral lung fields appears disproportionate compared to hilar vessels. Diaphragm is flattened with a slight downward concavity. In LL projection, marked increase of the AP thoracic diameter and clarity of retrosternal space would have been expected.

It is apparent that the relationship between emphysema and the chest radiograph is conflicting. Hyperinflation appears to be present in a higher proportion of cases with severe emphysema than arterial deficiency pattern is. However, it produces false positives, which occur only rarely when arterial deficiency is used as criterion. Arterial deficiency appears to be a difficult sign to recognize and varies considerably between observers, as the exact criteria for the recognition of arterial deficiency have never been agreed on. Variation in radiological criteria; patient selection based on pulmonary function testing as a basis of making an anatomical diagnosis; and limitation of determining parenchymal changes in terms of density changes seen on plain chest radiograph may explain in part variation in supposed sensitivities. Studies quoting sensitivity are difficult to understand in that the emphysema does not really lend itself to quantitative measurement along a single dimensional scale.

By the way, a reappraisal of the role of radiological techniques in the clinical assessment of emphysema has demonstrated that the chest radiograph helps to identify patients with functionally significant emphysema [12]. Furthermore, using the method originally described by Barnhard et al. [13] for the determination of total lung capacity, the volumetric analysis of discrete thoracic segments, such as giant bullas is obtained with the assumption that they are elliptical cylindroids [14]. The radiographic measurement of bulla volume to be resected predicts the surgical outcome, when used in the preoperative evaluation of patients undergoing elective bullectomy. The radiographic bulla volume was statistically the single most important factor determining the increase of $\Delta FEV_1\%$ (r=0.80,p< 0.0001), as expressed by the equation $\Delta FEV_1\%$= -5.83 + 0.028xbulla volume (ml), [14].

Giant emphysematous bulla, is a natural model of heterogeneity of emphysema distribution that has been defined as the predominance of the lesions in the upper lung lobe, and represents a criterion of emphysema severity. Thus, the extent of improvement in cases of heterogeneous emphysema may be predicted by means of quantitative assessment of the chest radiograph. This radiographic analysis may be of practical value when elective surgery is under consideration in patients with giant bullous emphysema

Computed tomography of the thorax has become a well-validated technique to diagnose emphysema *in vivo*, since Goddard et al. [15] demonstrated that "CT scan can detect the presence and distribution of pulmonary emphysema". Furthermore, in 1984 Hayrust et al. [16] reported the first pathological correlation and documented that "the frequency distribution curves of EMI numbers within the lung fields of patients who proved to have centriacinar emphysema differ significantly from those of the group who did not".

The CT qualitative evaluation is based on visual scoring of the size and extent of lung area with low attenuation value. This approach has been validated by comparing CT visual scores with emphysema graded according to the panel standard of Thurlbeck [11] or according modifications of the panel [17,18]. Panel Grading (PG) system is a method of ranking emphysema according to several categories of severity. Thus the CT qualitative evaluation reflects the severity of macroscopic emphysema.

Several CT – pathological studies published in literature [19-23] have compared the pathological scores obtained by PG in slices cut on the same plane of CT with CT visual scores. The high correlation coefficients indicate that CT and pathology results are linked. This does not imply that the percentage areas obtained by CT scan are equal to those obtained from pathology.

An objective evaluation of the extent of emphysema will provide quantitative results, if we identify areas of abnormally low attenuation within a threshold value, which defines emphysema. Once identified, this threshold needs to be validated with macroscopic and microscopic pathology.

In 1988 Muller et al. [24] introduced a CT scanner program the "Density mask" that highlights voxels within a given density range. They found that the density mask score highlighting all voxels with attenuation values -910 Hounsfield Units (HU) was closely related to the pathologic score. In 1995 Gevenois et al. [25], measured the relative area macroscopically occupied by emphysema on paper mounted lung sections using a computed assisted method. They compared the relative lung area macroscopically occupied by emphysema against the relative lung area occupied by CT attenuation values lower than different threshold values.

The authors documented that the only threshold for which there was no significant difference between the mean of the CT and the morphometric data was the -950 HU one. The mean, the standard error of the mean, and the 95% confidence interval on the differences between the relative area obtained with various thresholds and macroscopic morphometry were analyzed. The relative lung area at threshold lower than -950 HU (i.e. -970HU) underestimates emphysema, the relative lung area at threshold higher than -950 HU (i.e. -900HU) overestimates emphysema. In other words, the distribution of macroscopic measurements does not overlap the distribution of CT measurements except for the threshold -950HU. Data were calculated on HRCT obtained at full inspiration and at 1centimeter intervals. Also, in another paper Gevenois et al. [26] compared the CT relative lung areas at different threshold values with microscopic measurements of emphysema: the mean perimeter (MP) and mean interwall distance (MIWD). Again the relative lung area with attenuation values lower than -950 HU was the most closely related with the corresponding set of microscopic data, reflecting the enlargement of distal air spaces. Therefore, densitometry of computed tomography seems to provide an objective measurement of the extent of emphysema. However, it doesn't provide any information about heterogeneity of distribution of emphysematous lesions, i.e. to the severity of emphysema.

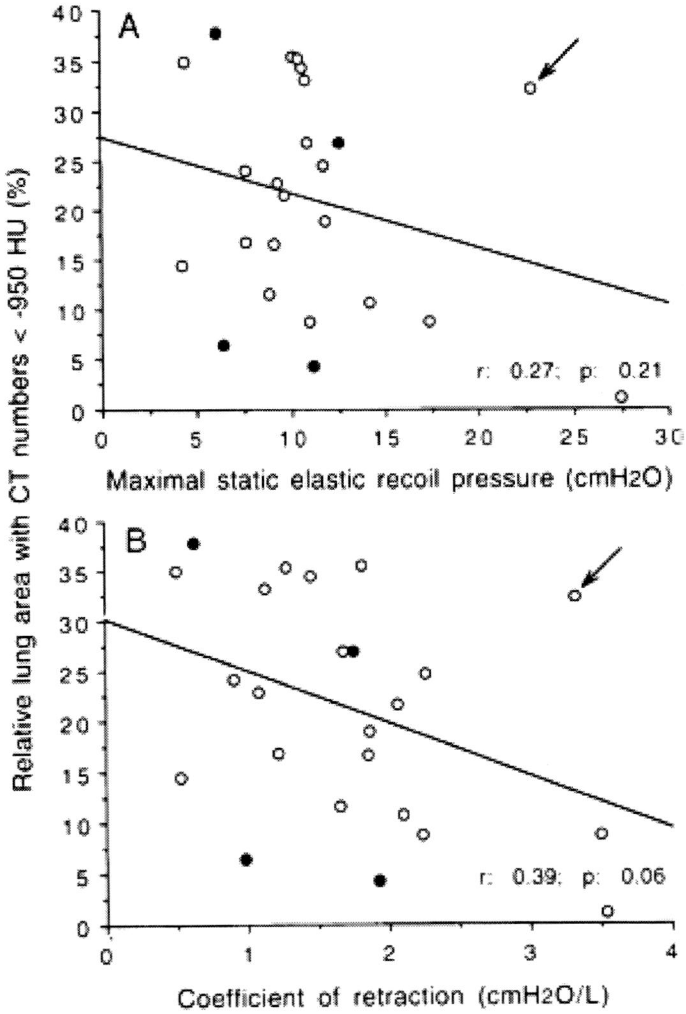

Figure 3. Extent of emphysema as assessed by HRCT quantitative analysis (RA_{950} plotted against $P_{st\,max}$ %predicted (panel A and, respectively coefficient of retraction i.e $P_{st\,max}$/TLC (panel B). Closed circled identify patients (no. 4) with change in post-bronchodilator FEV1 > 200 ml or >12%. Reproduced with permission from reference [28].

Studies from literature have documented reasonable correlation between mean lung density and both elastic recoil pressure and CO diffusing capacity [27, 28]. Nevertheless, the relationship between extent of emphysema as assessed by CT scan quantitative analysis and lung elastic recoil pressure is not statistically significant [28], see Figure 3. Thus, elastic properties seem to reflect the properties of lung tissue in between emphysematous spaces more than the emphysematous spaces themselves. On the other hand, the majority of studies from literature document that extent of emphysema bears from good to strong correlation with CO diffusing capacity (Figure 4), although spuriously low values of diffusing capacity have been reported in patients with very severe airflow limitation and without evidence of significant emphysema [27-31].

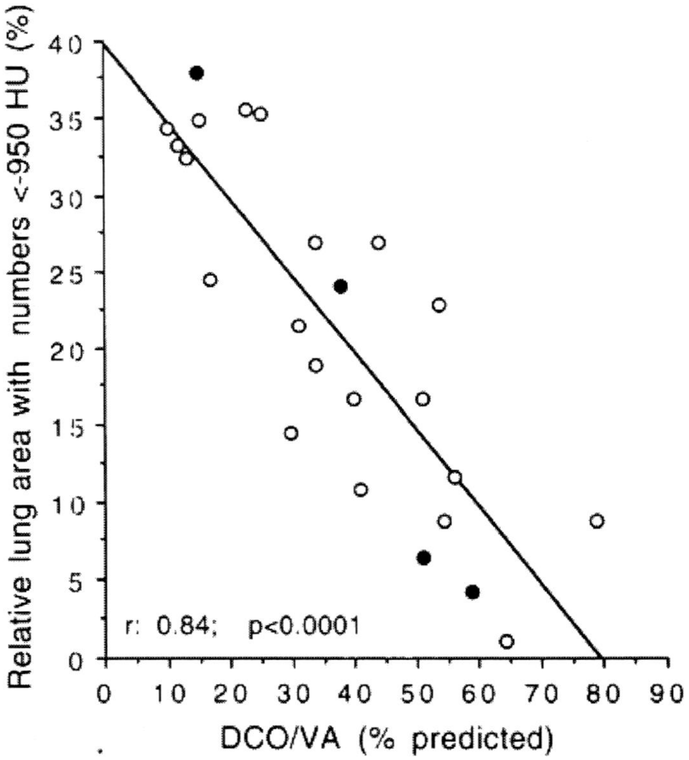

Figure 4. Extent of emphysema asassessed by HRCT quantitative analysis (RA 950) plotted against DCO/VA, % predicted. Closed circled identify patients (no. 4) with change in post-bronchodilator FEV1 > 200 ml or >12%. Reproduced with permission from reference [28].

Accuracy of lung imaging is greatly improved with advances in multi-detector row computed tomography (MDCT) that provides the ability to image the lung in 10 s or less with a theoretical *in vivo* resolution of 0.5 mm. Automated segmentation of the lungs [32], lobes [33], and airways tree to the fifth- through seventh generation bronchi [34-37] is today possible and accurate. Regional characterization of lung density, texture, ventilation and perfusion also make it possible functional imaging of emphysema. Parenchyma analysis permits differentiating population based on characteristics of the emphysema pattern without contrast material, when using the density mask approach [38-40]. Although, this technique alone is not sufficient to accurately distinguish normal from diseased lung [41-43], it is particularly useful in characterizing mild/moderate and severe emphysema, as demonstrated by NETT study where the technique has been used to identify subgroups of patients who benefit from LVRS [44].

Two representative cases of centrilobular (CLE) and panlobular emphysema (PLE) are shown in Figure 5, and respectively Figure 6. Holes of parenchymal destruction involving the center of pulmonary lobule characterize CLE that is prevailing to the lung upper lobe. Adjacent holes may combine in bigger ones, see Figure . Panlobular PLE results from destruction of pulmonary lobule. PLE is usually prevalent to the lower lung lobe. In Figure 5 the panlobular destruction is prevailing to the basal segments of left lung.

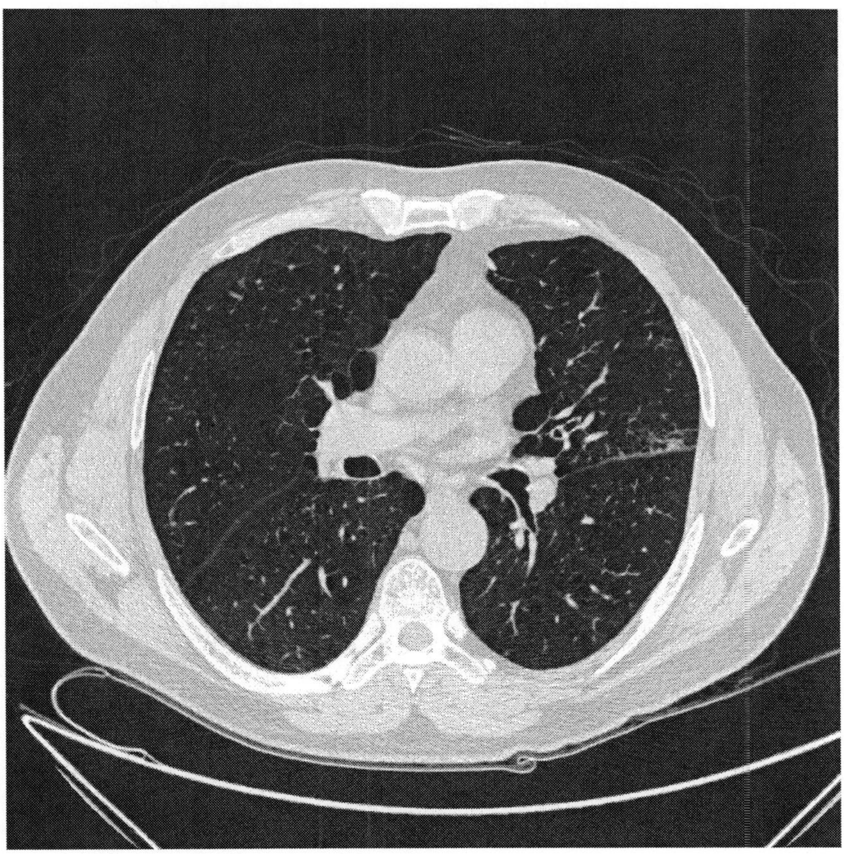

Figure 5. High Resolution Computed tomography : transverse thin section CT scan below the carena in a 64 year-old man, ex heavy smoker with occasional sputum, and chronic cough; (Courtesy of Dr. Paolo Poggi).

Paraseptal emphysema and a background of centrilobular emphysema. Paraseptal emphysema involves the alveolar ducts and sacs at the lung periphery. The emphysematous areas are often surrounded by interlobular septa (hence the name). It may be an incidental finding in young adults, and may be associated with spontaneous pneumothorax. It may also be seen in older patients with centrilobular emphysema (as in this case). Both centrilobular and paraseptal emphysema may progress to bulla formation. A bulla is defined as being at least 1cm in diameter, and with a wall less than 1mm thick. Bullae are thought to arise by air trapping in emphysematous spaces, causing local expansion.

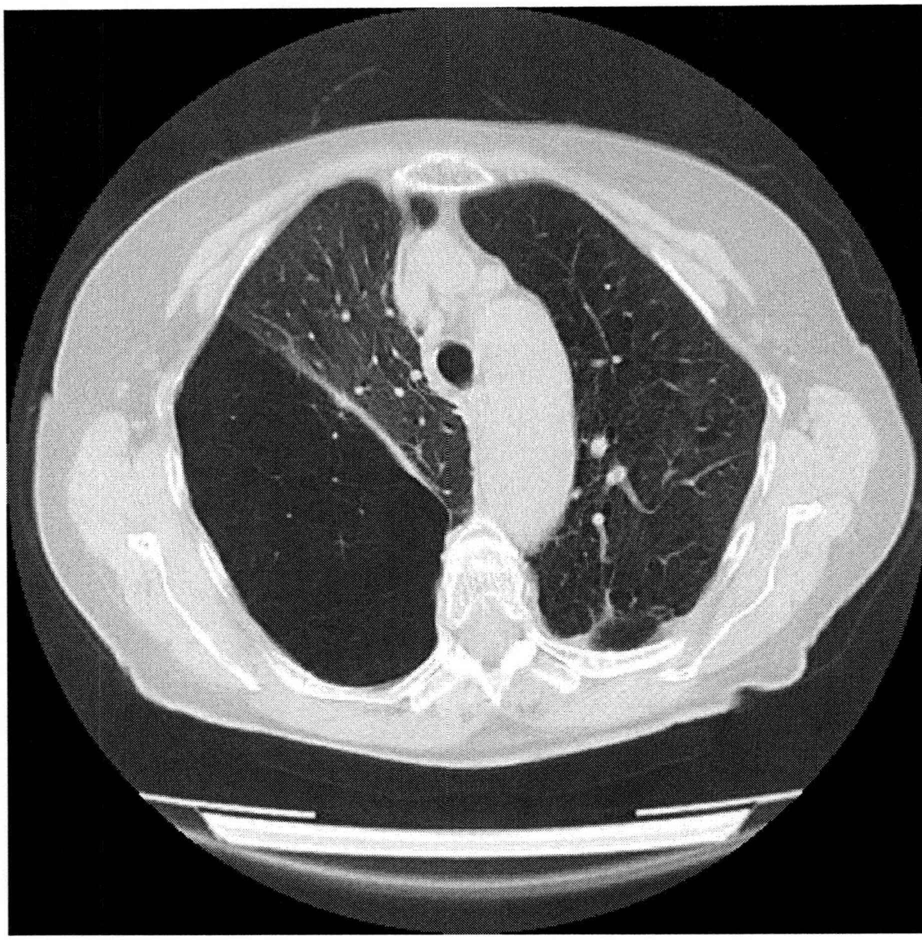

Figure 6. High Resolution Computed tomography: transverse thin-section CT scan at the level of aortic arc, obtained in a 65 year old woman with alpha$_1$-antitrypsin deficiency (Courtesy of Dr. Paolo Poggi). The long lines are the typical feature of advanced disease. The increased prevalence and extent of long lines is highly significant in patients with panlobular emphysema due to alpha$_1$-antitrypsin deficiency. There is coexisting centrilobular emphysema in the upper lobes. Typical features of panlobar emphysema (ie, mild bronchial dilatation, bronchial wall thickening, and panlobular pulmonary destruction) were seen in the lower zones of this patient.

Figure 7 give an example of CT scan quantitative parenchymal analysis by "Density Mask". A CT slice at level of aortic arc has been analyzed. The "Density Mask" program enables segmentation of lung fields, see panel b and panel C, determination of lung area with CT numbers lower than a predetermined threshold value, see panel D. The threshold value – 910 HU is selected by the operator.

As analysis methods have evolved, PC-based comprehensive lung image analysis packages have incorporated additional measurements of emphysema such as the index of complexity of airway geometry proposed by Mishima et al. [45]. The authors analyzed the statistical properties of clusters of contigous pixels with the same attenuation value < -960 HU, i.e. low atteunuation areas (LAA), in COPD and in heathy subjects. They documented that the cumulative size distribution of LAA clusters followed a power low characterized by an exponent D. The exponent D is assessed by the slope of log-log plot of hole size versus percentage of holes. Since with increasing severity of disease the small holes combines to form the bigger ones the dimension D, i.e., the slope of log-log plot, diminishes. Accordingly, COPD patients with percentage LAA similar to healthy subjects have smaller D values. The dimention D is correlated with CO diffusing capacity. Thus the power low analysis applied to the size distribution of LAA clusters reveals the pattern of progression of emphysema. The exponent D is a parameter sensitive to change in dimention of alveolar structure. Hence, D appears to be a powerful index for detection of terminal air space enlargement that occurs in early emphysema. In Figure 7, cluster distribution on a CT slice and the slope of log-log plot of hole size versus percentage of holes of a representative case of centrilobular (CLE) emphysema is shown.

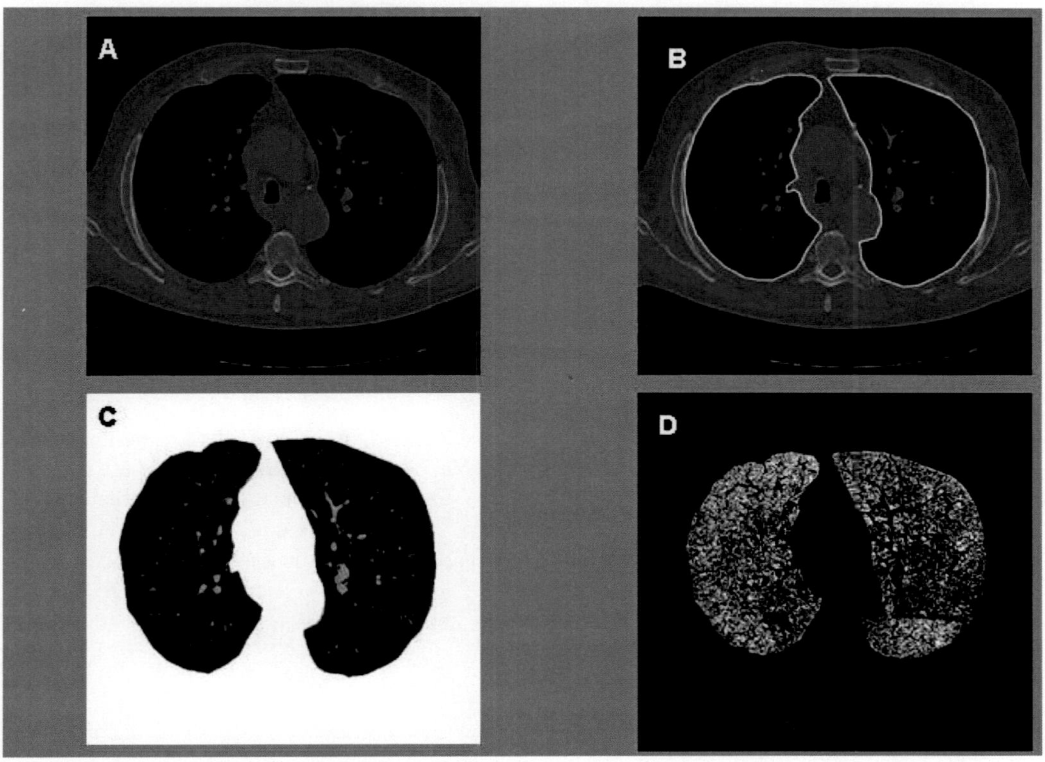

Figure 7. High Resolution Computed tomography: an example of CT scan image-processing program (Courtesy of Dr. Raffaele Dellaca'): A) transverse thin-section CT scan to be analyzed; B) manual lung segmentation. The areas occupied by trachea and stomach were manually erased, if required; C) extraction of boundaries of the lungs by using a subrange filter with a threshold of -400 HU, which distinguishes between lung tissue and adjacent tissue of the heart, diaphragm, and ribs; D) Lung cross-sectional areas and histograms of attenuation values (CT numbers) of individual highlighted sections were calculated. White areas represent the lung area with attenuation values lower than the threshold of emphysema. Values are expressed as percentage of the whole lung area.

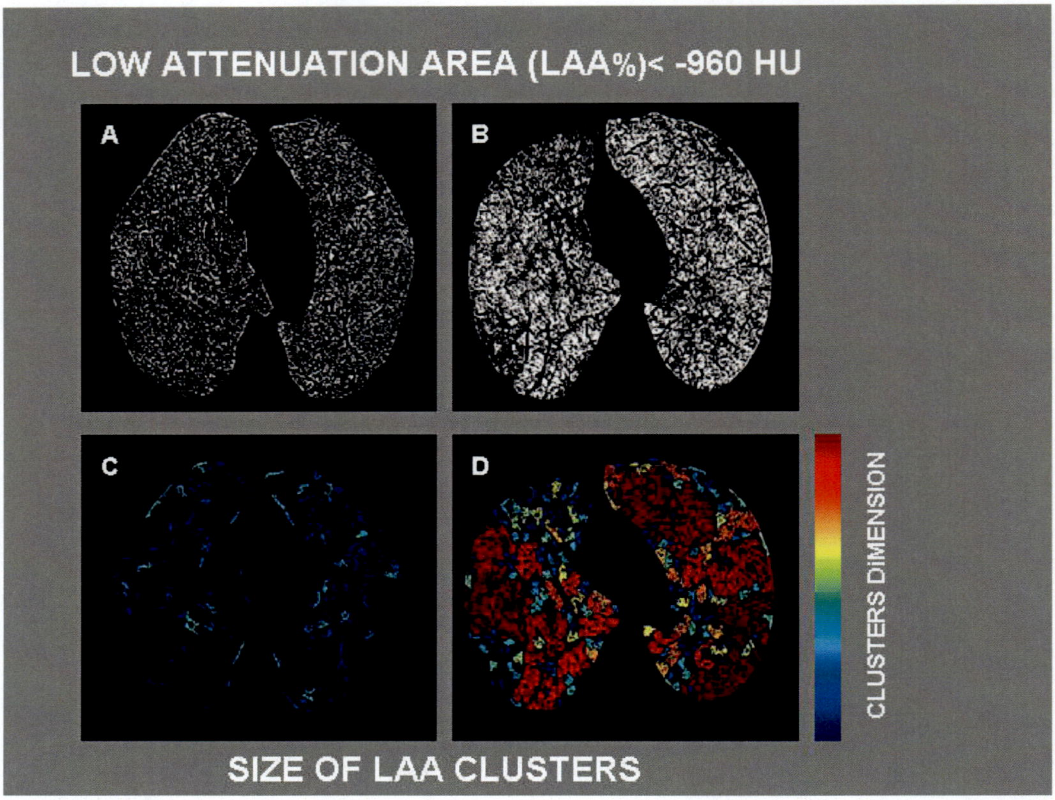

Figure 8. High Resolution Computed tomography: an example of CT scan image-processing program (Courtesy of Dr. Raffaele Dellaca'). Transverse thin-section CT scans at level of the aortic arc in two representative cases of centrilobular (CLE) emphysema. A and B) The percentage of low attenuation pixels (LAA%) was automatically calculated as in figure 5. C and D) The same images as in A and B, but the individual clusters comprising contiguous LAA regions are shown in contrasting colors. Cumulative frequency distributions of LAA sizes decrease linearly with the increase of clusters size on log–log plots. Values of the exponent *D* were obtained by linear regression in the log–log domain. A) LAA% = 22%; C) exponent D = 2.02; B LAA%= 45%; D) exponent D= 1.77.

High-resolution computed tomography (HRCT) enhances the resolving power of the image thus allowing detection of less severe emphysema [20, 23, 46-48]. Various computed assisted texture-based methods have successfully been used for tissue characterization [49]. Texture analysis relay on either region grey scale statistical measures, or textural measures. These techniques reveal useful in assessing early pathologic changes, mixed pathology, or complex pattern such as ground glass [50, 51]. Finally, CT protocols have been proposed to assess pulmonary ventilation and perfusion. Regional ventilation is measured from time course of CT density change during a multi-breath wash-in and washout of radio-dense Xenon gas [52]. Wash-in and washout times constant have been measured [53]. Dynamic imaging methods have been used to estimate arterial, venous and capillary transit times and capillary flow distribution [54]. Various approaches have been described for determining pulmonary blood flow and/or mean transit time.

All the above mentioned protocols are applied to better address the current research questions of phenotyping emphysema. CT parameters might provide answer to the question as to whether or not smoking cessation halts the progression of emphysema, as they have been shown more sensitive than pulmonary function tests to disease progression [55]. Up to date the results are still conflicting, because decline of lung function depends on either age or inflammation, and no reliable and specific biochemical markers are available to conclude definitely.

Weight loss is a clinical feature that has been acknowledged for at least one century to identify the emphysematous phenotype among patients with COPD [56]. British investigators have used weight loss together with functional and radiological criteria indicating presence of macroscopic emphysema to select patients with COPD as Type A i.e. prevailing emphysema, compared to Type B, i.e. prevailing chronic bronchitis, which have a plethoric habitus [57]. For a long time, the differences in gas exchange disturbance during exercise between the phenotypes have been related to the presence of emphysema [58]. Eventually, it became evident that in this condition responses to exercise are very variable and the attention was drifted to the complex picture of interrelationships between different causes of exercise intolerance [59] as well as to the assessment of systemic effects of COPD [50]. In particular, studies looking at systemic effects of COPD have analyzed the association between weight loss and COPD, especially the emphysematous type, as well as the multi-factorial mechanisms of muscle dysfunction. These studies were aimed at impacting patients centered outcomes through a comprehensive program that addresses pharmacological together with nutrition-rehabilitation interventions.

References

[1] Macklem PT. Airway obstruction and collateral ventilation. *Physiol Rev* 1971; 51: 368-436.

[2] Hogg JC, Macklem PT, Thurlbeck WM. Site and nature of airway obstruction in chronic obstructive lung disease. *N Engl J Med* 1968; 278: 1355-1360.

[3] Verbeken, EK, M. Cauberghs, KP Van De Woestijne. Membranous bronchioles and connective tissue network of normal and emphysematous lungs. *J Appl Physiol* 1996; 81: 2468-2480.

[4] Anthonisen NR, Connett JE, Kiley JP et al. Effect of smoking intervention and the use of an inhaled anticolinergic bronchodilator on the rate of decline of FEV1: the Lung Health Study. *JAMA* 1994; 272: 1497-1507.

[5] Laws JW, Heard BE. Emphysema and the chest film: A retrospective radiological diagnosis and pathological study. *Br J Radiol* 1962; 35: 750-761.

[6] Reid L, Millard FJC. Correlation between radiological diagnosis and structural lung changes in emphysema. *Clin Radiol* 1964; 15: 307-311.

[7] Sutinen S, Christoforidis AJ, Klugh GA et al. Roentgenographic criteria for the recognition of non symptomatic pulmonary emphysema. *Am Rev Respir Dis* 1965; 91: 69-76.

[8] Nicklaus TM, Stowell DW, Christiansen WR, et al. The accuracy of the roengenographic diagnosis of chronic pulmonary emphysema. *Am Rev Respir Dis* 1966; 93: 889-899.

[9] Katsura S, Martin CJ. The roentgenologic diagnosis of anatomic emphysema. *Am Rev Respir Dis* 1967; 96: 700-716.

[10] Thurlbeck WM, Dunill MS, Hartung W, et al. A comparison of three methods of measuring emphysema. *Human Pathol* 1970; 1: 215-226.

[11] Thurlbeck WM, Simon G. A radiographic appearance of the chest in emphysema. *Am Roentgenol* 1978; 130: 429-440.

[12] Miniati M, Filippi E, Falaschi F, Carrozzi L, Milne ENC, Sostman HD and Pistolesi M. Radiologic evaluation of emphysema in patients with chronic obstructive pulmonary disease. Chest radiography versus high resolution computed tomography. *Am Respir Crit Care Med.* 1995; 151: 1359-1367.

[13] Barnhard HJ, Pierce JA, Joyce JW and Bates JH. Roentgenographic determination of total lung capacity. A new method evaluated in health, emphysema and congestive heart failure. *Am J Med* 1960; 28:51-60.

[14] Baldi S, Palla A, Mussi A, Falaschi F, Carrozzi L, Giuntini C and Angeletti CA. Influence of bulla volume on post bullectomy outcome. *Can Respir* J 2001;8: 233-238.

[15] Goddard PR, Nicholson EM, Lazlo G, Watt I. Compuled tomography in pulmonary E. *Clin Radiol* 1982; 33:379-387.

[16] Hayhurst MD, Flenley DC, McLean A, et al. Diagnosis of emphysema by computerized tomography. *Lancet* 1984; 2: 320-322.

[17] Gough J, Wentworth J. Thin section of entire organs mounted on paper. *Harvey Lecture* 1957-58; 53: 182-185.

[18] Nagai A, Yamawaki I, Thurlbeck WM, Takizawa T. Assessment of lung parenchymal destruction using routine histological sections. *Am Rev Respir Dis* 1989; 139: 313-319.

[19] Bergin C, Muller N, Nichols DM, et al. The diagnosis of emphysema. A computed-pathologic correlation. *Am Rev Respir Dis* 1986; 133: 541-546.

[20] Miller RR, Muller N, Vidal S, Morrison NJ, Staples CA. Limitation of computed tomography in the assessment of emphysema. *Am Rev Respir Dis* 1989; 139: 980- 983.

[21] Morrison NJ, Abboud RT, Muller NL, et al. Pulmonary capillary blood volume in emphysema. *Am Rev Respir Dis* 1990; 141: 53-61.

[22] Spouge D, Mayo JR, Cardoso W, Muller NL. Panacinar emphysema: CT and Pathologic findings. *J Comput Assist Tomog* 1993; 17: 710-713.

[23] Hruban RH, Meziane MA, Zerhouni EA, et al. High resolution computed tomography of inflation-fixed human lungs. Pathologic-radiologic correlation of centrilobular emphysema. *Am Rev Respir Dis* 1987; 136:935-940.

[24] Muller NL, RR Miller, RT Abboud." Density mask". An objective method to quantitate emphysema using computed tomography. *Chest* 1988; 94: 782-787.

[25] Gevenois PA, De Maertelaer V, DeVuyst P, Zanen J, Yernault JC. Comparison of computed density and macroscopic morphometry in pulmonary emphysema. *Am J Respir Crit Care Med* 1995; 152:653-657.

[26] Gevenois PA, DeVuyst P, De Maertelaer V, Zanen J, Jacobovitz D, Cosio MG, Yernault JC. Comparison of computed density and microscopic morphometry in pulmonary emphysema. *Am J Respir Crit Care Med* 1996; 154:187-192.

[27] Gugger M, Gould G, Sudlow MF, Wraiht PK, MacNee W. Extent of pulmonary emphysema in man and its relation to the loss of lung elastic recoil. *Clin Sci* 1991; 80: 353-358.

[28] Baldi S, Miniati S, Bellina CR, Battolla L, Catapano G, Begliomini E, Giustini D, and Giuntini C. Relationship between extent of pulmonary emphysema by high-resolution computer tomography and lung elastic recoil in patients with chronic obstructive pulmonary disease. *Am J Respir Crit Care Med* 2001; 164: 585-589.

[29] Gelb AF, Schein M, Kuei J, Tashkin DP, Müller NL, Hogg JC, Epstein JD, Zamel N. Limited contribution of emphysema in advanced chronic obstructive pulmonary disease. *Am Rev Respir Dis* 1993; 147: 1157-1161.

[30] Gelb AF, Hogg JC, Müller NL, et al. Contribution of emphysema and small airways in COPD. *Chest* 1996; 109: 353-359.

[31] Gelb AF, Zamel N, Hogg JC, Müller NL, Schein M. Pseudophysiologic emphysema resulting from severe small-airways disease. *Am J Respir Crit Care Med* 1998; 158: 815-819.

[32] Hu S, Hoffman EA, Reinhardt JM. Automatic lung segmentation for accurate quantitation of volumetric X-ray CT images *IEEE Trans Med Imaging* 2001; 20: 490-498.

[33] Zhang L, Hoffman EA, Reinhardt JM. Lung lobar segmentation by graph search with 3D shape costrains. In Chen C-T, Clough AV, editors. Medical Imaging 2001. Physiology and function from multi-dimentional images; Feb 18-20, 2001 San Diego Bellingham, WA: *SPEI, Proceeding of SPIE*; vol 5031.

[34] Reinhardt JM, Raab SA, D'Souza ND, Hoffman E. Intrathoracic airways measurement: ex vivo validation. In Hoffman EA editor. *Medical imaging 1997. Physiology and function from multi-dimentional images*; Feb 23-25, 1997 San Diego Bellingham, WA: *SPIE, Proceeding of SPIE*; vol 3033.

[35] Saba O, Beck K, Chon D, Nixon E, Hoffman E. Lung volume measurement reproducibility using gated-axial and spatial multi-row detector CT (MDCT) [abstract]. *Am J Respir Crit Care Med* 2003; 167: A844.

[36] Tschirren J, Palàgyi K, Hoffman EA, Sonka M. Segmentation skeletonization, and branchpoint matching: a fully authomated quantitative evaluation of human intrathoracic airways trees. In: Dohi T, Kikinis R. editors. *Proceedings of the Fifth International Conference on Medical Image Computing and Computed Assisted Intervention, 2002.* Tokyo, Japan , Berlin Springer-Verlag ; 2002, pp.12-19.

[37] Tschirren J, Hoffman EA, Mc Lennan G, Sonka M. *Branchpoint labelling and matching in human airways trees Proceedings of the SPIE Medical Imaging*, 2003, San Diego, CA; 2003, pp. 187-194.

[38] Adams H, Bernard M, McConnokie K. An appraisal of CT pulmonary density mapping in normal subjects. *Clin Radiol* 1991; 43:238-242.

[39] Coxon HO, Rogers RM. Quantitative computed tomography of chronic obstructive pulmonary disease. *Acad Radiol* 2005; 12: 1457-1463.

[40] Newell JD Jr, Hogg JC, Snider GL. Report of a workshop: quantitative computed tomography scanning in longitudinal studies of emphysema. *Eur Respir J* 2004; 23: 769-775.

[41] Uppaluri R, Mitsa T, Sonka M, Hoffman EA, McLennan G. Quantification of pulmonary emphysema from lung CT images using texture analysis. *Am J Respi Crit Care Med* 1997; 156: 248-254.

[42] Uppaluri R, Hoffman E, Schwartz D, McLennan D, Hunninghake G, Dayton C, Hartley P. Quantitative analysis of the chest CT in asbestos-exposed subjects using an adaptive multiple feature method. *Am J Respi Crit Care Med* 1998; 157: A 276.

[43] Uppaluri R, McLennan G, Enright P, Hoffman E. AMFM a quantitative assessment of early parenchymal changes in smokers. *Am J Respi Crit Care Med* 1998; 157: A 788.

[44] Fishman A, Martinez F, Naunheim K, Piantadosi S, Wise R, Ries A, Weinmann G, Wood DE; National Emphysema Treatment Trial Research Group. A randomized trial comparing lung-volume-reduction surgery with medical therapy for severe emphysema. *N Engl J Med* 2003; 348: 2059-2073.

[45] Mishima M, Hirai T, Itoh H, Nakano Y, Sakai H, Muro I, Nishimura K, Oku Y, Chin K, Ohi M et al Complexity of terminal airspace geometry assessed by lung computed tomography in normal subjects and patients with chronic obstructive pulmonary disease. *Proc Nat Acad Sci USA* 1999; 96: 8829-8834.

[46] Murata K, Itoh H, Senda M, Yonekura Y, Nishimura K, Izumi T, Oshima S, Torizuka K. Stratified impairment of pulmonary ventilation in diffuse panbronchiolitis: PET and CT studies. *J Comput Assist Tomogr* 1989; 13: 48-53.

[47] Webb WR. High-resolution computed tomography of the lung: normal and abnormal anatomy. *Semin Roentgenol* 1991; 26: 110-117.

[48] Sanders C. Imaging of emphysema. *Semin Respir Crit Care Med* 1992; 13: 318-330.

[49] Sonka M, Hlavac V, Boyle R. *Image processing, analysis, and machine vision*. London Chapman and Hall; 1993.

[50] Uppaluri R, Hoffman EA, Sonka M, Hartley P, Hunninghake GW, McLennan. Computer recognition of regional lung disease patterns. *Am J Respi Crit Care Med* 1999; 160:648-654.

[51] Uppaluri R, Hoffman EA, Sonka M, Hunninghake GW, McLennan. Interstitial lung disease: a quantitative study using the adoptive multiple feature method. *Am J Respi Crit Care Med* 1999; 159: 519-525.

[52] Chon D, Simon BA, Beck KC, Shikata H, Saba OI, Won C, Hoffman EA. Differences in regional wash-in was-out time constantsfor Xenon-CT ventilation studies. *Respir Physiol Neurobiol* 2005; 148; 65-83.

[53] Chon D, Beck KC, Shikata H, Saba OI, Simon BA, Hoffman EA. Effect of reduced inhaled Xenon and krypton supplementation of signal-noise of regional CT-based ventilation measurements. *Am J Respir Crit Care Med* 2004; 167: A 547.

[54] Hoffman EA, Tajik JK. Dynamic and high resolution CT assessment of pulmonary blood flow distributions. *Am Rev Respir Dis* 1993; 147: A 201.

[55] Dirksen A, Dijkman JH, Madsen F, Stoel B, Hutchinson DC, Urlik Cs, Skovgaard LT, Kok-Jensen A, Rudolphus A, Seersholm N et al. A randomized clinical trial of a1.antitrypsin augmentation therapy. *Am J Respir Crit Care Med* 1999; 160: 1468-1472.

[56] Fowler J, Godlee R. Emphysema of the lungs. In: *Diseases of the lungs*. London: Longmans, green and Co., 1898; 171.

[57] Burrows B, Fletcher CM, Heard BE, Jones NL, Wootliff JS. The emphysematous and bronchial types of chronic airways obstruction. A clinico-pathological study of patients in London and Chicago. *Lancet* 1966; 16: 830–835.
[58] Jones NL. Pulmonary gas exchange during exercise in patients with chronic airflow obstruction. *Clin Sci* 1966; 31: 39-50.
[59] Jones NL, Jones G, Edwards RHT. Exercise tolerance in chronic airflow obstruction. *Am Rev Respir Dis* 1971; 103: 477-494.
[60] Hamilton AL, Killian KJ, Summers E, Jones NL. Muscle strength, symptoms intensity, and exercise capacity in patients with cardiorespiratory disorders *Am J Respir Crit Care Med* 1995; 152: 2021-2031.

3. The Contribution of Nutritional Status and Airflow Obstruction to Functional Emphysema

Body Mass Index (BMI), i.e. the ratio of body weight to height^2, is a crude index reflecting the complex metabolic disturbances that lead to weight loss in COPD [1]. Weight loss has been regarded as a determinant of course and prognosis of COPD [2-4], and a marker for more severely impaired lung function [5-7]. Eventually, several studies have provided evidence that nutritional abnormalities and weight loss are relevant contributors to disability and handicap experienced by the patients [8], and represent key points for better definition of rehabilitation program [9-11]. Therefore, the relationship between body mass index (BMI), severity of airflow obstruction and CO diffusing capacity (DL_{CO}), i.e. the functional hallmark of emphysema, is of paramount importance to the management of COPD phenotypes. Baldi et al. [12] reviewed a group of 104 patients with COPD with either emphysema or chronic bronchitis defined according to functional criteria in order to elucidate the pathophysiological significance of a low BMI in emphysema. Data indicate that DL_{CO}% was independently and significantly associated to both post-bronchodilator FEV_1 and BMI, according to the equation:

$DL_{CO} = -18.32 + 0.65 \cdot FEV_1 + 1.59 \cdot BMI$ ($R2 = 0.40$, $p < 0.0001$).

The association between CO diffusing capacity and BMI groups segregated by post-bronchodilator FEV_1 shows a significant difference between weight-stable and weight-loosing COPD patients for the same level of FEV_1 (Figure 1), and invites to look at weight loss as a systemic domain which may in and of itself contribute to the COPD wasting syndrome. In this contest weight loss and low BMI reflect complex metabolic alterations related to disturbed energy balance, systemic inflammation, hypoxic and metabolic adaptations targeting lung as well as skeletal and respiratory muscles in advanced COPD [13].

Recent studies [14-16] looking at systemic effects of COPD have analyzed the pathogenesis of differences in nutritional status in COPD phenotypes. They support the notion of a link between factors responsible for parenchymal destruction and nutritional abnormalities. Firstly, body weight and composition are substantially different between chronic bronchitis and emphysema [14]. The emphysematous type of COPD has lower values not only for BMI, but also for fat free mass index and fat mass index, compared to chronic bronchitis type [14]. Secondly, nutritional intervention studies have documented positive outcome of nutritional intervention in the majority of COPD patients [15]. Moreover, the fact that elevated systemic inflammatory response determines a non response to nutritional therapy [16] leads to speculate on the possibility that the systemic inflammatory response directly impacts on the metabolism. The resulting disturbed energy balance and wasting syndrome might contribute to emphysematous dysfunction independent of the severity of functional impairment.

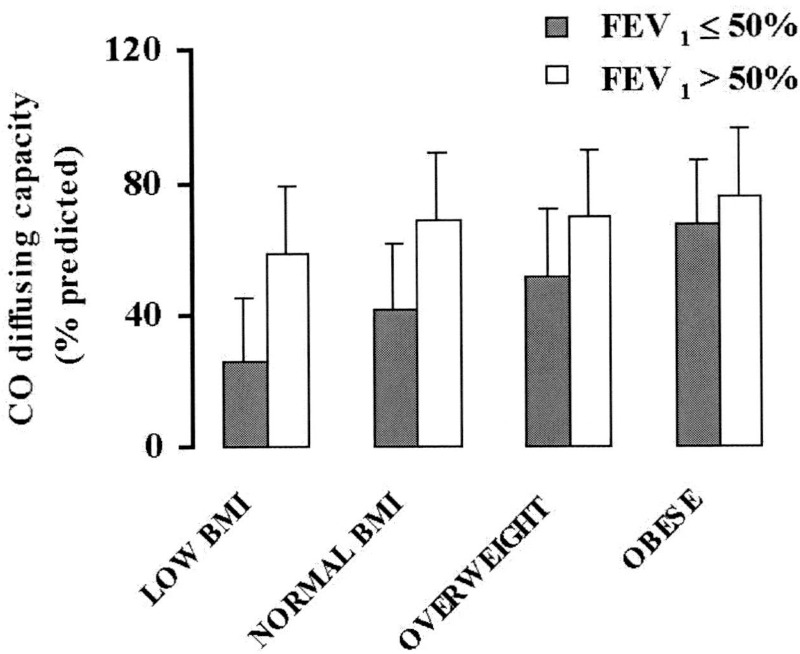

Figure 1. DLCO % predicted by categorised BMI (= 18.5; > 18.5 and = 25; > 25 and = 30; > 30) and post-bronchodilator FEV1(<50 % predicted vs = 50% predicted). No interaction was found between BMI and FEV1 (p=0. 30). Both factors were highly significant (p <0.0001). Rproduced with permission.

Besides differences in energy balance between emphysema and chronic bronchitis types, the relationship between CO diffusing capacity and BMI may also reflects differences in muscular adaptation, consequent to reduced availability of oxygen or tissue hypoxia. The negative correlation between diffusing capacity and fast myosin heavy chain isoform content in musculus vastus lateralis of COPD patients [17], and the occurrence of arterial oxygen desaturation in patients with emphysema as reflected by impaired diffusing capacity [18], lead to speculate on this hypothesis. Furthermore, the relationship between BMI and DLCO would suggests a decrease in oxygen supply and nutrients to muscles, especially during exercise, due to loss of capillary bed and inability to accommodate cardiac output without increasing pulmonary artery vascular pressure [19]. Therefore, these finding reinforce the idea that metabolic impairment as assessed by BMI may contribute to emphysematous dysfunction. In this contest BMI is an index of paramount importance to phenotype the wasting syndrome of COPD.

References

[1] Agusti AGN, Noguera A, Sauleda J, Sala E, Pons J, Busquets X. Systemic effects of chronic obstructive lung disease. *Eur Respir J 2003*; 21: 347 – 360.

[2] Burrows B, Earle RH. Course and prognosis of chronic obstructive lung disease. *N Engl J Med*. 1969; 280:397- 404.

[3] Anthonisen NR, Wright EC, Hodgkin JE. IPPB Trial Group. Prognosis in chronic obstructive pulmonary disease. *Am Rev Respir Dis* 1986; 133: 14-20.

[4] Landbo C, Prescott E, Lange P, Vestbo J, Almdal TP. Prognostic value of nutritional status in chronic obstructive pulmonary disease. *Am J Respir Crit Care Med* 1999; 160: 1865-1861.

[5] Vanderburg E, Van De Woestigne K, Gyselen A. Weight changes I the terminal stages of chronic obstructive lung disease. *Am Rev Respir Dis* 1967; 96: 556 – 565.

[6] Wilson DO, Rogers RM, Hoffman RM. Nutrition and chronic lung disease. *Am Rev Respir Dis* 1985; 132: 1347-1365.

[7] Wouters EF. Nutrition and metabolism in COPD. *Chest* 2000; 117: 274S -280S.

[8] Anonymus. Skeletal muscle dysfunction in chronic obstructive pulmonary disease. *Am J Respir Crit Care Med* 1999; 159; S1 – S40.

[9] Goldstein RS, Gort EH, Stubbing D, Avendano MA, Guyatt GH. Randomised controlled trial of respiratory rehabilitation. *Lancet* 1994; 1394 -1397.

[10] Ries AL Kaplan RM, Limberg TM, Prewitt LM. Effects of pulmonary rehabilitation on physiologic and psychosocial outcomes in patients with chronic obstructive pulmonary disease. *Ann Int Med* 1995; 122: 823- 832.

[11] Griffiths TL, Burr ML, Campbell IA et al. Results at I year of outpatients multidisciplinary pulmonary rehabilitation: a randomized controlled trial. *Lancet* 2000; 355: 362 -368.

[12] Baldi S, Pinna GD, Crotti P, Montemartini S, Dacosto E, Fanfulla F, Fracchia c and Bruschi C. Nutritional status and airflow obstruction: two independent contributors to CO diffusing capacity impairment in COPD. *Monaldi Arch Chest Dis* 2005; 63: 13-16.

[13] Pauwels RA, Buist AS, Calvelrly PM, Jenkins CR, Hard SS. Global strategy for the diagnosis, management and prevention of chronic obstructive pulmonary disease. NHLBI/WHO Global Initiative for chronic obstructive lung Disease(GOLD) Workshop Summary. *Am J Respir Crit Care Med* 2001; 163: 1256-1276.

[14] Engelen MPKJ, Schols AMWJ, Lamers RJS, Wouters EFM. Different patterns of chronic tissue wasting among patients with chronic obstructive pulmonary disease. *Clin Nutr* 1999; 18: 275-280.

[15] Schols AMWJ, Slangen J, Volovics L, Wouters EFM. Weight loss is a reversible factor in the prognosis of chronic obstructive pulmonary disease. *Am J respire Crit Care Med*.1998; 157: 1792-1797.

[16] Creutzberg E, Schols AMWJ, Welin-Scheepers et al. Characterization of non response to high caloric oral nutritional therapy in depleted patients with COPD. *Am J Respir Crit Care Med* 2000; 161: 745-752.

[17] Satta A, Migliori GB, Spanevello A et al. Fiber types in skeletal muscles of chronic obstructive pulmonary disease patients related to respiratory function and exercise tolerance. *Eur Respir J* 1997; 10 2583-2860.

[18] Owens GR, Rogers RM, Pennock BE et al. The diffusing capacity as a predictor of arterial oxygen desaturation during exercise in patients with chronic obstructive pulmonary disease. *N Engl J Med* 1984; 310: 1218-1221.

[19] Filley GF, Beckwitt HJ, Reeves JT, Mitchell R. Chronic obstructive bronchopulmonary disease. II. Oxygen transport in the two clinical types. *Am J Med* 1968; 44: 26-38.

4. Metabolic Derangements in Chronic Lung Diseases

Loss of muscle mass is a systemic effect accompanying the emphysematous type of COPD. Skeletal muscle wasting is associated with reduction in exercise capacity that reflects the shift from oxidative metabolism to glycolytic metabolism. Morphologic and metabolic abnormalities contribute to skeletal muscles dysfunction and are multifactorially determined; hypoxia, oxidative stress, inflammation, deconditioning, medication, nutritional depletion are involved. Among them, hypoxia has a big impact on muscle function. An inadequate oxygen delivery produces fatigue as documented from studies in animal muscles deprived of oxygen [1]. Chronic as well as intermittent hypoxia impact on glucose, protein and lipid metabolism [2]. Hypoxia itself contribute to oxidative stress as documented in animal exposed to intermittent hypoxia and in patients exposed to acute hypoxia, since the shift to glycolytic metabolism reduces muscles oxidative capacity [2].

Skeletal muscles undergo adaptive response to both chronic and intermittent hypoxia (IH). The term intermittent hypoxia describes conditions of repeated transient reduction in O_2 that applied to tissues with high metabolic rate relative to blood flow, such as cardiac or exercising skeletal muscle. In these contests IH may exist also in the absence of reductions in arterial PaO_2 and may trigger unique adaptation [2].

For skeletal muscles, IH can occur in condition of obstructive sleep apnea [3], transient altitude exposure (with or without exercise) [4-6], intermittent claudication [7-9], cardiopulmonary resuscitation [10], exercise in disease with compromised oxygen delivery such as chronic heart or lung disease [11], obstruction of placental blood flow [12] and the diving responses of marine animals [13]. In such cases capillary O_2 supply fails to match metabolic demands, resulting in transient localized hypoxia in the muscle cells or in the mitochondrial microenvironment.

Our understanding of IH or even chronic hypoxia in skeletal muscles at the present is sketchy, and so far there are no qualitative distinctions between metabolic adaptation to IH, and respectively to chronic hypoxia in muscles. In many cases it is likely that the responses overlap. However, whereas long term exposure to severe hypoxia can progress to cell injury and deterioration [14, 15], short term exposure may initiate adaptive responses, and unique physiological signals associated with transitions between hypoxia and re-oxygenation. As an example formation of reactive oxygen species (ROS) [12, 16-18] or facilitation of sympathetic outflow [19-21] and other reflex pathways [22, 23] can induce peculiar physiological responses.

A systematic analysis of ultrastructural and metabolic adaptations to hypoxia is beyond the aims of this review. However, the analysis of metabolic hypoxic derangements in COPD is appealing to answer the question as to whether they impact the progression of other co-morbid diseases. Recently interest has arisen because of the association of COPD with other systemic diseases including cardiovascular disease [32], diabetes [33], osteoporosis [34], and peptic ulceration [35] that enhance the severity of systemic inflammation.

Studies allowing for common etiological factors such as cigarette smoking, and steroid usage have identified an unexplained link.

In this scenario the analysis of glucose uptake and utilization is intriguing, since under hypoxic conditions it involves pathways that are activated somewhat differently from insulin or contractile dependent changes in uptake [24, 25]. Furthermore, hypoxia-induced transcription factors (HIF-1a) upregulate glucose transport proteins (Glut1 and Glut3) [26]. It is also worth mentioning that hypoxia-induced glucose uptake during contraction is in part adenosine dependent, which means that regulatory signal may be different under condition of IH where adenosine washout is high [27] compared to intermittent ischemia where adenosine would accumulate in tissues [28].

Diabetes mellitus has been associated with a reduced level of pulmonary function [29-35], but these findings have been inconsistently documented [36-39].

On the other hand, diabetes mellitus has been associated with markers of systemic inflammation [40], as well as with increased risk of other disease in which inflammation play a role, such as cardiovascular disease. Several epidemiological studies have demonstrated an association between type II diabetes and higher levels of markers of systemic inflammation [40-42]. Also, a variety of mediators of inflammation, including IL-1 and IL-6, and tumor necrosis factor that are implicated in the pathogenesis of COPD have also been associated with insulin resistance (43, 44). Therefore, the systemic inflammatory process related to different systemic co-morbidities might influence lung function independent of pulmonary inflammation related to COPD. The observation of that only a minority of smokers develops clinically significant COPD [45], and the persistence of inflammation following smoking cessation is consistent with this idea [46 - 47].

The association between glycemic state and lung function has been documented in the 3,254 members of the Framingham Offspring Cohort [48]. The study strongly support the evidence that adverse effect of diabetes and glycemic state on lung function was stronger among ever smokers than never smokers, suggesting an interaction between the level of fasting glycemia and tobacco smoking.

A reduction in serum markers of inflammation was documented with treatment of diabetes [49], further supporting the idea that diabetes may itself be a cause of systemic inflammation.

Several clues into the possible co-morbid enhancement of systemic inflammation and ventilatory impairment due to the association of tobacco smoking and proinflammatory effects of glycemic control are offered by the advanced glycation end products (AGEs). AGEs that result from the interaction between decomposing saccharides and polysaccharides have a pro-inflammatory effect. They alter matrix protein, affect the expression of cytokines and growth factors by macrophages and mesangial cells, alter the expression of inflammatory mediators by endothelial cells [50] and induce apoptosis [51]. Their trans-membrane receptors are seen in the lung, preferentially localized to the basal face of type I pneumocytes [52].

The progressive decrement in level of both residual FEV_1, i.e. predicted minus measured value, and residual FVC with increasing level of blood glucose documented in the Framingham study suggests that altered glucose metabolism is linked to more obstructive lung damage. Few other larger studies have documented some impairment of pulmonary function in subjects with diabetes [53, 54], as well as an association between a new diabetes diagnosis and annual decline of pulmonary function [55].

Glucose metabolism has hardly been studied in patients with COPD. The available data are inconclusive.

COPD is a chronic and irreversible disease. As a chronic disease, it could mostly induce insulin resistance. On the other hand, patients with COPD, above all those in the end-stage suffer from chronic hypoxaemia and/or hypercapnia, and acute respiratory failure is commonly seen during acute exacerbations requiring hospitalization. Long-term oxygen therapy is prescribed if resting arterial oxygen is < 55 mmHg. Despite normal blood gases at rest, COPD patients, in particular the emphysematous type, experience intermittent hypoxia during low-intensity activities of daily living such as walking, eating, dressing. Theoretically, hypoxia, as in healthy subjects exposed to chronic altitude, could stimulate glucose production and mostly reduce hepatic insulin sensitivity, while stimulating peripheral insulin sensitivity [55].

Data published by Hjalmarsen et al. [56] in normo-oxemic vs. hypoxaemic COPD patients, all with a normal BMI, indicate that COPD has no influence on glucose metabolism as long as arterial oxygen concentration is normal. In patients on LTOT, after glucose loading, plasma glucose increases despite a massive increase of plasma insulin. Data could have been influenced by glucocorticoid treatment. However, glucose tolerance was impaired also in COPD patients not on LTOT. Thus, hypoxia in COPD seems to have an effect opposite to the effect of hypoxia in healthy subjects.

Jacobsson et al. [57, 58] performed euglycemic hyperinsulinemic clamp studies in stable hypoxic COPD patients with a rather wide range of body weight and matched controls. They concluded that insulin sensitivity was normal in hypoxic COPD patients, because the rate of glucose infusion did not differed from controls. This conclusion may not be correct since it was based on the assumption that endogenous glucose production was suppressed to the same degree in COPD and healthy control [55]. In a further study Jacobsson et al. [59] infused insulin and glucose during an hyperinsulinemic euglicemic clamp in six COPD with low BMI < 21 kg/m2 and very severe airflow obstruction. After 90 minutes of room air breathing, the patients started breathing oxygen and lasted for 60 minutes. The authors documented a 32% increase in glucose uptake during oxygen breathing compared to room air breathing.

Cystic Fibrosis (CF) is a disease leading to progressive damage to many organs including the pancreas as a consequence of abnormal chloride channels activity and hyper-viscosity of ductular secretion. Many patients have severe fibrosis of the pancreas. Pancreatic endocrine dysfunction is also common. Glucose intolerance occurs in about 50-70% of adult patients with CF, while 5-9% develops overt diabetes with fasting hyperglycemia [60]. Exocrine insufficient CF patients without diabetes have impaired insulin secretion, but maintain normoglycemia, suggesting increased insulin sensitivity [60]. Moran et al. [60] tested different CF patients subgroups with euglicemic clamp. He documented a normal insulin sensitivity in exocrine sufficient patients, insulin resistance in diabetic CF patients, probably related to hyperglycemia-induced insulin resistance [61], and increased peripheral insulin sensitivity in exocrine insufficient patients without diabetes [60]. Despite the increase of peripheral insulin sensitivity, hepatic insulin sensitivity was reduced expressed in increased glucose production in the basal state and during insulin infusion [62]. Although the increase in peripheral insulin sensitivity has been confirmed by some authors [63], but not from others [64, 65], a similar picture resembles the changes induced by hypoxia in healthy subjects. If the same holds true for COPD patients, total peripheral glucose uptake will be underestimated in the COPD patients. Also in the study of Jacobsson et al. [58] glucose infusion rates were consistently, albeit not significantly higher in COPD patients. These data support the idea of higher total glucose uptake in COPD, suggesting increased peripheral insulin sensitivity in COPD patients.

The role of systemic inflammation in COPD and in comorbid diseases is not fully acknowledged yet. However, it seems a plausible mechanistic link between ventilatory impairment and insulin resistance mechanisms.

References

[1] Hill AV, Lupton H. Muscular exercise lactic acid , and the supply and utilization of oxygen. *QJM* 1923; 16: 135-171.

[2] Clanton TL, and Klawitter PF. Physiological and genomic consequences of intermittent hypoxia. Invited review: Adaptive responses of skeletal muscles to intermittent hypoxia: the known and the unknown. *J Appl Physiol* 2001; 90: 2476-2487.

[3] Redline S and Strohl KP. Recognition and consequences of obstructive sleep apnea hypopnea syndrome. *Clin Chest Med* 1998; 19: 1-18.

[4] Green HJ, MacDougall J, Tarnopolsky M, and Melissa NL. Downregulation of -Na^+ -K^+ -ATPase pumps in skeletal muscles with training to normobaric hypoxia. *J Appl Physiol* 1999; 86: 1745-1748.

[5] Mizuno M, Juel C Bro-Rasmussen T, Mygind E, Schibye B, Rasmussen B, and Saltin B. Limb skeletal muscle adaptation in athletes after training at altitude. *J Appl Physiol* 1990; 68: 496-502.

[6] Young AJ, Evans WJ, Fisher EC, Sharp RL, Costill DL, and Maher JT Skeletal muscle metabolism at sea level natives following short-term high altitude residence. *Eur J Appl Physiol* 1984; 52: 463-466.

[7] Bylund-Fellenius AC, Idstrom JP, and Holm S. Muscle respiration during exercise. *Am Rev Respir Dis*. 1984; 129:S10-S12.

[8] Elander A,, Idstrom JP, Schersten T, and Bylund-Fellenius AC. Metabolic adaptation to reduced muscle blood flow. I. Enzyme and metabolite alterations. *Am J Physiol Endocrinol Metab*. 1985; 249: E70-E76.

[9] Katayama K, Sato Y, Mrotome Y, Shima N, Ishida K, Mori S, and Miyamura M. Ventilatory chemosensitive adaptations to intermittent hypoxic exposure with endurance training and detraining. *J Appl Physiol* 1999; 86: 1805-1811.

[10] Gasser R, Schafhalter-Zoppoth I Schwarz T, Eber B, Koppel H, Lechleitner P, Pushendorf B, Dienstl F, and Klein W. Cyclic phenomena in early myocardial infarction. *Acta Med Austriaca* 1995; 22: 69-72.

[11] Gosker HR, Wouters EF, van der Vusse GJ, and Schols AM. Skeletal muscle dysfunction in chronic obstructive pulmonary disease and chronic heart failure; underlying mechanism and therapy perspectives. *Am J Clin Nutr* 2000; 71: 1033-1047.

[12] Tan S, Zhou F, Nielsen VG, Wang Z, Gladson CL, and Parks DA. Increased injury following intermittent fetal hypoxia-reoxygenation is associated with increased free-radical production in nfetal rabbit brain. *J Neuropathol Exp Neurol* 1999; 972-981.

[13] Elsner R, Oyasaeter S, Almaas R, and Saugstad OD. Diving seals, ischemia-reperfusion and oxygen radicals. *Comp Biochem Physiol* 1998; 119: 975-980.

[14] Ceretelli P. Muscle energetics and ultrastructure in chronic hypoxia. *Respiration* 1009; 59: 24-29.

[15] Green HJ, Sutton JR, Cymerman A, Young PM, and Houston CS. Operation Everest II: adaptations in human skeletal muscles. *J Appl Physiol* 1989: 2454-2461.

[16] Duranteau J, Chandel NS, Kulisz A, Shao Z, and Shumacker PT. Intracellular signaling by reactive oxygen species during hypoxia in cardiomyocytes. *J Biol Chem* 1998; 273: 11619-111624.

[17] Sirsjo A, Arstrand K, Kagedal B, Nylander G, and Gidlof A. In situ microdialysis for monitoring of extracellular gluthatione levels in normal , ischemic and post-ischemic skeletal muscle. *Free Radic Res* 1996; 25:385-391.

[18] Vanden Hoch TL, Becker LB Shao ZH, Li CQ and shumaker PT. preconditioning in cardiomyocytes protects by attenuating oxidant stress at reperfusion. *Circ Res* 2000; 86: 541-548.

[19] Fletcher EC. Effects of episodic hypoxia on sympathetic activity and blood pressure. *Respir Physiol* 2000; 119:189-197.

[20] Sica AL, Greenberg HE, Ruggiero DA, and Scharf SM. Chronic intermittent hypoxia : a model of sympathetic activation in the rat. *Resp Physiol* 2000; 121: 173- 184.

[21] Smith ML, and Muenter NK. Effect of hypoxia on sympathetic neural control in humans. *Respir Physiol* 2000; 121: 163-171.

[22] Narckievicz K, van de Borne PJ, Pesek CA, Dyken ME, and Somers VK. Selective potentiation of peripheral chemoreflex sensitivity in obstructive sleep apnea. *Circulation* 1999; 99: 1183-1189.

[23] Philips BG, Kato M, Narkiewicz K, Choe I, and Somers VK. Increases in leptin levels, sympathetic drive, and weight gain in obstructive sleep apnea. *Am J Physiol Heart Circ Physiol* 2000; 279: H234- H237.

[24] Wojtaszewski JFP, Lausten JL, Derave W and Ritcher EA. Hypoxia and contractions do not utilize the same signaling mechanism in stimulating skeletal muscle glucose transport. *Biochim Biophys Acta* 1998; 1380: 396-404.

[25] Youn JH, Gulva EA, Henriksen EJ, and Holloszy JO. Interactions between effects of W-7, insulin, and Hypoxia on glucose transport. *Am J Physiol Regulatory Integrative Comp Physiol* 1994; 267: R888-R894.

[26] Bunn HF and Poyton RO. Oxygen sensing and molecular adaptation to hypoxia. *Physiol Rev* 1996; 76: 839-895.

[27] Kasalicky J, Ressl J, Urbanova D, Widimsky J, Ostadal B, Pelouch V, Vizek M, Prochaska J. Relative organ blood flow in rats exposed to intermittent high altitude hypoxia. *Pflügers Arch* 1977; 368: 111-115.

[28] Derave W and Hespel P. Role of adenosine in regulating glucose uptake during contractions and hypoxia in rat skeletal muscle. *J Physiol* (Lond) 1999; 515: 255-263.

[29] Bell D, Collier A, Matthews DM, Cooksey EJ, Mc Hardy GJ, Clarke BF. Are reduced lung volumes in IDDM due to defect in connective tissue? *Diabetes 1988;* 37: 829 - 831.

[30] Schnack C, Festa A, Schwarzmaier-D'Assie A, Harber P, Schernthaner G. Pulmonary dysfunction in type 1 diabetes in relation to metabolic long-term control and to incipient diabetic nephropathy. *Nephron* 1996; 74: 395 - 400.

[31] Innocenti F, Fabbri A, Anichini R, Tuci S, Pettina G, Vannucci F, De GL, Seghieri G. Indications to reduced pulmonary function in type 1 (insulin-dependent) diabetes mellitus. *Diabetes Res Clin Pract* 1985; 1: 95 – 101.

[32] Primhak RA, Whincup G, Tsanakas JN,Milner RD.Reduced vital capacity in insulin-dependent diabetes. *Diabetes* 1987;36:324–326.

[33] Matsubara T, Hara F. The pulmonary function and histopathological studies of the lung in diabetes mellitus. *Nippon Ika Daigaku Zasshi* 1991;58:528–536.

[34] Sandler M, Bunn AE, Stewart RI. Cross-section study of pulmonary function in patients with insulin-dependent diabetes mellitus. *Am Rev Respir Dis* 1987;135:1223–1229.

[35] Strojek K, Ziora D, Sroczynski JW, Oklek K. Pulmonary complications of type 1 (insulin-dependent) diabetic patients. *Diabetologia* 1992; 35: 1173–1176.

[36] Schernthaner G, Haber P, Kummer F, Ludwig H. Lung elasticity in juvenile-onset diabetes mellitus. *Am Rev Respir Dis* 1977;116:544–546.

[37] Maccioni FJ, Colebatch HJ. Lung volume and distensibility in insulin dependent diabetes mellitus. *Am Rev Respir Dis* 1991;143:1253–1256.

[38] Katoh J, Hara Y, Kurusu M, Miyaji J, Narutaki K. Cardiorespiratory function as assessed by exercise testing in patients with non-insulin- dependent diabetes mellitus. *J Int Med Res* 1996;24:209–213.

[39] Schmidt MI, Duncan BB, Sharrett AR, Lindberg G, Savage PJ, Offenbacher S, Azambuja MI, Tracy RP, Heiss G. Markers of inflammation and prediction of diabetes mellitus in adults (Atherosclerosis Risk in Communities study): a cohort study. *Lancet* 1999; 13: 211-215.

[40] Duncan BB, Schmidt MI, Offenbacher S, Wu KK, Savage PJ, Heiss G. Factor VIII and other hemostasis variables are related to incident diabetes in adults: Atherosclerosis Risk in Communities (ARIC) Study. *Diabetes Care* 1999; 22: 767-772.

[41] Rodrigues-Moran M, Guerrero-Romero F. Increased levels of C-reactive Protein in noncontrolled type II diabetic subjects. *J Diabetes Complications* 1999; 13: 211-215.

[42] Bloomgarden ZT. American Diabetes Association Annual meeting, 1999: more on cardiovascular disease. *Diabetes Care* 2000; 23: 845-852.

[43] Moller DE. Potential role of TNF-alpha in the pathogenesis of insulin resistance and type 2 diabetes. *Trends Endocrinol Metab* 2000; 11: 212-217.

[44] Higgins M, Keller J, Becker M, Howatt W, Landis JR, Rotman H, Weg J, Higgins I. An index of risk for obstructive airways disease. *Am Rev Respir Dis* 1982; 125: 144-151.

[45] Turato G, Di Stefano A, Maestrelli P. et al. Effects of smoking cessation on airways inflammation in chronic bronchitis. *Am J Respir Crit Care Med* 1995; 152; 1262-1267.

[46] Rutgers SR, Postma DS, ten Hacken NH et al. Ongoing airway inflammation in patients with COPD who do not currently smoke. *Thorax* 2000; 55: 12-18.

[47] Walter RE, Beise A, Givelber RJ, O'Connor GT, Gottlieb DJ. Association between glycemic state and lung function. The Framingham Heart Study. *Am J Respir Crit Care Med* 2003; 167: 911-916.

[48] Arnalich F, Hernanz A, Lopez-Maderuelo D, Pena JM, Camacho J, Mader R Vazquez JJ, Montiel C. Enhanced acute-phase response and oxidative stress in older adults with type II diabetes . *Horm Metab Res* 2000; 32: 407-412.

[49] Brownlee M. Biochemistry and molecular cell biology of diabetic complications. *Nature* 2001; 414: 813-820.

[50] Roehlecke C, Kuhnt AK, Fehrenbach H, Werner C, Funk RH, Kasper M. Resistance of L132 lung cell clusters to glyoxal-induced apoptosis. *Histochem Cell Biol* 2000; 114: 283-292.

[51] Fehrenbach H, Kasper M. Tschering T, Shearman MS, Schuh D, Muller M. Receptor for advanced glycation end-products (RAGE) exhibits highly differential cellular and subcellular localization in rat and human lung. *Cell Mol Biol* 1998; 44: 1147-1157.

[52] Lange P, Groth S, Kastrup J, Mortensen J, Appleyard M, Nyboe J, Jensen G, Schnohr P. Diabetes mellitus, plasma glucose and lung function in a cross-sectional population study. *Eur Respir J* 1989; 2: 14-19.

[53] Lange P, Groth S, Mortensen J, Appleyard M, Nyboe J, Schnohr P, Jensen G. Diabetes mellitus and ventilatory capacity: a five years follow-up study. *Eur Respir J.* 1990; 3: 288-292.

[54] Enright P, Kronmal R, Higgins M, Schenker M, Haponik E. Spirometry reference values for women and men 65 to 85 years of age *Am Rev Respir Dis* 1993; 147: 125-133.

[55] Sauerwein HP, Schols AMW. Glucose metabolism in chronic lung disease. *Clin Nutr.* 2002; 21:367-371.

[56] Hjalmarsen A, Asebo U, Birkeland K, Sager G, Jorde R. Impaired glucose tolerance in patients with chronic hypoxic pulmonary disease. *Diabetes Metab* 1996; 22: 37-42.

[57] Jakobsson P, Jorfeldt L, von Schenck H. Fat metabolism and its response to infusion of insulin and glucose in patients with advanced chronic pulmonary disease. *Clin Physiol* 1995; 15: 319-329.

[58] Jakobsson P, Jorfeldt L, von Schenck H. Insulin resistance is not exhibited by advanced chronic pulmonary disease patients. *Clin Physiol.* 1995; 15: 547- 555.

[59] Jakobsson P, Jorfeldt L. Oxygen supplementation increases glucose tolerance during euglycemic hyperinsulinemic glucose clamp procedure in patients with severe COPD and Chronic hypoxaemia. *Clin Physiol Funct Imag* 2006; 26: 271-274.
[60] Moran A, Pyzdrowski KL, Weinreb J, Kahn BB, Smith SA, Adams K, Seaquist ER. Insulin sensitivity in Cystic Fibrosis. *Diabetes* 1994; 43: 1020-1026.
[61] Monauni T, Zenti MG, Cretti A, Daniels MC Targher G, Caruso G, Caputo M, McClain D, Del Prato S, Giaccari A, Muggero M, Bonora E, Bonadonna RC. Effect of glucosammine infusion on insulin secretion and insulin actions in humans. *Diabetes* 2000; 49; 926-935.
[62] Ahmad T, Nelson R, Taylor R. Insulin sensitivity and metabolic clearance rate of insulin ib cystic fibrosis. *Metabolism* 1994; 43: 163-167.
[63] Hardin DS, LeBlanc A, Lukenbaugh S, Seilnheimer DK. Insulin resistance is associated with decreased clinical status in cystic fibrosis. *J Pediatr* 1997; 948-956.
[64] Hardin DS, LeBlanc A, Para L, Seilnheimer DK. Hepatic insulin resistance and defects in substrate utilization in cystic fibrosis. *Diabetes* 1999; 48: 1082-1087.
[65] Cucinotta D, De Luca F, Gigante A, Arrigo T, Di Benedetto A, Tedeschi A, Lombardo F, Romano G, Sferlazzas C. No changes of insulin sensitivity in cystic fibrosis with different d*egrees of glucose tolerance: an epidemiological and longitudinal study.* Eur J Endocrinol 1994; 130: 253-258.

5. Skeletal Muscle Dysfunction in Cardio-Pulmonary Disorders

Research has shown that impaired skeletal muscle function is an important predictor of exercise limitation in cardiopulmonary disorders, independent of the primary ventilatory and/or cardiac limitations [1-3]. In an extensive study on the effects of muscle weakness on exercise capacity in cardio-respiratory disorders Hamilton et al. (1995) [3] documented, that in healthy subjects as well as in patients with COPD or CHF the sense of leg effort is one of the main reasons to stop exercising. These data suggest that reduced endurance, i.e. fatigue, might be the limiting factor of peripheral muscle performance in both COPD and CHF patients. This is one of the first studies that stresses the striking similarities between chronic obstructive pulmonary disease and chronic heart failure, as well as the co-morbid association of the two disorders.

Cardiopulmonary disorders are associated with muscle weakness [4-10]. Strength, i.e. the capacity of the muscle to develop maximal force, and endurance i.e. the capacity of the muscle to maintain a certain force over time, are both involved in the limitation of muscle performance. This has been shown to be the result of early lactic acidosis of lower exercising limbs, as animal muscle deprived of oxygen rapidly fatigues and produce lactic acid [11]. On the other hand, it is unlikely that respiratory muscles of exercising COPD patients contribute to the lactic acidosis response [12], because their force component is presumably the most important characteristic to operate against high impedances of the respiratory system [13]. In CHF it has been documented that respiratory muscle strength, not fatigability correlates with the degree of dyspnea [14]. Thus, it seems that strength limits the performance in respiratory muscles, whereas endurance limits the performance in peripheral muscles.

Muscle wasting has also been documented in cardiopulmonary disorders and plays an important role in exercise intolerance [3, 15-24]. However, no direct relationship has been shown between skeletal muscles morphologic alteration and exercise performance. A detailed revision of morphology of peripheral and respiratory muscles is beyond the aim of present chapter. We remand the reader to more specific review. Here it is worth to say that data analyzing capillary density [25, 26], and morphometry of mitochondria suggest alteration of oxidative capacity of peripheral muscles in cardiopulmonary disorders [26].

Skeletal muscle metabolism may be investigated by using 31P-nuclear magnetic resonance (31P-NMR). Direct and non invasive assessment of high-energy phosphates and pH indicates impaired energy metabolism in skeletal muscles of COPD and CHF. It seems that anaerobic metabolism is enhanced in these diseases, and because this process yields far less ATP than does complete oxidative degradation of glucose, this could explain the reduced high-energy phosphate concentrations.

Mechanisms related to oxygen delivery to peripheral and respiratory muscles are considered the main factors determining exercise capacity. In both COPD and CHF oxygen delivery to peripheral muscles may be reduced as a result of hypoxaemia, reduced blood supply or both.

The relation between convectional-diffusional oxygen transport to the tissues and the prognosis of chronic obstructive pulmonary disease has been scanty documented. Clarification of this point is crucial since disturbance in tissue oxygenation may be critical in determining the outcome.

Kawakami et al. [27] demonstrated that with respect to oxygen supply to tissues, mixed venous oxygenation, i.e. the diffusional component, is one of the prognostic factors in COPD, whereas the coefficient of oxygen deliver, i.e. the convectional components in the vascular system do not differentiate survivors from non-survivors. Mixed venous oxygenation approximates mean tissue oxygen tension, which is a statistical abstraction that represents an overall index of the state of tissue oxygenation [28]. A convenient non-invasive estimation of tissue oxygenation is represented by oxygen extractivity.

The term "oxygen extractivity", originally proposed by Siggaard-Andersen (29) indicates the property which allows tissues to extract the usual amount of oxygen without a fall in oxygen tension below the usual venous level. This is measured along the shape of the oxygen-binding curve, and quantified as oxygen extraction tension (PaO_{2x}) (30). PaO_{2x} describes disturbances in oxygen availability depending on arterial oxygen tension, hemoglobin oxygen affinity and hemoglobin oxygen capacity, and reflects adjustments of cardiac output to maintain normal venous oxygen tension, if oxygen consumption is normal (31, 32). A disturbance in one of those parameters and compensatory changes in both of the other two summarize complex interactions related to either intrapulmonary oxygen transport and blood supply, or systemic regulatory aspect of hemoglobin oxygen transport.

Does tissue hypoxia initiate the events leading to metabolic wasting in patients with advanced COPD?"

Previous studies (33, 34) indicated that COPD patients with a low cardiac output pattern experience oxygen desaturation during exercise, and that tissue hypoxia may account at least in part for muscle weakness and impaired performance during physical activity. This issue has been further addressed by Schols et al. (35) who suggested the notion of a link between CPR and impaired exercise capacity and distress due to respiratory symptoms. Moreover, Broekhuizen et al. (36) regarded to high sensitivity C_Reactive Protein (CRP) as a marker for metabolic and functional impairment in patients with advanced COPD. Surprisingly however, the authors found no significant difference in arterial oxygen tension (PaO_2) between the groups with normal, and respectively raised CRP levels.

Baldi et al. (unpublished observation) found a close relationship between CRP and PaO_{2x} (r=0.72), as assessed by the Siggaard-Andersen's algorithm in 44 patients with stable COPD. No relationship between CRP and PaO_2 (r=0. 21). The strong association finding argues for a pathogenetic link between systemic inflammation and reduced oxygen extractivity at tissue level. These data deserve further attention to unravel molecular responses elicited by tissue hypoxia within the lung, the systemic circulation, and the muscles. Hence, they invite to speculate on a general system of sensing and signaling of hypoxia to the transcriptional machinery in the nucleus of cells. In this contest CRP might also have a regulatory role on the hypoxic sensing and signaling system. Further investigation on this field is needed.

Tissue hypoxia and oxygen flux to skeletal and cardiac muscles is also a modulator of oxidative stress. Oxidative stress is supposed to be another factor contributing to muscle cell damage via reactive oxygen species, as documented by increased plasma concentration of lipid peroxidation products in both COPD and CHF patients [37, 38].

The main source of these oxygen free radicals is mitochondria because 2–5% of the oxygen consumed is not fully reduced in the electron transport chain and may leak away as superoxide radicals [39, 40]. An alternative source of free radicals is immune cells activated during inflammation [41]. Monocytes and macrophages produce the cytokine tumor necrosis factor alfa (TNF-a), which may in turn induce oxidative stress in myocytes [42]. Indeed, elevated TNF-a blood concentrations have been found in both COPD [43-45] and CHF [46-50] patients, particularly in those patients with weight loss or muscle wasting.

Susceptibility to these free radicals depends largely on the antioxidant status of tissues [40]. Repeated exposure to oxidative stress, during long-term physical training for example, stimulates the increase of antioxidant scavengers and enzymes such as reduced glutathione, vitamin E (in cell membranes), superoxide dismutase, glutathione peroxidase, and catalase against oxygen free radicals [39, 40, 51-53]. Oxygen flux to muscles and the resulting oxidative stress can increase tremendously during exercise [40, 54] and the disuse of muscles thus may take away this antioxidant-stimulating trigger and result in low antioxidant status. Chronic hypoxia probably acts in the same way because less oxygen is available to form reactive oxygen species. Limitations of oxygen supply are indeed found to be associated with reductions in superoxide dismutase activity in mammalian tissues like brain, lungs, and heart, although this change was not found in skeletal muscle tissue [55, 56]. In addition, in myocytes obtained from chronically hypoxic human myocardium cultured at low oxygen tension, antioxidant enzyme activities were lower than in myocytes cultured at a higher oxygen tension, illustrating the direct modulatory effect of oxygen [57]. In vivo and in vitro hypoxia-reoxygenation studies showed that oxygen oversupply after a period of oxygen shortage may give rise to free radical formation in myocytes [55, 58, 59]. Accordingly, in COPD and CHF patients, chronic hypoxia may result in reduced antioxidant status and occasional bouts of exercise may cause a burst of free radicals that exceeds the capacity of the defense system [39]. It is also possible that the patients' reduced oxidative capacity itself leads to enhanced oxidative stress because the sudden oversupply of oxygen during exercise is inefficiently metabolized.

Reactive oxygen species are capable of damaging lipids and proteins [39, 40, 51, 60]. Radicals that react with fatty acyl moieties in membrane phospholipids cause a chain reaction of peroxidations that increase the membrane permeability [60]. Maintenance of membrane integrity is crucial for adequate functioning of the respiratory chain because the driving force for oxidative ATP synthesis is the electrochemical proton gradient over the inner membrane of the mitochondrion, which is generated during the electron transfer from NADH to oxygen [61]. Leakage of ions through a more permeable mitochondrial inner membrane may thus impair mitochondrial function by uncoupling oxidative phosphorylation. Indeed, rats with an inherited overproduction of oxygen free radicals showed a higher degree of lipid peroxidation and protein damage in combination with impaired respiratory chain function in liver mitochondria than did control rats [2]. Furthermore, a marked decrease in ATP concentrations was observed in cultured endothelial cells exposed to reactive oxygen species [63]. In addition, there is evidence that an intracellular calcium overload, probably caused by a damaged sarcoplasmic reticulum membrane in combination with impaired activity of calcium ATPases, accompanies oxidative stress in animal myocytes [39, 55, 58, 59, 64-66], which may further uncouple respiration from ATP production through extensive depolarization of the inner membrane [67].

Protein oxidation by oxygen free radicals leads to formation of carbonyl groups on amino acid residues, which may modify the structure or chemical properties of the proteins affected [68]. These alterations may cause a decline in protein function or even complete protein unfolding. The latter gives rise to enhanced susceptibility to proteinases. These modified proteins may also be recognized as foreign substances and, hence, be attacked by the immune system. Whether radical-induced protein damage plays a role in the abnormalities in muscles of COPD and CHF patients is unclear. It was shown in animal studies that oxidative stress induced in vivo caused myofibrillar muscle protein modification and that these proteins were rapidly degraded by proteases [69]. Thus, theoretically, muscle atrophy can be enhanced by radical-induced protein damage. Indeed, it was shown that a calcium overload is involved in muscle atrophy [70] and that vitamin E deficiency facilitates muscle wasting and necrosis [71], both probably mediated by oxidative damage to proteins. Also, in human skeletal muscle it was shown that mitochondria and mitochondrial proteins were more susceptible to oxidative damage than were other subcellular components [72], which suggests that protein damage may cause impaired oxidative metabolism.

As opposed to necrosis, which is the result of exogenous damage, apoptosis of muscle cells is an active process of cell death, which has also been associated with oxidative stress [73]. In this study, the exposure of rat myoblasts to nitric oxide or hydrogen peroxide led to apoptotic cell death. Because these chemical stimuli are also released by immune cells, we cannot exclude the possibility that apoptosis underlies muscle wasting during inflammation.

References

[1] Cotes JE, Zejda J, King B.Lung function impairment as a guide to exercise limitation in work-related lung disorders. *Am Rev Respir Dis* 1988; 137: 1089-1093.

[2] Schols AM, Mostert R, Soeters PB, Wouters EF. Body composition and exercise performance in patients with chronic obstructive pulmonary disease. *Thorax* 1991; 46:695-699.

[3] Hamilton AL, Killian KJ, Summers E, Jones NL. Muscle strength, symptom intensity, and exercise capacity in patients with cardiopulmonary disorders *Am J Respir Crit Care Med*; 1995; 152: 2021-2031.

[4] Sullivan MJ, Hawthorne MH. Exercise intolerance in patients with chronic heart failure. *Prog Cardiovasc Dis* 1995; 38: 1-22.

[5] Decramer M, Gosselink R, Troosters T, Verschueren M, Evers G. Muscle weakness is related to utilization of health care resources in COPD patients. *Eur Respir J* 1997; 10: 417- 423.

[6] Bernhard S, LeBlanc P, Whittom F et al. Peripheral muscles weakness in patients with chronic obstructive pulmonary disease. *Am J Respir Crit Care Med* 1998; 158: 629-634.

[7] Gosselink R, Troosters T, Decramer M. Peripheral muscle weakness contributes to exercise limitation in COPD. *Am J Respir Crit Care Med* 1996; 153: 629-634.

[8] Zhattara-Hartmann MC, Badier M, Guillot C, Tomei C Jammes Y. Maximal force and endurance to fatigue of respiratory and skeletal muscles in chronic hypoxemic patients: the effects of oxygen breathing. *Muscle Nerve* 1995; 18: 945-502.

[9] Chua TP, Anker SD, Harrington D, Coats AJ. Inspiratory muscle strength is a determinant of maximum oxygen consumption in chronic heart failure. *Br Heart J* 1995; 74: 381-385.

[10] McParland C, Resch EF, Krishnan B, Wang Y, Cujec B, Gallagher CG. Inspiratory muscle weakness in chronic heart failure: role of nutrition and electrolyte status and systemic myopathy. *Am J Respir Crit Care Med*; 1995; 151: 1101-1107.

[11] Douglas CG. Coordination of the respiration and circulation with variation of bodily activity. *Lancet* 1927; 2: 213 - 30.

[12] Engelen MP, Casaburi R, Rucker R, Carithers E. Contribution of the respiratory muscles to the lactic acidosis of heavy exercise in COPD. *Chest* 1995; 108: 1246-1251.

[13] O'Donnell DE, Webb KA. Exertional breathlessness in patients with chronic airflow limitation. The role of lung hyperinflation. *Am Rev Respir Dis* 1993; 148: 1351-1357.

[14] Mancini DM, Henson D, LaManca J, Levine S. Respiratory muscle function and dyspnea in patients with chronic congestive heart failure. *Circulation* 1982; 86: 909-918.

[15] Harrington D, Anker SD, Chua TP et al. Skeletal muscle function and its relation to exercise tolerance in chronic heart failure. *J Am Coll Cardiol* 1997; 30: 1758-1764.

[16] Wilson JR, Mancini DM. The mechanism of extertional fatigue in heart failure. *Cardioscience* 1990; 1: 13-17.

[17] Shepard RJ. Exercise for patients with congestive heart failure. *Sport Med* 1997; 23: 75-92.

[18] Miyagi K, Asanoi H, Ishizaka S et al. Importance of total leg muscle mass for exercise intolerance in chronic heart failure. *Jpn Heart J* 1994; 35: 15-26.
[19] Engelen MP, Schols AM, Baken WC, Wesseling GJ, Wouters EF. Nutritional depletion in relation to respiratory and peripheral skeletal muscle function in out-patients with COPD. *Eur Respir J* 1994; 7: 1793- 1797.
[20] Whittom F, Jobin J, Simard PM et al. Histochemical and morphological characteristics of the vastus lateralis muscle in patients with chronic obstructive pulmonary disease. *Med Sci Sports Exerc* 1998; 30: 1467-1474.
[21] Wuyam B, Payem JF, Levy P et al. Metabolism and aerobic capacity of skeletal muscle in chronic respiratory failure related to chronic obstructive pulmonary disease. *Eur Respir J 1992*; 5: 157-162.
[22] Rochester DF. Body weight and respiratory muscle functionin chronic obstructive pulmonary disease. *Am Rev Respir Dis* 1986; 134: 646-648.
[23] Morrison WL, Gibson JN, Scrimgeour C, Rennie MJ. Muscle wasting in emphysema *Cli Sci* 1988; 75: 415-420.
[24] Sato Y, Asoh T, Honda Y, Fujimatsu Y, Higushi I, Oizumi K. Morphologic and histochemical evaluation of muscle in patients in patients with chronic pulmonary emphysema, manifesting generalized emaciation. *Eur Neurol* 1997; 37: 116-121.
[25] Sauleda J, Garcia-Palmer F, Wiesner RJ, Tarraga S, Harting I, Tomas P, Gomez C, Saus C, Palou A, Agusti AG. Cytochrome oxidase activity and mitochondrial gene expression in skeletal muscle of patients with chronic obstructive pulmonary disease. *Am J Respir Crit Care Med* 1998;157(5 Pt 1):1413-1417.
[26] Chance B, JS Leigh, J Kent, K McCully, S Nioka, BJ Clark, Maris JM. Multiple controls of oxidative metabolism in living tissue as studied by phosphorus magnetic resonance. *Proc Natl Acad Sci U.S.A.* 1986; 83: 9548-9462.
[27] Kawakami Y, Kishi F, Yamamoto H, Miyamoto K. Relation of oxygen delivery, mixed venous oxygenation and pulmonary hemodynamics to prognosis in chronic obstructive pulmonary disease. *N Engl J Med* 1983; 308: 1045-1049.
[28] Tenney SM, Mithoefer JC. The relationship of mixed venous oxygen transport: with special reference to adaptations to high altitude pulmonary disease. *Am Rev Respir Dis 1982*; 125: 474 - 479.
[29] Siggard-Andersen O, Fogh-Andersen N, Gøthgen IH, Larsen VH. Oxygen status of arterial and mixed venous blood. *Crit Care Med* 1995; 23:1284-1293.
[30] Siggaard-Andersen O, Wimberley PD, Gøthgen IH, Siggaard-Andersen M. A mathematical model of the haemoglobin-oxygen dissociation curve of human blood and of the oxygen partial pressure as a function of temperature. *Clin Chem* 1984; 30: 1646-1651.
[31] Ringsted C, Eliasen K, Gothgen IH, Siggaard-Andersen O. Positive correlation between 'the arterial oxygen extraction tension' and mixed venous pO2 but lack of correlation between 'the oxygen compensation factor' and cardiac output in 38 patients.*Scand J Clin Lab Invest Suppl.* 1990;203:67-73.
[32] Radwan L, Daum S. Evaluation of mixed venous oxygenation on the basis of arterial oxygen tension in chronic lung diseases. *Respiration* 1980;40(4):194-200.

[33] Filley GF, Beckwitt HJ, Reeves JT, Mitchell R. Chronic obstructive bronchopulmonary disease. II. Oxygen transport in the two clinical types. *Am J Med* 1968; 44: 26-38.

[34] Burrows B, LJ Kettel, AH Niden, M Rabinowitz, Diener CF. Patterns of cardiovascular dysfunction in chronic obstructive lung disease. *N Engl J Med* 1972; 27: 912-918.

[35] Schols AM, Buurma WA, Staal van den Brekel AJ, Dentener MA, Wouters EF. Evidence for a relation between metabolic derangements and increased levels of inflammatory mediators in a subgroup of patients with chronic obstructive pulmonary disease. *Thorax* 1996; 51: 819-824.

[36] Broekhuizen R, Wouters EFM, Creutzberg EC, Schols AM. Raised CRP levels mark metabolic and functional impairment in advanced COPD. *Thorax* 2006; 61: 17-22.

[37] Rahman I, Morrison D, Donaldson K, MacNee W. Systemic oxidative stress in asthma, COPD, and smokers. *Am J Respir Crit Care Med* 1996; 154: 1055-1060.

[38] Keith M, Geranmayegan A, sole MJ,et al. Increased oxidative stress in patients with congestive heart failure. *J Am Coll Cardiol* 1998; 31: 1352-1356.

[39] Giuliani A, Cestaro B. Exercise, free radical generation and vitamins. *Eur J Cancer Prev* 1997;6:S55–67.

[40] Ji LL. Exercise, oxidative stress, and antioxidants. *Am J Sports Med* 1996;24:S20–4.

[41] Reid MB. Reactive oxygen and nitric oxide in skeletal muscle. *News Physiol Sci* 1996;11:114–9.

[42] Buck M, Chojkier M. Muscle wasting and dedifferentiation induced by oxidative stress in a murine model of cachexia is prevented by inhibitors of nitric oxide synthesis and antioxidants. *EMBO J* 1996;15:1753–65.

[43] de Godoy I, Donahoe M, Calhoun WJ, Mancino J, Rogers RM. Elevated TNF-a production by peripheral blood monocytes of weight-losing COPD patients. *Am J Respir Crit Care Med* 1996;153:633–7.

[44] Schols AM, Buurman WA, Staal van den Brekel AJ, Dentener MA, Wouters EF. Evidence for a relation between metabolic derangements and increased levels of inflammatory mediators in a subgroup of patients with chronic obstructive pulmonary disease. *Thorax* 1996;51:819–24.

[45] Di Francia M, Barbier D, Mege JL, Orehek J. Tumor necrosis factor-a levels and weight loss in chronic obstructive pulmonary disease. *Am J Respir Crit Care Med* 1994;150:1453–5.

[46] Ferrari R, Bachetti T, Confortini R, et al. Tumor necrosis factor soluble receptors in patients with various degrees of congestive heart failure. *Circulation* 1995;92:1479–86.

[47] Katz SD, Rao R, Berman JW, et al. Pathophysiological correlates of increased serum tumor necrosis factor in patients with congestive heart failure. Relation to nitric oxide-dependent vasodilation in the forearm circulation. *Circulation* 1994;90:12–6.

[48] Levine B, Kalman J, Mayer L, Fillit HM, Packer M. Elevated circulating levels of tumor necrosis factor in severe chronic heart failure. *N Engl J Med* 1990;323:236–41.

[49] McMurray J, Abdullah I, Dargie HJ, Shapiro D. Increased concentrations of tumour necrosis factor in "cachectic" patients with severe chronic heart failure. *Br Heart J* 1991;66:356–8.

[50] Anker SD, Clark AL, Kemp M, et al. Tumor necrosis factor and steroid metabolism in chronic heart failure: possible relation to muscle wasting. *J Am Coll Cardiol* 1997;30:997–1001.
[51] Clarkson PM. Antioxidants and physical performance. *Crit Rev Food Sci Nutr* 1995;35:131–41.
[52] Sen CK, Hänninen O. Physiological antioxidants. In: Sen KC, Packer L, Hänninen O, eds. *Exercise and oxygen toxicity*. Amsterdam: Elsevier Science BV, 1994:89–126.
[53] Ohishi S, Kizaki T, Nagasawa J, et al. Effects of endurance training on superoxide dismutase activity, content and mRNA expression in rat muscle. *Clin Exp Pharmacol Physiol* 1997;24:326–32.
[54] Jackson MJ. Exercise and oxygen radical production by muscle. In: Sen KC, Packer L, Hänninen O, eds. *Exercise and oxygen toxicity*. Amsterdam: Elsevier Science BV, 1994:49–57.
[55] Ferrari R, Ceconi C, Curello S, Alfieri O, Visioli O. Myocardial damage during ischaemia and reperfusion. *Eur Heart J* 1993;14:25–30.
[56] Liu J, Simon LM, Phillips JR, Robin ED. Superoxide dismutase (SOD) activity in hypoxic mammalian systems. *J Appl Physiol* 1977; 42:107–10.
[57] Li RK, Mickle DA, Weisel RD, et al. Effect of oxygen tension on the anti-oxidant enzyme activities of tetralogy of Fallot ventricular myocytes. *J Mol Cell Cardiol* 1989;21:567–75.
[58] Gardner TJ. Oxygen radicals and myocardial stunning. *J Card Surg* 1994;9:422–4.
[59] Smith DR, Stone D, Darley-Usmar VM. Stimulation of mitochondrial oxygen consumption in isolated cardiomyocytes after hypoxia-reoxygenation. *Free Radic Res* 1996;24:159–66.
[60] Haramaki N, Packer L. Oxidative stress indices in exercise. In: Sen KC, Packer L, Hänninen O, eds. *Exercise and oxygen toxicity*. Amsterdam: Elsevier Science BV, 1994:77–87.
[61] Stryer L. *Biochemistry*. New York: WH Freeman and Company, 1988.
[62] Salganik RI, Shabalina IG, Solovyova NA, Kolosova NG, Solovyov VN, Kolpakov AR. Impairment of respiratory functions in mitochondria of rats with an inherited hyperproduction of free radicals. *Biochem Biophys Res Commun* 1994;205:180–5.
[63] Spragg RG, Hinshaw DB, Hyslop PA, Schraufstätter IU, Cochrane CG. Alterations in adenosine triphosphate and energy charge in cultured endothelial and P388D1 cells after oxidant injury. *J Clin Invest* 1985;76:1471–6.
[64] Astier C, Rock E, Lab C, Gueux E, Mazur A, Rayssiguier Y. Functional alterations in sarcoplasmic reticulum membranes of magnesium-deficient rat skeletal muscle as consequences of free radical-mediated process. *Free Radic Biol Med* 1996;20:667–74.
[65] Wang SY, Clague JR, Langer GA. Increase in calcium leak channel activity by metabolic inhibition or hydrogen peroxide in rat ventricular myocytes and its inhibition by polycation. *J Mol Cell Cardiol* 1995;27:211–22.
[66] Xu KY, Zweier JL, Becker LC. Hydroxyl radical inhibits sarcoplasmic reticulum Ca^{2+}-ATPase function by direct attack on the ATP binding site. *Circ Res* 1997;80:76–81.

[67] Minezaki KK, Suleiman MS, Chapman RA. Changes in mitochondrial function induced in isolated guinea-pig ventricular myocytes by calcium overload. *J Physiol* (Lond) 1994;476:459–71.
[68] Dean RT, Fu SL, Stocker R, Davies MJ. Biochemistry and pathology of radical-mediated protein oxidation. *Biochem J* 1997;324:1–18.
[69] Nagasawa T, Hatayama T, Watanabe Y, Tanaka M, Niisato Y, Kitts DD. Free radical mediated effects on skeletal muscle protein in rats treated with fe nitrilotriacetate. *Biochem Biophys Res Commun* 1997;231:37–41.
[70] Soares JM, Duarte JA, Carvalho J, Appell HJ. The possible role of intracellular Ca^{2+} accumulation for the development of immobilization atrophy. *Int J Sports Med* 1993;14:437–9.
[71] Thomas PK, Cooper JM, King RH, et al. Myopathy in vitamin E deficient rats: muscle fibre necrosis associated with disturbances of mitochondrial function. *J Anat* 1993;183:451–61.
[72] Haycock JW, Jones P, Harris JB, Mantle D. Differential susceptibility of human skeletal muscle proteins to free radical induced oxidative damage: a histochemical, immunocytochemical and electron microscopical study in vitro. Acta *Neuropathol* (Berl) 1996;92:331–40.
[73] Stangel M, Zettl UK, Mix E, et al. H_2O_2 and nitric oxide-mediated oxidative stress induce apoptosis in rat skeletal muscle myoblasts. *J Neuropathol Exp Neurol* 1996;55:36–43.

6. Therapeutic Targeting of Emphysema

Despite the explosion of knowledge based upon multidisciplinary research, mechanisms leading to the unique pattern of alveolar destruction in emphysema are not adequately understood. Consequently, the lack of novel or even currently effective treatment remains a significant challenge stimulating the search for new pharmacological, surgical and rehabilitative strategies. On the bottom line, the optimal therapeutic management of pulmonary emphysema recapitulates to treatment of COPD.

Emphysema therapy shares with COPD several domains: pharmacological strategies, rehabilitation strategies, and long-term oxygen therapy (LTOT). Among those, only two domains are specifically dedicated to the treatment of pulmonary emphysema: surgical strategies aimed at lung volume reduction, and nutritional interventions aimed at counteracting weight loss.

Therapeutic Pharmacologic Strategies

The available treatments for the management of stable COPD are used to prevent and control symptoms, reduce the exacerbations, increase exercise tolerance, and improve health status [1].

Long-acting β_2-agonists such as Salmeterol combine symptom control with improvement in lung function, and provide clinical relevant improvements in health status. Inhaled corticosteroids are recommended for the treatment of patients with the more severe disease and frequent exacerbations, and inhalation of the combination of long acting β_2-agonists and inhaled corticosteroids is more effective in improving lung function and symptoms and reducing exacerbations than either drug alone [2-4].

No currently available treatments have been reported to reduce the exaggerated airway wall inflammation of chronic obstructive lung disease, before the report of the SCO30005 Study Group [5].

To test the hypothesis that combined inhaled long acting β_2-agonists and corticosteroids reduce inflammation, the authors took bronchial biopsies and induced sputum samples from 140 current and former smokers with moderate to severe disease. Patients were randomized in a 13 weeks double blind study to placebo or salmeterol/fluticasone propionate 50/500 mg twice daily. This is the largest multicentric clinical trial involving repeat bronchial biopsies and sputum sample in COPD patients in stage II and III, according to GOLD guidelines. Data demonstrate a broad spectrum of anti-inflammatory effects of currently available combination therapy on several key parameters biopsy, $CD8^+$ cells, and sputum neutrophils. These findings support the consideration that combination treatment applied earlier than currently proposed guidelines may be helpful. They also provide a rationale for further investigation on combination therapy in disease progression and survival.

The TORCH (Toward a Revolution in COPD Health) trial [6] is currently investigating the effect of Salmeterol/Fluticasone propionate combination on all causes of mortality in COPD.

Thus, bronchodilators remain an active area for both basic and clinical investigation although they have been in use for several decades. Both β_2-agonists and anticholinergic agents seem to have important clinical benefits that are mediated through non-bronchodilator effects. All the three classes of bronchodilators are reported to have both anti-inflammatory effect and effect on tissue remodeling. Finally, rethinking the means by which bronchodilator effects are assessed could be a new promising therapeutic strategy, as it is well documented that effect on lung volume and in particular effects that occur with tachypnoea are crucial physiological features [7,8].

Prevention and symptom control involves also treatment with mucolytic and antioxidant drugs. Phlegm resulting from inflammation and mucociliary clearance impairment is a cardinal sign causing symptoms and predisposing to bacterial infection. In addition oxidant and antioxidant imbalance has been shown to be present in the pathogenesis of COPD, and especially of pulmonary emphysema.

Physiotherapy and rehidratation, in order to facilitate expectoration of mucus, have been cornerstones in COPD therapy and rehabilitation. Many drugs with supposed mucolytic properties have been tried. However, the efficacy of mucolytics is controversial.

Data indicate that at least acetylcystein 200 mg three times daily seems to have some effect on the sputum production and its viscosity [9]. A Thiol derivate erdostine has also shown effects on sputum production and symptoms [10]. Studies that measure mucus transport rate *in vivo* have provided conflicting results [11-13]. Hence, the mode of action resulting in the mucolytic effect is not fully known.

On the other hand, a treatment for emphysema that involves stimulating the lung to grow new alveoli has been considered a remote possibility. However, a report by Gloria and Donald Massaro suggests there may be a flicker of hope that this approach might be successful in the future (14). The authors showed that treatment with all-trans retinoic acid (RA) reversed the increase in lung volume, while maintaining number, average volume, and surface area of the alveoli after the induction of emphysema in rats using the proteolytic enzyme, elastase. Their hypothesis that RA might prevent elastase-induced emphysematous destruction was based on previous evidence that retinoids play a regulatory role in the formation of alveoli during fetal development. The Massaro's results should stimulate new experiments to confirm this finding, and fully investigate it as a form of therapy for emphysema. A recently published paper demonstrated safety and feasibility of all trans-retinoic acid administration in humans, but no effects on the emphysematous lesions progression assessed by means of CT scan [15]. Up to date the efficacy of antioxidants has not been satisfactorily established.

Other relevant pharmacological interventions in COPD address treatment and prevention of exacerbation by intensification of bronchodilator treatment, use of oxygen therapy [16], and management of nosocomial pneumonia to obtain the best use of available antimicrobial treatments and minimize the increase in microbial resistances [17]. These events greatly increase the economic burden imposed by COPD, and the hospital mortality [18], also they worse long-term outcome, with 40% mortality in the first years [19, 20].

Therapeutic Surgical Strategies

Many studies published in literature confirm that bullectomy improves dyspnea and airflow obstruction in patients with giant bullas with or without the association of functionally significant emphysema [21-27]. To date, surgery for bullous emphysema is regarded as a lesson learned for the surgery of end-stage emphysema. A bulla contributes to airflow obstruction that is reversible after bullectomy, independent of the presence of coexisting emphysema, and may predict postoperative improvement in ventilatory function with a simple and clinically useful formula [28].

Dr. Otto Brantingan, who claimed significant clinical improvements in small series of patients but had no physiologic studies to validate his clinical impression (29), introduced lung volume reduction surgery (LVRS) more than 40 years ago. Subsequently, it was shown that operation indeed improved airway function (30), but this improvement was transient (i.e., less than two years duration), (31). In the early 1990s, LVRS was reintroduced (32-34). Among the reasons for the renovated enthusiasm there are, on one hand, the extensive publicity released to the press extolling the merits of LVRS and the desperate plight of severely dyspnoeic patients with end-stage emphysema, improved surgical techniques including the use of surgical staples, thoracoscopic surgery, and improved critical care medicine facilities, on the other, improved pre- and postoperative evaluation and management of patients, due to widespread availability of sophisticated pulmonary function testing and vastly improved thoracic imaging.

HRCT of the chest enormously increased our ability to both discern the type of emphysema (panlobular, centrilobular, or paraseptal emphysema) and determine its location. Densitometry is an innovative technique that utilizes the actual X-ray attenuation values for the entire lung and allow an objective identification of extent of emphysema (35,36).

Up to now many preoperative assessment and surgical treatment for emphysema have been applied. Our understanding of the procedure and its effects however, have mostly stimulated more questions than answers. The National Emphysema Treatment trial (NETT), a multicentric clinical trial has involved both intervention and control group (pulmonary rehabilitation only) aimed at investigating the unanswered question about LVRS [37]: who is the best candidate for this procedure? How long do beneficial effects last? What is the true risk of the procedure? Is LVRS better than pulmonary rehabilitation? Do the benefits persist long enough to justify the risk and the cost of surgical intervention?

Unfortunately, most emphysema patients are poor candidates for any surgical intervention. A meticulous selection process is favored in which indications and contraindications are considered and the best solution is devised for each patient. Patients with hyperinflation, heterogeneous distribution of destruction, forced expiratory volume in 1 second (FEV_1) >20%, and a normal carbon dioxide tension (PCO_2) are offered LVRS while patients with diffuse disease, lower FEV_1, hypercapnia, and associated pulmonary hypertension are directed towards transplantation that has worked successfully for a limited number of patients with emphysema but it is severely limited by the lack of donor lungs [38-40].

Nutrition - Rehabilitation Strategies

The scientific roles of rehabilitation medicine were only discovered in 1994 [41]. As a consequence pulmonary rehabilitation remained an art for a long time rather than science based medicine. Rehabilitation interventions have largely been supportive and directed at patient education, changes in lifestyle, particularly smoking cessation, or changes directed to improve self management, exercise training muscle training, prevention of infections by immunization. As the disease advances, oxygen therapy and mechanical ventilation can offer further support (42).

Nowadays the scientific evidence for the effectiveness of pulmonary rehabilitation is overwhelming [43,44] and transplantation and LVRS have contributed to strengthen the interest around rehabilitation programs.

The components of a rehabilitation program are commonly tailored to improve exercise tolerance, to improve specific skeletal muscle resistance training, e.g. ventilatory and/or peripheral skeletal muscles, and to chest physiotherapy.

Exercise training improves muscular performance because strength, endurance, or both improve [45]. Disuse has been suggested to be an important factor responsible for the alterations in muscle metabolism in COPD and CHF. Disuse abnormalities possibly are reversed from training of the affected muscles. Indeed, exercise training improves exercise capacity in both COPD [46,47] and CHF [48-50] patients. Furthermore, increased cross-sectional areas of oxidative fibers and elevated oxidative enzyme activities in the quadriceps muscle in combination with less arterial lactate accumulation during exercise have been found in trained COPD patients [51, 52]. Training-induced increases in oxidative capacity and muscle mass of the quadriceps muscle have also been reported for CHF patients [53, 54]. Thus, in peripheral muscles, training induces a partial improvement of the oxidative capacity in combination with increased exercise performance, and higher fatigue resistance. Therefore, considering that fatigue is the main limiting factor in peripheral muscle performance, an endurance training protocol may be most suitable for improving the exercise capacity of limb muscles in COPD patients.

Improvement of oxidative capacity with training is not documented for respiratory muscles. However, the differences between respiratory and peripheral muscles in COPD and CHF suggest that different training approaches are required to effectively improve their performances. Whereas respiratory muscle training in CHF remains an unexplored field, a variety of studies have been performed for COPD [55]. Although training of respiratory muscle may improve its performance, there is little evidence of real clinical benefit. The best results are probably obtained with so-called resistance training [55], in which the inspiratory muscles are subjected to an increased pressure load. The fact that this is a kind of power training affecting respiratory muscle strength especially suggests that training of the diaphragm should be more focused on strength than on endurance [56, 57].

Another possible positive effect of exercise training is the increase in antioxidant status. As disuse has a negative effect on antioxidant status, and may therefore promote oxidative damage during occasional exercise, regular physical exercise involves a regular increase in exposure of muscle tissue to oxygen and training thus probably reduces the risk of oxidative stress [58].

All training programs must be integrated with nutritional support as nutritional status itself impact on quality of life, disability and handicap of COPD.

Nutritional disturbances and weight abnormalities in COPD are related to being either underweight or overweight. Although, the latter condition is not associated with increased mortality rate, it is worth to be treated by hypocaloric regimens together with physical training in order to improve the physical status. On the contrary weight loss, a condition present in about 20-30% of COPD patients [59, 60], impacts survival. Several retrospective studies have shown that weight loss [61, 62] and low body weight [63] are related to reduced survival rate, while weight gain is related to improved survival [61, 64].

More recently three studies one from Canada [65], one from the Netherlands [66] and one from Denmark [66] showed that depletion of FFM is particularly related to reduced survival rate, independent of body weight.

Reversal of weight loss in patients with COPD is not simply a matter of caloric supplementation, as malnutrition in COPD results from increased energy requirement [67]. Other factors may contribute to weight loss such as an inadequate caloric intake due to dyspnea, as well as gastrointestinal symptoms while eating, suppressed appetite from medications (e.g., theophylline), or malabsorption resulting in poor utilization of calories. Hence, psychosocial factors such as depression, poverty, cigarette smoking, eating and living arrangements may all contribute to poor nutrition. Resting energy expenditure (REE), as well as total daily energy expenditure (TDE) [68, 69] is increased depending on different mechanisms. While TDE seems to be dependent on increased oxygen consumption for activities [70], the REE has been related to persistent slow grade of inflammation [71, 72].

Evidence for a relation between metabolic derangements and increased levels of inflammatory mediators raise the question of an adequate assessment of energy requirements in COPD as well as of adherence to supplement prescription, which must be a supplement not a substitute of meals. Poor adherence to supplement prescription as well as an inadequate assessment of energy requirements may contribute to disappointing results obtained with nutritional intervention in outpatients [69]. On the contrary, placebo controlled randomized trials in clinically stable in-patients with COPD show a significant effect of oral nutritional support after 4 and 8 weeks on body weight, body composition and functional performance [73--75].

Nutrition and ventilation are intimately related, as oxygen is required for energy metabolism. Several randomized controlled trials compared the effects of high and low carbohydrate formulae in patients with stable COPD on immediate postprandial energy metabolism [76-79]. These data document adverse effects only in studies that used huge amount of oral nutritional supplement (ONS), i.e. 916 Kcal, that exceed the energy content of a normal meal. Delay of gastric emptying time is one reason, while post-prandial dyspnea is reported with high-fat ONS. Compared to macronutrient intake the portion size and daily distribution seem to be more relevant to avoid adverse effect of ONS.

When the goal of rehabilitation program is the increase of muscle mass, the combination of nutritional support and specific muscle stimulation by either exercise training or anabolic agents appear a relevant option. In a large clinical trial Schols et al. [80] documented significant weight gain, increase of fat free mass, and respiratory muscle strength with nutritional support combined to a general exercise program. The additional treatment with anabolic steroids provides similar increase in body weight, but a larger increase in fat free mass and muscles strength [80]. Other studies [81-83] confirm a positive effect of supplementation of anabolic steroids, although a substantial proportion of non-responders exists [84].

Several studies have shown that nutritional supplementation can improve both respiratory and peripheral muscle function in nutritionally depleted patients with COPD [85-87], but it is unclear, however, to what extent this improvement in muscle function is related to the increase in muscle mass [88]. Indeed, a substantial subgroup of COPD patients did not gain weight in response to high-energy nutritional therapy [89]. This subgroup was characterized by an elevated systemic inflammatory response, as evidenced by high concentrations of acute phase proteins and soluble TNF receptors. As mentioned earlier, systemic inflammation is associated with protein catabolism and probably plays a role in the loss of muscle mass. This suggests that antiinflammatory therapy might be beneficial in this particular subgroup. Many COPD patients receive inhaled or oral corticosteroids to treat local inflammation and acute infections. Systemic inflammation, however, is not reversed during this treatment [90]. In addition, oral steroids may have a negative effect on skeletal muscle as mentioned above.

A possible way to modulate systemic inflammation is through ingestion of polyunsaturated fatty acids (PUFAs). PUFAs are incorporated into the phospholipids of the cell membrane and play an important role in the regulation of inflammatory processes. Indeed, fish-oil supplementation reduced inflammatory mediators and had an anticachectic effect in pancreatic cancer patients [91]. No studies are yet available regarding PUFA supplementation in COPD .

COPD patients may have increased oxidative stress, in either muscle or lung tissue. Furthermore, vitamin E deficiency is associated with the pathogenesis of the wasting and weakness in thalassemia major [92]. Therefore, another mode of nutritional intervention might be supplementation with antioxidants such as vitamins, glutathione, and *N*-acetylcysteine. Several studies indeed showed a beneficial effect on wasting of antioxidant supplementation [93]. For example, vitamin E protects human skeletal muscle from damage during surgical ischemia-reperfusion [94] and vitamin C supplementation reduces exercise-induced oxidative stress [95]. Although antioxidant supplementation does reduce physical exercise–induced oxidative stress, it remains unclear whether exercise performance is enhanced [93,96]. In addition, there are some indications that vitamin supplementation may improve lung function [97, 98]. Antioxidant administration COPD therefore deserves further investigation.

A very promising field is represented by nutritional modulation of energy and substrate metabolism by so-called "nutriceuticals", although not yet recommended. Polyunsaturated fatty acid replacement [99] and Creatine replacement [100] have shown functional and structural effect on muscles function when added to classical pulmonary rehabilitation.

References

[1] Global Initiative for chronic obstructive lung disease. Global strategy for the diagnosis, management, and prevention of chronic obstructive lung disease. NHLBI/WHO workshop report. Bathesda, National Heart Lung Blood Institute, April 2001; update of the management section, GOLD website. Available from: *goldcopd.com* (accessed March 2, 2005).

[2] Calverly P, Pauwels R, Vestbo J, Jones P, Pride N, Gulsvik A, Anderson J, Maden C. Combining salmeterol and fluticasone in the treatment of chronic obstructive pulmonary disease. *Lancet* 2003; 361: 449-456.

[3] Szafranski W, Cukier A, Ramirez R, Menga G, Sansores R, Nahabedian S, Peterson S, Olsson H. efficacy and safety of budesonide/formoterol in the management of of chronic obstructive pulmonary disease. *Eur Respir J* 2003; 21: 74-81.

[4] Mahaler Da, Wire P, Horstman D, Chang C-N, Yates J, Fisher T, Shah T. effectiveness of fluticasone propionate and salmeterol combination delivered via the Diskus device in the treatment of chronic obstructive pulmonary disease. *Am J Respir Crit Care Med* 2002; 166; 449-456.

[5] Barnes NC, Qiu YS, Pavord ID, Parker d, Davis PA, Zhu J, Johnson M, Thomas NC, and Jeffery PK, on behalf of the SCO30005 Study Group. Anti-inflammatory Effects of salmeterol/fluticasone propionate in chronic obstructive lung disease. *Am J Respir Crit Care Med* 2006; 173: 736-743.

[6] Vestbo J and the TORCH Study Group. The TORCH (Toward a Revolution in COPD Health) survival study protocol. *Eur respire J* 2004; 24: 206-210.

[7] O'Donnell DE, Webb KA. Exertional breathlessness in patients with chronic airflow limitation. The role of lung hyperinflation. *Am Rev Respir Dis* 1993;148:1351-1357.

[8] Cerveri I, Pellegrino R, Dore R, Corsico A, Fulgoni P, van de Woestijne KP, Brusaso V. Mechanisms for isolated volume response to a bronchodilator in patients with COPD. *J Appl Physiol*. 2000;88:1989-1995.

[9] Aylward M, Maddock J, Dewland P. Clinical evaluation of acetylcysteine in the treatment of patients with chronic obstructive bronchitis: a balanced double blind trial with placebo control. *Eur J Respir Dis* 1980; 61 Suppl: 111: s81-s89.

[10] Dechant KL, Noble S. Erdostine. *Drugs* 1996; 52: 875-882.

[11] Santolicandro AM, Baldi S, and Giuntini C. The effect of a new expectorant drug on mucus transport in chronic bronchitis. *J Aerosol Med* 1995; 8: 33-42.

[12] Todisco T, polidori R, Rossi F et al. Effect of N-acetylcysteine in subjects with slow pulmonary mucocyliary clearance. *Eur J Respir Dis* 1985; 66 Suppl 139: s136-s141.

[13] Olivieri D, Marisco SA, Illiano A, del Donno M. In vivo measurement of drug effect on mucociliary transport. *Eur J Respir Dis* 1983; 64 Suppl 128: s551-s553.

[14] Massaro GD, Massaro D. retinoic acid treatment abrogates elastase-induced pulmonary emphysema in rats. *Am J Physiol* 1996; 270: L305-L310.

[15] Mao JT, Goldin JG, Dermand J, Ibrahim G, Brown MS, Emerick A, McNitt-Gray MF, Gjertson DW, Estrada F, Tashkin DP, Roth MD. A pilot study of all-trans-retinoic acid for the treatment of human emphysema. *Am J Respir Crit Care Med.* 2002;165: 718-723.

[16] Celli BR, MacNee W, ATS/ERS Task Force. Standard for the diagnosis and treatment of patients with COPD: a summary of the ATS/ERS position paper. *Eur Resp J* 2004: 23:932-946.

[17] Siafakas NM. Definition of acute exacerbation of chronic obstructive pulmonary disease. In Siafakas NM , Anthonisen NR, Georgopoulos D eds. *Management of acute exacerbations of COPD*. New York Marcel DekkerInc., 2004; pp. 1-4.

[18] Hagedorn SD. Acute exacerbation of COPD. How to evaluate severity and treat the underlying cause. *Postgrad Med* 1992; 91: 105-112.

[19] Fuso L, Incalzi RA, Pistelli R, et al. Predicting mortality of patients hospitalized for acutely exacerbated chronic obstructive pulmonary disease. *Am J Med* 1995; 98: 272-277.

[20] Senef MG, Wagner DP, Wagner RP, Zimmermann JE, Knaus WA. Hospital and 1-year survival of patients admitted to intensive care units with acute exacerbation of chronic obstructive pulmonary disease. *JAMA* 1995; 274: 1852- 1857.

[21] Pride NB, Hugh-Jones P, O'Brien EN, et al. Changes in lung function following the surgical treatment of bullous emphysema. *Q J Med* 1969; 39: 49-69.

[22] Potgieter PD, Benatar SR, Hewitson RP, Ferguson AD. Surgical treatment of bullous lung disease. *Thorax* 1981; 36: 885-890.

[23] Connolly JE, Wilson A. The current status of surgery of bullous emphysema. *J Thorac Cardiovasc Surg*. 1989; 97: 351-361.

[24] Boushy SF, Kohen R, Billig DM et al. Bullous emphysema: clinical, roentgenologic and physiologic study of 49 patients. *Dis Chest* 1968; 54: 17-24.

[25] Foreman S, Weill H, Duke R, et al. Bullous disease of the lung: physiologic improvement after surgery. *Ann Int Med* 1968; 69: 757-767.

[26] Viola AR, Zuffardi EA. Physiologic and clinical aspects of pulmonary bullous disease. *Am Rev Respir Dis* 1966; 95: 574-580.

[27] Morgan MDL, Edwards CW, Morris J, Mattews HR. Origin and behaviour of emphysematous bullae. *Thorax* 1989; 44: 533-538.

[28] Baldi S, Palla A, Mussi A, Falaschi F, Carrozzi L, Giuntini c and Angeletti CA. Influence of bulla volume on post bullectomy outcome. *Can Respir J* 2001;8: 233-238.

[29] Brantingan OC, Mueller E, Kress MB. A surgical approach to pulmonary emphysema. *Am Rev Respir Dis* 1959; 80: 194-202.

[30] Rogers RM Effect of removal of bullae on airway conductance and conductance volume ratios. *J Clin Invest* 1968; 47: 2569-2579.

[31] Rogers RM Lung reduction surgery in chronic obstructive lung disease. *Med Clin North Am* 1996; 80: 623–636.

[32] Wakabayashi A. Thoracoscopic laser pneumoplasty in the treatment of diffuse bullous emphysema. *Ann Thoracic Surg* 1995; 60: 936-939.

[33] Wakabayashi A. Thoracoscopic carbon dioxide laser treatment of bullous emphysema. *Ann Thoracic Surg* 1995; 337: 881-883.

[34] Cooper JD, Trulock EP, Tafillou AN. Bilateral pneumonectomy (volume reduction) for chronic obstructive pulmonary disease. *J Thorac Cardiovasc Surg* 1995; 109: 106-119.

[35] Gevenois PA, DeVuyst P, De Maertelaer V, Zanen J, Jacobovitz D, Cosio MG, Yernault JC. Comparison of computed density and macroscopic morphometry in pulmonary emphysema. *Am J Respir Crit Care Med* 1996;154:187–192.

[36] Müller NL, Staples CA, Miller RR, Abboud RT."Density mask". An objective method to quantitate emphysema using computed tomography. *Chest* 1988;94:782–787.

[37] Fishman A, Martinez F, Naunheim K, Piantadosi S, Wise R, Ries A, Weinmann G, Wood DE; National Emphysema Treatment Trial Research Group. A randomized trial comparing lung-volume-reduction surgery with medical therapy for severe emphysema. *N Engl J Med* 2003; 348: 2059-2073.

[38] Mal H, Andreasian B, Pamela F. Unilateral lung transplantation in end stage pulmonary emphysema. *Am Rev Respir Dis* 1989;140:797–802.

[39] Patterson GA, Cooper JD, Goldman B, *et al.* Technique of successful clinical double-lung transplantation. *Ann Thorac Surg* 1988;45:626–33.

[40] Pasque MK, Cooper JD, Kaiser LR, et al. An improved technique for bilateral lung transplantation: rationale and initial clinical experience. *Ann Thorac Surg* 1990;49:785–91.

[41] Fishman AP. Pulmonary rehabilitation research. *Am J Respir Crit Care Med* 1994;149: 825-833.

[42] Ferguson GT, Cherniack RM. Management of chronic obstructive pulmonary disease. *N Engl J Med* 1993; 328: 1017-1022.

[43] Celli BR. Pulmonary rehabilitation in patients with COPD. *Am J Respir Crit Care Med* 1995; 152: 861-864.

[44] Troosters T, Casaburi R, Gosselink R, Decramer M. Pulmonary rehabilitation in chronic obstructive pulmonary disease. *Am J Respir Crit Care* Med 2005; 1752: 19-38.

[45] McComas AJ. Skeletal muscle: form and function. Champaign, IL: *Human Kinetics*, 1996.

[46] Serres I, Varray A, Vallet G, Micallef JP, Préfaut C. Improved skeletal muscle performance after individualized exercise training in patients with chronic obstructive pulmonary disease. *J Cardiopulm Rehabil* 1997;17:232–8.

[47] O'Donnell DE, McGuire M, Samis L, Webb KA. General exercise training improves ventilatory and peripheral muscle strength and endurance in chronic airflow limitation. *Am J Respir Crit Care Med* 1998;157:1489–97.

[48] Shephard RJ. Exercise for patients with congestive heart failure. *Sports Med* 1997;23:75–92.

[49] Sullivan MJ, Hawthorne MH. Exercise intolerance in patients with chronic heart failure. *Prog Cardiovasc Dis* 1995;38:1–22.

[50] Adamopoulos S, Coats AJ. Peripheral abnormalities in chronic heart failure. *Postgrad Med J* 1991;67:S74–80.

[51] Wilson JR, Mancini DM. The mechanism of extertional fatigue in heart failure. *Cardioscience* 1990;1:13–7.

[52] Maltais F, LeBlanc P, Simard C, et al. Skeletal muscle adaptation to endurance training in patients with chronic obstructive pulmonary disease. *Am J Respir Crit Care Med* 1996;154:442–7.

[53] Hambrecht R, Fiehn E, Yu J, et al. Effects of endurance training on mitochondrial ultrastructure and fiber type distribution in skeletal muscle of patients with stable chronic heart failure. *J Am Coll Cardiol* 1997;29:1067–73.

[54] Kemp GJ, Thompson CH, Stratton JR, et al. Abnormalities in exercising skeletal muscle in congestive heart failure can be explained in terms of decreased mitochondrial ATP synthesis, reduced metabolic efficiency, and increased glycogenolysis. *Heart* 1996;76:35–41.

[55] Smith K, Cook D, Guyatt GH, Madhavan J, Oxman AD. Respiratory muscle training in chronic airflow limitation: a meta-analysis. *Am Rev Respir Dis* 1992;145:533–9.

[56] Rochester DF. The diaphragm in COPD. Better than expected, but not good enough. *N Engl J Med* 1991;325:961–2.

[57] Belman MJ, Botnick WC, Nathan SD, Chon KH. Ventilatory load characteristics during ventilatory muscle training. *Am J Respir Crit Care Med* 1994;149:925–9.

[58] Sen CK, Hänninen O. Physiological antioxidants. In: Sen KC, Packer L, Hänninen O, eds. *Exercise and oxygen toxicity*. Amsterdam: Elsevier Science BV, 1994:89–126.

[59] Engelen MP, Schols AM, Baken WC, Wesseling GJ, Wouters EF. Nutritional depletion in relation to respiratory and peripheral skeletal muscles function in out-patients with COPD. *Eur Respir J* 1994; 7: 1793-1797.

[60] Schols AM, Soeters PB, Dingemans AM, Mostert R, Frantzen PJ, Wouters EF. Prevalence and characteristics of nutritional depletion in patients with stable COPD eligible for pulmonary rehabilitation. *Am Rev Respir Dis* 1993; 147: 1151-1156.

[61] Prescott E, Aldmal T, Mikkelsen KL, Tofteng CL, Vestbo J, Lange P. Prognostic value of weight change in chronic obstructive pulmonary disease: results from the Copenhagen City Heart Study. *Eur Respir* J 2002; 20: 539 - 544.

[62] Vandenberg E, Van de Woestijne KP, Gyselen A. weight changes in the terminal stages of chronic obstructive pulmonary disease. Relation to respiratory function and prognosis *Am Rev Respir Dis* 1967; 95: 556-566.
[63] Wilson DO, Rogers RM, Wright EC, Anthonisen NR. Body weight in chronic obstructive pulmonary disease. The national institute of health intermittent positive pressure breathing trial. *Am Rev Respir Dis* 1989; 139; 1435-1438.
[64] Schols AM, Slangen J, Volovics L, Wouters EF. Weight loss is a reversible factor in the prognosis of chronic obstructive pulmonary disease. *Am J Respir Crit Care Med* 1998; 157; 1791 – 1797.
[65] Marquis K, Debigare R, Lacasse Y, et al. Midtight muscle cross sectional area is a better predictor of mortality than body mass index in patients with chronic obstructive pulmonary disease. *Am J Respir Crit Care Med* 2002; 166: 809-813.
[66] Schols AM, Broekhuizen R, Weling—Scheepers CA, Wouters EF. Body composition and mortality in chronic obstructive pulmonary disease *Am J Clin Nutr 2005*; 82: 53-59.
[67] Vestbo J, Prescott E, Almdal T et al. Body mass, fat-free body mass and prognosis in patients with chronic obstructive pulmonary disease from a ramdom population sample: finding from the Copenhagen city heart study. *Am J Respir Crit Care Med* 2006; 173: 79-83.
[68] Schols AM, Soeters PB, Mostert R, Saris WH, Wouters EF. Energy balance in chronic obstructive pulmonary disease. *Am Rev Respi Dis* 1991; 143; 1248-1252.
[69] Baarends EM, Schols AM, Pannemans DL, Westerterp KR, Wouters EF. Total free living energy expenditure in patients with severe chronic obstructive pulmonary disease. *Am J Respir Crit Care Med*; 1997; 155: 549-554.
[70] Schols AM, Fredrix EW, Soeters PB, Westerterp KR, Wouters EF. Resting energy expenditure in patients with chronic obstructive pulmonary disease *Am J Clin Nutr* 1991; 54: 983-987.
[71] Broekuizen R, Wouters EF, Creutzberg EC, Schols AM. Raised CRP levels marks metabolic and functional impairment in advanced COPD. *Thorax* 2006; 61: 17-22.
[72] Schols AM, Buurman WA, Staal van den Brekel AJ, Dentener MA, Wouters EF. Evidence for a relation between metabolic derangements and increased levels of inflammatory mediators in a subgroup of patients with chronic obstructive pulmonary disease. *Thorax* 1996; 51: 819-824.
[73] Efthimiou J, Fleming J, Gomes C, Spiro SG. The effect of supplementary oral nutrition in poorly nourished patients with chronic obstructive pulmonary disease. *Am Rev Respir Dis* 1988; 137: 1075-1082.
[74] Rogers RM, Donahoe M, Costantino J. Physiologic effects of oral supplemental feeding in malnourished patients with chronic obstructive pulmonary disease. A randomized control study. *Am Rev Respir D*is 1992; 146: 1511-1517.
[75] Whittaker JS, Ryan CF, Buckley PA, Road JD. The effects of refeeding on peripheral and respiratory muscle function in malnourished chronic obstructive pulmonary disease patients. *Am Rev Respir Dis* 1990; 142: 283-288.
[76] Vermeeren MA, Wouters EF, Nelissen LH, van Lier A, Hofma Z, Schols AM. Acute effects of different nutritional supplements on symptoms and functional capacity in

patients with chronic obstructive pulmonary disease. *Am J Clin Nutr* 2001; 73: 295-301.

[77] Efthimiou J, Mounsey PJ, , Benson DN, Madgwick R, Coles SJ, Benson MK. Effects of carbohydrate rich versus fat rich loads on gas exchange and walking performance in patients with chronic obstructive pulmonary disease. *Thorax* 1992; 47: 451-456.

[78] Brown SE, Nagendran RC,McHugh JW, Stansbury DW, Fisher CE, Light RW. Effects of a large carbohydrate load on walking performance in chronic air-flow obstruction. *Am Rev Respir Dis* 1985; 132: 960-962.

[79] Frankfort JD, Fisher CE, Stansbury DW, McArthur DL, Brown SE, Light RW. Effects of high- and low-carbohydrates meals on maximum exercise performance in chronic airflow obstruction. *Chest* 1991; 100: 792-795.

[80] Schols AM, Soeters PB, Mostert R, Pluymers RJ, Wouters EF. Physiologic effects of nutritional support and anabolic steroids in patients with chronic obstructive pulmonary disease. A placebo-controlled randomized trial. *Am J Respir Crit Care Med* 1995; 152: 1268-1274.

[81] Debigare R, Marquis K, Cote CH, Tremblay RR, Michaud A, LeBlanc P, Maltais F. Catabolic/anabolic balance and muscle wasting in patients with COPD. *Chest.* 2003;124:83-89.

[82] Creutzberg EC, Wouters EF, Mostert R, Pluymers RJ, Schols AM. A role for anabolic steroids in the rehabilitation of patients with COPD? A double blind, placebo-controlled, randomized trial. *Chest* 2003; 124: 1733-1742.

[83] Ferreira JM, Verreschi IT, Nery LE et al. The influence of 6 months of oral anabolic steroids on body mass and respiratory muscles in malnourished COPD patients. *Ches*t 1998; 114: 19-28.

[84] Schols AM, Mostert R, Cobben N, Soeters PB, Wouters EF. Transcutaneous oxygen saturation and carbon dioxide tension during meals in patients with chronic obstructive pulmonary disease. *Chest* 1991; 100: 1287-1292.

[85] Efthimiou J, Fleming J, Gomes C, Spiro SG. The effect of supplementary oral nutrition in poorly nourished patients with chronic obstructive pulmonary disease. *Am Rev Respir Dis* 1988;137: 1075–82.

[86] Rogers RM, Donahoe M, Costantino J. Physiologic effects of oral supplemental feeding in malnourished patients with chronic obstructive pulmonary disease. A randomized control study. *Am Rev Respir Dis* 1992;146:1511–7.

[87] Whittaker JS, Ryan CF, Buckley PA, Road JD. The effects of refeeding on peripheral and respiratory muscle function in malnourished chronic obstructive pulmonary disease patients. *Am Rev Respir Dis* 1990;142:283–8.

[88] Schols AM, Soeters PB, Mostert R, Pluymers RJ, Wouters EF. Physiologic effects of nutritional support and anabolic steroids in patients with chronic obstructive pulmonary disease. A placebo-controlled randomized trial. *Am J Respir Crit Care Med* 1995;152:1268–74.

[89] Creutzberg EC, Schols AMWJ, Weling-Scheepers CAPM, Buurman WA, Wouters EFM. Characterization of nonresponse to high caloric oral nutritional therapy in depleted patients with chronic obstructive pulmonary disease. *Am J Respir Crit Care Med* 2000;161:745–52.

[90] Keatings VM, Jatakanon A, Worsdell YM, Barnes PJ. Effects of inhaled and oral glucocorticoids on inflammatory indices in asthma and COPD. *Am J Respir Crit Care Med* 1997;155:542–8.
[91] Wigmore SJ, Ross JA, Falconer JS, et al. The effect of polyunsaturated fatty acids on the progress of cachexia in patients with pancreatic cancer. *Nutrition* 1996;12:S27–30.
[92] Shapira Y, Glick B, Finsterbush A, Goldfarb A, Rosenmann E. Myopathological findings in thalassemia major. *Eur Neurol* 1990; 30:324–7.
[93] Goldfarb AH, Sen CK. Antioxidant supplementation and the control of oxygen toxicity during exercise. In: Sen KC, Packer L, Hänninen O, eds. *Exercise and oxygen toxicity*. Amsterdam: Elsevier Science BV, 1994:163–89.
[94] Novelli GP, Adembri C, Gandini E, et al. Vitamin E protects human skeletal muscle from damage during surgical ischemia-reperfusion. *Am J Surg* 1997;173:206–9.
[95] Alessio HM, Goldfarb AH, Cao GH. Exercise induced oxidative stress before and after vitamin C supplementation. *Int J Sport Nutr* 1997;7:1–9.
[96] Clarkson PM. Antioxidants and physical performance. *Crit Rev Food Sci Nutr* 1995;35:131–41.
[97] Paiva SA, Godoy I, Vannucchi H, Favaro RM, Geraldo RR, Campana AO. Assessment of vitamin A status in chronic obstructive pulmonary disease patients and healthy smokers. *Am J Clin Nutr* 1996;64:928–34.
[98] Dow L, Tracey M, Villar A, et al. Does dietary intake of vitamins C and E influence lung function in older people? *Am J Respir Crit Care Med* 1996;154:1401–4.
[99] Broekhuizen R, Wouters EF, Creutzberg EC, Weeling-Scheepers CA, Schols AM. Polyunsaturated fatty acids improve exercise capacity in chronic obstructive pulmonary disease. *Thorax* 2005; 60: 376-382.
[100] Fuld JP, Kilduff LP, Neder JA, et al. Creatine supplementation during pulmonary rehabilitation in chronic obstructive pulmonary disease. *Thorax* 2005;60:531-537.

7. Comprehensive Clinical Assessment Tailored to Nutrition-Rehabilitation Intervention

The studies dealing with the pathogenesis of nutritional differences between COPD phenotypes have tended to deflect some attention away from the impact of nutritional status itself on quality of life, disability and handicap of COPD. In 1955 Dornhorst et al. [1] pointed out that changes in body habitus accompanies advanced emphysema. Filley et al. in [2] classified COPD patients according to disease process and body habitus.

The association between severity of airflow obstruction and weight loss was stressed in following clinical studies [3, 4]. Subsequently, it was demonstrated that COPD patients with weight loss have a shorter survival rate than those patients without weight loss [5, 6]. However, it was unclear whether poor nutritional status was the cause or just a marker of other factors intrinsic to the disease process.

More recently, studies demonstrating that nutritional status marks emphysematous process independent of severity of airflow obstruction have suggested complex metabolic alterations related to disturbed energy balance, systemic inflammation, hypoxia and metabolic adaptation targeting lung as well as skeletal and respiratory muscle [7, 8]. In this scenario it becomes of paramount importance to understand whether nutritional intervention can prevent or even reverse deterioration of the lung disease.

Weight loss ensues when energy intake does not meet energy need. In these conditions energy for the metabolic process is initially supplied from endogenous glycogen stores. Glycogenolysis and gluconeogenesis occur in liver as well in skeletal muscles. However, while muscle glycogen will be available only to muscles, liver glycogen will supply glucose for all other organ and system. These stores last for approximately 24 hours. Subsequently, fats are transformed into fatty acid and ketone bodies, and proteins (lean body mass) come to carbon chains suitable for gluconeogenesis. If this process is not halted by administration of exogenous calories, the result is an autocannibalization.

The negative effects of metabolic wasting syndrome involve limb skeletal muscles, respiratory muscles, immune system, and lead to loss of structural integrity of the lung and to multiple organ system failure.

Adverse effects on ventilatory control, metabolic rate and hypoxic ventilatory response have been documented after 10 days of a 500-Kcal carbohydrates diet. They returned to normal after 5 days of refeeding [9].

To the extent that weight loss is a factor associated to morbidity and mortality of patients with COPD, the assessment of possible causes and the corrective intervention become central to rehabilitation program.

The different possible causes for weight loss, as listed in Table 1. As discussed in the previous section, an adequate refeeding seems to halt or improve metabolic wasting in COPD if a proper nutrition assessment is part of rehabilitative management. Therefore the clinical assessment of patients with COPD should take into consideration body mass index, metabolic and systemic markers along with respiratory function parameters, such as residual volume and forced expiratory volume in one second (FEV1) which almost exclusively targets the lung.

The performance of a full nutritional assessment depends on the ability to make measurements, to relate these measurement to exercise performance parameters, available clinical markers of inflammation and oxidative stress as well as to the duration of nutritional support.

Table 1. Mechanisms and Causes for weight loss in COPD patients

⇐ Increased REE ⇒ increased work of breathing
⇐ Low caloric intake ⇒ dyspnea and/or gastrointestinal symptoms while eating, suppressed appetite from medications
⇐ Malabsoption ⇒ poor calories utilization
⇐ Psychosocial factors ⇒ depression, poverty, cigarette smoking, eating and living arrangements

The diet history should be the first step in the assessment of nutritional profile, looking for dietary habit, factors as bloating or early satiety, as well as the usual weight and the history of weight loss.

Anthropometric measurements are a simple way to assess body's basic fuel reserve. They should include: the actual weight, expressed as percentage of ideal body weight; triceps skin-fold (TSF) to represent fat stores and arm muscle circumference, and creatine height index (CHI) to estimate skeletal (lean muscle mass. Although the method is well-described [10], the interpretation of the measurement is less well standardized.

These measurements are not sensitive to short term changes, but are useful in serial assessment when beginning a rehabilitation and nutrition program or in collecting data for nutritional studies.

Assessment of visceral protein status in absence of a parenchymal liver disease reflects a decrease in protein synthesis because of limited substrate availability [11]. Their value is limited by their half-lives as shown in table 2.

Table 2. Visceral protein half-lives

Albumin	21 days
Transferrin	10 days
Thyroxyne-binding prealbumin	2 days
Retinol-binding protein	12 hours

Depressed total lymphocyte counts and delayed hypersensitivity skin testing are not enough specific indicators of poor protein-calorie intake as they are affected by many other factors.

Determination of 24-hour urine urea nitrogen (UNN) is a good indicator of lean body mass breakdown and can serve to assess whether an anabolic state has been achieved in response to therapy. This evaluation is interesting above all in acute clinical situations.

Determination of resting energy expenditure (REE) is basic for design of each patient actual diet. REE can be measured by indirect calorimetry with measurement of Oxygen consumption (VO_2) and CO_2 production (VCO_2) under standardized conditions [12, 13].

The measured REE in COPD may be expressed as percentage of predicted value according to the Harris-Benedict equation [14]. Studies that have compared HBE with indirect calorimetry have found the HBE to underestimate REE by as much as 40% [15-18]. Furthermore, REE was adjusted for fat free mass estimated by single frequency bioelectric impedance analysis [19]. Schols et al. [20] based on REE as % of HBE and adjusted for FFM stratified COPD patients into normometabolic and hypermetabolic. To adjust for FFM the authors calculated the REE as the group mean REE plus measured minus predicted REE, which was the calculated REE obtained by using the individual FFM in the linear regression equation of REE on FFM.

Another promising technique to study body composition is Dual energy x-ray absorptiometry (DEXA) that measures bone mineral content (BMC), bone mineral density (BMD), fat-free mass (FFM), and provides estimate of percent body fat. Hartmann et al. [20] evaluated the accuracy of this technique and the influence of scan mode in older adults, and pointed out the importance of using a single DEXA scan mode for clinical investigation and particularly for longitudinal studies.

Hayes et al. [21] tested the hypothesis that tissue-organ components can be derived from DEXA measurements, and in turn, REE can be calculated from the summed heat productions of DEXA-estimated brain, skeletal muscle mass (SM), adipose tissue, bone and residual mass (RM) in adults < 50 years of age. The results of the study are useful for educational purposes since they support the overall concept that predictable relations exist between major tissue-organ level components and heat production at rest. Obviously limitations exists mainly related to the validity of assumed tissue- and organ-specific metabolic rates, above all in elderly.

In 24 japanese males Nishimura et al. [22] documented that respiratory muscle strength is closely associated with body weight and lean body mass as assessed by DEXA.

Yoshikawa et al. [23] examined the effect of body composition on maximal exercise performance in 27 patients with COPD. They found that lean body mass as assessed by DEXA is an important determinant of maximal exercise performance. In another paper Yoshikawa et al. [24] studied 38 outpatients with COPD measuring regional lean body mass in arm, legs, trunk expressed as percentage of IBW. They documented significant depletion of each body region in patients with very severe airflow obstruction (FEV_1 <35%) compared to patients with mild-to-moderate airflow obstruction (mean FEV_1 64%). By stepwise regression the authors also found that leg lean mass/IBW is a significant predictor of VO_{2max} only in group with mild-to moderate airflow obstruction, not in patients with very severe airflow obstruction. These results suggest rethinking the rehabilitative approach of strength training of leg muscles in advanced disease. DEXA thus appears to be a promising tool for clinical investigation in a rehabilitative setting.

The need for a clinical assessment that is comprehensive of functional and systemic domains in COPD is demonstrated by the use of the BODE index, a recently proposed score system to measure performance status of COPD patients. The BODE index has been demonstrated better than FEV_1 at predicting the risk of death from any cause, and the risk of death for respiratory causes among patients with COPD [24].

BODE index is a multidimensional grading system that assesses respiratory and systemic expression of COPD. Its calculated based on: 1) the measurement of body mass index (BMI, Kg/m^2); 2) FEV_1, % predicted; 3) degree of dyspnea, measured with the Modified Medical Research Council (MMRC) dyspnea scale; and 4) the evaluation of exercise tolerance, as reflected by the distance walked at the 6 minute walking test (6MWD) [24]. Thus, it is a powerful clinical tool easily accessible in any clinical and rehabilitation setting incorporating functional, nutritional, and metabolic information.

References

[1] Dornhorst A. Respiratory insufficiency. *Lancet* 1955; 268: 1185.

[2] Filley GF, Beckwitt HJ, Reeves JT, Mitchell R. Chronic obstructive bronchopulmonary disease. II. Oxygen transport in the two clinical types. *Am J Med* 1968; 44: 26-38.

[3] Renzetti AD, McClement JH, Litt BD. The Veterans Administration cooperative study of pulmonary function. Mortality in relation to respiratory function in chronic obstructive pulmonary disease. *Am J Med* 1966; 41: 115-129

[4] Vandenbrug E, van de Woestigne K, Gyselen A. Weight changes in the terminal stages of chronic obstructive lung disease. *Am Rev Respir* Dis 1967; 96: 556-566.

[5] Driver AG, McAlevy MT, Smith VL. Nutritional assessment of patients with chronic obstructive pulmonary disease and acute respiratory failure. *Chest* 1982; 82: 568-571.

[6] Openbrier DR, Irwin MM, Rogers RM, Gottlieb GP, Dauber JH, Van Thiel DH, Pennock BE. Nutritional status and lung function in patients with emphysema and chronic bronchitis. *Chest* 1983; 83:17-22.

[7] Intermittent Positive Pressure Breathing Trial Group. Intermittent positive pressure breathing therapy of chronic obstructive pulmonary disease: a clinical trial. *Ann Intern Med* 1983; 99:612-620.

[8] Broekuizen R, Wouters EF, Creutzberg EC, Schols AM. Raised CRP levels marks metabolic and functional impairment in advanced COPD. *Thorax* 2006; 61: 17-22.

[9] Wilson DO, Rogers RM, Wright EC, Anthonisen NR. Body weight in chronic obstructive pulmonary disease. The national Institute of Health intermittent positive pressure breathing trial. *Am Rev Respir Dis* 1989; 139: 1435-1438.

[10] Doekel RC Jr, Zwillich CW, Scoggin CH, Kryger M, Weil JV. Clinical semi starvation: depression of hypoxic ventilatory response. *N Engl J Med* 1976; 295:358-361.

[11] Blackburn GL, Bistrian BR, Maini BS, Schlamm HT, Smith MF. Nutritional and metabolic assessment of hospitalized patients. *JPEN* 1977; 1: 11-22.

[12] Tavill AS. The synthesis and degradation of liver produced proteins.. *Gut* 1972; 13:225-241.

[13] Long CL, Schoeffer N, Geiger J, Schuler WR, Blackmore AS. Metabolic response to injury and illness estimation of energy and protein needs from indirect calorimetry and nitrogen balance. *JPEN* 1979; 3: 452-456.

[14] Schols AMWJ, Schoffelen P, Ceulemans H, Wouters EFM, Saris WH. Measurements of resting energy expenditure in patients with COPD in a clinical setting. *JPEN* 1992; 16: 364-368.

[15] Openbrier DR, Irwin M, Dauber JH, Owens GR, Rogers RM. Factors affecting nutritional status and the impact of nutritional support in patients with emphysema. *Chest* 1984; 85: 67s.

[16] Braum SR, Keim NL, Dixon RM, Claganz P, Anderegg A, Shrago ES. The prevalence and determinants of nutritional changes in chronic obstructive pulmonary disease. *Chest* 1984; 86: 558-563.

[17] Wilson DO, Rogers RM, Sanders MH, Pennock BE, Reilly JJ.Nutritional intervention in malnourished patients with emphysema. *Am Rev Respir Dis*. 1986;134:672-677.

[18] Moore JA, Angelillo VA. Equations for the prediction of resting energy expenditure in chronic obstructive lung disease. *Chest* 1988; 94: 1260-1263.

[19] Rochester DF. Body weight and respiratory muscle function in COPD. *Am Rev Respir Dis* 1986; 134: 646-648.

[20] Ravussin E, Bogardus C. Relationship of genetics, age and physical fitness to daily energy expenditure and fuel utilization. *Am J Clin Nutr* 1989; 49:968-975.

[21] Hartman CJL. Kanaley J, Wideman L, Teates CD, Bouchard C, Wetman A. Body composition by DEXA in older adults: accuracy and influence of scan mode. *Med Sci Sports Exerc* 1997; 29: 560-567.

[22] Nishimura Y, Tsutsumi M, Nakata H, Tsunenari T, Maeda H, Yokoyama M. Relationship between respiratory muscles strength qand lean body mass in men with COPD.*Chest* 1995; 107: 1232-1236.

[23] Yoshikawa M, Yoneda T, Kobayashi A, Fu A, Takenada H, Narita N, Nezu K. Body composition analysis by dual energy X-ray absortiometry and exercise performance in underweight patients with COPD. *Chest* 1999; 115: 371-375.

[24] Yoshikawa M, Yoneda T, Takenada H, Kobayashi A, Fukuoka A, Okamoto Y, Narita N, Nezu K. Diustribution of muscle mass and maximal exercise performance in patients with COPD. *Chest* 2001; 119; 93-98.

[25] Celli BR, Cote CG, Marin JM, Casanova C, Montes de Oca M, Mendez RA, Pinto Plata V, Cabral HJ. The body-mass index, airflow obstruction, dyspnea, and exercise capacity index in chronic obstructive pulmonary disease. *N Engl J Med 2004*; 350: 1005-1012.

Conclusion

Emphysema, chronic bronchitis and COPD have overlapping features. The interaction of host and environmental factors produces clinical pictures, which reflect these features to a greater and lesser extent from patient to patient. At the end of the day we have emphysema, which is a structural entity, COPD, which is largely a functional entity, and chronic bronchitis which is largely based on a clinical history. There is overlap and there are differences between these conditions.

The mechanical characteristics of the lungs can be measured. The functional characteristics such as flow rates, gas transfer capacity, communicating gas volume, total lung capacity and its subdivisions can be measured. The clinical consequences can be measured. The interrelationships between all these features is substantial and their contribution to a systemic inflammatory process involving lung, skeletal muscles, endothelial function, and metabolic derangements becomes apparent despite the overlay simplistic explanations which are often forwarded.

Given this complex background and despite the explosion of knowledge based upon multidisciplinary research, the prominence of different pathophysiologic mechanisms of airflow limitation in the course of the disease and their link to systemic inflammation is not adequately understood to the point that a uniform satisfactory answer is possible.

Up to date, a large body of evidence enables definition of several key points for better definition of rehabilitation programs. They point out the importance to assess performance status as a result of body mass index, metabolic and systemic inflammatory markers along with respiratory function parameters, which almost exclusively targets the lung.

A tailor-made comprehensive clinical assessment of nutrition rehabilitation intervention for COPD patients in the middle age and elderly is requested to address the priority of therapeutic and/or surgical intervention strategies. Thus, Rehabilitation becomes the hub of all diagnostic and preventive interventions in middle-aged and elderly aimed at controlling exaggerated inflammatory response to un-repaired organ injury that results from specific organ pathological process, together with co-morbid disease association and nutritional habitus.

In: Nutrition for the Middle Aged and Elderly
Editors: N. E. Bernhardt, A. M. Kasko, pp. 447-458
ISBN: 978-1-60456-146-3

Chapter XVII

The Role of Dietary Fatty Acids and Acyl-Coa Synthetases in the Development of Colorectal Cancer

Nikolaus Gassler*[*1], Andrea Reinartz[1], Elke Kaemmerer[2], Dieter Enders[3] and Wolfgang Bettray[3]
[1]Institute of Pathology, RWTH Aachen University, Aachen, Germany
[2]Department of Pediatrics, RWTH Aachen University, Aachen, Germany
[3]Institute of Organic Chemistry, RWTH Aachen University, Aachen, Germany

Abstract

Major dietary constituents like fatty acids, glucose and amino acids have been shown to be involved in gene expression and cellular reactivity mediated by signalling cascades in a hormonal-independent manner. Previous studies have confirmed a strong association between intake of saturated fatty acids and colon cancer risk. Diets particularly high in saturated fatty acids are generally associated with an increased risk of developing colorectal cancer, whereas diets high in omega-3 polyunsaturated fatty acids reduce this risk. This article focuses on molecular mechanisms by which fatty acids are assumed to regulate the behaviour of intestinal epithelia via acyl-CoA synthetase (ACSL) mediated synthesis of acyl-CoA derivatives. ACSL4 and ACSL5 variants might be involved in activation of dietary and endogenous provided free fatty acids by synthesis of acyl-CoA derivatives including ceramide and reduction of free arachidonic acids in an intestinal cellular environment. In general, there is increasing experimental evidence suggesting that disturbances of acyl-CoA synthetase-associated pathways could contribute to intestinal disorders and carcinogenesis in a dietary-dependent manner.

* Corresponding author: Prof. Dr. med. N. Gassler, Institute of Pathology, University Hospital RWTH Aachen, Pauwelsstrasse 30, 52074 Aachen; Germany, e-mail: ngassler@ukaachen.de. Phone: +49 241 8088897. Fax: +49 241 8082439

Introduction

Colorectal cancer (CRC) is one of the most frequent malignancies in the world (Saunders and Iveson, 2006). Its development is based on a sequence of events including molecular disturbances, especially gene mutations, aberrant signalling in several pathways, and execution of modifier genes in a susceptible person. The molecular injuries determining CRCs are associated with the development of histomorphological lesions comprising intraepithelial neoplasia, i.e. aberrant crypt foci (ACF) or adenomas, and mucosa-invasive (early) colorectal cancer. Moreover, the differences in cellular morphology of such lesions are summarized in the tumour-grading which is suggested as a well-suitable indicator for tumour prognosis and molecular changes behind tumour growth. The sentinel molecular events occurring early in progression from adenoma to carcinoma have been integrated into a coherent adenoma-carcinoma sequence by molecular research (Fearon and Vogelstein, 1990). This sequence is a time-consuming process. It is assumed that the great number of CRC's has a natural history of transition from precursor to malignant lesions that spans approx. 15 – 20 years (Dvory-Sobol and Arber, 2007).

CRCs comprise a heterogeneous group of malignancies including hereditary forms and so-called sporadic tumours (Jass et al., 2002). At present, the autosomal dominant condition, familial adenomatous polyposis (FAP) has been characterized as the counterpart of sporadic CRCs. Mutations in the *APC* gene are founder lesions in CRCs of FAP-type. In hereditary nonpolyposis colorectal cancer (HNPCC), the stepwise progression of tumours following the step of initiation is accelerated by an injured expression of mismatch repair genes. Consequently, HNPCC is not a hereditary form of CRC by its own (Jass et al., 2002). By defining subsets of colorectal cancer, it should be possible to characterize additional founder or modifying pathways and to develop more targeted approaches to tumour prevention and treatment.

In the last years, nutrition has been suggested as a fundamental factor in modifying initiation and progression of CRCs. Epidemiological data are indicating a link between the intake of dietary lipids and development of (sporadic) CRCs (Granados et al., 2006; Yeh et al., 2006). Among dietary lipids fatty acids are assumed to be the main component interfering with development of intestinal neoplasia. However, pathways of fatty acid metabolism intervening in the adenoma-carcinoma sequence are not well elucidated so far. The association of fatty acids like n-3 polyunsaturated fatty acids or long-chain saturated fatty acids and inhibition or promotion of colorectal carcinogenesis is in discussion (Balk et al., 2007; Chapkin et al., 2007). Despite this discrepancy, development of a diet that provides adequate nutrition and effective cancer prevention is an important goal in nutrition and cancer research.

Here we provide a short overview about the putative role of dietary free fatty acids activated by acyl-CoA synthetases in the development of intestinal neoplasia.

ACSL5 and Intestinal Metabolism of Dietary Lipids

Lipids comprise a heterogeneous group of chemical substances broadly defined as any hydrophobic, fat-soluble molecule. Fatty acids and their derivatives, e.g. glycerides and phospholipids as well as sterol-derivatives are important subgroups of lipids involved in diverse cellular pathways and functions. Evidence is given that activated fatty acids affect gene expression in hepatocytes and enterocytes through various mechanisms including changes in membrane composition, intracellular calcium levels, second messenger synthesis, and direct interaction with coding sequences in the nucleus (Sampath and Ntambi, 2005). Experimental evidence is given that dietary fatty acids and sphingoid bases are physiologically metabolised by enterocytes generating a multitude of cellular functions. Such activated lipid intermediates are precursor molecules in the formation of complex lipids and are involved in signal transduction, transcriptional activation, and modulation of a variety of cellular functions including membrane fusion, ion transportation, and cellular survival. Main pathways of dietary, apically incorporated fatty acids are illustrated in Figure 1. It is assumed that basolateral incorporated lipids initiate functions different from the dietary-induced phenomena (Murota and Storch, 2005). However, this issue is not well elucidated as yet and at present, dietary – not endogenous – fatty acids are assumed being critical in colorectal carcinogenesis (Granados et al., 2006).

An important step in the activation of long chain fatty acids is the synthesis of thiolester derivatives by addition of coenzyme-A (CoA). This biochemical synthesis is catalyzed by several enzymes including acyl-CoA synthetases (ACSL) (Mashek et al., 2004). Acyl-CoA derivatives are used in several biochemical pathways including the *de novo* synthesis of ceramides (Figure 2). Ceramides are central metabolites of bioactive sphingolipids, which can be synthesized either in response to the activation of sphingomyelinases or *de novo*. Fatty acids activated by ACSLs are necessary in the *de novo* ceramide synthesis. Here, sphinganine is modified by the enzyme dihydroceramide synthase catalysing the N-acylation of dihydrosphingosine to dihydroceramide. Finally, dihydroceramide desaturase catalyses the subsequent introduction of a *trans* double bond at C4-C5 to generate ceramides. Several inhibitors of the *de novo* ceramide synthesis have been identified including L-cycloserine, myriocin, fumonisin, D-*threo*-1-phenyl-2-palmitoylamino-3-morpholino-1-propanol (PPMP), and D-*threo*-1-phenyl-2-decanoylamino-3-morpholino-1-propanol (PDMP) (Pyne and Pyne, 2000; Ruvolo, 2003; Marasas et al., 2004).

The metabolic conversion of ceramide into sphingosine 1-phosphate is assumed to switch cells from an apoptotic state to a proliferative one. Ceramidases catalyse the deacylation of ceramide to produce non-esterified fatty acid and sphingosin (Bernardo et al., 1995). Condensation of serine and palmitoyl-CoA producing 3-oxosphinganine is the initial step in the intracellular *de novo* ceramide synthesis (Pyne and Pyne, 2000). Intracellular sphinganine (dihydrosphingosine) is generated from 3-oxosphinganine by rapid reduction catalyzed by a NAD(P)H reductase stereospecific for the D-isomer. Evidence is given that dietary sphinganine is absorbed by cellular systems and is able to interfere with the metabolism of sphingolipids (Ahn and Schroeder, 2002; Sugawara et al., 2003; Sugawara et al., 2004).

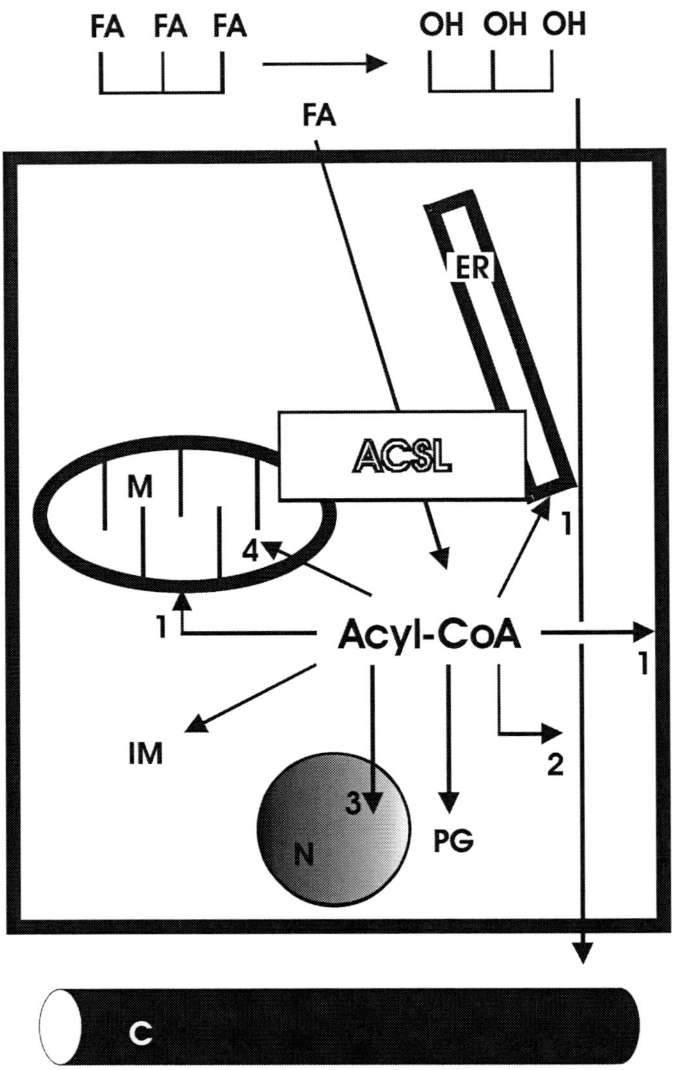

Figure 1. Main pathways in dietary long chain fatty acid metabolism of enterocytes. Dietary triglycerides are digested in free fatty acids and glycerol. The constituents are absorbed by enterocytes. Activation of free fatty acids to acyl-CoA derivatives is performed by several enzymes including acyl-CoA synthetases (ACSL) localized in endoplasmic reticulum (ER), mitochondria (M), and cytoplasm. Acyl-CoA derivatives are used for several biochemical pathways and cellular functions including configuration/ modification of cellular membranes (1), synthesis of triglycerides (2) for exocytosis in adjacent lymphatics or capillaries (C), nuclear transcription (3), beta-oxidation and mitochondrial behaviour (4), prostaglandin synthesis (PG), and other diverse functions in intermediary metabolism (IM).

Strong evidence is given that the sphingosine-based lipid ceramide is involved in apoptosis of tumour as well as non-tumour cells by different pathways (Ruvolo, 2003; Ahn and Schroeder, 2006).

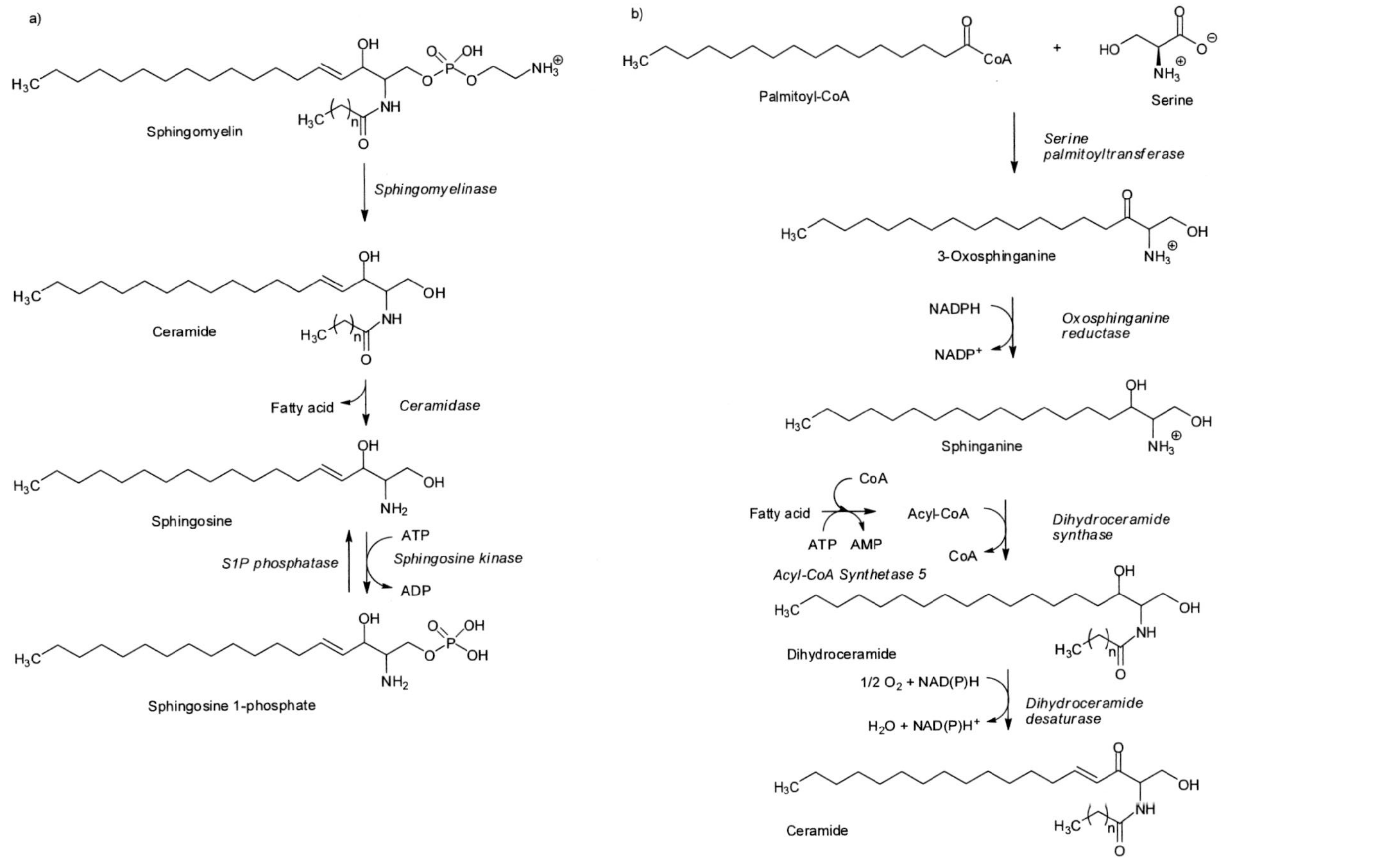

Figure 2. Sphingolipid metabolism. a) Central role of ceramide in sphingosine 1-phosphate metabolism and its synthesis by activation of sphingomyelinases. The amount of ceramide is further balanced by the *de novo* synthesis shown in more detail right hand. b) Ceramide *de novo* synthesis. In the scheme, the important role of acyl-CoA generating enzymes like acyl-CoA synthetase 5 (ACSL5) is addressed. Especially palmitoyl-CoA is used for the synthesis of the ceramide precursor 3-oxosphinganine, whereas several acyl-CoA derivatives are enzymatically added to sphinganine forming dihydroceramide. The acyl-CoA-forming enzyme ACSL5 is also located in mitochondrial membranes where ceramide synthesis is assumed to be highly important for the initiation of apoptosis.

The release of ceramide from sphingomyelin by stress stimuli like irradiation or heat shock is mediated by the acid sphingomyelinase, which is expressed in the cell surface membrane after stimulation with apoptotic triggers (Gulbins, 2003). Several apoptotic stimuli have been shown to induce apoptosis *via* an increase in mitochondrial ceramide levels probably mediated by both, release from sphingomyelin as well as *de novo* ceramide synthesis, because mitochondria contain enzymes capable of generating ceramide as ceramide synthase and reverse ceramidase (Bionda et al., 2004; Birbes et al., 2001; Siskind, 2005). Recent evidence indicates that the proapoptotic activity of ceramide depends on its ability to form large protein permeable channels, especially in mitochondria outer membranes (Siskind et al., 2006). It is assumed that the molecular basis of channel forming by ceramide is determined by the molecular structure of the ceramide backbone, especially the presence of the C4-C5 *trans* double-bound (Brockman et al., 2004). Given the interference of dietary sphinganine and sphinganine derivatives with intracellular ceramide *de novo* synthesis, this class of molecules provides numerous opportunities for indirect modulation of channel formation by ceramide.

In small intestinal mucosa, where fatty acids are preferentially absorbed, isoform 5 of the ACSL family is abundantly expressed by enterocytes (Yamashita et al., 2000, Gassler et al., 2004). ACSL5 is found in a spatial distribution with high amounts of ACSL5 mRNA and protein in villus or plateau-lining epithelia when compared with crypts. Consequently, expression of ACSL5 is stronger in small than large intestinal mucosa reflecting the differences in cellular lipid metabolism. ACSL isoforms other than ACLS5 are additionally found in intestinal surface epithelia; their function in pathophysiological pathways has been investigated (Cao et al., 2001). Using an inducible cell expression system, prevention of apoptosis is found after over-expression of ACSL4 probably due to reduction of free arachidonic acid signaling apoptosis (Cao et al., 2000). In the majority of CRCs, ACSL4 and cyclooxygenase-2 (COX-2) are up-regulated and interference with arachidonic acid metabolism is suggested (Cao et al., 2001). The additive effect of the enzymes in lowering free arachidonic acid levels is suggested as an important mechanism in prevention of cellular apoptosis and driving tumour progression.

However, it is suggested that in addition to ACSL4 ACSL isoform 5 plays a central role in intestinal lipid metabolism and probably in cellular differentiation (Yeh et al., 2006). This hypothesis is initiated by spatial distribution of ACSL5 along the crypt-villus axis and cloning of two ACSL5 variants from human small intestinal or gastric mucosa (accession no. AB033899; AM262166).

The sequences differ in a 72 bp region corresponding to exon 20 of the *ACSL5* gene. Biochemical analysis of both recombinant proteins, ACSL5-fl and ACSL5-Δ20, shows a significant shift in pH dependency of enzyme activities. Whereas ACSL5-fl is active in a strong bimodal dependency at pH 7.5 and pH 9.5, ACSL5-Δ20 shows a more uniform performance over a broad pH spectrum with minor peaks at pH 7.5 and 8.5. The phenomenon is determined by molecular differences in organization of the fatty acid activation 1 domain (FAA1) encoded by exon 20. *In situ*, ACSL5 proteins show a spatial distribution along the crypt-villus axis (CVA) in human small intestinal mucosa. ACSL5-fl is preferentially found in the villus-lining epithelia, whereas ACSL5-Δ20 is expressed throughout the CVA.

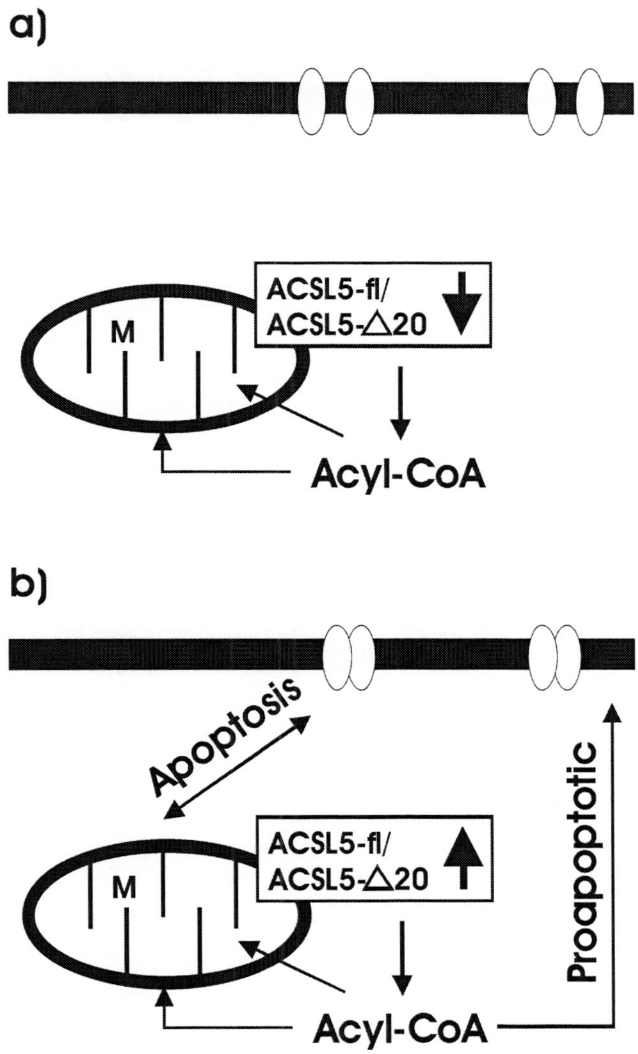

Figure 3. Main aspects of the putative ACSL5-fl/ ACSL5-Δ20 pathway. **a)** Low ACSL5-fl/ ACSL5-Δ20 ratio is associated with insensitivity to apoptosis or antiapoptotic behaviour. This scenario might favour cellular proliferation. **b)** High ACSL5-fl/ ACSL5-Δ20 ratio is associated with sensitivity to apoptosis probably mediated by mitochondrial and extramitochondrial activities via acyl-CoA derivatives like ceramide.

It is suggested by this data that the ACSL5-fl/ ACSL5-Δ20 ratio has some input to the development of apoptosis/ senescence of enterocytes, because overexpression of ACSL5-fl sensitizes enterocytes to TRAIL-mediated apoptosis accompanied by surface expression of TRAIL-receptors and increased caspase 3-like activity (Gassler et al., 2007). In such TRAIL-sensitive cells, expression of the FLICE-inhibitory protein (FLIP) is substantially decreased. However, treatment of ACSL5-fl transfectants with fumonisin B1, a specific inhibitor of the ceramide synthase, restores FLIP-expression levels. Main aspects of the putative pathway are illustrated in Figure 3.

The Concept of Modifier Genes in CRC Development

It is assumed that the search for further key modifier genes underlying carcinogenesis has not been highly successful, because alleles of modifier genes have a moderate-to-high population frequency with a low penetrance (Samuelson et al., 2007). However, using whole-genome linkage studies in inbred animal cancer models in addition to functional studies is suggested as a modern approach to define potential cancer susceptibility genes. Consequently, an increasing number of studies focussed on gene – environment interactions and cancer predisposition has led to the identification of so-called tumour modifiers (Dragani and Manenti, 1997; Papanikolaou et al., 2000). Important modifier genes identified in intestinal and colorectal carcinogenesis are DNA methyltransferase (*Dnmt*), *COX-2*, and the modifier of Min1 (*Mom1*) that decreases the number of tumour nodules in the *Min* (*Multiple Intestinal Neoplasia*) – mouse model (Dietrich et al., 1993; Laird et al., 1995; Oshima et al., 1996). *Min* mice develop numerous tumour nodules, predominantly in the small intestine, and die by about 5 month of age with anemia and intestinal obstruction from polyps and tumours. It was shown that tumour progress and tumour multiplicity in mice depend on the inbred strain in which the *Min* mutation was analyzed. This observation is paralleled by findings in humans. Patients carrying the same mutation in the *APC* gene [human ortholog of *Min* (Shoemaker et al., 1997)] can have dramatic differences in disease expression (Crabtree et al., 2002). However, the genes responsible for this variable expression of the FAP phenotype are widely unknown.

In the *Min – Mom1* scenario secretory phospholipase A2 was discussed as a molecule involved in modifying tumour progression as its expression was induced by the carcinogen azoxymethane (Papanikolaou et al., 2000). However, functional variants of phospholipase A2 have not been isolated so far, suggesting that other genetic loci might act as modifiers of the phenotype observed in CRC. From the data it is assumed that the number of so-called modifier genes is much higher, and that alleles acting in this manner comprise the majority of genetic risk for many common diseases including CRC (Reich and Lander, 2001). Moreover, it is speculated that interindividual differences in susceptibility for colorectal tumours and modification in well-characterized pathways of colorectal carcinogenesis like the APC- or the so-called 'serrated-type' pathway is determined by the genetic polymorphism of modifiers in the epithelial and/or mesenchymal compartment.

In addition to *APC* and phospholipase A2, which are expressed by epithelial cells, *Foxl1* was identified as the first mesenchymal modifier gene of *Min* (Perreault et al., 2005). *Foxl1* encodes a winged helix transcription factor expressed in the mesenchyme of the gastrointestinal tract. The factor is an important regulator of the Wnt/APC/beta-catenin pathway influencing accumulation of nuclear beta-catenin. Loss of *Foxl1* was shown to increase tumour multiplicity in *Min* mice caused by accelerated loss of heterozygosity at the *Min* locus (Perreault et al., 2005). The data underline the important hypothesis that other genes, or even environmental conditions, that favour increased turnover of intestinal epithelial cells will likewise accelerate tumour initiation and tumour progression.

At present, regulation of modifier gene expression by environmental conditions, especially dietary components, is suggested (Perreault et al., 2005). This point of view is for example favoured by the coincidence of CRCs and an increased alimentary supply of fatty acids or *COX-2* expression as discussed above. Concerning putative modifiers, dietary-induced changes in the expression of ACSL isoforms have been recorded for rat liver (Lewin et al., 2001). In high alimentary feeding both ACSL1 and ACSL4 expression increased, whereas ACSL5 expression decreased. The opposite constellation was found in fasting animals. In a more subtle study however, induction of ACSL5 expression in rat hepatocytes was found after feeding with a diet enriched with sucrose, whereas a fatty acid diet did not induce any change in ACSL5 expression (Oikawa et al., 1998). In contrary to a fatty acid enriched diet, ACSL5 expression was lowered by both, a cholesterol-enriched diet as well as fasting. The strong inductive effect of carbohydrate re-feeding on ACSL5 expression in rat hepatocytes recorded by Oikawa and colleagues was corroborated recently by another study (Achouri et al., 2005). In these experiments regulation of ACLS5 expression by dietary components was shown in cultured hepatocytes as well as in rats. The minor dietary effects of intestinal ACSL5 expression recorded in the Oikawa-study are probably due the analysis of total bowel tissue preparations instead of dissected enterocytes. Therefore regulation of intestinal ACSL isoforms, especially ACSL5 variants, is not really investigated as yet. Under the supposition that intestinal ACSL expression is similarly changed by dietary effects as it was found in liver tissues, the pathways shown in Figures 1 and 3 could be of high relevance for a better understanding of dietary-induced changes of putative modifier genes in CRC.

Acknowledgements

The authors are grateful to P. Akens for typing and proofreading the manuscript.

References

Achouri Y, Hegarty BD, Allanic D, Bécard D, Hainault I, Ferré P, Foufelle F. Long chain fatty acyl-CoA synthetase 5 expression is induced by insulin and glucose: involvement of sterol regulatory element-binding protein-1c. *Biochimie* 87:1149-1155;2005.

Ahn EH, Schroeder JJ. Sphinganine causes early activation of JNK and p38 MAPK and inhibition of AKT activation in HT-29 human colon cancer cells. *Anticancer. Res.* 26:121-127;2006.

Ahn EH, Schroeder JJ. Sphingoid bases and ceramide induce apoptosis in HT-29 and HCT-116 human colon cancer cells. *Exp. Biol. Med.* 227:345-353;2002.

Balk EM, Horsley TA, Newberry SJ, Lichtenstein AH, Yetley EA, Schachter HM, Moher D, MacLean CH, Lau J. A collaborative effort to apply the evidence-based review process to the field of nutrition: challenges, benefits, and lessons learned. *Am. J. Clin. Nutr.* 85:1448-1456;2007.

Bernardo K, Hurwitz R, Zenk T, Desnick RJ, Ferlinz K, Schuchman EH, Sandhoff K. Purification, characterization, and biosynthesis of human acid ceramidase. *J. Biol. Chem.* 270:11098-11102;1995.

Bionda C, Portoukalian J, Schmitt D, Rodriguez-Lafrasse C, Ardail D. Subcellular compartmentalization of ceramide metabolism: MAM (mitochondria-associated membrane) and/or mitochondria? *Biochem. J.* 382:527-533;2004.

Birbes H, El Bawab S, Hannun YA, Obeid LM. Selective hydrolysis of a mitochondrial pool of sphingomyelin induces apoptosis. *Fed. Am. Soc. Exp. Biol. J.* 15:2669-2679;2001.

Brockman HL, Momsen MM, Brown RE, He L, Chun J, Byun HS, Bittman R. The 4,5-double bond of ceramide regulates its dipole potential, elastic properties, and packing behavior. *Biophys. J.* 87:1722-1731;2004.

Cao Y, Dave KB, Doan TP, Prescott SM. Fatty acid CoA ligase 4 is up-regulated in colon adenocarcinoma. *Cancer Res.* 61:8429-8434;2001.

Cao Y, Pearman AT, Zimmerman GA, McIntyre TM, Prescott SM. Intracellular unesterified arachidonic acid signals apoptosis. *Proc. Natl. Acad. Sci. USA* 97:11280-11285;2000.

Chapkin RS, McMurray DN, Lupton JR. Colon cancer, fatty acids and anti-inflammatory compounds. *Curr. Opin. Gastroenterol.* 23:48-54; 2007.

Crabtree MD, Tomlinson IP, Hodgson SV, Neale K, Phillips RK, Houlston RS. Explaining variation in familial adenomatous polyposis: relationship between genotype and phenotype and evidence for modifier genes. *Gut* 51:420-423;2002.

Dietrich WF, Lander ES, Smith JS, Moser AR, Gould KA, Luongo C, Borenstein N, Dove W. Genetic identification of Mom-1, a major modifier locus affecting Min-induced intestinal multiple neoplasia in the mouse. *Cell* 75:631-639;1993.

Dragani TA, Manenti G. Mom1 leads the pack. *Nature Genet.* 17:7-8;1997.

Dvory-Sobol H, Arber N. Cyclooxygenase-2 as target for chemopreventive interventions: new approaches. *Cancer Biomark.* 3:153-161;2007.

Fearon ER, Vogelstein B. A genetic model for colorectal tumorigenesis. *Cell* 61:759-767;1990.

Gassler N, Kopitz J, Tehrani A, Ottenwälder B, Schnölzer M, Kartenbeck J, Lyer S, Autschbach F, Poustka A, Otto HF, Mollenhauer J. Expression of acyl-CoA synthetase 5 reflects the state of villus architecture in human small intestine. *J. Pathol.* 202:188-196;2004.

Gassler N, Roth W, Funke B, Schneider A, Herzog F, Tischendorf JJ, Grund K, Penzel R, Bravo IG, Mariadason J, Ehemann V, Sykora J, Haas TL, Walczak H, Ganten T, Zentgraf H, Erb P, Alonso A, Autschbach F, Schirmacher P, Knüchel R, Kopitz J. Regulation of enterocyte apoptosis by acyl-CoA synthetase 5 splicing. *Gastroenterology* 133:587-598;2007.

Granados S, Quiles JL, Gil A, Ramirez-Tortosa MC. Dietary lipids and cancer. *Nutr. Hosp.* 2:42-52, 44-54;2006.

Gulbins E. Regulation of death receptor signaling and apoptosis by ceramide. *Pharmacol. Res.* 47:393-399;2003.

Jass JR, Whitehall VL, Young J, Leggett BA. Emerging concepts in colorectal neoplasia. *Gastroenterology* 123:862-876;2002.

Laird PW, Jackson-Grusby L, Fazeli A, Dickinson SL, Jung WE, Li E, Weinberg RA, Jaenisch R. Suppression of intestinal neoplasia by DNA hypomethylation. *Cell* 81:197-205;1995.

Lewin TM, Kim JH, Granger DA, Vance JE, Coleman RA. Acyl-CoA synthetase isoforms 1, 4, and 5 are present in different subcellular membranes in rat liver and can be inhibited independently. *J. Biol. Chem*. 276:24674-24679;2001.

Marasas WF, Riley RT, Hendricks KA, Stevens VL, Sadler TW, Gelineau-van Waes J, Missmer SA, Cabrera J, Torres O, Gelderblom WC, Allegood J, Martinez C, Maddox J, Miller JD, Starr L, Sullards MC, Roman AV, Voss KA, Wang E, Merrill AH Jr. Fumonisins disrupt sphingolipid metabolism, folate transport, and neural tube development in embryo culture and in vivo: a potential risk factor for human neural tube defects among populations consuming fumonisin-contaminated maize. *J. Nutr.* 134:711-716;2004.

Mashek DG, Bornfeldt KE, Coleman RA, Berger J, Bernlohr DA, Black P, DiRusso CC, Farber SA, Guo W, Hashimoto N, Khodiyar V, Kuypers FA, Maltais LJ, Nebert DW, Renieri A, Schaffer JE, Stahl A, Watkins PA, Vasiliou V, Yamamoto TT. Revised nomenclature for the mammalian long-chain acyl-CoA synthetase gene family. *J. Lipid. Res.* 45:1958-1961;2004.

Murota K, Storch J. Uptake of micellar long-chain fatty acid and sn-2-monoacylglycerol into human intestinal Caco-2 cells exhibits characteristics of protein-mediated transport. *J. Nutr.* 135:1626-1630;2005.

Oikawa E, Iijima H, Suzuki T, Sasano H, Sato H, Kamataki A, Nagura H, Kang MJ, Fujino TT, Suzuki H, Yamamoto TT. A novel acyl-CoA synthetase, ACS5, expressed in intestinal epithelial cells and proliferating preadipocytes. *J. Biochem*. 124:679-685;1998.

Oshima M, Dinchuk JE, Kargman SL, Oshima H, Hancock B, Kwong E, Trzaskos JM, Evans JF, Taketo MM. Suppression of intestinal polyposis in Apc delta716 knockout mice by inhibition of cyclooxygenase 2 (COX-2). *Cell* 87:803-809;1996.

Papanikolaou A, Wang QS, Mulherkar R, Bolt A, Rosenberg DW. Expression analysis of the group IIA secretory phospholipase A(2) in mice with differential susceptibility to azoxymethane-induced colon tumorigenesis. *Carcinogenesis* 21:133-138;2000.

Perreault N, Sackett SD, Katz JP, Furth EE, Kaestner KH. Foxl1 is a mesenchymal modifier of Min in carcinogenesis of stomach and colon. *Genes Dev.* 19:311-315;2005.

Pyne S, Pyne NJ. Sphingosine 1-phosphate signalling in mammalian cells. *Biochem. J.* 349:385-402;2000.

Reich DE, Lander ES. On the allelic spectrum of human disease. *Trends Genet* 17:502-510;2001.

Ruvolo PP. Intracellular signal transduction pathways activated by ceramide and its metabolites. *Pharmacol. Res*. 47:383-392;2003.

Sampath H, Ntambi JM. The fate and intermediary metabolism of stearic acid. *Lipids* 40:1187-1191;2005.

Samuelson DJ, Hesselson SE, Aperavich BA, Zan Y, Haag JD, Trentham-Dietz A, Hampton JM, Mau B, Chen KS, Baynes C, Khaw KT, Luben R, Perkins B, Shah M, Pharoah PD, Dunning AM, Easton DF, Ponder BA, Gould MN. Rat Mcs5a is a compound quantitative trait locus with orthologous human loci that associate with breast cancer risk. *Proc. Natl. Acad. Sci. USA* 104:6299-6304;2007.

Saunders M, Iveson T. Management of advanced colorectal cancer: state of the art. *Br. J. Cancer* 95:131-138;2006

Shoemaker AR, Gould KA, Luongo C, Moser AR, Dove WF. Studies of neoplasia in the Min mouse. *Biochim. Biophys. Acta* 1332:F25-F48;1997.

Siskind LJ, Kolesnick RN, Colombini M. Ceramide forms channels in mitochondrial outer membranes at physiologically relevant concentrations. *Mitochondrion* 6:118-125;2006.

Siskind LJ. Mitochondrial ceramide and the induction of apoptosis. *J. Bioenerg. Biomembr.* 37:143-153;2005.

Sugawara T, Kinoshita M, Ohnishi M, Nagata J, Saito M. Digestion of maize sphingolipids in rats and uptake of sphingadienine by Caco-2 cells. *J. Nutr.* 133:2777-2782;2003.

Sugawara T, Kinoshita M, Ohnishi M, Tsuzuki T, Miyazawa T, Nagata J, Hirata T, Saito M. Efflux of sphingoid bases by P-glycoprotein in human intestinal Caco-2 cells. *Biosci. Biotechnol. Biochem.* 68:2541-2546;2004.

Yamashita Y, Kumabe T, Cho YY, Watanabe M, Kawagishi J, Yoshimoto T, Fujino T, Kang MJ, Yamamoto TT. Fatty acid induced glioma cell growth is mediated by the acyl-CoA synthetase 5 gene located on chromosome 10q25.1-q25.2, a region frequently deleted in malignant gliomas. *Oncogene* 19:5919-5925; 2000.

Yeh CS, Wang JW, Cheng TL, Juan CH, Wu CH, Lin SR. Fatty acid metabolism pathway play an important role in carcinogenesis of human colorectal cancers by microarray-bioinformatics analysis. *Cancer Let.* 233:297-308;2006.

Index

A

Aβ, 457
abdomen, 396
Abdullah, 425
AC, 9, 104, 106, 185, 233, 247, 249, 317, 368, 394, 415
access, 280, 290, 301
accidents, 144
accounting, 130
accuracy, x, 214, 218, 219, 221, 223, 226, 227, 244, 395, 405, 441, 444
acetonitrile, 138
acetylcholine, 338
acetylcholinesterase, 233
acetylcholinesterase inhibitor, 233
acid, viii, 63, 73, 75, 79, 94, 95, 96, 98, 102, 103, 104, 105, 109, 111, 113, 116, 117, 118, 125, 130, 131, 133, 135, 136, 137, 141, 144, 146, 153, 160, 161, 164, 165, 171, 172, 173, 174, 178, 181, 183, 185, 186, 188, 190, 192, 194, 275, 293, 298, 322, 324, 337, 344, 348, 357, 361, 362, 363, 367, 377, 419, 429, 448, 449, 450, 452, 455, 456, 457, 458
acidic, 138, 160, 161
acidity, 337
acidosis, 161, 419
activation, 7, 41, 48, 49, 58, 103, 109, 116, 138, 192, 339, 362, 379, 416, 447, 449, 451, 452, 455
active oxygen, 142
active site, 127
active transport, 357
acute infection, 363, 432
acute lung injury, 321, 326
acute respiratory distress syndrome, 326
acylation, 449
adaptation, 29, 390, 391, 410, 412, 415, 417, 436, 440
addiction, 144
additives, 112, 132, 188
adenocarcinoma, 456
adenoma, 122, 126, 136, 148, 149, 153, 154, 448
adenosine, 8, 140, 340, 413, 417, 426
adenosine triphosphate, 340, 426
adhesion, 68, 130, 137, 166, 272
adhesives, 334
adipocyte, 28, 68
adipocytes, 38, 41, 49, 50, 57, 59, 60, 70
Adipocytokines, 85
adiponectin, 85
adipose, 37, 49, 67, 68, 69, 70, 84, 85, 86, 89, 90, 91, 112, 230, 323, 325, 365, 442
adipose tissue, 37, 49, 67, 68, 69, 70, 84, 85, 86, 89, 90, 91, 112, 230, 323, 365, 442
adiposity, viii, 37, 55, 63, 67, 68, 70, 72, 84, 90, 91, 111, 366
adjustment, 45, 46, 136, 272, 303
administration, 47, 48, 78, 105, 133, 145, 189, 192, 335, 342, 350, 351, 357, 369, 393, 429, 433, 440
adolescence, 158
adolescents, 29, 77, 93, 100, 186, 201, 316
adrenaline, 161
adult onset diabetes, 148
adult population, 39, 79, 111
adulthood, 102, 159, 161, 354, 357, 363, 364
adults, xii, 36, 38, 42, 44, 47, 53, 54, 55, 60, 66, 67, 83, 84, 85, 90, 92, 94, 95, 97, 99, 103, 106, 124, 145, 148, 149, 162, 163, 167, 171, 173, 175, 180, 183, 185, 188, 189, 196, 199, 200, 201, 204, 207, 210, 211, 216, 217, 223, 226, 227, 228, 231, 232, 236, 246, 247, 254, 257, 265, 269, 272, 273, 281,

285, 286, 289, 290, 291, 293, 294, 296, 297, 300, 316, 321, 322, 326, 327, 328, 330, 331, 335, 338, 348, 351, 357, 364, 365, 366, 417, 442
adventitia, 272
advertisements, 254, 265
aerodigestive tract, 358, 367
aetiology, 64, 82
Africa, 4, 110, 127, 130, 159
African American(s), 38, 45, 54, 90, 160, 203, 208, 275, 280
African American women, 39
ageing, ix, 64, 65, 76, 82, 101, 157, 167, 229, 232, 286, 293, 294, 328, 335, 336, 345, 346, 354, 367, 369, 394
agent, 7, 9, 53, 75, 126, 131, 138, 177, 333, 338
aggregates, 380
aggregation, 3, 4, 7, 8, 68, 78
aggression, 116
aggressiveness, 326
aging, vii, xii, 37, 64, 65, 66, 67, 68, 70, 72, 76, 82, 83, 85, 89, 90, 93, 96, 97, 99, 102, 111, 124, 145, 191, 214, 215, 217, 219, 226, 227, 229, 230, 232, 233, 236, 242, 248, 249, 285, 290, 291, 296, 297, 298, 320, 321, 323, 326, 328, 329, 335, 336, 337, 338, 345, 346, 348, 351, 353, 354, 355, 359, 360, 363, 364, 365, 366, 367, 368, 369, 389, 392, 393, 394
aging population, 82
aging process, vii, xii, 64, 67, 111, 236, 285, 291, 335, 336, 345, 354, 360, 366, 369, 393
agonist, 140, 339
AIM, 342
airflow obstruction, 390, 391, 395, 409, 411, 414, 429, 438, 439, 442, 444
airway inflammation, 418
airways, 400, 407, 409, 418
albino, 185
albumin, x, 12, 24, 25, 26, 213, 214, 219, 221, 222, 223, 226, 227, 230, 237, 320, 325, 344, 373, 374, 375, 377, 381, 383, 384, 385, 387
alcohol, ix, 8, 27, 55, 74, 75, 96, 97, 114, 126, 137, 144, 150, 157, 160, 200, 293, 302, 313, 342
alcohol abuse, 160
alcohol consumption, 27, 74, 75, 96, 97, 144, 200
alcohol use, 75, 97
alcoholics, 335
alcoholism, 347
aldosterone, 381
alfalfa, 140
algorithm, 421
alimentation, 220
alkaline, 161, 175, 180, 181, 193
alkaline phosphatase, 175, 180, 193
alkaloids, 5
alkalosis, 334, 335, 346
allele(s), 50, 51, 87, 454
alloys, 333
alpha1-antitrypsin, 402
alpha-tocopherol, 77, 104
alternative, x, 51, 195, 206, 214, 227, 292, 315, 364, 378, 381, 421
alters, xii, 95, 147, 285
aluminium, 78, 101
aluminum, 101, 102
alveoli, 320, 392, 429
Alzheimer's disease (AD), x, 64, 65, 67, 68, 69, 72, 76, 77, 78, 79, 80, 82, 83, 85, 87, 89, 92, 93, 94, 95, 96, 97, 98, 99, 99, 100, 101, 102, 104, 105, 106, 177, 192, 220, 222, 230, 233, 293, 245, 248, 251, 252, 293, 298, 345, 357,434, 436, 443
ambivalence, 197
American Diabetes Association(ADA), 89, 316, 341, 348, 350, 364, 418
American Heart Association, 351, 364
American Indian(s), 275
American Psychiatric Association, 81
amines, 114, 128
amino acid(s), 75, 126, 160, 296, 322, 381, 422, 447
Amsterdam, 426, 436, 439
amyloid beta, 76, 102
amyloid plaques, 82
AN, 327, 435
anabolic steroid(s), 432, 438
anaemia, 2
anatomy, 408
androgen(s), 112, 126, 151
androstenedione, 112
anemia, 125, 239, 361, 374, 377, 454
aneurysm, 338, 348
angina, 356
angiogenesis, 6, 140, 155
angiotensin II, 3
animal models, 7, 48, 49, 77, 132, 142
animals, 40, 41, 72, 76, 101, 110, 123, 130, 140, 143, 164, 172, 174, 178, 335, 353, 364, 412, 455
anion, 171
anorexia, xii, 215, 218, 229, 248, 285, 286, 294, 351, 376
anoxia, 65
antagonists, 338

antibiotic(s), 177, 378
antibody, 239, 252, 323
anti-cancer, 126, 127, 143
anticancer activity, 125
anticholinergic, 428
anticoagulant, 177
anticonvulsants, 160
antidiuretic hormone, 381
antigen, 380
anti-inflammatory, 5, 77, 113, 143, 145, 164, 272, 374, 428, 456
antioxidant(s), xii, 4, 5, 7, 9,63, 71, 74, 75, 76, 77, 78, 79, 80, 100, 101, 105, 111, 112, 127, 128, 129, 130, 131, 133, 135, 136, 142, 152, 153, 154, 155, 158, 180, 181, 194, 273, 282, 300, 319, 322, 323, 328, 329, 330, 336, 337, 344, 349, 353, 354, 355, 356, 357, 358, 363, 364, 366, 367, 421, 425, 426, 428, 429, 431, 433, 436
antioxidant consumption, 356
antiretroviral, 232
Antitrypsin, 379
antitumor, 143, 151
anxiety, 215, 236, 249, 302, 344
anxiety disorder, 236
aorta, 339
AP, 90, 102, 146, 181, 185, 326, 396, 397, 435
APC, 448, 454
apoptosis, 98, 109, 116, 117, 125, 126, 127, 130, 137, 138, 142, 145, 151, 155, 273, 389, 393, 394, 414, 418, 422, 427, 450, 451, 452, 453, 455, 456, 458
apoptotic, 155, 422, 449, 452
apoptotic pathway, 155
appetite, 72, 215, 229, 232, 290, 294, 301, 377, 390, 391, 431, 440
aptitude, 215
AR, 85, 88, 94, 95, 147, 148, 185, 232, 283, 284, 295, 330, 348, 350, 367, 417, 426, 435, 456, 458
arachidonic acid, 73, 130, 447, 452, 456
Argentina, 252
arginine, 40, 58
Arizona, 127
aromatic hydrocarbons, 114
arrest, 137, 154
arrhythmia, 345
ARS, 187
arsenic, 296
arterial hypertension, 7, 70, 333, 342
arteries, 272, 338, 347
arteriosclerosis, 345
artery, 51, 61, 69, 86, 339, 342, 348, 356, 360, 410
arthritis, 302, 361
asbestos, 408
ascites, 151
ascorbic acid, 133, 178, 357, 362, 363, 367
ash, 160
Asia, 28, 56, 84, 110, 130, 140, 159, 232, 304, 305, 307
Asian countries, 39
aspartate, 160, 346
aspirate, 323
aspirin, 8, 103, 356, 365
assault, 128
assessment, x, xi, 27, 52, 64, 75, 98, 115, 122, 155, 158, 192, 198, 199, 203, 214, 217, 221, 222, 225, 226, 227, 228, 229, 230, 231, 232, 233, 235, 236, 237, 238, 239, 241, 242, 244, 245, 246, 247, 248, 250, 251, 252, 295, 296, 324, 325, 327, 330, 331, 346, 349, 365, 386, 390, 391, 398, 405, 406, 408, 420, 430, 432, 440, 441, 443
assessment techniques, 247
assimilation, 264
assumptions, 218
asthenia, 344
asthma, 333, 362, 425, 439
asymptomatic, 68
atherogenesis, 338, 347, 356, 357
atherosclerosis, 69, 88, 130, 141, 281, 330, 336, 337, 338, 347, 348, 351, 355, 360, 365, 366
Atherosclerosis Risk in Communities (ARIC), xi
athletes, 264, 415
atoms, 142
ATP, 34, 49, 50, 61, 338, 340, 420, 422, 426, 436
atria, 341
atrophy, 74, 76, 84, 88, 98, 345, 422, 427
attacks, 336, 346
attention, viii, 40, 63, 66, 67, 71, 73, 79, 80, 81, 117, 129, 238, 241, 254, 265, 322, 324, 325, 377, 390, 405, 421, 439
attitudes, 199, 236, 268, 269, 294
atypical, 236
AU, 246
Australia, 167, 297, 299, 300, 316, 317, 319, 328
autoantibodies, 378
autoimmune disease(s), 39, 40, 380
autonomy, 249
autosomal dominant, 448
autosomal recessive, 52
availability, 7, 23, 79, 118, 127, 164, 240, 376, 410, 420, 429, 441

avoidance, 238, 364
awareness, 27, 236, 242, 251, 321

B

B vitamins, 76, 99, 119, 289
back pain, 302
backlash, 269
bacteria, 141, 176, 380
bacterial infection, 428
barley, 119
Barrett's esophagus, 115
barriers, 199, 203, 315
Basa, 1
basal metabolic rate, 294, 320, 324, 327, 360
battery, 80
Bayesian, 274
BD, 145, 193, 394, 443, 455
beef, 124, 162, 181, 258, 259, 260, 262, 265, 266, 267, 329
beer, 8, 74, 258, 259, 260, 264, 266
behavior, ix, x, 109, 112, 130, 195, 196, 197, 198, 199, 200, 201, 202, 203, 204, 205, 206, 207, 208, 209, 210, 372, 456
behavioral intentions, 196
Beijing, 39
Belgium, 235, 250
beliefs, vii, xi, 1, 2, 215, 253, 254, 268, 294
beneficial effect, vii, 1, 2, 3, 7, 35, 47, 79, 81, 110, 129, 137, 140, 141, 142, 169, 170, 176, 178, 180, 300, 329, 335, 359, 360, 430, 433
benefits, 74, 80, 98, 128, 132, 140, 144, 155, 164, 169, 192, 226, 237, 238, 239, 265, 300, 315, 321, 323, 359, 428, 430, 455
benign, 344
beta-carotene, 132, 152, 153, 180, 347, 368
beverages, vii, 1, 2, 3, 4, 7, 15, 16, 17, 18, 23, 27, 126, 144, 171, 188, 256, 260, 289
bias, ix, 108, 276
bicarbonate, 173, 183, 189
bile, 109, 118, 120, 121
bile acids, 118, 120, 121
binding, 34, 40, 49, 57, 59, 112, 118, 121, 140, 155, 219, 281, 329, 363, 373, 374, 375, 378, 420, 426, 441, 455
binding globulin, 112
bioactive compounds, 113, 164
bioavailability, xii, 32, 35, 37, 55, 102, 144, 155, 319, 355
Bioelectrical Impedance Vector Analysis, BIVA, x
bioindicators, 372, 373, 376, 383
bioinformatics, 458
biological activity, 4, 109, 341
biological processes, 130
biological systems, 173, 355
biomarker(s), 8, 92, 117, 219, 272, 273, 359, 360, 365, 366
biomedical, vii, 1, 2
biomedical knowledge, vii, 1, 2
biopsy, 341, 428
biosphere, 369
biosynthesis, 73, 140, 186, 272, 338, 455
birth, xii, 38, 42, 45, 55, 120, 166, 299, 301, 304, 305, 307
black tea, 137
bladder, 109, 125, 129, 143
bladder cancer, 109
bleeding, 379
blood, 3, 5, 7, 9, 10, 12, 14, 24, 29, 32, 34, 35, 39, 41, 46, 56, 68, 69, 70, 72, 82, 83, 89, 95, 108, 111, 113, 119, 121, 124, 131, 132, 148, 152, 162, 164, 166, 170, 171, 176, 178, 180, 188, 190, 193, 204, 282, 284, 320, 330, 335, 337, 339, 341, 343, 344, 345, 346, 347, 350, 359, 360, 364, 366, 375, 376, 381, 382, 387, 394, 404, 406, 408, 412, 414, 415, 416, 417, 420, 421, 424
blood clot, 35, 113, 164, 166
blood flow, 320, 339, 404, 408, 412, 415, 417
blood plasma, 375
blood pressure, 7, 9, 10, 12, 14, 56, 69, 70, 83, 89, 170, 188, 282, 337, 346, 359, 360, 364, 416
blood stream, 32, 68
blood supply, 420
blood vessels, 82, 178
bloodstream, 32, 34, 37, 322
BMD, 159, 161, 165, 166, 169, 170, 177, 180, 441
BN, 101, 102, 150, 367
body composition, vii, x, xii, 67, 70, 84, 90, 93, 213, 215, 216, 217, 218, 219, 225, 226, 227, 228, 229, 230, 231, 237, 248, 252, 285, 289, 290, 320, 321, 322, 327, 329, 331, 372, 390, 432, 441, 442
body density, 217
body fat, 37, 68, 72, 73, 91, 93, 96, 202, 217, 232, 330, 359, 441
body fluid, 121, 166, 231
body mass index (BMI), x, xi, xii, 12, 28, 37, 38, 45, 47, 57, 65, 67, 70, 120, 84, 90, 111, 112, 144, 145, 182, 200, 201, 202, 203, 217, 221, 222, 223, 224, 226, 227, 228, 231, 232, 244, 246, 271, 274, 276, 278, 279, 286, 299, 303, 304, 309, 310, 321,

327, 359, 361, 397, 409, 410, 414, 437, 440, 442, 444
body size, 146, 148, 217
body weight, 12, 28, 37, 55, 67, 84, 106, 111, 120, 144, 158, 166, 171, 202, 217, 219, 230, 232, 244, 294, 298, 320, 321, 322, 325, 327, 385, 409, 414, 431, 432, 441, 442
bonds, 50, 116, 135
bone growth, 166, 344
bone marrow, 121, 166, 192, 194
bone mass, ix, 157, 158, 159, 160, 161, 173, 178, 181, 182, 183, 189, 192, 214, 323
bone mineral content, 120, 158, 166, 441
bone remodeling, 183
bone resorption, 162, 164, 165, 172, 174, 177, 180, 181, 183, 192, 193, 194, 334
borate, 178
boric acid, 178
Boron, 178, 189, 193, 288
bowel, 109, 115, 117, 146, 290, 315, 455
brain, 65, 68, 69, 72, 74, 75, 76, 78, 82, 83, 85, 86, 89, 93, 96, 97, 98, 101, 102, 121, 166, 177, 179, 334, 343, 367, 416, 421, 442
brain damage, 74, 76, 96, 343
brain development, 65, 96, 177
brain functioning, 78
Brassica oleracea, 138
Brazil, 4, 128, 169, 353, 361, 362, 365
breakdown, 160, 322, 441
breakfast, 117, 265
breast, viii, 107, 109, 110, 111, 112, 114, 115, 119, 120, 122, 124, 125, 126, 127, 128, 129, 131, 135, 136, 139, 140, 141, 143, 144, 145, 146, 147, 148, 149, 150, 151, 152, 153, 154, 155, 274, 283, 457
breast cancer, viii, 107, 110, 111, 112, 120, 125, 126, 127, 128, 131, 135, 136, 139, 143, 144, 145, 146, 147, 148, 149, 150, 151, 152, 153, 154, 155, 274, 283, 457
breathing, 302, 344, 414, 423, 437, 440, 443
breathlessness, 423, 434
Britain, 5
broccoli sprouts, viii
bronchioles, 390, 391, 405
bronchitis, 390, 395, 405, 409, 410, 418, 434, 443, 444
bronchodilator, 399, 400, 405, 409, 410, 428, 429, 434
buccal mucosa, 131, 153
buffer, 161

C

Ca^{2+}, ix, 33, 34, 35, 37, 41, 48, 49, 52, 58, 59, 60, 157, 161, 166, 426, 427
cabbage, 137, 138, 139
cachexia, 215, 218, 425, 439
caffeine, 4, 5, 9
calciferol, 57, 176
calcification, 172, 178
calciotropic hormones, 34, 35, 53
calcitonin, 34, 53, 166, 179
calcium, viii, ix, 23, 27, 31, 32, 33, 34, 35, 36, 37, 39, 40, 41, 46, 47, 48, 49, 52, 53, 55, 56, 57, 58, 59, 76, 79, 107, 114, 115, 120, 121, 122, 149, 157, 158, 160, 161, 162, 163, 164, 165, 166, 167, 168, 169, 170, 171, 172, 173, 174, 175, 176, 177, 178, 179, 180, 181, 182, 183, 184, 185, 186, 187, 188, 189, 190, 191, 192, 193, 274, 283, 289, 293, 330, 333, 337, 338, 339, 342, 343, 345, 347, 348, 349, 351, 422, 426, 427, 449
calcium channel blocker, 333
caliber, 395
calibration, 221
California, 31, 42, 45, 93
caloric intake, 40, 41, 72, 358, 360, 431, 440
caloric restriction, 72, 93, 359, 360, 366, 367, 368
calorie, x, 72, 124, 195, 201, 202, 206, 246, 250, 256, 291, 359, 360, 366, 441
calorimetry, 441, 443
Canada, 181, 431
cancer cells, 138, 142, 149, 455
cancer screening, 149, 203
cancerous cells, 108, 127
candidates, 430
capillary, 178, 381, 390, 392, 394, 404, 406, 410, 412, 420
carbohydrate(s), 23, 24, 27, 29, 72, 116, 119, 142, 147, 148, 149, 211, 256, 257, 261, 262, 264, 265, 291, 296, 340, 359, 432, 438, 440, 455
carbohydrate metabolism, 340
carbon, 65, 125, 135, 142, 161, 430, 435, 438, 440
carbon dioxide, 430, 435, 438
carbon monoxide, 65
carbonyl groups, 422
carcinogen(s), 109, 120, 128, 137, 138, 145, 154, 454
carcinogenesis, 108, 109, 125, 126, 128, 142, 144, 152, 153, 154, 272, 273, 281, 282, 386, 447, 448, 449, 454, 457, 458
carcinogenicity, 110

carcinoma, 151, 155, 281, 380, 448
cardiac muscle, 421
cardiac output, 410, 420, 424
cardiocirculatory system, vii
cardiology, 351
cardiopulmonary, 412, 419, 420, 423
cardiovascular disease, viii, 3, 6, 7, 9, 10, 39, 40, 54, 56, 63, 67, 68, 71, 81, 90, 91, 92, 95, 97, 110, 115, 132, 143, 153, 214, 249, 293, 299, 315, 316, 337, 346, 348, 355, 356, 367, 369, 413, 418
cardiovascular risk, 3, 68, 85, 87, 293, 365
cardiovascular system, 3, 4, 5, 6, 7, 9, 282, 337
caregivers, 80, 236
Caribbean, 361
carotene, viii, 77, 91, 107, 129, 130, 131, 132, 137, 152, 153, 180, 347, 357, 358, 368, 369
carotenoids, viii, 79, 107, 114, 129, 130, 132, 193, 194, 300, 358, 361, 365
carrier, 97
cartilage, 133, 190
case study, 230
casein, 322
caspase, 138, 393, 453
catabolism, xii, 75, 95, 319, 375, 381, 382, 384, 432
catalase, 421
catechins, 5, 6, 7, 137, 143
catecholamines, 338, 381
categorization, 35, 315
Catholic, 6
cation, 35, 52, 61, 171, 173, 174, 333, 334, 336, 338, 347
Caucasians, 38, 42, 51, 275
causal inference, 52
causality, 71, 359
CD8+, 428
CE, 82, 95, 106, 188, 228, 247, 326, 438
cell, 7, 9, 31, 33, 34, 42, 45, 48, 49, 52, 58, 61, 73, 75, 76, 78, 98, 102, 105, 108, 109, 113, 116, 118, 120, 121, 124, 125, 130, 135, 136, 137, 140, 141, 142, 143, 149, 150, 151, 154, 155, 164, 166, 175, 177, 178, 179, 180, 192, 193, 194, 218, 225, 227, 231, 272, 273, 281, 302, 310, 323, 334, 335, 366, 367, 376, 392, 393, 394, 412, 418, 421, 422, 432, 452, 458
cell adhesion, 7, 9, 137
cell culture, 192
cell cycle, 137, 154
cell death, 75, 76, 98, 109, 125, 422
cell differentiation, 137, 140
cell division, 108, 154
cell growth, 113, 164, 177, 272, 458
cell line, 116, 124, 142, 150, 151, 155
cell lines, 116, 142, 155
cell membranes, 136, 376, 421
cell signaling, 98
cell surface, 121, 166, 452
cellular immunity, 379
cellulose, 337
Central Europe, 127
central nervous system, 4, 98, 108
central obesity, 90
cereals, 15, 16, 17, 18, 23, 24, 71, 117, 124, 135, 141, 169, 291, 293
cerebral blood flow, 339
cerebrovascular disease, 74, 89, 282, 339, 348
ceruloplasmin, 179
cervical, 124, 125, 149
cervical carcinoma, 149
cervical dysplasia, 125
cervix, 111
Chalmers, 89
channel blocker, 333
channels, x, 48, 49, 52, 58, 61, 195, 205, 207, 338, 339, 414, 452, 458
CHAOS, 356, 368
chelating agents, 78, 101
chemical properties, 422
chemical reactions, 136
chemoprevention, 122, 131, 132, 145, 155, 281
chemopreventive agents, 129, 138, 155
Chicago, 409
chicken, 144, 257, 259, 260, 263, 264, 265, 266
childhood, 108, 158, 175, 228
children, 27, 29, 93, 160, 171, 172, 186, 188, 231, 290, 339, 349
Chile, 361, 369
China, 5, 23, 28, 127, 361
Chinese, 5, 114, 138, 139, 143, 168
chloride, 170, 173, 189, 190, 414
chlorophyll, 343
chocolate, vii, 1, 2, 4, 6, 7, 8, 9, 116, 143
cholecalciferol, 32, 36, 123, 174, 191
cholecystokinin, 215
cholesterol, 3, 4, 5, 7, 24, 25, 26, 29, 69, 70, 72, 73, 87, 95, 123, 130, 179, 186, 256, 261, 262, 263, 266, 267, 272, 291, 296, 335, 337, 338, 339, 347, 357, 360, 373, 375, 376, 377, 380, 382, 455
cholinesterase, 373, 375
chromium, 189, 288, 296, 349
chromosome, 50, 130, 150, 458

chronic cough, 396, 397, 401
chronic diseases, x, 40, 82, 110, 119, 149, 213, 226, 315, 328, 354, 364, 375
chronic hypoxia, 412, 416, 421
chronic illness, 241
chronic obstructive pulmonary disease, 361, 391, 395, 406, 407, 408, 411, 412, 416, 419, 420, 423, 424, 425, 433, 434, 435, 436, 437, 438, 439, 443, 444
cigarette smoke, 128, 136, 389, 392, 393
cigarette smokers, 136
cigarette smoking, 109, 413, 431, 440
circulation, 3, 4, 5, 141, 376, 423, 425
cirrhosis, 232, 361, 374
civil servants, 83
classes, 5, 142, 225, 257, 280, 428
classification, 64, 65, 216, 217, 219, 221, 222, 223, 227, 303, 348
claudication, 412
cleaning, 3
clinical assessment, 390, 391, 397, 440, 442, 444
clinical diagnosis, 67
clinical examination, 276, 325
clinical trials, 46, 47, 131, 161, 170, 177, 181, 356, 364
clinicians, 122, 238
cloning, 85, 452
cluster analysis, 71
clustering, 69, 80, 211
clusters, 402, 404, 418
C-N, 433
CO2, 441
coagulation, 3, 73, 176
cobalamin, 151, 330
cocoa, 6, 7, 9, 105, 185
cocoa butter, 185
coconut, 116
codes, 276
coding, 449
coefficient of variation, 275
coenzyme, 176, 178, 330, 376, 449
coffee, vii, 1, 2, 4, 5, 7, 8, 9, 178
cognition, 70, 76, 77, 86, 87
cognitive abilities, 81
cognitive activity, 83
cognitive deficit, 88
cognitive development, 64, 66
cognitive domains, 80
cognitive dysfunction, 76, 87, 105
cognitive function, 64, 67, 68, 70, 72, 76, 78, 79, 80, 82, 83, 84, 85, 88, 89, 90, 93, 96, 99, 100, 103, 104, 105, 245, 298, 324, 344
cognitive impairment, 64, 68, 77, 78, 81, 83, 96, 98, 99, 100, 103, 104, 105, 239, 246, 247, 293
cognitive performance, 73, 100, 103
cognitive process, 68
cohort, viii, xii, 38, 43, 45, 46, 55, 64, 69, 73, 83, 85, 87, 88, 90, 92, 94, 100, 111, 119, 120, 127, 129, 135, 136, 145, 146, 148, 149, 152, 176, 236, 258, 260, 264, 274, 275, 276, 297, 299, 303, 304, 309, 310, 313, 314, 315, 317, 326, 327, 356, 357, 366, 417
collaboration, 82, 280, 374
collagen, 133, 165, 175, 178, 179, 180, 357
collateral, 391, 405
college students, xi, 253, 254, 257, 260, 261, 262
colon, 54, 111, 114, 116, 117, 119, 120, 121, 122, 124, 125, 126, 128, 129, 131, 135, 136, 138, 140, 141, 143, 144, 145, 146, 147, 149, 152, 154, 155, 176, 203, 208, 274, 283, 447, 455, 456, 457
colon cancer, 117, 121, 122, 125, 126, 128, 131, 136, 144, 146, 147, 154, 155, 203, 208, 274, 283, 447, 455
colorectal, ix, 35, 92, 108, 110, 114, 117, 119, 120, 121, 122, 128, 131, 136, 146, 147, 148, 149, 150, 151, 153, 154, 170, 187, 203, 208, 229, 274, 282, 283, 380, 386, 447, 448, 449, 454, 456, 457, 458
colorectal cancer, ix, 35, 108, 114, 117, 119, 120, 121, 122, 128, 136, 146, 147, 148, 149, 150, 151, 170, 203, 208, 229, 274, 282, 283, 447, 448, 457, 458
colorectum, viii
coma, 326
combination therapy, 428
combined effect, 217, 344
commercial, 12, 123
commercials, 254
commodity, 118
communication, 137, 148, 205, 211
community, 51, 60, 79, 83, 84, 87, 89, 94, 99, 101, 199, 203, 204, 207, 209, 227, 228, 231, 240, 246, 248, 249, 286, 295, 297, 301, 316, 321, 327, 363, 387
comorbidity, 329
compensation, 424
compilation, 220
complement, 322, 378
complement system, 378
complex carbohydrates, 116

complex interactions, 420
complexity, 108, 402
compliance, 238, 244, 356, 392
complications, xii, 70, 72, 81, 217, 246, 319, 323, 340, 350, 354, 372, 381, 384, 417, 418
components, x, xii, 6, 11, 12, 24, 28, 71, 73, 119, 129, 136, 142, 197, 214, 273, 291, 299, 301, 314, 315, 323, 337, 364, 372, 383, 420, 422, 430, 442, 454
composition, vii, x, xii, 3, 9, 23, 67, 70, 84, 90, 93, 94, 112, 146, 158, 190, 213, 214, 215, 216, 217, 218, 219, 220, 225, 226, 227, 228, 229, 230, 231, 233, 237, 248, 252, 285, 289, 290, 320, 321, 322, 327, 329, 331, 360, 372, 391, 409, 423, 437, 444, 449
compounds, 76, 109, 113, 114, 116, 120, 122, 129, 130, 132, 133, 137, 138, 140, 142, 143, 164, 176, 356, 456
computed tomography, 70, 218, 343, 399, 400, 404, 406, 407, 408, 435
concentration, 29, 35, 36, 42, 45, 53, 60, 70, 76, 80, 111, 112, 113, 120, 121, 124, 129, 130, 136, 140, 164, 166, 171, 173, 174, 176, 178, 179, 189, 215, 281, 282, 334, 335, 337, 338, 340, 341, 347, 357, 374, 377, 380, 382, 384, 414, 421
concordance, x, 213, 216
conductance, 435
conduction, 334
conductor, 218
confidence, 170, 197, 219, 225, 302, 313, 393, 398
confidence interval, 170, 302, 393, 398
configuration, 158, 178, 450
conflict, 209, 265
confounders, 46, 72
confounding variables, 136
confusion, 239, 325
congestive heart failure, 335, 336, 361, 406, 423, 425, 436
conjugation, 109
connective tissue, 133, 177, 179, 391, 405, 417
consensus, 35, 97, 132, 226, 243
conservation, 334
constipation, 170, 257, 292, 302, 354
construction, 382
consultants, 239
consumers, 74, 124, 269, 291, 294
consumption, viii, ix, xii, 3, 4, 5, 6, 8, 9, 15, 17, 23, 27, 28, 32, 55, 72, 73, 74, 75, 76, 77, 92, 94, 96, 97, 105, 107, 110, 111, 116, 119, 128, 129, 143, 144, 160, 161, 163, 164, 167, 171, 177, 182, 189, 194, 195, 199, 200, 202, 203, 204, 206, 211, 268, 285, 289, 290, 300, 301, 303, 304, 314, 315, 316, 337, 356, 357, 364, 376, 382, 441
contact time, 120
contaminants, ix, 108, 110, 128
contamination, 239
contraceptives, 115
control, ix, 34, 35, 37, 41, 53, 67, 69, 70, 72, 78, 84, 108, 114, 119, 120, 125, 128, 129, 131, 135, 136, 144, 145, 147, 148, 152, 155, 161, 170, 171, 176, 177, 180, 188, 199, 203, 209, 215, 217, 229, 238, 239, 258, 265, 274, 276, 292, 321, 340, 345, 350, 356, 359, 360, 361, 362, 363, 364, 366, 413, 414, 416, 417, 422, 427, 428, 430, 434, 437, 438, 439, 440
control group, 41, 128, 199, 203, 238, 239, 360, 430
controlled trials, 29, 69, 71, 169, 188, 237, 251, 353, 356, 363, 365, 432
conversion, 75, 112, 118, 123, 133, 174, 379, 449
cooking, 119, 138, 215
cooling, 119
COPD, 389, 390, 391, 392, 393, 394, 395, 402, 405, 407, 409, 410, 411, 412, 413, 414, 415, 418, 419, 420, 421, 422, 423, 424, 425, 427, 428, 429, 430, 431, 432, 433, 434, 435, 436, 437, 438, 439, 440, 441, 442, 443, 444
Copenhagen, 96, 436, 437
copper, ix, 76, 78, 94, 101, 102, 158, 179, 181, 183, 193, 283, 296, 323, 347
coronary arteries, 272
coronary artery disease, 51, 61, 339, 342, 348, 356
coronary heart disease, 5, 8, 9, 71, 72, 74, 87, 90, 94, 97, 101, 144, 154, 159, 284, 295, 359, 366, 367, 368
correlation, x, 47, 120, 151, 180, 190, 214, 217, 221, 223, 227, 257, 260, 341, 350, 355, 357, 387, 398, 400, 406, 410, 424
correlation analysis, 221, 223
correlation coefficient, 398
correlations, 103, 143, 257, 329
corticosteroids, 160, 428, 432
cortisol, 161, 323, 329, 381
costs, 67, 200, 216, 219, 238
Council of Europe, 296
counseling, 209
coupling, 68, 333, 394
course work, 255
coverage, 254
covering, 39, 244
COX-2, 100, 112, 452, 454, 455, 457

Cranberry, 134, 141
C-reactive protein, 68, 86, 281, 272, 281, 282, 330, 360, 371, 372, 373, 374, 378, 380, 382, 383, 384
creatine, 385, 441
creatinine, 173, 219, 320, 344, 377, 380, 385, 386
credit, 255
Crete, 71
cretinism, 75
critical value, 384
cross-cultural comparison, ix, 108
cross-sectional study, 36, 37, 38, 93, 194, 273
CRP, 68, 272, 273, 374, 378, 421, 425, 437, 443
crystals, 178, 192
CT scan, 398, 400, 401, 402, 403, 404, 429
cultural factors, x, 213
culture, 39, 151, 192, 457
cumulative frequency, 222
CVD, viii, 63, 68, 69, 72, 73, 75, 81, 300, 356, 357, 359
cyanocobalamin, 126
cycling, 154
cyclooxygenase, 100, 452, 457
cyclooxygenase-2, 100, 452
cyclophosphamide, 375
cystic fibrosis, 419
cystine, 160
cytochrome, 109, 130, 138, 179
cytokines, 68, 70, 86, 164, 165, 166, 272, 281, 330, 374, 381, 413
cytoplasm, 450
cytosine, 126
Cytotoxic, 151
cytotoxic agents, 126
cytotoxicity, 282
Czech Republic, 371

D

Daidzein, 141
daily living, 236, 238, 250, 301, 414
dairy, ix, 15, 16, 17, 18, 23, 32, 73, 107, 115, 117, 135, 167, 170, 187, 261, 264, 265, 291, 293
dairy products, ix, 15, 16, 17, 18, 23, 73, 107, 115, 117, 135, 167, 170, 264, 265, 293
danger, 384
data collection, 256
data set, 243, 244, 275
database, 301, 368
dating, 286, 294
DBP, 12, 13, 14
DD, 104, 329, 427
death(s), xii, 6, 67, 72, 75, 76, 83, 98, 103, 108, 109, 110, 111, 112, 125, 128, 195, 200, 275, 283, 285, 286, 301, 303, 339, 342, 348, 351, 354, 355, 356, 358, 366, 367, 422, 442, 456
death rate, 111
decision making, 197, 251
decisions, 144
defects, 52, 111, 125, 334, 419, 457
defense, 140, 152, 236, 355, 358, 368, 378, 422
defense mechanisms, 355, 358
deficiency, ix, 27, 35, 37, 38, 39, 41, 46, 49, 54, 56, 57, 58, 59, 65, 75, 78, 81, 102, 103, 121, 125, 127, 135, 150, 151, 157, 164, 172, 174, 175, 177, 179, 187, 190, 192, 193, 232, 272, 273, 282, 290, 293, 294, 296, 323, 334, 335, 336, 338, 340, 344, 345, 346, 347, 349, 350, 361, 364, 377, 397, 402, 422, 433
deficit(s), 88, 98, 99, 248, 290, 322, 333, 335, 336, 344, 345, 374, 375, 376
definition, xi, 5, 227, 235, 302, 303, 354, 355, 390, 391, 409, 444
degradation, 34, 75, 160, 381, 382, 385, 420, 443
dehydration, 218, 290, 375
delayed gastric emptying, 215
delirium, 237
delivery, x, 111, 195, 205, 294, 302, 320, 325, 412, 420, 424
demand, x, 181, 213, 215, 268, 322, 324
dementia, viii, 63, 64, 65, 67, 69, 71, 73, 74, 76, 77, 78, 80, 82, 83, 84, 85, 86, 87, 88, 89, 90, 92, 94, 96, 97, 98, 99, 100, 101, 102, 103, 105, 215, 223, 228, 232, 236, 245, 297, 298, 302
demography, 361
demyelination, 87
Denmark, 431
density, ix, 39, 87, 95, 105, 130, 136, 157, 159, 162, 165, 170, 173, 174, 176, 181, 182, 185, 187, 189, 190, 191, 192, 193, 194, 217, 218, 246, 289, 301, 335, 344, 357, 360, 397, 398, 400, 404, 406, 407, 420, 435, 441
dental caries, 178
dentate gyrus, 93
dentures, 290
Department of Agriculture, 128, 186, 269
Department of Health and Human Services, 82
dependent variable, 261
dephosphorylation, 49
depolarization, 422
deposition, 70, 76, 77, 86, 100, 165, 166

deposits, 64
depression, 228, 237, 249, 250, 252, 302, 354, 361, 431, 440, 443
depressive symptoms, 245
deprivation, 97, 175, 189, 193, 334, 344, 376
derivatives, 116, 135, 176, 447, 449, 450, 451, 452, 453
dermis, 37
destruction, 355, 389, 390, 393, 394, 401, 402, 406, 409, 427, 429, 430
detection, x, xi, 201, 213, 216, 226, 235, 403, 404
detoxification, 127
developed countries, 110, 130, 300, 363
developing countries, viii, 11, 39, 107, 110, 300, 354, 361
deviation, 224, 363
dexamethasone, 160
DG, 84, 98, 104, 326, 328, 368, 457
DHA, 73, 79, 95, 116
diabetes (mellitus), viii, xi, 31, 32, 39, 40, 41, 46, 47, 48, 50, 51, 52, 56, 57, 58, 59, 60, 61, 63, 65, 69, 81, 83, 85, 88, 89, 91, 119, 120, 148, 149, 204, 209, 211, 237, 272, 280, 282, 284, 286, 289, 294, 299, 302, 315, 316, 330, 337, 338, 339, 340, 341, 342, 348, 349, 350, 356, 357, 360, 361, 365, 413, 414, 417, 418
diabetic nephropathy, 417
diabetic patients, 46, 51, 58, 335, 340, 341, 349, 350, 417
diabetic retinopathy, 349
Diagnostic and Statistical Manual of Mental Disorders (DSM), 81, 220
diagnostic criteria, 159
dialysis, 323
diaphragm, 60, 403, 431, 436
diarrhea, 343, 354
diastolic blood pressure, 12, 14, 69, 359
dielectric, 218
dietary behaviour, 300, 315
dietary fat, viii, 29, 63, 72, 73, 96, 112, 122, 163, 164, 198, 199, 201, 202, 205, 206, 209, 265, 269, 449
dietary fiber, 116, 117, 118, 119, 120, 146, 292, 337
dietary habits, 71, 286, 316
dietary intake, 11, 53, 73, 77, 93, 121, 146, 163, 171, 199, 231, 249, 293, 297, 314, 316, 336, 337, 339, 340, 343, 347, 357, 363, 439
dietary supplementation, 165
dieting, 264
differentiation, 34, 137, 140, 166, 175, 180, 193, 314, 368, 384, 452
diffusion, 4, 64, 75
digestibility, 142
digestion, xii, 119, 319, 328
digestive enzymes, 142
digestive tract, 119, 147
digitalis, 335, 346
digitalis toxicity, 335
digoxin toxicity, 342
dilation, 4
dioxin, 138
dipole, 456
disability, 89, 220, 239, 248, 252, 290, 291, 301, 327, 390, 391, 409, 431, 439
discharges, 237, 238
discs, 177
disease progression, 69, 405, 428
disease rate, 115
disequilibrium, 51
disinfection, 3
disorder, 39, 52, 68, 78, 82, 108, 158, 286, 294, 333, 336, 340
displacement, 171, 225
dissociation, 424
distress, 161, 202, 394, 421
distribution, 57, 70, 72, 91, 93, 140, 154, 155, 172, 228, 230, 231, 260, 290, 302, 336, 398, 402, 404, 430, 432, 436, 452
diuretic, 4, 5, 7, 335, 342
diversity, 95, 154
division, 108, 154
dizziness, 302, 344
DNA, 50, 75, 76, 78, 98, 108, 109, 111, 116, 125, 126, 128, 130, 137, 140, 150, 151, 273, 281, 282, 335, 355, 360, 454, 456
DNA breakage, 76, 137
DNA damage, 98, 109, 128, 360
DNA polymerase, 282
DNA repair, 127, 335
Docosahexaenoic (acid), 73, 96, 116, 186
doctors, 67, 257
dosage, 3, 7, 171, 290, 356
dose-response relationship, 132
dosing, 145, 368
double blind study, 104, 428
double bonds, 116, 135
double-blind trial, 104, 190
down-regulation, 172

drinking pattern(s), 8
drinking water, 78, 101, 173, 178, 274, 280, 283, 339, 348
drug interaction, 239, 297
drug metabolism, 290, 354
drug reactions, 237
drug resistance, 6
drug therapy, 240, 354
drug use, 336
drugs, 69, 78, 79, 209, 215, 236, 245, 272, 290, 336, 340, 342, 428
DSM-IV, 81
duodenum, 133, 143, 336
durability, 81
duration, 32, 47, 65, 75, 80, 276, 342, 381, 429, 440
DXA, 37, 218
dyslipidemia, 69, 70, 88, 286, 289, 294, 364
dysphagia, 354, 364
dysplasia, 125
dyspnea, 420, 423, 429, 431, 432, 440, 442, 444
dysuria, 302

E

E. coli, 119
ears, 264
earth, 127
eating, ix, 27, 81, 160, 195, 196, 201, 204, 206, 207, 215, 242, 254, 256, 268, 290, 294, 296, 301, 303, 313, 315, 359, 414, 431, 440
echocardiogram, 344
economic change, xii, 285
economic status, 65, 357
edema, 218, 335, 381
education, xi, xii, 64, 81, 82, 90, 106, 186, 203, 205, 207, 208, 209, 210, 239, 242, 244, 271, 276, 277, 278, 279, 294, 299, 300, 301, 303, 304, 305, 307, 313, 315, 364, 430
educational programs, 27
Eel, 124
EGCG, 143
egg(s), xi, 23, 73, 113, 115, 120, 130, 135, 164, 173, 253, 258, 260, 262, 263, 265, 266, 291, 359
Egypt, 2, 349
eicosanoids, 7, 101, 113, 164
eicosapentaenoic acid, 185
elaboration, 272
elasticity, 417
elastin, 392
elderly population, ix, 64, 85, 99, 157, 181, 217, 222, 231, 232, 244, 249, 293, 298, 316, 330, 336
elders, 68, 86, 229, 354
electrical properties, 218
electrochemical, 422
electrodes, 341, 342
electrolysis, 333
electrolyte(s), 172, 289, 333, 335, 338, 342, 423
electron(s), 111, 135, 142, 421, 422, 427
email, 253, 299
embryo, 457
embryonic, 108
emotional distress, 201
emphysema, 389, 390, 391, 392, 393, 394, 395, 396, 397, 398, 399, 400, 401, 402, 403, 404, 405, 406, 407, 408, 409, 410, 424, 427, 428, 429, 430, 434, 435, 439, 443, 444
employees, 208
encoding, 52
endocrine, 32, 34, 38, 52, 53, 55, 59, 60, 68, 70, 85, 215, 336, 342, 345, 414
endocrine disorders, 342
endocrine system, 32, 38, 52, 53, 55, 60
endocrinology, 146
endometrium, viii
endoplasmic reticulum, 450
endoscopic, 246, 249
endothelial cells, 34, 282, 414, 422
endothelial dysfunction, 73, 92, 95, 360
endothelium, 71, 338
end-stage renal disease, 172
endurance, 416, 419, 423, 426, 430, 431, 436
energy, x, xii, 23, 24, 27, 37, 65, 67, 68, 73, 76, 93, 96, 98, 110, 111, 119, 124, 136, 174, 179, 213, 215, 218, 226, 230, 232, 233, 239, 243, 246, 249, 251, 265, 289, 291, 294, 296, 297, 319, 324, 325, 328, 331, 334, 336, 339, 360, 361, 362, 364, 366, 368, 369, 377, 381, 387, 390, 391, 409, 410, 420, 426, 431, 432, 433, 437, 439, 440, 441, 443, 444
energy consumption, 111
England, 5, 82, 83, 86, 87, 89, 91, 92, 94, 95, 96, 98, 103, 104
enlargement, 390, 392, 399, 403
enthusiasm, 80, 429
environment, 52, 108, 109, 119, 181, 290, 294, 447, 454
environmental chemicals, 109
environmental conditions, 454
environmental factors, 64, 354, 390, 395, 444
environmental influences, 65

enzyme(s), 35, 75, 79, 108, 109, 113, 123, 127, 133, 137, 138, 140, 142, 147, 155, 164, 179, 180, 272, 290, 338, 339, 340, 373, 375, 377, 421, 426, 430, 449, 450, 451, 452
EPA, 73, 79, 95, 104, 116, 185
epidemic, 36, 40, 52, 53, 64, 196, 212, 215, 233, 361
epidemiologic studies, ix, 41, 79, 108, 117, 144, 243, 284, 359
epidemiology, 60, 71, 72, 75, 84, 96, 182, 326
epidermis, 37
epigallocatechin gallate, 5, 137
epilepsy, 65
epithelia, 52, 108, 447, 452
epithelial cells, 121, 125, 150, 272, 341, 454, 457
epithelium, 118, 121, 151, 167
equipment, 341
ergocalciferol, 32
ergosterol, 123
ERS, 434
erythrocyte membranes, 94
erythrocytes, 334, 341, 345, 373, 378, 380
esophageal, 109, 115, 125, 131, 143, 272, 274, 283
esophageal cancer, 274, 283
esophagus, viii, 107, 111, 114, 115, 129, 135, 143
essential fatty acids, ix, 96, 146, 158, 184, 185, 186, 353, 363
ester, 69
estimating, 325, 331
estradiol, 112, 140, 146, 154
estrogen, 115, 129, 137, 139, 140, 146, 151, 154, 155, 158, 179, 193
ethanol, 74, 96, 97
Ethanol, 96
ethnic groups, 38, 45, 217
ethnicity, 46, 56, 67, 90
etiology, 82, 110, 154, 160, 162, 378
euphoria, 4
Europe, 4, 5, 6, 39, 56, 71, 89, 122, 125, 127, 158, 159, 243, 293, 296, 300, 304, 305, 307, 316
European, ix, 6, 8, 9, 83, 86, 93, 96, 101, 132, 135, 140, 148, 149, 154, 157, 162, 173, 187, 220, 268, 297, 300, 351, 359, 365, 368
European Community, ix, 157, 173, 187
European Union, 162
evening, 164
event-related potential, 104
evolution, 81, 233, 244, 349
examinations, 122, 275, 276, 372, 373, 377
excess body weight, 111
excitability, 334
excitotoxicity, 98
exclusion, 236, 377
excretion, 47, 109, 160, 161, 162, 163, 164, 165, 166, 171, 172, 173, 183, 185, 188, 189, 237, 290, 336, 340, 345, 347, 364, 385, 386
execution, 448
executive function, 80
exercise, xi, 110, 144, 180, 183, 194, 201, 202, 204, 208, 211, 249, 256, 257, 265, 271, 276, 278, 279, 291, 322, 328, 339, 348, 390, 391, 405, 409, 410, 412, 415, 417, 419, 420, 421, 423, 424, 426, 427, 430, 431, 432, 433, 436, 438, 439, 440, 442, 444
exercise performance, 420, 423, 431, 433, 438, 440, 442, 444
exocytosis, 450
exons, 50
expectorant, 434
expenditures, 208
Expert System, 211
expert systems, 211
exposure, 32, 36, 37, 39, 56, 74, 78, 79, 96, 98, 108, 109, 123, 125, 128, 132, 144, 145, 176, 190, 211, 264, 322, 324, 393, 412, 416, 421, 422, 431
Exposure, 115, 167
external environment, 108
extracellular matrix, 348
extraction, 403, 420, 424
extrasystoles, 344
eyes, 256

F

failure, 237, 325, 342, 364, 393, 440
faith, 203, 209
false positive, 397
family, ix, 52, 61, 73, 108, 112, 126, 135, 138, 141, 148, 158, 237, 239, 244, 257, 290, 294, 298, 334, 452, 457
family history, 108, 126, 148, 158
FAO, 188, 232, 315
fast food, 260, 289
fasting, 12, 27, 42, 44, 45, 47, 51, 57, 59, 70, 120, 171, 173, 180, 340, 413, 414, 455
fasting glucose, 42, 45, 70, 120
fat, ix, x, 23, 24, 27, 29, 32, 37, 55, 64, 67, 68, 70, 72, 73, 74, 86, 90, 91, 93, 94, 95, 96, 106, 108, 114, 115, 116, 121, 122, 124, 131, 147, 153, 164, 167, 169, 176, 185, 195, 196, 198, 199, 200, 201, 202, 203, 204, 205, 206, 207, 209, 211, 214, 217, 218, 226, 230, 231, 232, 254, 256, 259, 261, 262,

263, 265, 266, 267, 268, 269, 290, 291, 296, 321, 322, 330, 345, 359, 372, 377, 409, 432, 437, 438, 441, 449
fat reduction, 96, 199, 201, 202, 205, 206
fatigue, 5, 273, 344, 345, 412, 419, 423, 431, 436
fatty acid(s), ix, 27, 29, 72, 73, 80, 92, 94, 95, 96, 102, 104, 112, 113, 114, 116, 118, 121, 141, 146, 158, 160, 161, 163, 164, 165, 184, 185, 186, 296, 353, 355, 363, 376, 381, 433, 439, 440, 447, 448, 449, 450, 452, 455, 456, 457
fear, 236
feedback, 32, 34, 35, 37, 112, 198, 199, 201, 202, 204, 206, 207, 377
females, 12, 23, 24, 38, 39, 44, 47, 54, 178, 231
femoral bone, 187, 334
femur, 169, 184, 247
fermentable carbohydrates, 116
fermentation, 2, 117, 146
fertility, 6, 127
fever, 5
fiber, viii
fiber content, 261
fibers, 117, 119, 178, 392, 430
fibrils, 101, 179
fibrin, 379, 380
fibrinogen, 3, 68, 280, 284, 344, 373, 378, 379, 380
fibroblasts, 102, 178, 379
fibromyalgia, 345
fibrosis, 414, 419
Filipino, 131
film, 405
filtration, 160, 167, 320
Finland, 93, 136, 155, 176, 300
fish, 23, 27, 32, 71, 73, 94, 95, 113, 114, 116, 135, 144, 164, 165, 173, 174, 181, 186, 265, 291, 292, 293, 432
fish oil, 27, 113, 164, 165, 186
fitness, 293, 297
flavonoids, vii, 2, 4, 5, 7, 77, 79, 101, 114, 140, 142, 143, 155, 156
flexibility, 204
flora, 119, 141, 146, 147, 177
fluid, 3, 121, 134, 166, 169, 172, 174, 225, 231, 289, 290, 296, 297, 322, 334, 379
fluid balance, 297
Fluoride, 178, 184, 192, 288
fluoride, ix
fMRI, 105
focusing, 300
folate, 65, 75, 76, 97, 98, 99, 103, 114, 125, 126, 144, 150, 151, 291, 287, 293, 296, 297, 324, 330, 457
folic acid, viii, 63, 75, 79, 98, 103, 125, 144, 293, 298, 348, 361, 377
folklore, 254
food, ix, xi, 3, 6, 15, 17, 23, 24, 27, 28, 29, 32, 40, 41, 55, 71, 72, 79, 81, 83, 84, 93, 95, 108, 110, 114, 119, 120, 122, 124, 127, 128, 129, 132, 133, 137, 142, 173, 178, 180, 186, 188, 202, 211, 215, 240, 249, 253, 254, 255, 256, 257, 258, 259, 260, 261, 262, 263, 264, 268, 269, 273, 274, 287, 288, 289, 290, 291, 294, 296, 297, 300, 301, 304, 316, 343, 354, 355, 362, 364, 385
Food and Drug Administration (FDA), 169
food additives, 132, 188
food descriptions, 256, 258, 259, 260, 262, 264
food industry, 264
food intake, xi, 27, 28, 29, 41, 84, 93, 120, 180, 215, 249, 253, 264, 289, 294, 354, 362
food names, xi, 253, 254, 255, 256, 257, 258, 260, 261, 262, 263, 264, 269
food products, 268
food stereotypes, 255
forgetfulness, 344
fortification, 80
fractures, ix, 36, 39, 54, 157, 158, 159, 161, 162, 166, 170, 176, 177, 181, 182, 184, 187, 191, 192, 237, 239, 293
fragility, ix, 39, 157, 158, 159, 166, 182
fragmentation, 392
Framingham study, 414
France, 6, 74, 152, 167, 213, 215, 229, 233, 361
free radical scavenger, 79
free radicals, 129, 135, 136, 142, 193, 281, 322, 339, 342, 354, 355, 367, 368, 421, 422, 426
freedom, 302
frequency distribution, 398, 404
Friedmann, 248
fructooligosaccharides, 119
fructose, 282
fruits, 23, 76, 128, 129, 131, 132, 133, 135, 137, 140, 141, 143, 144, 161, 196, 200, 257, 260, 289, 291, 293, 300, 301, 315, 353, 359, 362, 364
fuel, 117, 441, 443
functional changes, 355
functional imaging, 400
fusion, 449

G

gallbladder, 111
Gamma, 101
gamma-tocopherol, 77, 101, 136
gases, 116, 414
gastric, 119, 133, 135, 147, 156, 215, 272, 274, 283, 294, 323, 324, 379, 432, 452
gastric mucosa, 452
gastritis, 289, 290
gastrocnemius, 366
gastrointestinal tract, ix, 34, 107, 133, 174, 289, 290, 296, 334, 376, 381, 454
gender, xi, 70, 204, 205, 222, 226, 244, 256, 271, 276, 278, 279, 357, 361, 367
gender differences, 367
gene, 32, 34, 48, 49, 50, 51, 52, 60, 61, 76, 85, 86, 89, 95, 116, 117, 125, 150, 175, 282, 329, 334, 366, 393, 424, 447, 448, 449, 452, 454, 457, 458
gene expression, 49, 50, 89, 125, 329, 366, 393, 424, 447, 449, 454
gene therapy, 85
gene transfer, 86
generation, 7, 116, 130, 220, 360, 400, 425
genes, 32, 50, 51, 52, 126, 151, 448, 454, 455, 456
genetic factors, 72, 74
genetic instability, 335
genetic mutations, 128
genetics, 269, 443
Geneva, 233, 315
Genistein, 140, 141, 143
genome, 454
genomic instability, 125
genotype, 51, 69, 73, 74, 87, 88, 95, 174, 190, 456
geriatric, xi
geriatricians, xi
Germany, 4, 42, 127, 167, 209, 361, 447
Ginkgo biloba, 80, 105
girls, 39, 186
gland, 33, 35, 53, 143, 377
glass, vii, 2, 3, 8, 124, 404
glasses, 3, 292
glial, 97
glioma, 458
glucagon, 53, 58, 339, 349, 381
glucocorticoids, 160, 439
gluconeogenesis, 381, 440
glucose, vii, viii, 4, 29, 31, 32, 39, 40, 41, 42, 44, 45, 46, 47, 48, 49, 50, 51, 52, 55, 57, 58, 59, 60, 69, 70, 72, 83, 88, 107, 119, 148, 179, 204, 315, 322, 333, 339, 340, 349, 350, 366, 381, 412, 413, 414, 415, 416, 417, 418, 419, 420, 440, 447, 455
glucose metabolism, viii, 32, 45, 46, 48, 52, 107, 120, 179, 315, 333, 339, 414
glucose tolerance, vii, 31, 41, 42, 44, 48, 57, 58, 83, 340, 349, 414, 418, 419
glucose tolerance test, 42, 349
glucose-induced insulin secretion, 40
glucosidases, 141
GLUT, 49, 59
glutamate, 98, 160, 173
glutamine, 381
glutathione, 75, 109, 127, 145, 344, 362, 366, 421, 433
glutathione peroxidase, 127, 366, 421
glycerol, 450
glycogen, 265, 440
glycolysis, 340
glycoprotein, 458
glycosides, 155
goals, 254, 288, 369, 389, 395
gold, 220, 221, 373
government, 264
G-protein, 339
grading, 229, 233, 247, 252, 330, 442, 448
grains, 113, 116, 117, 119, 120, 128, 140, 146, 164, 289, 291, 341, 353, 356, 364
granules, 119, 379
graph, 218, 225, 231, 407
Great Britain, 5
Greece, 333
green tea, vii, 2, 4, 5, 6, 9, 143
Greenland, 94, 145
group size, 302
groups, x, 12, 27, 36, 38, 39, 45, 67, 71, 75, 93, 113, 135, 142, 164, 199, 202, 203, 205, 214, 217, 219, 221, 223, 224, 227, 238, 239, 241, 242, 256, 294, 300, 335, 347, 361, 363, 381, 409, 421
growth, ix, 34, 64, 75, 76, 108, 111, 113, 116, 121, 125, 126, 127, 138, 140, 143, 145, 155, 161, 162, 164, 166, 175, 177, 178, 179, 184, 190, 219, 254, 257, 269, 272, 273, 282, 331, 344, 359, 394, 395, 414, 448, 458
growth factor, ix, 108, 111, 140, 145, 162, 178, 184, 219, 272, 331, 359, 394, 395, 414
growth factors, ix, 108, 111, 178, 272, 359, 414
guanine, 126
guidance, 207
guidelines, ix, 29, 108, 143, 181, 182, 200, 230, 286, 291, 316, 342, 351, 353, 364, 428

gut, 34, 108, 117, 119, 165, 296, 298
gyrus, 93

H

haemoglobin, 424
half-life, 219, 373, 374, 375
hands, 123
hardness, 274, 283
harm, 131, 132
harmful effects, 3, 120
Harvard, 186, 346
hazards, 66, 239, 303, 394
Hcy, 70, 75, 76
HD, 79, 153, 356, 406
HDL, 3, 29, 69, 70, 73, 74, 338, 339, 373, 376
HE, 185, 416
head, 65, 321
head injury, 65
headache, 4, 5
healing, 5, 133, 324, 342, 357, 372, 379, 380, 384
Health and Human Services, 82
health care, 200, 294, 423
health care costs, 200
health education, 203
health effects, 39, 40
health problems, 5, 292, 302
health services, 286, 294
health status, 238, 245, 248, 296, 337, 347, 354, 427, 428
healthfulness, 269
Healthy eating, 160
heart, 8, 10, 88, 90, 91, 96, 177, 229, 326, 351, 356, 362, 364, 368, 369, 391, 416, 418, 423, 424, 425, 426, 433, 436
heart disease, 5, 8, 9, 68, 71, 72, 74, 87, 88, 90, 91, 94, 97, 98, 101, 115, 130, 144, 149, 154, 159, 284, 292, 295, 302, 356, 359, 366, 367, 368
heart failure, 335, 336, 361, 416, 419, 423, 424, 425, 426, 436
heart rate, 345, 348
heat, 116, 119, 236, 442, 452
heavy metals, 77
height, 12, 28, 67, 111, 115, 146, 214, 217, 218, 219, 232, 244, 276, 320, 321, 354, 385, 386, 441
Helicobacter pylori, 115
heme, 78, 102, 133
hemodynamics, 424
hemoglobin, 120, 148, 204, 420
Hemoglobin, 363
hemorrhage, 343, 351
hemostasis, 86, 417
hepatitis, 109, 144
Hepatitis B, 115
hepatocellular, 281
hepatocellular carcinoma, 281
hepatocytes, 367, 375, 449, 455
herbs, 161
heredity, 160
heterodimer, 50
heterogeneity, 77, 398, 399
heterozygosity, 454
high blood pressure, 12, 69, 364
high fat, 211, 262, 263
higher education, 300, 303, 304
higher quality, 321
hip, ix, 37, 54, 70, 90, 158, 159, 161, 162, 165, 166, 170, 176, 177, 178, 182, 184, 186, 191, 194, 203, 237, 239
hip fractures, 159, 162, 166, 170, 177, 184, 191, 237, 239
hippocampus, 68, 86
Hippocrates, 68
Hispanic, 45, 160, 247
histogram, 403
histone, 117
HK, 89, 97, 151, 182, 188, 297
homeostasis, viii, 31, 32, 33, 34, 35, 37, 47, 49, 50, 51, 52, 53, 55, 61, 68, 75, 78, 85, 102, 162, 173, 174, 175, 188, 236, 337, 339, 346, 349
homocysteine, 4, 10, 70, 75, 76, 79, 91, 97, 98, 99, 103, 151, 293, 297, 298, 339, 348
hormone, 32, 33, 34, 35, 37, 39, 50, 53, 54, 55, 68, 112, 121, 123, 125, 137, 140, 162, 166, 174, 175, 184, 187, 188, 190, 193, 290, 333, 334, 345, 377, 381
hospitalization, 85, 233, 237, 242, 247, 248, 250, 289, 328, 372, 414
hospitals, 239, 240, 243, 294, 295
host, 40, 179, 386, 390, 395, 444
hub, 394, 444
human immunodeficiency virus (HIV), 65, 105, 231, 232
Human Kinetics, 230, 268, 436
human neutrophils, 366
human subjects, 147, 192, 232
humoral immunity, 378
Huntington's disease, 65, 79, 104, 105
hydrocephalus, 65

hydrogen, 77, 78, 102, 135, 142, 273, 360, 366, 422, 426
hydrogen atoms, 142
hydrogen peroxide, 77, 78, 102, 273, 360, 366, 422, 426
hydrolysis, 138, 140, 154, 456
hydrolyzed, 138
hydrophilic, 109
hydrophobic, 449
hydroxyapatite, 120, 166, 334
hydroxyl, 128, 135, 142, 282
hydroxyl groups, 142
hydroxylation, 139, 178
hygiene, 354
hypercalcemia, 33
hypercalciuria, 160, 172, 176, 182, 184, 189
hypercapnia, 414, 430
hypercholesterolemia, 73, 205, 347
hyperglycemia, 41, 42, 45, 340, 345, 381, 414
hyperhomocysteinemia, 79, 98, 293, 297
hyperinflation, 423, 430, 434
hyperinsulinemia, 42, 59, 68, 120, 340
hyperparathyroidism, 34, 39, 54, 55, 162, 167, 175, 344
hyperphosphatemia, 171, 172
hyperphosphorylated tau protein, 64
hyperplasia, 272
hypersensitivity, 98, 358, 441
hypertension, viii, 7, 10, 39, 40, 56, 59, 60, 63, 65, 69, 70, 81, 86, 89, 90, 91, 237, 272, 281, 284, 282, 286, 289, 294, 302, 333, 336, 337, 338, 342, 344, 346, 348, 349, 360, 361, 362
hyperthyroidism, 344, 352, 375
hypertrophy, 86
hypokalemia, 336, 345
hypokalemic periodic paralysis, 345
hypomagnesemia, 52, 61
hypomethylation, 126, 456
hypoperfusion, 69
hypophosphatemia, 188
hypoplasia, 190
hypopnea, 415
hypotension, 344
hypothalamus, 67, 86
hypothesis, 8, 31, 37, 49, 69, 95, 100, 119, 160, 161, 173, 200, 254, 273, 394, 410, 428, 429, 442, 452, 454
hypoventilation, 372
hypoxia, 65, 69, 390, 391, 410, 412, 413, 414, 415, 416, 417, 420, 421, 426, 439
Hypoxia, 412, 416, 417

I

iatrogenic, 238, 337, 354
IB, 95, 101
id, 203, 217, 227, 300, 338, 343
identification, 40, 64, 158, 217, 229, 317, 325, 430, 454, 456
idiopathic, 172, 184, 189
IL-6, 68, 381, 413
ileum, 336
Iliad, 2
image analysis, 402
images, 404, 407, 408
imaging, 67, 70, 74, 97, 218, 389, 391, 395, 400, 404, 407, 429
imaging techniques, 67, 70, 391, 395
imbalances, 52
immigrants, 23, 29
immobilization, 162, 385, 427
immune function, 34, 137, 239, 323, 324, 358
immune response, 130, 239, 329, 358, 364
immune system, 40, 110, 127, 133, 161, 364, 422, 440
immunity, 85, 232, 281, 323, 324, 329, 336, 377, 378, 379
immunization, 430
immunodeficiency, 105, 231
immunoglobulins, 377
immunological, 358, 372, 373, 377
immunosuppression, 345
impaired energy metabolism, 420
impairments, 286, 321
implementation, 88, 247
in vitro, 40, 41, 48, 49, 58, 76, 77, 101, 177, 192, 194, 282, 421, 427
in vivo, 6, 7, 9, 57, 58, 76, 94, 101, 130, 151, 192, 355, 389, 390, 395, 398, 400, 422, 428, 457
incidence, viii, 36, 63, 64, 69, 74, 76, 82, 87, 91, 94, 99, 107, 109, 125, 128, 129, 131, 132, 140, 143, 146, 147, 150, 151, 152, 153, 161, 170, 176, 186, 191, 232, 241, 252, 280, 284, 321, 341, 343, 356, 358, 361, 367, 368
inclusion, viii, 65, 107, 196
income, 204, 205, 210, 244, 290, 291, 292, 294, 303, 304, 306, 308, 315
independence, 237, 238, 239
independent variable, 261
India, 29, 39, 56, 167, 361

Indian(s), 39, 50, 56, 60, 275, 282
indication, 119, 361, 384
indicators, 87, 90, 179, 186, 193, 216, 217, 219, 221, 223, 224, 226, 298, 325, 331, 371, 372, 386, 441
indices, 46, 83, 100, 268, 347, 372, 373, 383, 426, 439
indirect effect, 34
individualization, 198
Indonesia, 361
inducer, 138, 155
induction, 117, 138, 142, 145, 155, 175, 177, 272, 429, 455, 458
induration, 383
industrialized countries, viii, 107, 119, 337, 353
industry, 264
infancy, 108, 171, 205
infants, 39, 172, 186, 188
infarction, 8, 9, 103, 339, 342, 350, 351, 356, 380
infection, 109, 115, 133, 231, 324, 325, 329, 358, 363, 364, 372, 379, 386, 387
infectious disease(s), 11, 110, 380
inferences, 52
inflammation, xii, 5, 68, 70, 73, 76, 85, 86, 91, 92, 95, 101, 106, 113, 127, 164, 219, 272, 273, 281, 319, 322, 323, 324, 325, 330, 338, 360, 371, 372, 373, 376, 378, 379, 381, 382, 383, 384, 386, 387, 389, 390, 391, 392, 394, 405, 409, 412, 413, 415, 417, 418, 421, 422, 428, 432, 439, 440, 444
inflammatory, 5, 39, 40, 68, 70, 71, 73, 77, 78, 81, 96, 113, 115, 116, 143, 145, 146, 164, 165, 166, 224, 272, 273, 281, 322, 323, 329, 330, 359, 360, 363, 371, 372, 374, 375, 376, 378, 379, 380, 381, 382, 383, 384, 389, 410, 413, 414, 425, 432, 433, 437, 439, 444, 445, 456
inflammatory bowel disease, 115, 146
inflammatory disease, 374, 378, 380, 381, 382, 384
inflammatory mediators, 414, 425, 432, 437
inflammatory response, 116, 272, 322, 323, 329, 330, 360, 363, 410, 432, 445
inflation, 406
influenza, 8, 57, 249, 252
influenza a, 57
influenza vaccine, 252
ingest, 77
ingestion, 173, 178, 179, 188, 365, 432
inhibition, 41, 59, 89, 109, 116, 137, 138, 140, 178, 192, 322, 339, 342, 375, 394, 426, 448, 455, 457
inhibitor, 3, 10, 186, 233, 272, 453
inhibitory effect, 113, 129, 164, 180
initiation, 108, 142, 245, 322, 448, 451, 454
injury(ies), 65, 68, 158, 290, 321, 322, 324, 325, 326, 331, 342, 392, 393, 412, 416, 426, 443, 445, 448
innovation, 200
insomnia, 344
inspiration, 399
instability, 125, 130, 335
institutionalized individuals, 215, 222, 226
institutions, 238, 240, 250, 364
instruments, 64, 230, 242, 317
insulin, vii, viii, 4, 29, 31, 32, 34, 39, 40, 41, 42, 44, 45, 46, 47, 48, 49, 50, 51, 52, 56, 57, 58, 59, 60, 65, 68, 69, 70, 71, 73, 85, 91, 95, 107, 111, 119, 148, 162, 184, 215, 219, 282, 284, 322, 330, 331, 339, 340, 344, 345, 348, 349, 350, 359, 366, 381, 413, 414, 415, 417, 418, 419, 455
insulin dependent diabetes, 148, 417
insulin resistance, viii, 31, 32, 34, 41, 42, 45, 46, 47, 49, 50, 51, 52, 56, 57, 58, 59, 65, 68, 69, 70, 71, 73, 91, 95, 107, 148, 282, 330, 340, 345, 348, 349, 381, 413, 414, 415, 418, 419
insulin sensitivity, vii, 31, 42, 45, 47, 49, 50, 58, 59, 73, 95, 340, 344, 350, 359, 366, 414, 415, 419
insulin signaling, 68
insulinoma, 59
integration, 68
integrity, 73, 78, 158, 177, 179, 273, 334, 393, 422, 440
intellectual disabilities, 192
intelligence, 77, 100
intelligence quotient, 77
intensity, 254, 276, 409, 414, 423
intensive care unit, 249, 319, 322, 326, 327, 331, 434
intentions, 196
interaction(s), viii, 5, 32, 34, 35, 36, 40, 45, 52, 63, 64, 79, 93, 130, 150, 152, 154, 158, 163, 190, 215, 237, 239, 281, 289, 290, 297, 339, 365, 367, 376, 389, 390, 393, 394, 395, 410, 413, 444, 449, 454
intercellular adhesion molecule, 63
interdependence, 345
interference, 452
interferon, 379
interferon gamma, 379
interleukin(s), 68, 116, 186, 272, 329, 360, 365, 381
interleukin-1, 116, 272
internal mechanisms, 108
International Classification of Diseases, 276
internet, 257

interpretation, 232, 233, 237, 241, 242, 254, 371, 372, 383, 441
interrelations, 52
interrelationships, 405, 444
interval, 170, 196, 276, 342, 393
intervention, ix, 38, 41, 48, 49, 79, 80, 81, 132, 149, 153, 162, 176, 177, 180, 195, 197, 198, 202, 203, 204, 205, 206, 207, 209, 210, 237, 238, 239, 241, 244, 245, 250, 325, 358, 364, 369, 384, 390, 405, 410, 430, 432, 433, 440, 443, 444
interview, 46, 275
intestinal obstruction, 454
intestine, 34, 35, 50, 121, 146, 166, 175, 177, 334, 454, 456
intima, 91, 360, 379
introns, 51
inulin, 119, 146
iodine, 75, 189, 288, 296
ion channels, 52
ion transport, 449
ionized calcium level, 171
ionizing radiation, 109
ions, 52, 56, 79, 130, 142, 166, 338, 348, 422
IR, 42, 44, 45, 47, 51, 187, 188, 190, 232
Ireland, 285
iron, 2, 23, 28, 76, 101, 102, 133, 179, 181, 183, 289, 302, 329, 337, 361, 363, 374, 377
iron transport, 179
irradiation, 32, 37, 452
ischaemia, 323, 426
ischemia, 69, 347, 413, 416, 433, 439
ischemic stroke, 87, 97, 103, 115
Islam, 185
Islamic, 4
Islamic world, 4
Isoflavones, 105, 137, 140
isoflavonoid, 140
isolation, 215, 291, 323, 358
isoleucine, 381
isotope, 174, 190, 333, 350
Italian population, 82
Italy, x, 1, 3, 4, 5, 9, 42, 63, 93, 147, 213, 214, 216, 220, 221, 227, 295, 361

J

Japan, 11, 156, 158, 166, 177, 186, 243, 274, 317, 360, 407
Japanese women, 39, 56
jejunum, 57
joint pain, 5
joints, 302
Jordan, 9, 365
Jung, 360, 366, 456

K

K^+, 161, 415
Kant, 251
kidney(s), viii, 32, 34, 35, 37, 52, 53, 57, 107, 111, 114, 121, 122, 123, 124, 125, 160, 161, 166, 173, 175, 187, 189, 334, 336, 337
kidney stones, 122, 173, 187, 189
killer cells, 127
kinase, 48, 49, 50, 57, 60, 98, 137, 154, 340
kinase activity, 50, 60, 137, 340
kinetic model, 174, 190
kinetics, 328, 346, 376
King, 153, 273, 281, 423, 427
Kobe, 28
krypton, 408
kyphosis, 396

L

LAA, 402, 404
lactation, 175
lactic acid, 415, 419, 423
large intestine, 146
larynx, viii, 107, 114
laser, 101, 435
latency, 71
later life, 79, 81, 87, 358
Latin America, 110, 159, 361
Latino, 99
LDL, 3, 4, 5, 69, 70, 73, 74, 95, 130, 136, 338, 348, 356, 357, 360, 373, 376
leaching, 160
lead, x, 32, 34, 36, 39, 41, 49, 50, 52, 68, 69, 78, 116, 126, 128, 130, 170, 173, 213, 214, 215, 218, 236, 286, 289, 290, 323, 325, 335, 338, 340, 342, 344, 353, 354, 355, 409, 410, 440
leaks, 360
lean body mass, xii, 67, 84, 229, 250, 289, 319, 320, 321, 322, 325, 440, 441, 442, 444
learning, vii, 2, 8, 98
lecithin, 338
legumes, 71, 117, 128, 140, 141, 143, 144, 181, 292, 293, 343

leisure, 276
leisure time, 276
leptin, 68, 70, 85, 86, 215, 229, 329, 373, 377, 416
lesions, 64, 69, 76, 77, 87, 131, 281, 290, 339, 343, 398, 399, 429, 448
leucine, 381
leukemia, 126
leukocyte(s), 116, 281, 379
leukoplakia, 131, 153
leukotrienes, 113, 164
life expectancy, 110, 159, 359
life quality, 363, 364
life satisfaction, 317
life span, 68, 85, 93, 111, 222, 335, 353, 355, 358, 359, 364, 393
life style, 132
lifespan, ix, 195, 236, 359, 360
lifestyle, ix, 5, 56, 81, 109, 110, 114, 154, 157, 200, 202, 205, 211, 215, 289, 297, 316, 354, 357, 430
lifestyle behaviors, 200, 205
lifestyle changes, 202
lifetime, ix, 65, 75, 81, 157, 159, 174, 334
ligand(s), 50, 52, 58, 155, 341, 378
lignans, 114, 137, 140, 141, 155
likelihood, 161, 175, 200, 241, 242, 272, 273, 302, 321, 324
limitation, 80, 122, 217, 314, 390, 395, 397, 400, 419, 423, 434, 436, 444
linkage, 51, 454
links, 7, 65, 71, 100
lipase, 338
lipid(s), 25, 27, 28, 29, 69, 73, 77, 95, 97, 105, 113, 128, 130, 135, 136, 154, 164, 170, 184, 185, 186, 188, 204, 209, 293, 282, 336, 337, 338, 344, 347, 349, 355, 359, 363, 371, 372, 373, 376, 386, 412, 421, 422, 448, 449, 450, 452, 456, 457
lipid metabolism, 371, 376, 412, 452
lipid peroxidation, 77, 136, 337, 355, 363, 421, 422
lipid peroxides, 130
lipid profile, 69, 73, 344, 359
lipolysis, 55, 342, 376, 381
lipopolysaccharides, 376
lipoprotein(s), 29, 69, 71, 73, 87, 95, 97, 130, 136, 171, 335, 338, 347, 357, 360, 372, 373, 376, 380, 382, 383, 386
literature, x, xi, 52, 64, 80, 165, 207, 214, 216, 218, 219, 222, 233, 235, 241, 242, 243, 316, 326, 328, 336, 353, 355, 359, 380, 398, 400, 429
lithium, 375
liver, viii, 32, 107, 108, 111, 114, 123, 127, 130, 143, 192, 232, 237, 272, 273, 274, 283, 323, 367, 371, 373, 374, 375, 376, 377, 378, 379, 381, 422, 440, 441, 443, 455, 457
liver cancer, 274, 283
liver cirrhosis, 232, 374
liver disease, 375, 441
living arrangements, 431, 440
localization, 57, 70, 418
location, 32, 193, 430
locus, 454, 456, 457
London, 9, 46, 58, 145, 155, 189, 229, 346, 349, 391, 408, 409
loneliness, 215
longevity, 65, 69, 73, 86, 88, 92, 145, 286, 293, 294, 295, 335, 354, 359, 360, 363, 366
longitudinal studies, 64, 69, 76, 79, 407, 442
longitudinal study, 28, 314, 327, 419
Los Angeles, 31
loss of appetite, 215
loss of heterozygosity, 454
low risk, 47, 143, 383, 384
low-density lipoprotein, 95, 136, 357, 360
LPS, 366
lumbar spine, 173
lung, 105, 109, 121, 124, 125, 128, 129, 130, 131, 132, 133, 135, 136, 143, 150, 152, 153, 166, 233, 284, 320, 321, 326, 368, 389, 390, 391, 392, 393, 394, 395, 397, 398, 400, 401, 402, 403, 405, 406, 407, 408, 409, 411, 412, 413, 414, 417, 418, 421, 423, 424, 427, 428, 429, 430, 433, 434, 435, 439, 440, 443, 444
lung cancer, 105, 109, 124, 128, 131, 132, 135, 136, 150, 152, 153, 233, 284, 368
lung disease, 392, 408, 411, 412, 418, 424, 433, 434, 440
lung function, 133, 405, 409, 413, 418, 428, 433, 434, 439, 443
lutein, viii, 107, 130, 137
lycopene, viii, 107, 130, 137, 180, 193, 358
lymph, 379
lymphocyte, 219, 323, 358, 387, 441
lymphocytes, 341, 373, 377, 378, 379, 381, 385
lymphoma, 125
lysine, 178
lysosomes, 379

M

machinery, 421

macromolecules, 57, 142, 355
macronutrients, viii, 34, 63, 81, 83, 290, 354
macrophages, 91, 272, 378, 379, 381, 382, 414, 421
magazines, 203, 254, 256, 257, 265
magnesium, viii, ix, xi, 4, 31, 32, 35, 39, 40, 46, 48, 50, 52, 53, 54, 56, 58, 59, 60, 61, 158, 161, 171, 174, 179, 180, 181, 183, 185, 188, 189, 190, 193, 271, 272, 273, 274, 275, 276, 277, 278, 279, 280, 281, 282, 283, 284, 333, 334, 335, 336, 337, 338, 339, 340, 341, 342, 343, 344, 345, 346, 347, 348, 349, 350, 351, 426
magnetic resonance, 97, 218, 273, 424
magnetic resonance imaging,(MRI), 76, 88, 97, 98, 104, 218
magnetic resonance spectroscopy, 273
Maintenance, 197, 199, 201, 202, 203, 204, 205, 207, 211, 422
maize, 18, 23, 457, 458
malabsorption, 215, 336, 354, 431
males, 12, 23, 24, 39, 44, 47, 178, 183, 190, 231, 442
malignant cells, 151
malnutrition, x, xi, xii, 27, 66, 84, 106, 110, 213, 214, 215, 216, 217, 219, 220, 221, 222, 224, 226, 227, 229, 230, 231, 233, 235, 237, 239, 240, 241, 243, 244, 245, 246, 248, 249, 250, 251, 252, 285, 286, 291, 294, 295, 297, 301, 323, 354, 358, 361, 362, 363, 364, 371, 372, 373, 374, 375, 376, 377, 378, 381, 382, 383, 384, 385, 386, 387, 431
malondialdehyde (MDA), 355, 362, 363
mammal, 130
mammalian cells, 457
mammalian tissues, 421
mammography, 201
management, ix, x, xi, 64, 72, 157, 158, 177, 180, 181, 195, 197, 201, 202, 203, 204, 205, 206, 207, 211, 231, 235, 237, 240, 285, 321, 342, 351, 391, 409, 411, 427, 429, 430, 433, 440
manganese, 777, 79, 102, 181, 183, 189, 288, 296, 323, 337
manipulation, 186
MAPK, 455
mapping, 407
marital status, xii, 204, 294, 299, 313
market, 169, 172
marrow, 121, 166, 192, 194
Maryland, 120, 126
masking, 338
matrix, 175, 334, 339, 348, 379, 413
matrix metalloproteinase, 339, 348
maturation, 179, 346, 389, 392, 394
maturation process, 346
MCP-1, 91
meals, 3, 71, 93, 170, 215, 290, 292, 294, 303, 364, 368, 432, 438
measurement, 71, 120, 218, 231, 243, 244, 245, 284, 341, 350, 367, 389, 392, 395, 397, 399, 407, 434, 440, 441, 442
measures, ix, xi, 37, 45, 76, 80, 157, 158, 167, 177, 181, 206, 232, 235, 238, 240, 301, 304, 314, 341, 364, 404, 441
meat, viii, 23, 71, 107, 110, 113, 114, 115, 116, 120, 121, 127, 144, 147, 162, 164, 173, 183, 257, 261, 265, 293, 359, 385
mechanical ventilation, 327, 430
mechanical ventilator, 240
media, xi, 91, 253, 254, 255, 257, 263, 264, 272, 360
media messages, xi, 253, 264
median, 276, 289, 356, 363
mediation, 92
medical care, 294
Medicare, 242, 295
medication, 204, 237, 290, 354, 377, 412
medicine, 2, 6, 7, 10, 53, 129, 145, 154, 166, 216, 247, 316, 429, 430
Mediterranean, 3, 71, 72, 73, 76, 81, 92, 106, 211, 286, 293, 297
Mediterranean countries, 3, 286, 293
melanin, 38
membrane permeability, 422
membranes, 73, 78, 94, 136, 174, 376, 426, 450, 451, 452, 457, 458
memory, 68, 80, 98, 99, 103, 302
memory performance, 68, 103
men, ix, 3, 8, 37, 42, 45, 55, 56, 57, 84, 85, 90, 91, 92, 93, 94, 95, 99, 100, 104, 106, 111, 115, 120, 128, 136, 144, 148, 149, 157, 159, 160, 165, 166, 171, 174, 176, 177, 182, 184, 188, 190, 191, 214, 215, 220, 221, 222, 223, 224, 225, 229, 230, 232, 243, 255, 265, 269, 275, 284, 293, 297, 300, 322, 327, 329, 330, 339, 343, 347, 348, 356, 357, 359, 361, 368, 377, 380, 385, 418, 444
menarche, 115
meningitis, 65
menopause, 115, 158, 159, 169, 182, 187
mental disorder, 82
mental impairment, 80
mercury, 79, 102
mesangial cells, 414
mesenchyme, 454

messages, xi, 204, 205, 208, 253, 254, 255, 256, 257, 264, 265, 315
messenger RNA, 34, 178
meta-analysis, 5, 9, 29, 51, 94, 97, 98, 196, 198, 205, 209, 244, 251, 315, 341, 350, 357, 358, 365, 436
metabolic acidosis, 161
metabolic disorder, 86, 339
metabolic disturbances, 409
metabolic pathways, 273, 323
metabolic syndrome, viii, 43, 46, 55, 57, 60, 63, 70, 71, 86, 88, 89, 90, 91, 95, 229, 281, 282, 330, 349
metabolites, 58, 98, 133, 155, 185, 449, 457
metabolizing, 130
metal ions, 79, 130, 142, 348
metalloproteinase, 339, 348
metals, 77, 78, 79, 101, 102, 142, 333
metastasis, 143
methionine, 75, 125, 150, 160
methyl group, 75, 135
methyl groups, 75, 135
methylation, 75, 125, 126, 151
methylenetetrahydrofolate reductase, 126
Mexican Americans, 45
Mexico, 6, 167
Mg^{2+}, 39, 49, 50, 52, 60, 61, 161
mice, 78, 86, 100, 102, 126, 151, 359, 394, 454, 457
microarray, 458
microbial, 116, 429
microdialysis, 416
microenvironment, 412
micrograms, 144
micronucleus, 153
micronutrients, viii, ix, 46, 63, 75, 79, 81, 83, 129, 136, 157, 273, 290, 291, 300, 322, 323, 324, 328, 353, 354, 358, 361, 363, 367, 369
micro-organisms, 130
Middle East, 39
migration, 272
mild cognitive impairment, 77, 78, 83, 96, 98, 100, 103, 104
military, 268
milk, 6, 7, 23, 113, 115, 116, 122, 124, 130, 164, 167, 169, 170, 171, 172, 187, 256, 258, 260, 266, 267, 291
milligrams, 135
mineral water, 172, 335
minerals, viii, xii, 32, 40, 52, 75, 107, 111, 119, 161, 174, 179, 180, 184, 188, 193, 256, 261, 262, 289, 319, 322, 323, 333, 337
Mini Nutritional Assessment, MNA, x
Minnesota, 322, 328
minority, 413
mitochondria, 166, 337, 342, 353, 364, 367, 420, 421, 422, 426, 450, 452, 456
mitochondrial DNA, 111
mitochondrial membrane, 451
mitosis, 109
mitral valve prolapse, 344
mixing, 6
mobility, 37, 245, 246, 251, 289, 292, 321, 358, 372
model system, 250
modeling, 166, 274, 302
models, 7, 48, 49, 50, 76, 77, 81, 101, 110, 130, 132, 142, 196, 203, 218, 272, 302, 303, 358, 454
modifier gene, 448, 454, 456
moieties, 142, 422
mole, 174
molecular changes, 448
molecular mechanisms, 6, 394, 447
molecular oxygen, 130, 179
molecular structure, 452
molecules, 7, 8, 9, 34, 71, 79, 109, 127, 130, 135, 136, 142, 178, 360, 380, 449, 452
molybdenum, 296
Mongolia, 23, 28
monkeys, 366
monoclonal antibody, 239
monocytes, 175, 425
monotherapy, 170
monounsaturated fat, 72, 95
monounsaturated fatty acids, 72
mood, 6, 103, 345
morbidity, x, xii, 12, 28, 66, 176, 213, 215, 219, 220, 226, 243, 246, 248, 274, 280, 286, 294, 319, 320, 322, 334, 354, 440
morning, 161
morphology, 91, 188, 420, 448
morphometric, 398
mortality, x, xi, xii, 3, 9, 12, 27, 23, 66, 71, 83, 94, 110, 125, 128, 132, 145, 148, 149, 150, 153, 213, 215, 219, 220, 222, 226, 231, 233, 236, 237, 238, 239, 243, 246, 249, 251, 271, 274, 275, 276, 277, 278, 279, 280, 282, 283, 284, 286, 293, 294, 295, 297, 301, 319, 322, 323, 326, 327, 328, 329, 330, 334, 342, 354, 357, 359, 366, 367, 369, 372, 380, 381, 386, 387, 428, 429, 431, 434, 437, 440
mortality rate, 12, 125, 150, 153, 219, 282, 342, 357, 431
mortality risk, 323, 387
motivation, 198, 238

mouse model, 93, 454
movement, 103, 197, 379
mRNA, 49, 59, 70, 85, 90, 426, 452
mucosa, 108, 117, 126, 131, 151, 153, 448, 452
mucus, 428, 434
multidimensional, 295, 442
multiple myeloma, 125
multiple sclerosis, 65
multiples, 237
multiplicity, 454
murmur, 344
muscle atrophy, 345, 422
muscle biopsy, 341
muscle cells, 33, 49, 140, 272, 338, 347, 348, 412, 422
muscle contraction, 166, 334
muscle mass, 161, 214, 219, 265, 268, 289, 322, 324, 327, 390, 412, 424, 431, 432, 441, 444
muscle performance, 345, 419, 431
muscle strength, 36, 321, 419, 423, 431, 432, 436, 442
muscle tissue, 50, 431
muscle weakness, 419, 421, 423
muscles, 39, 50, 60, 108, 257, 321, 345, 372, 381, 385, 389, 390, 391, 409, 410, 412, 419, 420, 421, 422, 423, 430, 431, 432, 433, 438, 440, 442, 444
muscular mass, 372, 377, 385, 386
muscular tissue, 385
Muslims, 39
mutant, 86
mutation, 61, 454
mutations, 61, 111, 118, 126, 128, 448
myeloma, 125
myoblasts, 422, 427
myocardial infarction, 8, 9, 103, 339, 342, 350, 351, 356, 380, 416
myocardium, 342, 421
myopathy, 423
myosin, 410

N

Na^+, 58, 415
NaCl, 173
NAD, 449
NADH, 422
naringin, 137
nasopharynx, 114
National Health Interview Survey, 208
National Institutes of Health, 187, 218, 231, 367
National Research Council, 67, 84, 163, 184
native population, 6
natural evolution, 349
natural food, 132, 173
natural killer cell, 127
nausea, 354
neck, 173, 176, 177, 247
necrosis, 68, 116, 186, 272, 379, 381, 422, 425, 426, 427
neoplasia, 117, 145, 282, 448, 456, 458
neoplasm, xi, 271, 276, 279, 280
Neoplastic, 65
Nepal, 11, 12, 27, 28, 29
nephrocalcinosis, 172
nephrolithiasis, 184, 185, 336
nephron, 54
nerve, 293
nervous system, 4, 75, 83, 84, 85, 98, 108, 191, 344
Netherlands, 93, 167, 283, 300, 431
network, 391, 392, 405
neurobiology, 81
neurodegeneration, 67, 79, 97, 101, 102, 141
neurodegenerative disease(s), 76
neurodegenerative disorders, 68, 72, 100
neuro-degenerative disorders, viii
neurofibrillary tangles, 64, 101
neuroinflammation, 101
neurologic disorders, 78
neurological disease, 76
neurological disorder, 215
neuronal cells, 75
neuronal death, 72
neuronal degeneration, 78
neurons, 34, 64, 76, 78, 79, 98
neuropathy, 349
neuropeptide, 377
neuroprotective, 3, 72, 339, 351
neuroscience, 77
neurotoxicity, 78, 98, 102
neurotransmitter(s), 75, 166
neurotrophic factors, 72
neutrophils, 366, 428
New England, 82, 83, 86, 87, 89, 91, 92, 94, 95, 96, 98, 103, 104
New York, 8, 145, 146, 182, 209, 210, 268, 269, 366, 426, 434
New Zealand, 42, 46
Newton, 347
NHS, 296
niacin, 65

nickel, 296
NIH, 363
nimodipine, 343
nitrate, 173, 283
nitric oxide, 3, 7, 8, 76, 79, 128, 130, 282, 422, 425, 427
nitric oxide synthase, 76, 79
nitrogen, 129, 179, 183, 321, 322, 327, 374, 441, 443
nitrosamines, 114, 133
nitroso compounds, 133
NMDA receptors, 339
NMR, 341, 420
nocturia, 302
nodules, 454
noise, 408
non-human primates, 359
non-institutionalized, 243
non-insulin dependent diabetes, 148
Norfolk, 120, 148
normal aging, 232, 355, 368
normal development, 165
normal distribution, 172
North America, 39, 88, 105, 119, 159, 165, 181, 244, 295, 296, 330
North Carolina, 276
Norway, 4
nosocomial pneumonia, 429
nuclear magnetic resonance, 420
nuclear receptors, 34
nucleic acid, 174, 336, 355, 378
nucleic acid synthesis, 174, 336
nucleus, 166, 421, 449
nurses, 43, 239
nursing, 36, 228, 232, 237, 238, 240, 243, 246, 247, 249, 250, 251, 252, 286, 294, 298
nursing home, 36, 228, 237, 238, 240, 243, 246, 247, 249, 250, 251, 252, 286, 294, 298
nutraceuticals, 102
nutrient descriptions, xi, 253, 254, 255, 262, 263
nutrients, ix, x, xi, 23, 24, 27, 65, 71, 72, 79, 83, 100, 126, 133, 144, 158, 164, 178, 180, 181, 187, 189, 213, 215, 249, 253, 255, 257, 262, 263, 268, 286, 289, 290, 291, 294, 300, 359, 361, 364, 376, 390, 391, 410
nutritional assessment, x, xi, 214, 221, 227, 228, 231, 232, 233, 235, 241, 242, 245, 247, 248, 252, 324, 325, 440
nutritional deficiencies, 80, 325, 361, 363, 364
nutritional screening, 223, 232, 242, 324, 325, 387
nutritional supplements, 27, 437
nuts, 113, 127, 128, 133, 135, 141, 144, 164, 169, 172, 181, 265, 291, 341, 343, 356, 359

O

Obese, 54
obese patients, 69, 286
obesity, viii, xii, 28, 36, 37, 38, 54, 55, 56, 59, 60, 63, 65, 66, 67, 68, 69, 72, 73, 83, 84, 86, 87, 88, 89, 90, 91, 92, 93, 95, 96, 106, 111, 112, 114, 115, 124, 145, 196, 212, 218, 229, 282, 285, 286, 289, 294, 295, 315, 338, 361, 364, 369
observations, 77, 222, 229, 356
obstruction, 391, 405, 409, 412, 429, 438, 442, 454
obstructive lung disease, 391, 405, 411, 425, 428, 433, 435, 443
obstructive sleep apnea, 86, 412, 415, 416
occlusion, 339
Odyssey, 2
oedema, 325
offenders, 335
oil, 71, 77, 95, 113, 116, 124, 164, 165, 185, 186, 293, 432
oils, 15, 16, 17, 18, 27, 113, 135, 164, 174, 176, 356, 359
old age, 96, 185, 236, 249, 293, 295, 330, 371, 372, 373, 380, 385
older adults, xii, 60, 66, 84, 90, 94, 97, 103, 106, 162, 185, 211, 228, 231, 232, 246, 247, 254, 257, 285, 286, 290, 291, 293, 294, 297, 327, 328, 335, 364, 365, 366, 418, 441, 444
older people, xii, 81, 103, 104, 219, 220, 230, 233, 248, 289, 290, 291, 301, 317, 319, 321, 322, 323, 324, 327, 328, 336, 369, 439
olfactory, 215
oligofructose, 119, 146
oligomers, 100
Oligosaccharides, 119
olive oil, 71, 293
omega-3, viii, ix, 102, 106, 107, 113, 141, 146, 158, 164, 185, 447
omega-6, viii
oncogene(s), 126, 458
Oncology, 145, 151, 281, 282
operator, 221, 402
optimal health, 165
oral cavity, viii, 107, 114, 129, 135, 290
oral health, xii, 290, 299, 317, 364, 367
oral leukoplakia, 153
orange juice, 167, 169

organ, 68, 69, 70, 85, 108, 121, 273, 279, 280, 319, 321, 324, 336, 359, 372, 392, 393, 394, 417, 440, 442, 445
organelles, 339
organism, 5, 354, 355, 360, 371, 372, 373, 374, 376, 377, 378, 380, 381
organization, 239, 257, 452
ornithine, 137
orthostatic hypotension, 344
osmolality, 173
ossification, 175
osteoclastogenesis, 192
osteoclasts, 162, 165, 172, 175, 180, 193
osteomalacia, 175
osteoporosis, ix, 34, 67, 141, 149, 157, 158, 159, 160, 161, 162, 164, 165, 166, 167, 174, 176, 177, 178, 180, 181, 182, 183, 184, 185, 186, 187, 188, 190, 191, 192, 193, 214, 236, 237, 293, 302, 330, 344, 345, 413
osteoporotic fractures, ix
osteosarcoma, 58
outpatients, 249, 252, 411, 432, 442
ovarian cancer, 125, 147, 149, 150, 274, 282, 283
ovariectomy, 164
ovaries, 112, 374
overeating, 268
overload, 342, 422, 427
overproduction, 39, 422
overweight, 12, 37, 38, 67, 68, 73, 83, 84, 111, 112, 119, 196, 201, 202, 207, 223, 246, 248, 286, 294, 295, 323, 330, 361, 431
oxalate, 122, 170
oxidants, 323
oxidation, 3, 4, 5, 78, 109, 116, 127, 129, 130, 136, 180, 282, 350, 355, 356, 357, 360, 376, 381, 422, 450
oxidative damage, 72, 111, 128, 273, 322, 328, 346, 355, 422, 427, 431
oxidative stress, 72, 73, 76, 77, 97, 98, 100, 103, 111, 128, 180, 193, 194, 272, 273, 281, 282, 297, 323, 344, 355, 358, 360, 362, 363, 365, 367, 389, 393, 412, 418, 421, 422, 425, 427, 431, 433, 439, 440
oxide, 3, 7, 8, 76, 79, 128, 130, 282, 339
oxygen, 72, 116, 128, 129, 130, 133, 135, 142, 145, 179, 193, 194, 273, 282, 320, 334, 342, 353, 355, 358, 360, 364, 367, 410, 412, 414, 415, 416, 417, 419, 420, 421, 422, 423, 424, 425, 426, 427, 429, 430, 431, 432, 436, 438, 439, 441, 442
oxygen consumption, 420, 423, 426, 432
oxygenation, 412, 420, 424

P

p38, 455
Pacific, 28
packaging, 254
pain, 5, 116, 302, 344, 345, 348
palpitations, 344
pancreas, 40, 57, 58, 111, 129, 143, 380, 414
pancreatic, 31, 34, 40, 41, 48, 49, 57, 119, 120, 124, 125, 147, 149, 272, 433, 439
pancreatic cancer, 119, 120, 147, 149, 433, 439
paradox, 74, 97, 154, 366
paralysis, 345
parameter, x, 214, 376, 403
parasympathetic nervous system, 344
parathyroid (hormone), 33, 34, 37, 39, 53, 55, 57, 121, 162, 166, 174, 175, 182, 184, 187, 188, 190, 193, 345
parenchyma, 375, 378, 400
parenchymal changes, 397, 408
parents, 201, 211, 271
Paris, 8, 233, 250, 275, 280, 346
Parkinson's disease, 65
particles, 69, 70, 73, 74, 78, 193
passive, 336
pasta, 259, 266
pathogenesis, 40, 52, 68, 75, 77, 78, 140, 180, 185, 190, 335, 340, 359, 389, 390, 391, 392, 394, 395, 409, 413, 418, 428, 433, 439
pathogenic, 75, 76, 112
pathogens, 392
pathological aging, 219
pathology, 29, 68, 82, 216, 222, 392, 398, 404, 427
pathophysiology, 46, 52, 146, 231, 272, 344, 391
pathways, viii, 5, 31, 32, 52, 65, 68, 78, 123, 137, 140, 142, 155, 177, 273, 323, 392, 413, 447, 448, 449, 450, 452, 454, 455, 457
patient care, 29
pectin, 117
pediatric patients, 330
peers, 257
penetrance, 454
peptic ulcer, 413
peptides, 68
percentage of fat, 372
perception, 232, 236, 244
perceptions, 255

performance, 68, 73, 80, 100, 103, 179, 185, 215, 231, 268, 298, 345, 390, 420, 421, 426, 430, 431, 432, 436, 438, 439, 440, 442, 444, 452
perfusion, 40, 54, 69, 339, 400, 404
periodontal, 165
periodontal disease, 165
peripheral blood, 41, 425
peripheral vascular disease, 68, 87
permeability, 381
permit, 161
peroxidation, 77, 112, 116, 136, 154, 337, 355, 363
peroxide, 77, 78, 102, 273, 360
personal, 173, 198, 303, 305, 307, 315, 346
personal relevance, 198
pesticide, ix, 108
PET, 408
pH, 118, 161, 171, 337, 420, 452
phagocytosis, 378, 379
pharmaceutical(s), 200, 208, 281
pharmacokinetics, 236
pharmacological treatment, 81
pharmacology, 53
pharynx, viii, 107, 114, 129
phenolic acid(s), 142
phenotype(s), 82, 109, 247, 389, 390, 391, 394, 405, 409, 410, 439, 454, 456
phosphate(s), 34, 53, 122, 151, 161, 166, 170, 171, 172, 173, 175, 188, 189, 193, 385, 420, 449, 451, 457
phospholipids, 75, 116, 171, 422, 432, 449
phosphorous, ix, 34, 39, 157
phosphorus, 32, 34, 52, 53, 171, 172, 175, 180, 181, 182, 183, 188, 189, 424
phosphorylation, 50, 59, 192, 340, 422
physical activity, 65, 72, 81, 114, 136, 144, 145, 159, 200, 202, 203, 204, 205, 230, 247, 251, 256, 284, 291, 300, 304, 315, 322, 325, 327, 364, 385, 421
physical exercise, 431, 433
physical fitness, 443
physicians, 218, 231, 394
physiology, 32, 53, 56, 146, 164, 276, 296, 298
phytochemicals, viii, 107, 129, 135, 137, 140, 141, 181
pilot study, 434
pioglitazone, 60
placebo, 44, 47, 69, 103, 104, 105, 122, 131, 162, 176, 191, 329, 356, 428, 432, 434, 438
planning, 80, 238
plant sterols, 32
plants, 128, 130, 135, 138, 140, 142, 154, 176
plaque(s), 87, 338
plasma, 7, 32, 42, 44, 47, 49, 51, 53, 54, 59, 73, 75, 76, 86, 88, 92, 95, 97, 98, 99, 101, 103, 105, 123, 130, 150, 161, 171, 173, 179, 192, 194, 273, 282, 298, 329, 331, 334, 338, 339, 345, 350, 357, 359, 360, 365, 368, 371, 372, 373, 374, 375, 376, 377, 379, 381, 382, 383, 386, 387, 414, 418, 421
plasma levels, 73, 338, 383
plasma membrane, 32, 49, 97, 123, 334
plasma proteins, 329, 331, 371, 372, 373, 377, 381
plasminogen, 3, 380
plasticity, 72, 98
platelet aggregation, 3, 4, 68
platelets, 8, 59, 334, 341
plausibility, 71, 131
PM, 91, 97, 99, 102, 103, 153, 228, 246, 247, 249, 281, 297, 330, 350, 391, 394, 411, 416, 424, 426, 439
PN, 93
pneumonectomy, 435
pneumonia, 237, 250, 363
Poland, 107, 157, 274
policy initiative, 286
pollutants, 393
pollution, 128
polycyclic aromatic hydrocarbon, 114
polycystic ovarian syndrome, 42, 45
polymer, 142
polymerase, 282
polymerization, 119
polymorphism(s), 32, 50, 51, 60, 126, 150, 454
polyp, 126, 131
polypeptide, 375
polyphenols, vii, 2, 3, 4, 5, 8, 9, 74, 97, 129, 137, 142, 142, 143, 155, 156, 353, 363
polyps, 115, 122, 126, 131, 454
polysaccharide, 378
polyunsaturated fat(ty acids), 27, 72, 80, 95, 102, 104, 116, 185, 355, 432, 439, 447, 448
poor, x, 27, 37, 67, 69, 126, 128, 213, 215, 219, 224, 230, 237, 239, 242, 248, 272, 286, 290, 301, 302, 314, 324, 337, 340, 343, 357, 361, 364, 430, 431, 439, 440, 441
population, ix, 39, 45, 50, 51, 52, 55, 56, 58, 60, 64, 65, 66, 67, 79, 80, 82, 83, 84, 85, 87, 90, 94, 96, 99, 100, 110, 111, 112, 115, 119, 122, 126, 132, 140, 141, 148, 157, 159, 181, 182, 197, 200, 201, 204, 205, 211, 215, 217, 218, 222, 226, 227, 228, 231, 232, 239, 243, 244, 245, 246, 248, 249, 250,

251, 252, 286, 293, 298, 301, 316, 327, 330, 334, 336, 339, 340, 341, 353, 359, 360, 361, 363, 365, 366, 368, 381, 400, 418, 437, 454
pork, 115, 116, 162
portability, x, 213, 216
positive correlation, 257
positive relation, 78
positive relationship, 78
postmenopausal women, 9, 39, 57, 105, 112, 114, 146, 148, 159, 162, 171, 173, 174, 176, 179, 180, 181, 182, 183, 184, 187, 189, 190, 191, 193, 194, 211, 367
potassium, 49, 56, 59, 161, 172, 173, 181, 189, 190, 231, 336, 338, 345, 347, 348, 349, 351
potato(es), 23, 134, 143, 168, 172, 259, 260, 266, 267, 314, 315, 343
poultry, 181, 265, 291, 292
poverty, 361, 431, 440
power, 51, 77, 238, 402, 404, 431
prealbumin, 325, 373, 374, 375, 377, 381, 383, 384, 385, 386, 387, 441
prediction, 70, 247, 326, 417, 443
predictive accuracy, 218
predictors, 99, 158, 211, 230, 246
prednisone, 160
pregnancy, 115, 175
premature death, 195
premenopausal, 111, 112, 145, 152, 173, 189
premenopausal women, 111, 112, 173, 189
preschool, 27
pressure, 7, 9, 10, 12, 13, 14, 56, 69, 70, 83, 89, 130, 170, 188, 238, 239, 251, 282, 337, 360, 362, 363, 365, 392, 393, 400, 410, 424, 431, 437, 443
pressure sore, 362, 363, 365
prevention, ix, xii, 6, 8, 9, 10, 35, 52, 54, 64, 69, 72, 73, 76, 81, 89, 98, 111, 122, 128, 130, 131, 136, 137, 141, 145, 149, 151, 152, 153, 154, 156, 157, 165, 176, 177, 179, 180, 181, 182, 185, 187, 191, 201, 203, 208, 216, 217, 249, 250, 251, 281, 285, 286, 291, 300, 315, 316, 342, 349, 350, 351, 353, 354, 356, 357, 363, 367, 369, 391, 411, 429, 430, 433, 448, 452
prevention of infection, 430
prices, 268
prion diseases, 65
probability, 127, 205, 225, 244, 303, 389, 390, 395
probiotic, 177
problem behavior(s), 197, 210, 211
production, 4, 32, 34, 35, 37, 55, 75, 78, 102, 112, 113, 117, 118, 121, 125, 130, 160, 161, 164, 165, 177, 186, 189, 290, 323, 329, 334, 344, 348, 355, 358, 360, 366, 379, 414, 415, 416, 422, 425, 426, 428, 441, 442
productivity, 200, 208
profit, 69
prognosis, 229, 326, 351, 373, 384, 409, 411, 420, 424, 437, 448
program, 80, 81, 103, 106, 202, 203, 206, 208, 209, 211, 238, 247, 250, 298, 398, 402, 403, 404, 405, 432, 441
pro-inflammatory, 165, 272, 413
proinflammatory effect, 413
proliferation, 34, 108, 113, 118, 120, 121, 137, 138, 140, 141, 149, 150, 151, 164, 175, 180, 193, 272, 358, 367, 380, 453
promote, 32, 55, 65, 68, 72, 113, 118, 159, 164, 181, 245, 254, 264, 265, 268, 269, 301, 314, 431
promoter, 50
promoter region, 50
propagation, 355
prophylactic, 6
prostaglandin(s), 113, 116, 127, 164, 177, 186, 378, 450
prostate, ix, 108, 109, 111, 122, 124, 125, 128, 131, 135, 136, 140, 141, 143, 144, 149, 150, 152, 153, 155, 274, 281, 283, 358, 366
prostate cancer, ix, 108, 111, 115, 125, 128, 131, 135, 136, 140, 141, 144, 150, 153, 155, 274, 281, 283, 358, 366
proteases, 422
protective factors, 64, 125
protective mechanisms, 154
protective role, 73, 79, 185
protein aggregation, 78
protein function, 422
protein kinase C, 49, 57
protein oxidation, 78, 180, 427
protein synthesis, 322, 334, 441
proteins, 7, 23, 52, 68, 86, 128, 175, 177, 179, 191, 323, 325, 329, 330, 331, 335, 341, 355, 359, 371, 372, 373, 374, 377, 378, 381, 382, 383, 384, 386, 413, 422, 427, 432, 440, 443, 452
proteolysis, 381
proteolytic enzyme, 429
pro-thrombotic, 68, 70
protocol, 104, 201, 220, 244, 245, 431, 433
protocols, 243, 404
psychology, 255
psychosocial factors, 431
psychosocial variables, 203

puberty, 228
public health, 11, 27, 52, 64, 114, 195, 200
pulmonary function test, 397, 405, 429
pulmonary hypertension, 430
pulmonary rehabilitation, 411, 430, 433, 436, 439
pulses, 135, 161
pumps, 415
pyridoxal, 151

Q

QT interval, 342
quadriceps, 430
quality assurance, 239
quality control, 217, 245
quality of life, xii, 105, 106, 200, 203, 207, 216, 226, 239, 246, 247, 249, 251, 294, 298, 299, 301, 302, 313, 314, 321, 325, 326, 327, 348, 354, 358, 364, 365, 372, 390, 391, 431, 439
quartile, 42, 43, 45, 46, 135, 136, 275
Quercetin, 143
questionnaire, 220, 221, 242, 274, 276, 284
quinone, 155

R

race, 37, 70, 205, 231, 275, 276
radiation, 37, 109, 123, 150, 366
radical formation, 421
radical reactions, 356
radio, 199, 404
radiography, 395, 406
range, 5, 24, 34, 38, 40, 49, 52, 59, 67, 127, 142, 143, 162, 171, 178, 197, 216, 217, 220, 223, 243, 254, 273, 291, 321, 333, 334, 337, 342, 359, 361, 362, 363, 373, 374, 375, 377, 378, 379, 380, 384, 385, 390, 391, 398, 414
ratings, xi, 206, 253, 254, 255, 257, 260, 261, 262, 263, 265
reactant, 380
reactants, 371, 381, 382
reaction mechanism, 152
reactive oxygen, 72, 116, 129, 130, 133, 145, 179, 193, 194, 273, 282, 355, 360, 364, 412, 416, 421, 422
reactivity, 109, 447
reality, 5
recall, ix, 11, 108, 256
receptors, 31, 32, 33, 34, 48, 49, 50, 57, 59, 60, 85, 121, 140, 155, 166, 339, 376, 394, 395, 414, 425, 432, 453
recognition, 6, 216, 236, 237, 243, 249, 364, 397, 405, 408
reconciliation, 248
reconstruction, 392
recovery, 321, 339
recruiting, 71
rectum, 111
recurrence, 92, 122, 149
recycling, 367
red blood cell, 171, 345
red blood cells, 171, 345
red meat, viii, 73, 107, 114, 121, 127, 144, 162
redox, 78, 154, 355
reduction, 7, 36, 41, 70, 71, 72, 76, 96, 102, 109, 122, 126, 127, 128, 131, 162, 170, 173, 176, 179, 199, 201, 202, 205, 206, 214, 215, 222, 223, 225, 238, 273, 284, 289, 298, 300, 324, 325, 342, 343, 356, 358, 360, 390, 395, 408, 412, 413, 427, 429, 435, 447, 449, 452
reflection, 73
refractory, 190
regional, 90, 91, 339, 408, 442
Registry, 350
regression, xi, 212, 218, 261, 271, 304, 404, 441, 442
regression analysis, 212
regression equation, 218, 441
regulation, 6, 34, 59, 60, 67, 68, 85, 96, 116, 117, 171, 172, 175, 189, 215, 229, 272, 289, 323, 378, 432, 454
regulators, 378
rehabilitation, xii, 10, 162, 238, 239, 246, 250, 251, 319, 322, 390, 391, 405, 409, 411, 427, 428, 430, 432, 435, 438, 440, 441, 442, 444
rehabilitation program, 239, 390, 391, 409, 430, 432, 440, 444
Reimann, 101
relationship(s), ix, xi, 28, 29, 40, 53, 55, 59, 67, 72, 74, 76, 78, 86, 88, 89, 108, 111, 115, 132, 145, 171, 180, 189, 208, 221, 254, 264, 271, 272, 274, 275, 280, 283, 291, 327, 338, 339, 347, 371, 390, 395, 397, 400, 409, 410, 420, 421, 424, 456
relatives, 237, 255
relaxation, 345, 347
relevance, vii, 1, 3, 198, 231, 243, 455
reliability, 220, 242, 244, 252, 391
remodel(l)ing, 158, 170, 172, 183 428

renal, 4, 52, 61, 125, 160, 163, 167, 171, 172, 175, 182, 183, 188, 190, 237, 272, 320, 323, 326, 334, 335, 342, 344, 345, 362, 374, 375, 385
renal disease, 172, 362, 374, 375
renal failure, 237, 342
renal function, 182, 188, 190, 320, 326, 375
renal replacement therapy, 323
renin, 4, 89
repair, 34, 72, 125, 126, 127, 128, 335, 393, 448
reparation, 173, 301, 376, 381
reperfusion therapy, 342
replication, 8, 71, 82, 118, 178, 192, 273
reproductive age, 39, 54
reproductive cells, 108
reputation, 254, 264
research design, 239
reserves, 161, 375, 382
residential, 294
residues, ix, 6, 108, 142, 422
resistance, viii, 6, 8, 31, 32, 34, 41, 42, 44, 45, 46, 47, 49, 50, 51, 52, 56, 57, 58, 59, 65, 68, 69, 70, 71, 73, 85, 91, 95, 107, 133, 148, 198, 218, 282, 330, 337, 340, 344, 345, 348, 349, 354, 381, 392, 415, 418, 419, 430, 431
resistin, 91
resolution, 400, 404, 406, 407, 408
resources, 292, 423
respiration, 72, 415, 422, 423
respiratory, vii, xi, 1, 4, 135, 215, 271, 276, 279, 280, 321, 326, 372, 389, 390, 391, 394, 409, 411, 412, 414, 419, 420, 421, 422, 423, 424, 426, 431, 432, 436, 437, 438, 440, 442, 443, 444
respiratory disorders, 419
respiratory distress syndrome, 326
respiratory failure, 414, 424, 443
responsiveness, 49, 59, 60, 167, 172
retardation, 190
retention, 161, 183, 186, 206, 341, 381
reticulum, 166, 422, 426, 450
retinoic acid, 131, 194, 429, 434
retinol, 28, 153, 219, 373, 374, 375, 441
retinopathy, 349
retirement, 83, 237
RF, 102, 281
rheumatic diseases, 378, 380
Rhode Island, 204, 208, 209
rhythm, 5
riboflavin, 324, 330
rice, 23, 117, 121, 178, 257, 258, 266
rickets, 39, 175
rings, 73
risk assessment, 155
risk behaviors, 201, 202
risk factors, viii, ix, 36, 38, 41, 46, 63, 64, 65, 69, 73, 81, 83, 84, 85, 87, 88, 89, 90, 92, 95, 99, 114, 126, 147, 157, 182, 200, 207, 208, 232, 349, 356
RL, 89, 90, 91, 97, 105, 185, 247, 248, 251, 284, 328, 350, 369, 415
RNA, 34, 59, 178, 282
rodents, 359
roentgen, 395, 396, 397
Royal Society, 189
rural areas, 11

S

SA, 27, 82, 87, 98, 101, 146, 147, 150, 156, 182, 189, 194, 227, 282, 330, 394, 407, 419, 434, 439, 457
safety, ix, 158, 238, 429, 433
salmon, 32
salt(s), 114, 161, 170, 173, 181, 182, 188, 189, 268, 269, 291, 334
sample, x, 37, 82, 162, 199, 201, 203, 204, 205, 214, 217, 220, 221, 223, 225, 226, 227, 254, 255, 257, 258, 259, 260, 262, 264, 303, 351, 366, 428, 437
sampling, 303, 306, 330, 341, 350
sarcopenia, 214, 229, 239, 289, 327, 372
SAS, 276, 302
satisfaction, 238, 294, 317, 321
saturated fat(ty acis), ix, 72, 73, 74, 78, 108, 164, 196, 199, 202, 291, 447, 448
saturation, 438
Saudi Arabia, 39
Scandinavia, 167
Schmid, 348
school, 244, 276, 305, 307
schooling, 276
science, 75, 79, 154, 291, 394, 430
sclerosis, 65
scores, 80, 198, 223, 231, 238, 260, 313, 314, 398
scurvy, 357, 366
sea level, 11, 415
search, 66, 210, 241, 368, 407, 427, 454
seasonality, 40
SEC, 141
secrete, 175
secretion, vii, 31, 32, 33, 35, 40, 41, 42, 44, 45, 46, 47, 48, 51, 52, 57, 58, 59, 60, 121, 171, 175, 178,

188, 290, 324, 333, 334, 339, 342, 344, 345, 349, 381, 414, 419
secular trend, 217
sedimentation, 372, 373, 378, 380
seed, viii, 107, 141
seeds, 6, 113, 117, 119, 128, 164, 169, 181, 343
segmentation, 400, 402, 403, 407
selenium, viii, 79, 102, 107, 114, 127, 128, 129, 132, 140, 151, 152, 154, 155, 323, 328, 329, 345
self-assessment, 203
self-efficacy, 196, 199
self-esteem, 317
self-monitoring, 204
senescence, 335, 346, 353, 354, 394, 453
senile dementia, 82
senile plaques, 102
sensation, 5, 344
sensing, 121, 166, 334, 417, 421
sensitivity, vii, 4, 31, 42, 45, 47, 49, 50, 58, 59, 73, 78, 95, 172, 215, 220, 221, 223, 227, 232, 244, 340, 341, 344, 350, 359, 366, 374, 380, 397, 414, 415, 416, 419, 421, 453
sepsis, 321, 323, 326, 331, 376, 385
septic shock, 329
Serbia, 333
series, 40, 50, 80, 116, 136, 196, 201, 203, 231, 315, 359, 376, 382, 429
serine, 160, 449
serum albumin, 219, 221, 227, 230, 237, 320, 373, 381, 385, 387
severe stress, 323
severity, 52, 233, 245, 321, 325, 327, 389, 390, 391, 395, 398, 399, 403, 409, 410, 413, 434, 439
sex, 23, 46, 47, 93, 146, 182, 217, 218, 222, 225, 227, 228, 230, 231, 233, 323, 359, 362, 372, 383
sex differences, 222
sex hormones, 146, 323
sexual behavior, 109, 112
SGA, 219, 227
shape, 178, 407, 420
shares, 79, 427
sharing, 4
sheep, 59, 349
shock, 329, 452
shortage, 421
side effects, 337
sign, 344, 395, 397, 428
signal transduction, 5, 96, 137, 333, 449, 457
signal(l)ing, 8, 52, 68, 85, 93, 98, 394, 416, 421, 447, 448, 452, 456, 457
signals, 389, 392, 412, 456
signs, 64, 325, 344, 383, 384, 389, 390, 395, 396, 397
silicon, 296
similarity, 380
sine, 344
sites, viii, 107, 108, 110, 111, 112, 128, 136, 169, 170, 281, 338
skeletal muscle, 49, 50, 230, 289, 321, 327, 328, 334, 390, 412, 415, 416, 417, 419, 420, 421, 422, 423, 424, 425, 426, 427, 430, 432, 433, 436, 439, 440, 442, 444
skeleton, 161, 163, 166, 171, 174, 175
skin, 32, 36, 37, 38, 54, 55, 118, 121, 123, 124, 128, 133, 143, 151, 166, 167, 174, 177, 211, 259, 267, 324, 325, 330, 377, 383, 385, 441
skin cancer, 128, 211
skinfolds, 217, 228
sleep apnea, 86
sleep disorders, 344
small intestine, 35, 50, 175, 334, 454, 456
small vessel disease, 98
smoke, 128, 144, 275, 389, 392, 418
smoke exposure, 392
smokers, 77, 128, 132, 136, 153, 180, 200, 201, 210, 275, 276, 368, 408, 413, 425, 428, 439
smoking, ix, xi, 9, 109, 115, 157, 160, 200, 201, 203, 204, 205, 208, 210, 211, 212, 271, 275, 276, 278, 279, 284, 300, 303, 304, 313, 315, 357, 364, 365, 405, 413, 418, 430
smoking cessation, 200, 201, 203, 204, 205, 208, 210, 405, 413, 418, 430
smooth muscle, 140, 272, 338, 347, 348
smooth muscle cells, 140, 272, 338, 347, 348
social change, 289
social class, 357
social costs, 216
social factors, 236, 300
social isolation, 291
social network, 203
social norms, 196
social support, 196, 197, 203
society, 5, 390, 391
socioeconomic conditions, 23, 337, 347
socioeconomic status, 294
sodium, ix, 145, 158, 161, 171, 173, 189, 193, 256, 261, 262, 266, 267, 291, 337, 338, 345, 347, 367, 381
soft drinks, 171, 188
software, 227, 231

soil, 127, 128, 178
solar, 123, 150
solubility, 109, 118, 178
sounds, 241
South America, 4
South Carolina, 271
soy isoflavones, 141
soybean(s), 77, 137, 140, 141, 176, 178, 191, 343
Spain, 4, 6, 295
spatial learning, 98
species, 72, 78, 116, 128, 129, 130, 138, 145, 193, 194, 273, 282, 355, 358, 360, 364, 412, 416, 421, 422
specificity, 71, 155, 193, 216, 219, 220, 221, 223, 227, 344, 374, 380
spectroscopy, 273, 341
spectrum, 192, 216, 389, 390, 428, 452, 457
speed, 117
sperm, 127
sphingolipids, 449, 458
sphingosine, 449, 450, 451
spices, 6, 161
spine, 169, 173, 187, 361
spine fractures, 187
spirometry, 396
spontaneous pneumothorax, 401
sports, 276
sputum, 396, 397, 401, 428
St. Louis, 188
stability, 125, 127, 131, 135, 200, 229, 273, 282, 335, 346
stages, 108, 128, 142, 196, 197, 198, 208, 223, 273, 374, 411, 437, 443
standard deviation, 224, 363
standard error, 398
standardization, x, 213, 216, 243
standards, 217, 218, 244, 314
starch, 114, 116, 119, 143, 144, 146
starch granules, 119
starch polysaccharides, 114, 144
starvation, 328, 342, 377, 381, 443
statin, 88, 281
statins, 10, 272
Statins, 88
statistics, 145, 223, 224
stereotype, 264
stereotypes, 255, 268, 269
steroid(s), 53, 54, 56, 376, 432
steroid hormone, 33, 137
sterols, 32
stimulus, 333
stochastic, 393, 394
stomach, 5, 110, 111, 114, 125, 129, 131, 133, 135, 138, 143, 215, 274, 282, 403, 457
storage, 37, 70, 116, 166, 290
strain, 162, 454
strategies, xii, 197, 198, 207, 237, 285, 286, 325, 364, 369, 427, 444
stratification, 244
strength, xi, 36, 114, 121, 158, 161, 166, 179, 193, 203, 237, 238, 253, 254, 255, 256, 257, 258, 259, 260, 261, 262, 263, 264, 265, 321, 344, 409, 420, 423, 430, 431, 432, 442, 444
stress, 72, 73, 76, 93, 97, 98, 100, 103, 111, 128, 140, 180, 193, 194, 215, 237, 239, 272, 273, 281, 282, 297, 319, 323, 329, 330, 333, 336, 344, 345, 353, 354, 355, 358, 360, 362, 363, 364, 365, 367, 368, 375, 376, 380, 381, 382, 385, 394, 412, 416, 421, 426, 433, 452
stroke, 9, 40, 56, 68, 69, 72, 74, 76, 87, 88, 94, 97, 98, 103, 115, 130, 141, 293, 299, 302, 315, 338, 339, 343, 348, 351, 356, 366
students, xi, 253, 254, 255, 257, 260, 262, 264
subacute, 251
subarachnoid hemorrhage, 343, 351
subgroups, 119, 205, 223, 225, 401, 415, 449
substitutes, 96
substitution, 115, 151, 339
substrates, 146, 324
sucrose, 120, 455
sugar, 119, 120, 140, 142, 147, 268, 269, 315
sugars, viii
sulfate, 109, 189
sulfur, 75, 160, 188
sulfuric acid, 141
summer, 123
Sun, 98, 186, 205, 212
sunflower, 95, 128
superoxide, 128, 129, 179, 360, 393, 421, 426
superoxide dismutase, 179, 393, 421, 426
supply, x, 75, 102, 113, 123, 127, 130, 135, 164, 190, 211, 213, 215, 347, 358, 380, 381, 410, 412, 415, 420, 421, 440, 455
support services, 302
suppression, 35, 138, 172, 175, 376
surface area, 429
surgeons, 327
surgical intervention, 430, 444
surrogates, 70

survival, xii, 3, 67, 71, 92, 126, 151, 231, 239, 246, 286, 290, 294, 297, 299, 301, 302, 314, 321, 322, 326, 327, 359, 381, 394, 428, 431, 433, 434, 439, 449
survival rate, 67, 431, 439
survivors, 301, 321, 326, 327, 420
susceptibility, ix, 50, 60, 109, 157, 196, 273, 336, 354, 422, 427, 454, 457
susceptibility genes, 454
swallowing, 290
Sweden, 232
sweets, 72, 116, 289
swelling, 116
symptom(s), xi, 64, 116, 127, 141, 174, 219, 230, 235, 236, 239, 245, 313, 315, 325, 344, 345, 381, 409, 421, 423, 428, 431, 437, 440
synapse, 96
synaptic plasticity, 98
synbiotics, viii
syndrome, viii, 28, 42, 43, 45, 46, 53, 55, 57, 60, 63, 65, 70, 71, 86, 88, 89, 90, 91, 95, 148, 216, 229, 281, 282, 329, 330, 344, 349, 364, 409, 410, 415, 440
synthesis, 4, 7, 33, 34, 37, 38, 75, 78, 116, 123, 124, 125, 133, 150, 165, 172, 174, 175, 177, 192, 322, 323, 324, 334, 336, 344, 357, 374, 375, 376, 378, 379, 381, 382, 422, 425, 436, 443, 447, 449, 450, 451, 452
Syphilis, 65
systemic circulation, 421
systems, 3, 4, 48, 75, 77, 133, 140, 142, 173, 211, 257, 272, 320, 336, 344, 354, 355, 364, 372, 426, 449
systolic blood pressure, 7, 14, 69

T

T lymphocyte, 323
tachycardia, 342
Tailored materials, 198
Taiwan, 274, 283
tamoxifen, 140
tangles, 64, 101
tannins, 142
target behavior, 204, 206
targets, x, 9, 195, 199, 207, 355, 440, 444
tau, 64
tea, vii
Tea, 1, 2, 5, 143, 156
teachers, 257
technology, 154, 208, 239, 247
teeth, 34, 35, 120, 133, 166, 256, 302, 303
telephone, 204
television, 254, 257
temperature, 424
tenosynovitis, 362
tension, 320, 420, 421, 424, 426, 430, 438
ternary complex, 282
tertiary education, 301
test scores, 80
testosterone, 215
tetrachlorodibenzo-p-dioxin, 138
tetralogy, 426
thalassemia, 433, 439
theory, 145, 196, 203, 208, 209, 354, 355, 366, 368
therapeutic approaches, 351
therapeutic interventions, 220
therapeutics, 237
therapy, 6, 85, 88, 101, 103, 127, 177, 179, 193, 240, 323, 326, 330, 337, 342, 346, 348, 351, 354, 356, 374, 378, 408, 410, 411, 414, 416, 427, 428, 429, 430, 432, 435, 438, 441, 443
thiazide, 336, 340
thiazide diuretics, 340
thinking, xi, 253, 260, 264, 268, 269
thiobarbituric acid, 344
Thomson, 151, 268
thorax, 398
threonine, 160
threshold, x, 120, 176, 184, 213, 221, 232, 244, 398, 402, 403
thresholds, 398
thrombosis, 130, 281, 293, 302, 342
thromboxanes, 113, 164, 381
thrombus, 380
thymidine, 125
thyroid, 35, 50, 344, 377
thyroid gland, 35, 377
thyroxin, 374
trend, 38, 42, 45, 46, 51, 159, 171, 217, 314, 361, 374
Triacylglycerol, 25, 26
trial, viii, 46, 47, 64, 79, 89, 103, 104, 105, 106, 122, 128, 131, 149, 151, 152, 153, 162, 177, 187, 188, 190, 191, 201, 204, 208, 210, 211, 237, 246, 247, 248, 249, 251, 252, 268, 294, 298, 323, 329, 343, 350, 351, 356, 357, 365, 367, 368, 408, 411, 428, 430, 432, 434, 435, 437, 438, 443
tricarboxylic acid, 111
tricarboxylic acid cycle, 111

triceps, 228, 383, 385, 441
triggers, 452
triglyceride(s), 7, 70, 95, 282, 335, 338, 360, 450
tuberculosis, 361, 362, 380
tumor, 68, 108, 109, 110, 116, 126, 127, 130, 142, 143, 151, 155, 186, 272, 282, 379, 380, 381, 413, 421, 425
tumor cells, 126, 155
tumor growth, 126, 127, 143, 282
tumor necrosis factor, 68, 116, 186, 272, 381, 413, 421, 425
tumor proliferation, 380
tumorigenesis, 143, 145, 456, 457
tumors, 109, 110, 140, 273
tumour growth, 448
tumours, 65, 448, 454
turnover, ix, 158, 179, 180, 186, 188, 190, 331, 344, 350, 454
twins, 88
type 1 diabetes, 50, 60, 149, 349, 417
type 2 diabetes, vii, 31, 32, 39, 40, 41, 46, 47, 48, 50, 51, 52, 57, 58, 59, 60, 61, 83, 88, 91, 211, 282, 284, 341, 349, 350, 418
Type I error, 258
tyrosine, 50, 60, 137, 192, 340

U

UG, 230, 248, 250
UK, 155, 167, 248, 300, 427
ulcer, 247
ultrastructure, 416, 436
ultraviolet, 32, 37, 56, 123, 150, 174
ultraviolet irradiation, 32
ultraviolet light, 32, 56, 174
undergraduate, 255
underlying mechanisms, 71, 81, 222, 226
undernutrition, 226, 228, 246, 248, 251, 285, 289, 294, 316
uniform, 392, 444, 452
United Kingdom, 135, 243, 361
United Nations, 182, 360, 368
United States, 7, 36, 39, 54, 128, 147, 148, 149, 151, 184, 211, 212, 231, 243, 357, 366
univariate, 225, 227
urban areas, 23
urea, 441
urine, 35, 109, 160, 161, 165, 336, 344, 372, 373, 378, 379, 380, 385, 441
USDA, 118, 128, 163, 184, 186, 187, 256, 265, 291, 292
users, 100, 356, 367
USSR, 150
uterus, 111
UV(light), 37, 123, 128, 150
UV radiation, 37

V

vaccinations, 239
vaccine, 252
validation, 218, 242, 252, 328, 407
validity, 231, 242, 442
valine, 381
values, x, 3, 7, 12, 24, 147, 179, 180, 213, 216, 217, 218, 221, 223, 226, 227, 228, 231, 244, 261, 262, 268, 269, 286, 341, 362, 372, 373, 374, 375, 376, 377, 378, 379, 380, 383, 384, 385, 386, 398, 399, 400, 403, 409, 418, 430
vanadium, 296
variability, 162, 218, 244
variable, 79, 80, 110, 127, 173, 183, 196, 260, 261, 276, 405, 454
variables, 136, 161, 196, 203, 212, 217, 218, 219, 226, 227, 261, 268, 273, 276, 302, 304, 305, 307, 357, 417
variance, 261, 262, 321
variation, ix, 38, 52, 60, 80, 169, 195, 202, 205, 206, 217, 231, 273, 275, 282, 300, 350, 397, 423, 456
vascular cell adhesion molecule, 7, 9
vascular dementia, 69, 78, 86, 87, 99, 102, 298
vascular diseases, 347
vascular system, vii, 1, 68, 420
vasoconstriction, 4, 339
vasoconstrictor, 338
vasodilation, 7, 425
vasospasm, 343, 351
vastus lateralis, 410, 424
VAT, 70
vector, 218, 221, 225, 227, 228, 231, 233
vegetable oil, 113, 135, 164, 176, 186, 356
vegetables, viii, xii, 23, 27, 71, 76, 107, 114, 120, 122, 126, 128, 129, 131, 132, 133, 135, 137, 138, 139, 140, 143, 144, 152, 154, 161, 168, 170, 172, 173, 176, 181, 196, 197, 199, 200, 202, 204, 206, 257, 260, 289, 291, 293, 299, 300, 301, 302, 303, 304, 309, 311, 312, 313, 314, 315, 316, 341, 343, 353, 356, 357, 359, 362, 364
VEGF, 393, 394, 395

Venezuela, 127
ventilation, 323, 327, 391, 400, 404, 405, 408, 432
ventricular arrhythmia(s), 342, 351
ventricular tachycardia, 342
versatility, 220
vertebrates, 336, 378
vessels, 4, 7, 76, 82, 178, 281, 339, 379, 395, 397
village, 11, 12, 17, 18, 21, 22, 23, 27, 28
villus, 452, 456
virus, 8, 105, 231
virus infection, 231
virus replication, 8
viruses, 109
visceral adiposity, viii, 63, 70, 90, 91
viscosity, 414, 428
vision, 408
vitamin A, 23, 27, 114, 130, 131, 153, 296, 344, 361, 365, 369, 375, 439
vitamin B1, 23, 75, 76, 99, 126, 150, 151, 293, 298, 324, 330, 361, 377
vitamin B12, 75, 76, 99, 126, 150, 151, 293, 298, 324, 330, 361, 377
vitamin B2, 361
vitamin B6, 75, 151, 293, 323, 324
vitamin C, 23, 77, 100, 114, 133, 134, 135, 136, 153, 177, 178, 180, 181, 194, 300, 330, 347, 357, 361, 364, 365, 368, 369, 433, 439
Vitamin C, 19, 20, 21, 22, 129, 133, 134, 154, 177, 178, 192, 194, 357, 362, 365, 366
vitamin D, vii, ix, 31, 32, 33, 34, 35, 36, 37, 38, 39, 40, 41, 43, 44, 45, 46, 47, 48, 49, 50, 52, 53, 54, 55, 56, 57, 58, 60, 61, 108, 122, 123, 124, 125, 149, 150, 157, 158, 160, 167, 172, 174, 176, 180, 181, 185, 189, 190, 191, 192, 293, 324, 344
Vitamin D, 31, 32, 33, 35, 36, 37, 38, 39, 40, 41, 42, 43, 44, 45, 48, 49, 50, 53, 54, 55, 56, 57, 58, 60, 120, 122, 123, 149, 164, 174, 175, 176, 184, 190, 191, 297, 324
vitamin D deficiency, ix, 36, 38, 39, 41, 46, 54, 56, 57, 58, 157, 175, 190
vitamin D receptor (VDR), viii
vitamin E, 57, 77, 80, 100, 104, 105, 119, 132, 133, 135, 136, 153, 289, 300, 316, 344, 355, 356, 358, 361, 365, 368, 369, 421, 422, 427, 433
vitamin K, 181, 191, 192, 296
vitamin supplementation, 76, 300, 433
vitamins, viii, ix, xii, 63, 75, 76, 97, 99, 103, 107, 111, 114, 119, 129, 130, 131, 152, 153, 158, 180, 181, 184, 191, 194, 256, 261, 262, 289, 293, 316, 319, 322, 323, 337, 353, 355, 361, 363, 364, 365, 367, 425, 433, 439
VLDL, 376
volumetric changes, 76
vomiting, 323
vulnerability, 81, 335

W

Wales, 83
walking, 80, 103, 245, 414, 438, 442
war, 240, 359, 361
Warsaw, 107, 157
Washington, 81, 84, 120, 126, 145, 146, 149, 169, 181, 184, 186, 188, 189, 194, 211, 268, 269, 275, 296
weakness, 80, 345, 423, 433
wealth, 357
wear, 39
web, 198, 206, 210
weight changes, 55, 437
weight control, 72, 114, 144
weight gain, 38, 41, 55, 244, 252, 254, 264, 268, 269, 290, 416, 431, 432
weight loss, xi, 67, 68, 81, 85, 106, 203, 207, 209, 214, 215, 216, 217, 226, 228, 233, 235, 239, 242, 244, 246, 249, 252, 257, 268, 286, 294, 364, 365, 389, 390, 396, 405, 409, 421, 425, 427, 431, 439, 440, 441
weight management, x, 195, 201, 202, 203, 206, 207, 211
weight status, 106
well-being, 103, 238, 301, 316, 365
western diet, 146
wheat, 23, 117, 119, 127, 131, 146, 359
wheat germ, 119
white matter, 76, 87, 98
whole grain, 116, 119, 120, 128, 140, 141, 146, 291, 341, 343, 353, 356, 364
Wilson's disease, 65, 78
wine, vii, 1, 2, 3, 4, 7, 8, 10, 71, 74, 77, 137, 143, 293
winter, 36, 39, 125
withdrawal, 301, 302, 303, 343
workers, 203, 208
World Health Organization, (WHO), 82, 154, 159, 182, 188, 200, 217, 223, 233, 244, 300, 315, 391, 411, 433
World War, 359
wound healing, 357, 372, 379, 380

writing, 256

X

x-ray, 37, 218, 396, 397, 407, 430, 441, 444

Y

yeast, 121, 128, 358
yield, 109
yogurt, 169, 258, 259, 260, 266, 293
yolk, 124
young adults, 36, 54, 167, 171, 188, 199, 210, 293, 401
young men, 182, 188
young women, 162, 169, 186, 188

Z

zinc, viii, ix, 77, 78, 79, 101, 102, 107, 114, 158, 181, 183, 189, 283, 288, 289, 296, 323, 328, 329, 330, 337, 347, 361, 369, 374